Essentials *for the* Canadian Medical Licensing Exam

REVIEW AND PREP FOR MCCQE PART I

Jeeshan H. Chowdhury BSc, MSc (Oxon)

Joint MD/DPhil Student
University of Alberta
Edmonton, Alberta

University of Oxford
Oxford, United Kingdom

Shaheed Merani PhD

Joint MD/PhD Student
University of Alberta
Edmonton, Alberta

 Wolters Kluwer | Lippincott Williams & Wilkins
Health

Philadelphia · Baltimore · New York · London
Buenos Aires · Hong Kong · Sydney · Tokyo

Acquisitions Editor: Charley Mitchell
Managing Editor: Kelly Horvath, Kelley Squazzo
Marketing Manager: Emilie Moyer
Production Editor: Julie Montalbano
Designer: Stephen Druding
Compositor: Laserwords Private Limited, Chennai, India

9 8 7 6 5 4 3 2 1

Library of Congress Cataloging-in-Publication Data

Essentials for the Canadian medical licensing exam : review and prep for MCCQE / [edited by] Jeeshan Chowdhury, Shaheed Merani.
    p. ; cm.
  Includes bibliographical references and index.
  ISBN 978-0-7817-7650-9 (alk. paper)
  1. Physicians—Licenses—Canada—Examinations—Study guides. I. Chowdhury, Jeeshan. II. Merani, Shaheed.
  [DNLM: 1. Medicine—Canada—Examination Questions. W 18.2 E78 2010]
  RC58.E87 2010
  610.71′171—dc22

                                                              2009000750

DISCLAIMER

Care has been taken to confirm the accuracy of the information present and to describe generally accepted practices. However, the authors, editors, and publisher are not responsible for errors or omissions or for any consequences from application of the information in this book and make no warranty, expressed or implied, with respect to the currency, completeness, or accuracy of the contents of the publication. Application of this information in a particular situation remains the professional responsibility of the practitioner; the clinical treatments described and recommended may not be considered absolute and universal recommendations.

The authors, editors, and publisher have exerted every effort to ensure that drug selection and dosage set forth in this text are in accordance with the current recommendations and practice at the time of publication. However, in view of ongoing research, changes in government regulations, and the constant flow of information relating to drug therapy and drug reactions, the reader is urged to check the package insert for each drug for any change in indications and dosage and for added warnings and precautions. This is particularly important when the recommended agent is a new or infrequently employed drug.

Some drugs and medical devices presented in this publication have Food and Drug Administration (FDA) clearance for limited use in restricted research settings. It is the responsibility of the health care provider to ascertain the FDA status of each drug or device planned for use in their clinical practice.

To purchase additional copies of this book, call our customer service department at (800) 638-3030 or fax orders to (301) 223-2320. International customers should call (301) 223-2300.

Visit Lippincott Williams & Wilkins on the Internet: at http://www.lww.com. Lippincott Williams & Wilkins customer service representatives are available from 8:30 AM to 6 PM, EST.

Dedicated to my parents and brothers
—Jeeshan H. Chowdhury

Dedicated to my family, especially my grandmother
—Shaheed Merani

The Medical Council of Canada Qualifying Examination (MCCQE) Part I is an important milestone for medical students, signifying a culmination of years' of training in basic science and clinical medicine. The Medical Council of Canada (MCC) recommends numerous separate texts as reference for this exam preparation. Such a vast reading list is neither a practical nor a feasible means of approaching this critical exam for most candidates. The singular intent of this text is to provide a succinct yet complete review for the MCCQE Part I using the most efficient and effective means.

This book is based entirely on the MCC's *Objectives for the Qualifying Examination* "that lay out **exactly what you have to know** for any of the MCC examinations." This text contains only the specific and essential information required to meet the *Objectives*—all extraneous information has been deliberately omitted.

This text avoids time-wasting prose and effusive lists. Information is presented only in concise and easily assimilated visual formats. A focus on tables and flow charts allow complex and detailed concepts to be swiftly and effectively reviewed for comprehension and retention. Text within boxes signals the reader to key competencies highlighted by the *Objectives*.

This text is a collaborative project that combines the perspective and insights of students preparing for the examination with the experience of residents and acumen of faculty. The result is a novel and innovative resource to aid in the process of preparing for the MCCQE Part I. As medical school curricula are becoming more tailored to the exam, we believe it will also prove useful in your general studies as well.

We would appreciate your feedback on how to improve this resource and wish you the best success in the MCCQE Part I.

**Jeeshan H. Chowdhury and
Shaheed Merani**

Please read the following carefully:

This publication is provided to assist you in preparing for the Medical Council of Canada Licensing Examination, Part I. Under no circumstances should the information contained in this publication be relied upon for any other purpose.

Although the authors have made reasonable efforts to ensure the accuracy of the information contained herein, the authors, editors, and publisher do not guarantee or represent that this information is accurate, complete, current, or suitable for any particular purpose or jurisdiction.

The authors, editors, and publisher make no warranty whatsoever, whether express or implied, with respect to this publication and its contents, and in no event will the authors, editors, or publisher be liable for any loss, damage, or injury arising from or connected to use of this publication, including without limitation loss of profits, direct, indirect, special, incidental, consequential, or punitive damages.

This exclusion of liability will apply whether such loss, damage, or injury is based in contract, tort, or negligence (including without limitation gross negligence).

Contributing Editor

Aleem M.F. Bharwani, MD, FRCP(C)
General Internal Medicine Fellow
Department of Medicine
University of Calgary
Calgary, Alberta
Specialist in Internal Medicine
Alberta Health Services;
Master in Public Policy
Harvard Kennedy School
Cambridge, Massachusettes, USA

Contributors

Al'a Abdo
Medical Student
Université de Montréal
Montreal, Quebec

Hernish Jayant Acharya, MD
Resident
Department of Physical Medicine and
Rehabilitation
Glenrose Rehabilitation Hospital, University of
Alberta
Edmonton, Alberta

Martha Ainslie, MD, FRCPC
Clinical Assistant Professor
Department of Medicine
University of Calgary
Calgary, Alberta;
Respirologist, Division of Respiratory Medicine
Department of Medicine
Peter Lougheed Hospital
Calgary, Alberta

François Bénard, MD, FRCSC
Program Director
Department of Urology
Université de Montréal
Montreal, Quebec

Fraser R. Brenneis, MD, CCFC, FCFP
Senior Associate Dean (Education)
Faculty of Medicine & Dentistry
Department of Family Medicine
University of Alberta
Edmonton, Alberta

Meghan Brison, MD
Resident
Department of Emergency Medicine
University of British Columbia
Vancouver, British Columbia

Michael F. Byrne, MD (Cantab), BA, MA, MRCP (UK), FRCPC
Clinical Associate Professor
University of British Columbia
Vancouver, British Columbia

Michelle L. Catton, MD
Resident
Department of Internal Medicine
University of Saskatchewan
Saskatoon, Saskatchewan

Andrea Cheung, MD
Family Medicine Resident
Toronto East General Hospital
University of Toronto
Toronto, Ontario

Oliver Haw For Chin, MD, FRCPC
Assistant Professor
Division of General Internal Medicine
Department of Medicine
University of Calgary
Calgary, Alberta

Jeeshan H. Chowdhury, BSc, MSc (Oxon)
Joint MD/DPhil Student
University of Alberta, Edmonton
Alberta, Canada;
University of Oxford
Oxford, United Kingdom

Raiyan Chowdhury, BSc, MD
Resident
Division of Otolaryngology
Head and Neck Surgery
University of Alberta
Edmonton, Alberta

John Crossley, MD, CCFP(EM), FRCPC
Assistant Professor;
Program Director
Royal College Training Program in Emergency
Medicine
Division of Emergency Medicine
Department of Medicine
McMaster University
Hamilton, Ontario

Yen Dang, MD
Resident
Division of General Surgery
Department of Surgery
Queen's University
Kingston, Ontario

Niloofar Dehghan
Medical Student
University of Ottawa
Ottawa, Ontario

Myriam Farah, MD
Chief Medical Resident
Department of Medicine
University of British Columbia
Vancouver, British Columbia

Robert J. Feibel, MD, FRCSC
Associate Professor
Department of Orthopaedic Surgery
The Ottawa Hospital
Ottawa, Ontario

W.L. Alan Fung, MD, MPhil, ScM
Resident Physician
Department of Psychiatry
University of Toronto, Toronto
Ontario, Canada;
Department of Epidemiology
Harvard University, Boston
Massachusetts, USA;
Gerontology Research Unit
Massachusetts General Hospital
Harvard Medical School
Boston, Massachusetts, USA

Ahmed Galal, MD, FRCP
Director
McGill Stem Cell Transplant Program
Montreal, Quebec;
Attending Staff
Division of Hematology, Department of Medicine
Royal Victoria Hospital
Montreal, Quebec;
Associate Professor
Faculty of Medicine
McGill University
Montreal, Quebec

Stephane Michel Gauthier, MD
Resident
Department of Internal Medicine
University of Ottawa
Ottawa, Ontario

Ralph George, MD, FRCS
Medical Director
CIBC Breast Centre
St. Michael's Hospital
Toronto, Ontario

Nicholas Giacomantonio, MD, FRCPC
Associate Professor of Medicine
Department of Medicine
Dalhousie University
Halifax, Nova Scotia;
Cardiologist
Department of Medicine
QE II Health Sciences Centre
Halifax, Nova Scotia

Jeremy Gilbert, MD, FRCPC
Department of Medicine
Division of Endocrinology
University of Toronto
Toronto, Ontario

Andrée Gruslin, MD, FRCS
Associate Professor
Faculty of Medicine
Department of Obstetrics and Gynecology
University of Ottawa
Ottawa, Ontario;
Maternal Fetal Medicine Specialist
Department of Obstetrics and Gynecology
The Ottawa Hospital
Ottawa, Ontario

Mohamed Shahul Hameed, MD
Attending Physician
Eastern Maine Medical Centre
Bangor, Maine, USA

Christopher Hall, MD
Resident
Emergency Medicine Training Program
McMaster University Hamilton, Ontario

Leora Horn, MD, MSC
Clinical Fellow in Oncology
Department of Medicine
University of Toronto
Toronto, Ontario

Scott Edward Jarvis, MD, PhD
Resident
Department of Neurology
University of Calgary
Calgary, Alberta

Michelle-Lee Jones, MD
Resident
Department of Neurology
McGill University
Montreal, Quebec

Jaskaran Kang
Medical Student
Queen's University
Kingston, Ontario

Janna Kasumovic, MD
Resident
Department of Family Medicine
University of Alberta
Edmonton, Alberta

Ahmed Kayssi, MSc
Medical Student
Queen's University
Kingston, Ontario

James L. Kennedy, MD, FRCPC
Professor
Department of Psychiatry and Institute of Medical
Science
University of Toronto
Toronto, Ontario;
Head of Neurogenetics Section
Director, Department of Neuroscience
Centre for Addiction and Mental Health
Toronto, Ontario

Hisham Khalil, MD
Resident
Department of Obstetrics and Gynecology
University of Ottawa and The Ottawa
Hospital
Ottawa, Ontario

Stephen Kingwell, MD
Resident
Department of Orthopaedic Surgery
University of Ottawa
Ottawa, Ontario

Valerie G. Kirk, MD, FRCPC
Associate Professor
Department of Pediatrics
University of Calgary
Calgary, Alberta;
Pediatric Respirology
Department of Pediatrics
Alberta Children's Hospital
Calgary, Alberta

Radha P. Kohly, BSc, PhD, MD
Resident
Department of Ophthalmology
University of Toronto
Toronto, Ontario;
Resident
Department of Ophthalmology
Toronto Western Hospital
Toronto, Ontario

Tehseen Ladha, MD
Resident
Department of Pediatrics
University of Calgary
Alberta Children's Hospital
Calgary, Alberta

Wai-Ching Lam, MD, FRCSC
Associate Professor
Department of Ophthalmology and Vision Sciences
University of Toronto
Toronto, Ontario;
Staff Ophthalmologist
Department of Ophthalmology
Toronto Western Hospital
Toronto, Ontario

Darren Lau
Joint MD/PhD Student
University of Alberta
Edmonton, Alberta

Grace Li
Medical Student
Undergraduate School of Medicine
University of British Columbia
Vancouver, British Columbia

Thierry Lebeau, MD
Resident
Department of Urology
Université de Montréal
Montreal, Quebec

Brendan Leier, PhD
Assistant Professor
John Dosseter Health Ethics Centre
University of Alberta
Edmonton, Alberta;
Clinical Ethicist
Stollery Children's Hospital
University of Alberta
Edmonton, Alberta

Natasha B. Leighl, MD, MMSc, FRCPC
Assistant Professor
Department of Medicine
University of Toronto
Toronto, Ontario;
Staff Physician
Department of Oncology and Hematology
Princess Margaret Hospital—UHN
Toronto, Ontario

Julien Letendre, MD
Resident
Department of Urology
Université de Montréal
Montreal, Quebec

Richard Liu, MD, FRCPC
Program Director
Division of Otolaryngology
Head and Neck Surgery
University of Alberta
Edmonton, Alberta

Harvey Lui, MD, FRCPC
Professor and Head
Department of Dermatology and Skin Science
Vancouver General Hospital
University of British Columbia
Vancouver, British Columbia

Shaheed Merani, PhD
Joint MD/PhD Student
University of Alberta
Edmonton, Alberta

Nisha Mistry, MD
Dermatology Resident
Department of Dermatology and Skin
Science
University of British Columbia
Vancouver, British Columbia

Rajeev H. Muni, BSc, MD
Resident
Department of Ophthalmology
University of Toronto
Toronto, Ontario;
Resident
Department of Ophthalmology
Toronto Western Hospital
Toronto, Ontario

Mohamed Firdaus Bin Mohamed Mydeen, MD
Research Associate
Department of Pathology
Dalhousie University
Halifax, Nova Scotia

Julian J. Owen, BHSc, MD
Resident
Department of Emergency Medicine
McMaster University
Hamilton, Ontario

Lamide Oyewumi, MD, PhD
University of Ottawa
Ottawa, Ontario

Erika Dianne Penz, SM, MD
Pulmonary Medicine Fellow
Division of Respiratory Medicine
Department of Medicine
University of Calgary
Calgary, Alberta

Farah Ramji, B.Sc., M.H.Sc., MD
Resident
Division of Respiratory Medicine
Department of Medicine
University of British Columbia
Vancouver, British Columbia

Sapna Rawal, MD
Resident
Department of Diagnostic Radiology
McGill University
Montreal, Quebec

Surabhi Rawal, BSc
Medical Student
McGill University
Montreal, Quebec
Faculty of Medicine

Theodore Elgin Roberts, MD
Assistant Professor
Director, Adult Neurology Residency
Department of Internal Medicine
(Neurology)
University of Alberta
Edmonton, Alberta;
Staff
Clinical Neurosciences Program
Capital Health, University of Alberta
Hospitals
Edmonton, Alberta

Naminder K. Sandhu, MD
Resident
Department of Pediatrics
University of Calgary
Alberta Children's Hospital
Calgary, Alberta

C. Douglas Smith, MD
Associate Professor
Department of Medicine
University of Ottawa
Ottawa, Ontario;
Chief, Division of Rheumatology
Department of Medicine
The Ottawa Hospital—Riverside Campus
Ottawa, Ontario

Ning Zi Sun, MD
Resident
Department of Medicine
McGill University
Montreal, Quebec

Sharla Kae Sutherland, MD, PhD
Vice President, Regulatory and Scientific Affairs
CV Technologies, Inc.
Edmonton, Alberta

Tomoko Takano, MD, PhD
Associate Professor
Department of Medicine
McGill University
Montreal, Quebec;
Nephrologist
Department of Medicine
McGill University Health Centre
Montreal, Quebec

Lilly Teng, MD
Resident
Department of Diagnostic Imaging
University of Toronto
Toronto, Ontario

John Teshima, MD, FRCPC, MEd
Assistant Professor
Department of Psychiatry
University of Toronto
Toronto, Ontario;
Staff Psychiatrist
Department of Psychiatry
Sunnybrook Health Sciences Centre
Toronto, Ontario

Yi Zhen Ting
Medical Student
Dalhousie University
Halifax, Nova Scotia;
Clinical Clerk
Department of Medicine
Capital Health District Authority
Halifax, Nova Scotia

Michael Tso, BScH
Medical Student
Undergraduate School of Medicine
University of British Columbia
Vancouver, British Columbia

Kaylyn Kit Man Wong, HBSc
Medical Student
Faculty of Medicine
University of Toronto
Toronto, Ontario

René Wong, MD, MEd, FRCPC
Assistant Professor, University
of Toronto
Department of Medicine
Division of Endocrinology
University of Toronto
Toronto, Ontario

Brandie Laurel Walker, PhD, MD
Pulmonary Medicine Fellow
Division of Respiratory Medicine
Department of Medicine
Calgary, Alberta

Evelyn Wu, MSc
Medical Student
Undergraduate School of Medicine
University of British Columbia
Vancouver, British Columbia

Daphne Yau, MSc
Medical Student
Queen's University
Kingston, Ontario

Eric M. Yoshida, MD, MHSc, FRCP(C), FACP, FACG
Professor of Medicine
Head, Division of Gastroenterology
University of British Columbia
Vancouver, British Columbia

Clement Zai, MSc
Institute of Medical Science
University of Toronto
Toronto, Ontario;
Neurogenetics Section
Centre for Addiction and Mental Health
Toronto, Ontario

Gwyneth Zai, MD, MSc
Resident Physician
Department of Psychiatry
University of Toronto
Toronto, Ontario;
Neurogenetics Section
Centre for Addiction and Mental Health
Toronto, Ontario

Jay Zhu, MD
Resident
Division of Otolaryngology
Head and Neck Surgery
University of Alberta
Edmonton, Alberta

We would like to thank Kelly Horvath and Donna Balado of Lippincott Williams & Wilkins for their editorial support and guidance in taking this project from a mere scheme to a reality. We would also like to thank Jennifer Clements for the illustrations and figures that are such a key aspect to this project. Dhanya Ramesh and Julie Montalbano are to be thanked for guidance through the production and publication process; and Corey Wolfe and Emilie Moyer for that with marketing.

We would also like to extend our appreciation to the dedicated contributors to this book, the medical students who incorporated their own experiences in preparing for the exam, residents who were able to look back on their experiences and shared advice and insights they only wished were available to them, and the faculty who not only supervised and reviewed the chapters but shared their knowledge and expertise.

CONTENTS

CHAPTER 1

Introduction

Jeeshan H. Chowdhury and Shaheed Merani

WHAT IS THE MCCQE PART I?

The MCC examines medical school graduates and grants licensure to legally practice medicine in Canada. Licensure in Canada is formally obtained through the LMCC, which requires successful completion of the MCCQE Part I and II. In general, medical students in Canada complete the MCCQE Part 1 at the end of their undergraduate medical education (just before graduation from medical school) and before beginning their postgraduate medical training (i.e., residency training program).

The MCCQE Part I is a two-part computer-based test. The first section, of 3.5 hours, consists of 196 MCQs and is completed the morning of the examination day (Table 1.1). The afternoon component consists of the CDM section, a 4-hour section of approximately 60 cases, each associated with one to four short-menu or short-written answer style questions. For both portions of the examination, a table of normal values is provided (see appendix).

The MCQ section of the examination is divided into 7 subsections of 28 questions each. Each question is in the format of a question stem followed by a list of five answer choices. Only one answer choice is correct for each question. Each question may be accompanied by an image or table.

The CDM section of the examination consists of approximately 80 questions, and focuses on CDM and problem-solving skills. Questions in the realm of differential diagnosis, diagnostic test selection, clinical data collection and patient management should be expected. In this section, there are short-menu questions, consisting of between 10 and 40 option choices; examinees are asked to either select one answer, a certain number of answer options, or as many answer options as are appropriate. Within the CDM section, short-written response ("write-in") questions should be expected. Responses should be specific, use generic drug names, and worded carefully as directed by the question.

Both sections of the MCCQE Part I are based on the *Objectives for the Qualifying Examination*. The latest version of the *Objectives* was established in 2003 by the MCC, and outlines the expectation of competent physicians, consisting of **General Objectives** and **Clinical Presentations**.

The **General Objectives** for the Part I outline history taking and physical exam skills. Competent candidates are expected to communicate effectively with patients, families, and other relevant persons. It is expected that a candidate will be able to collect data through history taking; conduct appropriate physical exams; select, interpret, and determine the reliability of clinical investigations; and use CDM strategies and judgment to arrive at a diagnosis and appropriate management strategy. To appropriately care for patients, the MCC recognizes that physicians must be versed in topics of health promotion and maintenance, critical appraisal of medical evidence, medical economics, and the C_2LEO aspects of medicine.

The **Clinical Presentations** of the MCCQE **Objectives** define the clinical competencies of the medical graduate specific to select common presentations. Within each clinical presentation, the MCC define the pertinent data collection, diagnostics, clinical problem-solving, and management strategies required of the competent examinee.

Table **1.1**	**Summary of MCCQE Sections**	
	MCQ	**CDM**
When	Morning	Afternoon
Time allotted	3.5 h	4 h
Style	Multiple choice	Cases with short menu or written response
Questions	196	60 cases × 1–4 questions

HOW TO USE THIS TEXT?

Essentials for the Canadian Medical Licensing Exam: Review and Prep for MCCQE Part I is written for medical students and international medical graduates who are preparing to write the MCCQE Part I. As a summative review for the MCCQE Part I *Objectives*, this text will also be of value to medical students through their training both in preclinical and clerkship years, and meet basic needs in postgraduate education.

All the content presented is based on the *Objectives* which "lay[s] out exactly what you have to know for any of the MCC examinations" and which "the MCC test committee use . . . when they are creating examination questions."

Content is also organized based on the *Objectives*. The text is divided into chapters, which address the main clinical specialties. Topics within each chapter correspond directly with **Clinical Presentations** of the MCCQE Part I *Objectives*. Many of the clinical presentations of the MCCQE Part I *Objectives* have a multispecialty scope, but for ease of reference we have avoided wherever possible to divide topics into separate chapters.

Chapter 2 is entirely dedicated to C_2LEO aspects. Although distinct from the format of the clinical chapters, this chapter forms a summative review of C_2LEO objectives from the MCC. C_2LEO content is covered in all chapters where appropriate to a specific presentation.

It is expected that students reading this text will already have a basic conceptual understanding of the material. This text organizes and presents material in a highly effective format to allow for a reliable study plan, rapid comprehension, and durable recall that is useful both for examination and during clinical practice.

CLINICAL PRESENTATION: OBJECTIVES BASED

Each chapter contains distinct topics based on the common **clinical presentations**, of which a list can be found in the Index. Taken directly from the list of MCCQE Clinical Presentations, these topics form the framework of this text. Each clinical presentation is organized into the categories used by the *Objectives* that will detail the differential diagnosis, relevant physical exam characteristics and diagnostic tests, treatment and patient consultation techniques, as well as fundamental ASC and relevant C_2LEO aspects which require understanding for the qualifying examination candidate. Each topic is further divided into the following subtopics.

DEFINITION/RATIONALE

Outlines the fundamental definitions, scope, and epidemiologic facts of the clinical presentation.

CAUSAL CONDITIONS

Present a systems-based approach for differential diagnosis.

APPROACH/MANAGEMENT

Provides overview of physical exam, investigations, diagnosis, and management of the clinical presentation.

APPLIED SCIENTIFIC CONCEPT

Reviews basic scientific concepts pertinent to the clinical management of the clinical presentation.

EFFECTIVE VISUAL LEARNING TOOLS

In addition to the clinical presentation and objective-based design of the topics, a number of highly effective visual learning tools are used. These tools succinctly display complex and detailed concepts for swift and highly effective review.

CLINICAL DECISION-MAKING ALGORITHMS

More complex clinical presentations will have diagrammatic CDM trees that focus student attention on clinical approach.

TABLES AND CHARTS

Details and lists are presented in system-based tables that organize information for improved retention and recall.

CLINICAL BOXES

Highlights ranging from key concepts, high-yield points, mnemonics, and clinical pearls.

C_2LEO BOXES

Specific applications of C_2LEO aspects of medicine are identified.

ASC BOXES

Emphasize fundamental basic scientific concepts of clinical importance.

RED FLAGS

Underscore emergent matters or potential clues to serious medical conditions.

RECOMMENDED READING

For further in depth study of the concepts that are reviewed, a list of effective texts and study material is recommended as an online compendium to this text.

INTERACTIVE ONLINE QUESTION BANK

A compilation of 100 MCCQE-style multiple choice questions is presented online to assist in preparation for the exam. Use the access code provided on the inside front cover.

Cultural-Communication, Legal, Ethical, and Organizational Aspects of Medicine

Darren Lau, Brendan Leier, and Sharla Kae Sutherland

All medical care is provided against the backdrop of the patient–physician relationship. This relationship, the duties and entitlements it entails, and the organizational backdrop supporting it comprise the MCCQE's *Considerations of the* C$_2$LEO objectives. C$_2$LEO relates the social aspects of the medical enterprise that are essential to sound clinical practice.

Ethics concerns the values, customs, and notions of right and wrong behavior that underlie clinical relationships. Three approaches to ethics are dominant: **Consequentialist ethics** defines actions as right or wrong by the nature of their consequences. **Virtue ethics** considers the personal characteristics, i.e., virtues or vices, underlying the action.

MCCQE C$_2$LEO Essentials
The Four-Principles Approach

In 1989, Beauchamp and Childress popularized a four-principle approach to medical ethics: **respect for patient autonomy, beneficence, nonmaleficence**, and **justice**.
- **Respect for patient autonomy** means realizing the patient's right to make decisions with regard to their own lives and medical care.
- **Beneficence** obliges physicians to provide care, to do good by their patients, and to seek good outcomes.
- **Nonmaleficence** is the duty not to harm.
- **Justice** refers to fair allocations of, and fair processes for allocating medical resources.

These principles command broad acceptance, and have *prima facie* status: they are each meant to be binding unless they conflict with other significant moral values.

MCCQE C$_2$LEO Essentials
Patient–Physician Relationship

The patient–physician relationship is a fiduciary relationship. The physician is bound to:
- Serve the patient's interests with due care and diligence
- Refrain from conflicts of interest
- Resolve all conflicts of interest in the patient's favor

Moreover,

- The fiduciary relationship confers a legal duty of the utmost loyalty.
- Trust is essential to the patient–physician relationship. The patient is entitled to have faith in the relationship's integrity.
- The patient–physician relationship is **patient centered.**
- Physicians must provide continuous and accessible care, and never abandon their patient.

The relationship is terminated when:

- Care has been transferred
- Adequate notice has been given for the patient to make alternative arrangements

Duty-based or deontologic approaches define right or wrong by reference to primary duties that are valuable in and of themselves, regardless of their outcomes. Duties may be derived from professional codes, religious law, or philosophical principles. Elements of all three ethical approaches are incorporated in the well-accepted four-principles approach to medical ethics.

The first principle, **respect for patient autonomy**, refers to the right of the individual to make decisions about his or her own life and medical care. The principle of **beneficence** compels physicians to provide care, and to see to the well-being of his or her patient. The patient–physician relationship is therapeutic: its purpose is to promote patient welfare.

Nonmaleficence is the duty not to harm. Medical interventions come with risks, and often result in unintended consequences. Physicians should be aware of their limitations, and of the appropriate applications of medical technology, procedures, and pharmaceuticals.

The principle of **justice** refers to the fair allocation of scarce resources as well as the fair process through which this distribution occurs.

The ethical dimensions of clinical practice vary from situation to situation, and are topics of discussion and controversy. Where consensus is achieved regarding right and wrong behavior, ethical principles may find their way into Canada's formal system of rules. These are the legal aspects of clinical medicine. Some of these rules are statutes enacted by legislatures. On issues unaddressed in statute, the demands of the law may be created and refined by judicial precedents, which form a coherent body of common law; or by invoking and applying the general principles laid out in a **Civil Code**, as occurs in civil law jurisdictions. Principles of law referred to in this chapter are rooted in common law which is applicable across Canada except in Quebec, where civil law is observed. In many instances, common law and civil law formulations of physician duties and patient rights will be similar.

The law recognizes the patient as a person with human and other legal rights, including the right to security of person and inviolability, and the right to freedom from discrimination. These rights are formulated at a constitutional level, in the Canada **Charter of Rights and Freedoms**. In addition, both common and civil law recognize a fundamental right to self-determination. Rights are trumps that can normally be expected to take precedence over other considerations. However, rights may be legitimately limited for certain social interests. Specific instances under which individual rights must give way are recognized in various statutory and nonstatutory laws.

The law also recognizes the physician as a person to whom duties apply. Indeed, the patient–physican relationship has been described as a fiduciary relationship, imposing on physicians one of the highest standards of conduct recognized at law. In a fiduciary relationship, the physician is an agent acting on behalf of a vulnerable party, and is obliged to act solely in that party's interests at all times. Current physicians, as the stewards of trust inspired by generations of previous professionals, are obliged to honor and nurture this relationship for future generations of physicians.

Physicians must follow through on undertakings made to patients, must not exploit the relationship for personal advantage, and must maintain and respect professional boundaries at all times. Physicians are obliged to provide for continuous and accessible care, and never to abandon their patients. These basic duties arise from ethical and legal understandings of the patient–physician relationship, and are only terminated when care has been transferred, or after adequate notice has been given to allow the patient to make alternative arrangements. The patient–physician relationship, as the central fixture of medical practice, permeates medicine's legal, ethical, and organizational aspects.

CONSENT

Consent is the autonomous authorization of a medical intervention by individual patient. Valid consent—or refusal to consent—requires that a **capable** patient makes a **voluntary** decision regarding a **referable** procedure or treatment, in light of a physician's **disclosure** of information. Physicians are duty-bound to seek consent before any treatment or procedure. The treating physician is ultimately responsible for ensuring consent.

MCCQE C₂LEO Essentials

Consent

- Is required, ethically, by respect for patient autonomy, and legally, by the patient's common-law right to self-determination and by statute, where applicable
- Refers to specific interventions performed at particular times and places by certain personnel
- Requires
  - Disclosure
  - Voluntarism and
  - Capacity
- Is required whenever treatment or diagnostic options are recommended

The patient has the right to refuse consent, even when this may lead to death. Consent may be withdrawn at any time without prejudice on the level of clinical care provided.

ETHICAL AND LEGAL BASIS

Patient **self-determination** or **autonomy** is a fundamental right. Individuals' abilities to pursue various aims are contingent on their states of physical well-being. Control over one's body is therefore fundamental in determining the direction of one's own life. This is recognized in common law, under which physicians find themselves liable for battery if they treat a patient without consent, or for negligence, if they treat a patient under inadequately formed consent and patient harm occurs as a result. Certain provinces have taken the further step of legislating consent. Ontario's *HCCA*, e.g., "provides rules with respect to consent to treatment that apply consistently in all circumstances".

Physician colleges also recognize a professional duty to seek consent. Failure to adequately uphold these norms could lead to professional disciplinary action, including suspension or loss of licence.

DISCLOSURE

Meaningful decision making requires that individuals are apprised of information relevant to their circumstances. Only then can the decision be attributed to their authentic preferences.

In *Reibl v. Hughes*, the court decided that adequate disclosure should include **whatever a reasonable person in the patient's circumstances would want to know**. This **modified-objective** standard strikes a balance between objectivity and subjectivity in determining adequate disclosure on a case-by-case basis. An entirely subjective standard might read: **what the patient would have wanted to know**. However, this alternative is difficult to evaluate fairly. In the modified-objective standard, the reference to **a reasonable person**, a hypothetical legal construct, allows courts to infer the content of an adequate disclosure independent of a patient's whims, while remaining responsive to particular circumstances.

MCCQE C₂LEO Essentials

Disclosure

- What a reasonable person in the patient's circumstances would want to know
- Usually includes
  - Nature of the intervention
  - Gravity of the patient's situation and of intervention
  - Material risks and benefits, including special or unusual risks
  - Alternatives and consequences of nonconsent
  - Information regarding delegation of care
- Patient questions must be addressed
- The treating physician must ensure patient understanding

Supreme Court Chief Justice Laskin's formulation of the general content of an adequate disclosure in *Hopp v. Lepp* is instructive:

> " ... a surgeon, generally, should *answer any specific questions* posed by the patient as to the risks involved and should, without being questioned, disclose to him *the nature of the proposed operation, its gravity, any material risks and any special or unusual risks* ... However, having said that, it should be added that *the scope of the duty of disclosure and whether or not it has been breached are matters which must be decided in relation to the circumstances of each particular case.*" (*Hopp v. Lepp*, italics added by present authors.)

Information should be presented in broad terms and simple language. Translation services should be sought to address linguistic barriers. Information should account for extramedical (e.g., social and financial) circumstances. And the treating physician should check for patient understanding.

VOLUNTARISM

Voluntarism refers to freedom from coercion, so that a patient's authentic sense of what is best can guide medical decisions. Is the patient free to act "in character," in accordance with those values and interests formed throughout the patient's life?

In the clinic, voluntarism can be thought of as freedom from external interference. These include pain, a rushed environment, local resource scarcity, physical restraints, and coercive family dynamics. Medical staff should facilitate a voluntary decision by providing pain control; creating calm and supportive settings for discussing major decisions; ensuring that local resource scarcity does not restrict the patient's range of options, including arranging for patient transfer, as needed; using restraints only as necessary, and using the least restrictive modalities; and checking in with the patient regarding the role of the family. A family conference may be appropriate. Hospital ethicists should be consulted for difficult cases.

CAPACITY

Capacity refers to the ability to consent or refuse consent to medical treatment. According to the Ontario *HCCA*, the capable patient is "able to understand the information that is relevant to making a decision"; and "able to appreciate the reasonably foreseeable consequences of a decision or lack of decision."

There is no one-size-fits-all or easy way of assessing capacity. Capacity does not refer to global cognitive or affective status, as assessed, e.g., by the Folstein MMSE, although

MCCQE C₂LEO Essentials
Voluntarism and Capacity

Voluntarism
- Minimize coercive influences, or influences that interfere with decision making, e.g., provide adequate pain control.

Capacity
- A process standard of capacity applies: Is the patient able to understand and appreciate information? The consequences and alternatives to action or nonaction?
- Capacity is specific for each decision
- Capacity ≠ global cognitive status
- Capacity may fluctuate
- The patient should be allowed to direct treatment as much as possible
- Refusal to consent ≠ incapacity
- Minors and mentally disabled patients raise special issues for capacity
- If the patient is not competent, consent may be obtained from a court, parent, or SDM according to provincial law and specific circumstances
- At least two justifications for proxy or substitute decisions should be recognized: **what the patient would have wanted** and the **best interests** standards; the acceptability of the justification will depend on the circumstances

bad MMSE performance may lead a physician to suspect the patient's capacity. Capacity is specific. It refers to a patient's ability to make a particular decision. A patient incapable of making one decision is not necessarily incapable with respect to another. Capacity is also dynamic. It changes with time and circumstance. Capacity should be assessed and reassessed regularly, and for different sorts of decisions. Out of respect for autonomy, patients should direct their own care to the extent that they are capable. Where the stakes resting on a capacity determination are substantial, a formal assessment by a psychiatrist and/or an ethicist consultation should be sought.

Capacity can be affected by many factors, including disease, drug-use, and depression. Reversible factors should be addressed, and important decisions delayed until capacity is restored, if possible.

Capacity goes beyond simple understanding: to **appreciate** one's circumstances, the patient must **be able** to recognize that he or she has a condition to which the treatment and its consequences might apply. This is not to say that the patient must characterize his or her condition as pathological or as necessitating treatment. To presume this would be tantamount to saying that a patient is capable if he or she agrees with the medical opinion. **Nonconsent does not constitute evidence of incapacity** and medical staff must be open to idiosyncratic perceptions of health and wellness.

EXCEPTIONS TO CONSENT

When a patient presents in an urgent care setting, efforts should be undertaken to facilitate consent (e.g., find a translator for a capable non-English speaker, or locate a SDM for an incapable patient). This might not be feasible in emergencies, where delay could lead to significant bodily harm. In such situations, it would be better to err on the side of bodily integrity: treatment should occur without delay.

However, the emergency exception does not apply where there is reason to believe that the patient would refuse treatment if he or she were capable. In *Malette v. Shulman*, an emergency physician was held liable for initiating a life-saving transfusion on an incapable car accident victim, despite his awareness that a card declaring refusal of blood products for religious reasons had been found in the victim's purse.

Provincial public health statutes require compulsory diagnostic testing or treatment in suspected cases of certain infections. Mental health statutes may also provide for admission to hospital without consent. These vary from province to province. Legislation may also require that an SDM consent to diagnostic or therapeutic interventions, after admission.

THE INCAPABLE PATIENT

A patient may be unable to understand the medical problem, the proposed treatment, alternatives, or consequences of consent/nonconsent. The patient may be unable to appreciate his or her situation, i.e., unable to recognize that he or she has a condition to which this information applies. He or she may be unable to make a decision that is not substantially based on delusion or depression. This patient is incapable.

ETHICAL AND LEGAL CONSIDERATIONS

When patients are incapable, their decision making—or lack thereof—may subject them to undue harm. Moreover, decisions made in these states cannot meaningfully be said to be rooted in the values and beliefs that comprise a consistent self-identity. That is to say, decision making is no longer autonomous.

We protect incapable patients by making decisions on their behalf—but according to whose guiding values? Patients' illnesses should not deprive them of the right to live a full and complete life according to their own values. To ensure that their preferences continue to guide their care during illness, physicians rely on personal directives, and on SDMs **duty-bound to consider what the patient would have wanted if he or she were capable**. The right to control one's own body continues, even during a period of incapacity, even during a life-threatening emergency.

For some incapable patients, such as young children or patients who have had lifelong and severe mental handicap, respect for patient autonomy must be balanced against beneficence. Such a patient should be involved in decision making to the extent that

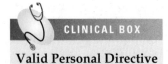

CLINICAL BOX

Valid Personal Directive

A valid personal directive written by or on behalf of a previously capable individual must be obeyed.

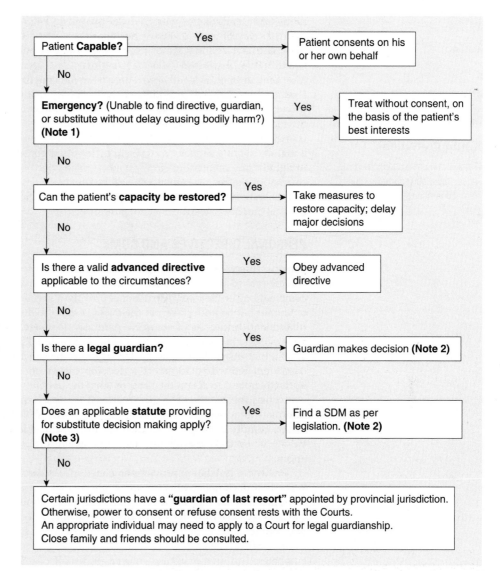

Figure 2.1 Consent algorithm for incapable patient.

Note 1: Evidence of a patient preference, even in the event of a life-threatening emergency, must nonetheless guide decision making (see, for e.g., *Malette v. Shulman*).

Note 2: SDMs are duty-bound to act on what the patient would have wanted, if he or she were capable. If the patient was never previously capable to make health care decisions, is a minor, or if the patient's wishes are unknown, substitutes should apply the best interests standard.

Note 3: Applicable statutes include child welfare statutes (e.g., Alberta's *Child, Youth, and Family Protection and Enhancement Act*), mental health statutes, and statutes concerning dependent adults.

maturity or disability permits, out of respect for nascent capacity and/or a burgeoning sense of selfhood. However, consent should be sought from the patient's guardian or an appropriate SDM, **who is obliged to act in the patient's best interests**. Here, the patient's circumstances privilege considerations of beneficence. Young children, lifelong severe mental handicap, and genuine uncertainty about a patient's preferences are examples of when the best interests standard should apply.

AGE AND CAPACITY

Age does not necessarily correlate with capacity. Under the common law doctrine of the mature minor, minors, like adults, are presumed capable, unless a specific assessment reveals incapacity. Extending the notion of capacity to encompass minors privileges their autonomy: The preferences of a capable minor must be respected.

For most minors, decision making will integrate medical opinion, the patient's preferences, and the family's preferences in varying degrees depending on the family's dynamics. It is therefore preferable to facilitate a therapeutic alliance inclusive of both the patient and his or her family. However, in the event that this is not feasible, the doctrine of the mature minor privileges the autonomy of a capable patient, age notwithstanding.

Statutory law may supercede common law. British Columbia's *Child Family and Community Services Act* allows the Director of Child Family and Community Services to appeal to the court, and for the court to order treatment, where a child—any individual younger than 19 years of age—or his or her guardians refuse to consent for treatment necessary to "preserve the child's life or to prevent serious or permanent impairment of the child's health" (B. [S.J.] v. British Columbia [Director of Child, Family and Community Services]). Therefore, a minor in BC is legally prevented from refusing life-saving care. This is *not* to say that a minor is incapable of providing consent, or of refusing treatment that is not necessary to preserve life or to prevent serious injury. In such instances, it is likely that the doctrine of the mature minor still applies. Other jurisdictions may have their own, unique, legislative frameworks. In general, a mature minor should be presumed capable. If the question of a mature minor's capacity to consent or to refuse consent becomes problematic, perhaps in light of life-threatening circumstances, the advice of child welfare authorities, hospital counsel, or the hospital ethicist should be sought.

In any case, physicians **must** report a parent's failure or refusal to seek necessary medical therapy to child protection authorities.

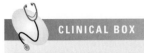

CLINICAL BOX

Child Protection

Failure to meet a child's medical needs must be reported to child protection agencies.

PERSONAL DIRECTIVES AND SDMs

Personal directives are mechanisms enabling a competent person to maintain control over clinical care in the event of future incapacity. Directives may be instructional, proxy, or combinations of the two. Instructional directives specify clinical interventions that should or should not be undertaken in the event of certain illnesses, such as the use of a feeding tube under conditions of complete paralysis or severe dementia. Instructional directives have pitfalls, in that they are unable to anticipate all possible situations that may arise, and in that instructions may be too vague to be practicable. Proxy directives appoint a competent individual to act as a decision maker on the patient's behalf. The proxy is normally bound to act on the basis of what the patient would have wanted. This approach overcomes the pitfalls of the instructional approach but requires that the proxy be well informed in advance. Notably, the proxy's powers are not absolute. Physicians cannot legally comply if the proxy's decisions are unjustifiable either by the patient's wishes or values, or by the patient's best interests, where the patient's wishes standard does not apply.

Provincial legislation provides an enabling framework for health care directives. Where legislation does not exist, case law suggests that written directives must nonetheless be respected because they express the patient's autonomous preferences.

If no personal directive can be discovered, or if no legal guardian with powers of agency over health care decisions can be found, consent can be obtained, where statutes permit, from an SDM. The Ontario HCCA, for example, provides a prioritized list of individuals empowered to give or refuse consent on behalf of an incapable patient. Depending on the circumstances, the SDM may be obliged either to consider what the patient would have wanted or to consider the patient's best interests. Where statutes do not provide for substitute decision making, power to consent or refuse consent on a patient's behalf rests with the Courts or with Court-appointed guardians. However, medical staff regularly consult and consider the views of close family members.

CONFIDENTIALITY

Confidentiality refers to the physician's duty to safeguard information disclosed by patients, i.e., never to divulge it in ways inconsistent with the understanding of the original disclosure, except as the patient directs or permits. Privacy refers to the patient's control over knowledge of his or her personal affairs. Confidentiality protects patients' privacy.

CONFIDENTIALITY—ETHICAL AND LEGAL CONSIDERATIONS

Confidentiality is essential to the patient–physician relationship. We perceive our bodies as intimate, private domains. Information about our bodies should be intimately kept, especially since it may affect the range of opportunities available in patients' lives. The knowledge that a patient has HIV/AIDS, for example, may subject the patient to stereotyping and discrimination if revealed unwittingly. Physicians are obliged to maximize

MCCQE C₂LEO Essentials

Confidentiality

- Underpinned ethically by autonomy and beneficence, and legally by fiduciary duty
- Facilitates trust in the patient–physician relationship
- Health information **must** be disclosed to a third party when
  - The law requires reporting
  - To prevent serious harm from befalling a third party, **i.e., duty to warn**
  - To prevent serious harm from befalling the patient
  - Where a valid court order requires disclosure
  - Where the patient requests or authorizes that health information be transferred
- The patient should be notified of a required disclosure
- Common mandatory disclosures with which physicians should be familiar vary from province to province, and may include:
  - Certain communicable diseases
  - Suspected child abuse or abandonment
  - Fitness to operate a motor vehicle
- Decision-capable minors are entitled to confidentiality
- Anonomized or deidentified information is generally not considered private, but should be created or used carefully nonetheless
- Confidentiality rules and exceptions are complicated—guidance should be sought from the professional college

autonomy, as well as defend the patient from potential harm, by observing confidentiality. Health information should go only where the patient would wish it. The patient–physician relationship is built on patients' trust that physicians will apply these moral standards in their activities.

Certain provinces have enacted statutes with the primary aim of regulating the treatment of health information (e.g., Alberta's *Health Information Act*). These statutes outline the responsibilities of health information custodians and patients' rights in respect of their information. At common law, the patient–physician relation can be modeled as a trust relationship, in which the physician is a fiduciary agent acting for his or her principal, the patient. A fiduciary (from Latin, *fides*, meaning "faith") is bound to further the interests of the beneficiary with the utmost loyalty. Fiduciaries are prohibited from allowing personal interests to supersede their duties to a principal, from being in a position where duties to multiple principals clash, and from profiting from their position of trust without their beneficiary's consent. Fiduciary duty is therefore a legal guarantee that the physician's position of power is never used for personal gain, third-party gain, or in a manner that harms the patient.

A patient has a continuing interest in his or her health information. Serving this interest means safeguarding the patient's information and disclosing it as directed. In practice, this means taking reasonable precautions to maintain confidentiality by:

- Limiting information disclosed over phone
- Avoiding the transmission of health information by fax or E-mail
- Securing charts and maintaining computer network security
- Deidentifying patient data for presentations or educational and research purposes

In general, anonomized, or deidentified, data is not considered private. Personal information may also be used or disclosed without the subject's knowledge or consent for statistical or scholarly purposes, where such ends cannot be achieved without patient information, and where it is impractical to obtain consent, subject to ethical research review.

There are instances in which, regardless of patient preferences, health information **must** be disclosed to a third party. For example, maintaining confidentiality may pose significant risk of substantial harm to the public. Disclosure of health information to the appropriate authorities may be necessary. Disclosure is also mandatory where statute requires it. In many cases, these laws (e.g., public health legislation) express a broader public interest that legitimately limits the exercise of individual rights. Confidentiality is not absolute, and it is important that physicians know the exceptions.

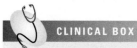

CLINICAL BOX

Danger to Others

" . . . the confidential character of patient-psychotherapist communications must yield to the extent that disclosure is essential to avert danger to others. The protective privilege ends where the public peril begins" (*Tarasoff v. Regents*).

CLINICAL BOX

Recent Disclosure Legislation—Two Examples of Emerging Issues

- In 2007, Saskatchewan became the second province to enact mandatory disclosure of gunshot and stabbing wounds. Medical staff must report, to local police, that such a wound has been treated, the name of the patient, and the location of the medical facility. Reporters are immune for liability for disclosure. Ontario has had similar legislation since 2005.
- In 2007, Alberta passed legislation requiring a "source individual" to submit to testing upon the request of an emergency services personnel who was exposed to the source individual's bodily fluids in the course of their work.

(Source: Rossall, Jonathan. "Mandating Disclosure – Where Art Thou?")

Table **2.1**	**Disclosures of Health Information**	
Keywords	**Scenario**	**Mandatory**
Nonstatutory		
Court order	Upon request of a court order	X
Executor of estate	To the executor of the estate, for a deceased patient; the executor represents the deceased legally, not the next-of-kin	X
Patient consents	With patient consent, any use or disclosure is permissible	
Parents, minor patient incapable	Upon request of a patient's parents, **but not** where the patient is a mature minor	X
Patient directs	Must disclose information to a third party as directed or authorized by the patient	X
Federal Jurisdiction		
Aviation safety[a]	Medical conditions of flight crews, air traffic controllers, and others where the conditions is a threat to aviation safety	X
Mental illness, violent[b]	Patients treated for mental illness associated with violence or threatened violence	X
Railway safety[c]	Medical conditions of railroad workers in safety critical positions, where the condition is a threat to public safety	X
Provincial Jurisdiction		
Animal bites	Animal bites in which rabies is suspected	X
Board, statutory	Upon request of a Board or Tribunal, empowered by statute to issue subpoena (e.g., Attendance Board, *School Act*)	X
CA	Pathological reports indicating malignancy	X
Care-giver	To a person responsible for providing continuing care and treatment to the patient	
Child abuse	Suspected child abuse	X
Deaths, suspicious	Deaths under certain conditions (e.g., unexplained deaths, or deaths consequent to negligent care)	X
Discipline, professional	To the College of Physicians and Surgeons of Alberta pursuant to an investigation	X
Diseases, communicable	Certain communicable diseases	X
Diseases, notifiable under OHS	Specific notifiable diseases (e.g., lead poisoning, asbestosis, and noise-induced hearing loss)	X
Family members	To family members or individuals close to the patient, or for purposes of contacting such individuals, **if** the information is in general terms and **not contrary to the patient's express wishes**	
Legal guardian	Upon request of patient's legal guardian, with documentation of appointment	X
Motor vehicles	Persons medically unfit to drive	
Persons in care	Suspected abuse of a "person in care"	X
WCB	Upon the request of the WCB, only information relevant to work–related injuries likely to disable the patient from work for more than 1d	X
Danger to others[d]	Patients who present a clear and substantial danger to society	?

This table is based on Alberta disclosures as of 2005. Disclosures not marked "mandatory" are meant to be considered "permissible" or "discretionary."

Where the table references a federal statute, the disclosure applies uniformly across Canada. Otherwise, disclosure obligations are developed in provincial statute or case law, and vary from province to province. Practitioners must be familiar with regulations in their own jurisdictions.

[a]Aeronautics Act (Federal Statute)

[b]Firearms Act (Federal Statute)

[c]Railway Safety Act (Federal Statute)

[d]The case-precedent suggesting a duty to disclose in this situation is an American case, *Tarasoff v. Regents*. This duty has not been tested in Canadian jurisprudence.

(College of Physicians and Surgeons of Alberta. *Release of Medical Information: A Guide for Alberta Physicians*, CPSA; 2005. http://www.cpsa.ca/)

CONFIDENTIALITY—DISCLOSURES TO THIRD PARTIES

Infectious disease reporting to public health officials often constitutes mandatory disclosures of health information. Notifiable diseases commonly include sexually transmitted infections such as HIV/AIDS, gonococcal infections, *C. trachomatis* infections, mucopurulent cervicitis, LGV, syphilis, and chancroid; and other infections such as hepatitis, tuberculosis, enteric pathogens, foodborne illnesses, epidemic gastroenteritides, small pox, anthrax, viral hemorrhagic fevers, etc. Practitioners should be familiar with local regulations. Additionally, it is usually desirable to notify the patient about the required disclosure. This practice may enlist the patient. At the least, it helps maintain the bond of trust and transparency underlying the patient–physician relationship.

In the absence of legislation requiring otherwise, medical staff need not report gunshot wounds, stabbings, admitted use of illegal drugs, or injuries suffered during the commission of a crime. Such information may be obtained by a police officer with a valid court order.

PATIENT ACCESS TO HEALTH INFORMATION AND THE MEDICAL RECORD

The medical record is subject to physician control and responsibility. Medical staff have professional duties to document clinical activities, observations, and interactions on a medical record; to maintain the integrity of the record, and keep it up-to-date; to ensure for its secure storage; and to facilitate continuity of care by transmitting copies of the record as appropriate. The physician-clinic maintains ownership over, control of, and responsibility for the medical record.

MCCQE C₂LEO Essentials

Patient Access and the Medical Record

- Physicians have a duty to maintain adequate records for each patient they treat.
- The law specifies minimum time frames for the preservation of medical records (10 yr in most jurisdictions.)
- Patients have a right of access to health information, including the contents of the medical record.

Patients should be allowed access and control over their health information. For example, a patient request that a medical record—or, rather, a copy thereof—be transferred to a new clinic must be respected. A patient should also be able to review his or her medical record on request. It is reasonable to recover costs incurred providing access to the medical record, perhaps with a small access fee.

TRUTH TELLING

ETHICAL AND LEGAL CONSIDERATIONS

Health information, and control thereof, is important in determining the direction of one's life. A patient's autonomy is furthered when health information is made available so that the patient can make an informed decision based on authentic preferences. Withholding or falsely representing health information has previously been justified under the physician's duty of beneficence. By this account, the doctrine of therapeutic privilege, the health information is said to be too complex, or too tragic for the patient to deal with. It may concern a terminal diagnosis, to which the patient might respond with despondency or cynicism. This might in turn lead the patient to self-harm, or to forgo further treatment. It is for the patient's well-being that the physician withholds information.

Therapeutic privilege presumes that the physician knows the patient's best interests better than the patient does. In a plural society of individuals, each pursuing unique ends,

MCCQE C₂LEO Essentials

Truth Telling

- Truth telling is based on respect for patient autonomy, and is important for the maintenance of faith in the patient–physician relationship
- Physicians must speak truthfully, and refrain from falsehood
- Provide patients with opportunities to know important health information, including
  - Purpose and implications of investigations
  - Diagnosis and prognosis
  - Risks and benefits of treatment
  - Risks to which the patient may have been exposed (e.g., by medical error)
- Respect the patient's right to know, or not to know: seek consent for disclosure, and ascertain patient preferences.
- The doctrine of therapeutic privilege has been discredited except in extraordinary circumstances

this presumption is untenable at best, paternalistic at worst. Therapeutic privilege serves a narrow set of interests determined by physicians, and may fail to account for complex circumstances or conceptions of wellness. This failure may do the patient harm. It certainly infringes on self-determination, by preventing the full range of patient preferences from expressing themselves.

Therapeutic privilege may usefully be invoked where a significant risk of substantial harm accompanies honest disclosure. However, means of mitigating the risk of harm should be explored first, including emotional support and counselling. The situations that remain will be extraordinary. Therapeutic privilege is, properly, a last resort.

There are consequential grounds for truth telling. Patients or their families will inevitably come to know information that was withheld or misrepresented. The consequent feelings of betrayal may jeopardize the patient–physician relationship. The importance of honesty should not be underestimated.

Of course, none of the foregoing should dismiss the psychological coping value of shunning information. A patient's way of dealing with illness will be affected by personal and cultural context. A decision to waive disclosure, if made voluntarily, is a valid decision, and should be respected.

Legally, patients have rights of access and control over their health information—these rights and the corresponding obligations they place on health information custodians can be found in health information statutes and in the fiduciary nature of the patient–physician relationship (see Confidentiality). Additionally, failure to disclose health information that leads to patient harm may be construed as negligence.

Medicine is best practiced within the patient's own conception of best interests—this requires honesty, frank discussion, and attentiveness to patient preferences.

A PATIENT-CENTERED PROTOCOL FOR BREAKING BAD NEWS

Patients should be provided with opportunities to know their health information. Admittedly, health information may be difficult to handle, and should be disclosed sensitively. Permission to disclose information should be sought first. The SPIKES protocol published by Baile et al. is useful.

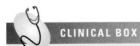

CLINICAL BOX

SPIKES Protocol for Breaking Bad News

S—Setting up the interview

P—Assessing patient's perceptions

I—Obtaining the patient's Invitation (i.e., to disclose information)

K—Giving Knowledge and information to the patient

E—Addressing the patient's Emotions

S—Strategy and Summary

NEGLIGENCE

Negligence is a tort: a private, as opposed to a public, wrong actionable through legal means, involving an injury to person or property. The usual remedy imposed by courts for physicians found liable for negligence is monetary compensation for damages and costs.

Professional colleges may also suspend or revoke license to practice. This occurs separately from the negligence suit.

At common law, the physician is liable for negligence when the plaintiff is able to prove the existence of a duty of care, a breach of that duty, causation, and consequent harm.

MCCQE C₂LEO Essentials

Negligence

Negligence requires that the plaintiff prove the existence of a duty of care, a breach of duty, causation, and consequent patient harm.

- Duty of care
  - Arises from the doctor–patient relationship
  - Duty is also owed to third parties in certain instances
  - The duty of care ends at the termination of the patient–physician relationship
- Standard of care
  - **The quality of care that can be expected of a reasonable practitioner of similar training and experience**
  - Specific to the time of alleged negligence
  - Different for specialists and generalists
  - Standard of care is the same for similar practitioners **regardless of location**
- Breach of duty
  - Breach of duty ≠ error of judgment
  - Key question: Could a reasonable practitioner with appropriate training commit this error or omission? If no, then breach of duty has likely occurred
- Causation
- Patient harm

Actions for negligence must be launched within certain time periods after treatment, with limits varying from province to province according to statute.

Robertson G. Negligence and malpractice, Chapter 3. In: Downie J, Caulfield T, Flood C, eds. *Canadian health law and policy*, 2nd ed. Markham: Butterworths Canada Ltd.; 2002.

DUTY OF CARE

A duty of care arises from the patient–physician relationship. Physicians also owe duties of care to individuals outside established patient–physician relationships. For example, there exists, in the United States, a duty to disclose health information when maintenance of confidentiality would result in significant risk of substantial harm to others (see Confidentiality). This responsibility is essentially a duty of care owed to third parties threatened with harm. The legal precedent establishing this duty is the US case, *Tarasoff v. Regents*. Case-law precedent has yet to be established in Canada, but it is likely that similar duties will be found to exist.

In the event of an emergency, a physician may be called upon to care for an individual with whom he or she has no patient–physician relationship. Whether or not Canadian law recognizes a duty of rescue, under which a physician-as-bystander would be obliged to act, is controversial. Nonetheless, if emergency care is provided, the provider may be obliged to exercise due diligence and to meet professional standards, to the extent that emergent circumstances make this possible. The physician may therefore owe a duty of care to the injured individual.

To those to whom a duty of care is owed, the medical practitioner is bound to provide adequate care, and to exercise **the degree of care and skill which could reasonably be expected of a normal, prudent practitioner of the same experience and standing**. This standard of care differs according to training; however, it should be noted that generalists performing procedures typically performed by specialists will be held to the specialist standard of care. Recognizing that medical knowledge changes quickly, the standard of care is also dynamic. In medical malpractice suits, the relevant standard is the set of expectations that existed at the time of the alleged negligence. Additionally, the standard of care is common to all equivalent practitioners, regardless of locality. Therefore, a rural emergency physician is held to the same standard as an urban emergency physician. And although physicians cannot be expected to provide services that are not locally available, there is a duty to disclose such services and how they might be accessed to the patient, and to arrange for appropriate referral or transfer.

In an era of health care reform, physicians may feel pressured to minimize referrals or transfers, or to reduce the utilization of expensive services. This pressure often relates to institutional cost-containment efforts. However, where medically appropriate services are available, physicians are required to disclose this fact, to discuss access with the patient, and to arrange access as appropriate, regardless of cost. Cost-containment is not a defence to negligence.

The specific content of the standard of care is usually based on the approved practices that exist at the time of care. These are to be determined at court by reference to, among other things, expert testimony, clinical practice guidelines, and hospital policies. However, there is some latitude for the courts to deviate from approved practice. This may occur when approved practices are fraught with obvious risk, or when the matter under consideration is of a nontechnical nature, such that an individual without clinical expertise may determine a minimum standard of care. These circumstances are limited, but they highlight the point that physicians should not accept approved practices unquestioningly.

BREACH OF DUTY

A breach of care occurs when a medical provider makes an error or omission that no reasonable physician of similar training and experience would make under the circumstances. Not all errors are breaches of duty. Physicians are not infallible, and circumstances can militate against diagnostic or therapeutic success. Errors in diagnosis and treatment, **i.e., errors of judgment**, will occur. These errors may lead to significant harm, but do not constitute negligence if the standard of the reasonable practitioner is met.

Notably, an error of judgment in the initial instance may become a breach of duty if, for example, medical staff fail to reevaluate a (mis-)diagnosis in light of nonresponse to treatment.

CAUSATION AND INJURY

A negligence suit requires that there be patient harm, and that the harm occurred as a result of the breach of duty. If injury or causation cannot be established, damages will not be awarded. Recently, certain claims have made thorny issues of causation and injury. A suit alleging wrongful life is brought by parents, **on behalf of a disabled child**, who is born, e.g., as a result of a physician's failure to recommend genetic screening. If the physician had fulfilled the standard of care and recommended genetic screening, the disability may have been detected, the parents would have terminated the pregnancy, and the child would have been saved from the harm of a life of disability. Wrongful life suits have not been well received by Canadian courts: establishing injury on behalf of the child would require comparing the child's life to nonexistence!

A wrongful birth suit, in contrast, is brought on behalf of the parents, and seeks compensation for costs and damages incurred in caring for the disabled child. Damages for the cost of raising the child have been awarded in such cases.

RESOURCE ALLOCATION

Resource allocation decisions concern questions of justice: How are resources fairly distributed among health needs? On what basis is it acceptable to make these decisions? The basis, whether intentional or unintentional, for differential access to health care goods and services among patients should meet ethical and legal standards for fairness.

Responsibilities for health care resource allocations occur, at three levels: macrolevel, mesolevel, and microlevel. Broadly speaking, global budgets are determined at the

MCCQE C₂LEO Essentials
Resource Allocation and Clinical Decision Making

- The physician owes a primary duty to the patient.
- Clinical care (i.e., **micro**level decision making) must not be compromised by cost constraints.
- Resources should be allocated fairly: on the basis of morally relevant criteria, i.e., need and potential benefit, using fair and publicly defensible procedures.
- The impact of **meso**level and **macro**level rationing decisions should be discussed with the patient in a supportive way.
- Resources should be deployed prudently.

Table **2.2**	Levels of Health Care Resource Allocation	
Macro	**Meso**	**Micro**
Government policy—federal and provincial (e.g., health insurance policy, taxation, federal transfer payments, physician fee-for-service regulations)	Health region/institutional policy (e.g., decision to add ICU beds, ICU admissions policy)	Physician—Patient clinical interaction (e.g., prescription decisions, aggressive vs. conservative approaches)

macrolevel. Services and access conditions are determined by mesolevel policy. Finally, clinical decision making occurs at the microlevel. While macrolevel and mesolevel decision makers must make decisions that incorporate considerations of costs and competing interests, the microlevel decision maker (e.g., the physician) must remain loyal to the patient's interests. The physician may—and should—advocate for the patient interests in macrolevel and mesolevel decisions. Ultimately, though, the physician's clinical work occurs **within** the resource frameworks and constraints determined at the upper levels. This division of responsibilities removes global cost considerations from the microlevel, freeing clinicians to focus on patient welfare. Clinical decisions should be driven entirely by patient need and potential benefit.

This section addresses clinical resource allocation, and focuses on three issues: fair access to health care, the obligation to seek the patient's best interests, and prudent use of health care resources.

FAIR ACCESS TO HEALTH CARE

Individuals are morally equal, and equally worthy of respect. This is not to say that equality of outcomes must follow: not all individuals who show up in hospital should receive equal quantities of morphine, for example. In medical decision making, the fundamental equality of individuals is observed when cases that are similar in morally relevant ways are treated similarly, and dissimilar cases dissimilarly.

The "morally relevant ways" usually boil down to need and potential benefit. Differential treatment on the basis of such properties as age, sex, and religion are tolerated **only insofar as** these properties can be demonstrably linked to need and potential benefit. Otherwise, these properties are irrelevant. All other things being equal, granting a white female differential access to reproductive health over a female of aboriginal descent—perhaps by providing better counselling or by providing access to services such as abortion more readily—represents a devaluation of the aboriginal female's interests on the grounds of race. This sort of discrimination fails to recognize the patient as a morally significant being worthy of equal respect.

Legally, equality rights are recognized in Section 15 of the Canadian *Charter of Rights and Freedoms*. Constitutional case law has conceptualized equality obligations into two sorts: nondiscrimination requires that individuals be treated alike; substantive equality requires that positive measures be undertaken to provide equal access for those whose special characteristics disadvantage them on the basis of race, religion, sex, disability, and so on. The *Charter of Rights and Freedoms* may apply to hospitals operating under a public mandate, or with public funds. Physicians may also be bound by professional codes of ethics, and by provincial human rights statutes that impose similar duties.

In clinical care, this means that discrimination is unacceptable. Resources should be allocated on the basis of morally relevant criteria, using fair and publicly defensible procedures. Positive measures (e.g., sign language or TTD services for the deaf, access to female physicians for female patients whose cultural beliefs prohibit care from a female physician, etc.) should be taken to ensure that the interests of all patients are equally served.

PRUDENT USE OF CLINICAL RESOURCES AND THE OBLIGATION TO SEEK THE PATIENT'S BEST INTERESTS

In the late 1980s and 1990s, governments, perceiving budget deficits and rising health care costs, embarked on a series of health care reform initiatives. As a side effect, physicians have felt pressure to contain costs, e.g., by minimizing the use of expensive modalities. In the negligence case, *Law Estate v. Simice et al.*, physicians accused of negligence in failing to provide a patient with a medically necessary CT scan mentioned cost constraints. In response, British Columbia Supreme Court Justice Spencer writes:

> "If it comes to a choice between a physician's responsibility to his or her individual patient and his or her responsibility to the Medicare system overall, the former must take precedence in a case such as this. The severity of the harm that may occur to the patient who is permitted to go undiagnosed is far greater than the financial harm that will occur to the medicare system if one more CT scan procedure only shows the patient is not suffering from a serious medical condition." (*Law Estate v. Simice*)

Cost constraints should not interfere with clinical care. First, physicians, owing a duty of care to their patients, must meet the standard of care that can be expected from a reasonable practitioner of similar training and experience. Cost constraints are no defence against negligence. Second, physicians are fiduciaries in a trust relationship with their relatively vulnerable patients. They are duty-bound to look after the interests of their patients with the utmost loyalty. Because the cost of physicians' services in Canada is borne by the Medicare system, allowing cost considerations into clinical reasoning amounts to the entry of a third-party interest. Physicians are duty-bound to resist this intrusion, and to maintain the independence of their clinical judgment. Where cost constraints do affect clinical decisions, perhaps because of limitations imposed at the mesolevel and macrolevel, physicians need to discuss, in a sensitive manner that avoids laying blame, the effects of cost constraints, available treatment alternatives, and the means of accessing them.

This does not mean, of course, that physicians should not use resources prudently. Physicians may need to mediate a common understanding of fair and prudent care with patients. Excessive treatment, or treatments of marginal benefit, may subject patients to more harm than good. Physicians, having many patients, are also fiduciaries to many beneficiaries. Moe Litman suggests that physicians might apply the legal concept of "keeping an even hand amongst beneficiaries" as a lens. Not to be applied literally, this principle is satisfied if "allocation decisions are made on a nonpersonalized, relatively objective basis, in accordance with appropriate principles intended to maximize the health care of patients". In the clinic, this means:

- Choosing interventions known to be beneficial on the basis of evidence
- Minimizing the use of marginally beneficial tests or interventions
- Seeking the tests or treatments that will accomplish the diagnostic or therapeutic goal for the least cost
- Advocating for one's own patients, but not manipulating the system to gain unfair advantage to them.

Physicians are not obliged to provide interventions that are harmful or futile, though the notion of futility needs to be approached with respect for alternative conceptions of "meaningfulness" in health care. The duty to seek consent, i.e., a duty not to treat patients against their will does not imply a positive duty to treat. Physicians **are** bound by professional ethics and by the law of negligence to provide a professional level of care, but not to satisfy every desire.

RESEARCH ETHICS

Research involves the use of formal methods, in a purposeful way, for the generation of generalizable knowledge. Ideally, medical research contributes to social welfare by increasing our capacity to detect, treat, and predict the course of disease. However, research that involves human subjects poses special considerations, given, among other things, the risk of doing harm to research subjects.

Physicians are often involved in human research. That physicians are also clinicians, expected to form treatment relationships with their patients, admits for some confusion. Whereas the goal of research is to develop generalizable knowledge, the purpose of a therapeutic relationship is to promote patient well-being and autonomy. Often, the two aims do not coincide. For instance, a clinical trial may require randomization of patient to treatment or treatment control groups. In a therapeutic relationship, treatments are matched to patients on the basis of need and potential benefit. Can a physician, in good conscience, permit randomized treatment? Another example: A chart review may require health

---

MCCQE C₂LEO Essentials
Research Ethics

- Ethical research involves a balance between patient welfare interests and the social benefits of research.
- Patient autonomy and the right of self-determination are privileged.
- Fully informed and voluntary consent is the default norm, but consent and disclosure standards vary for different sorts of research, and for research with different populations.
- Patients cannot consent to otherwise unethical research.
- Sound and ethical research meets a high standard of scholarly merit and minimizes the risk to which patients are exposed.
- Conflicts of interest must be disclosed.
- Human research should be approved by and accountable to an independent REB.

---

information to be accessed, in a way that confers no direct benefit to the patient whatsoever. The chart review would appear to contravene the physician's duty to further the patient's welfare, which normally rules against noneffective interventions, that is, those known to provide no benefits to the patient. Conflicts such as these are ubiquitous—they stem from a fundamental tension between the research and clinical roles physicians inhabit. The task of physician-researchers and regulators is to negotiate these tensions: first, by maintaining respect for autonomy as a touchstone; second, by negotiating a balance between them.

CANADA'S RESEARCH REGULATORY FRAMEWORK AND REBS

Canada lacks comprehensive human research legislation. Instead, there are a number of statutes that relate to various aspects of research, in patchwork fashion (e.g., provincial consent and health information laws). But the most comprehensive statements of researchers' duties and subjects' rights are quasi-legal guidelines and recommendations, which fall into two categories. First, ethical codes and conduct guidelines developed by professional organizations form a body of professional norms, adopted by members themselves, that professionals are obliged to uphold. These include the **CMA Code of Ethics** and the World Medical Association's **Helsinki Declaration**. Although they do not carry the force of statute, they have power nonetheless. Courts may invoke them to determine the standard of care in negligence suits, and professional colleges may discipline breaches as professional misconduct. Second, funding may be contingent on guidelines developed by research funders, the most notable of which is the tricouncil (i.e., joint CIHR, NSERC, and SSHRC) policy statement, **Ethical Conduct for Research Involving Humans**. Researchers who fail to observe these guidelines may be ineligible for public funding, or may have their funding revoked. This gives the tricouncil policy great clout for publicly funded research.

Additionally, protocols for clinical trials intended to demonstrate a drug, medical device, and biologic or natural product's safety and efficacy for regulatory purposes must undergo review and approval by various directorates of Health Canada before initiation. Health Canada's powers and mandates over these matters are provided by the federal *Food and Drug Act* and related federal regulation. These regulations also impose other ethics requirements.

This network of instruments is Canada's research regulatory framework. Among other things, it may be criticized for gaps in regulatory coverage. For example, obligations incumbent on privately funded research not aimed at regulatory approval with Health Canada are unclear.

Prominent in this system of regulation is the requirement for independent review. A history of ethical disasters in human research—the Nazi doctors and Tuskegee, to name two examples—suggests that research should be reviewed before projects are undertaken. Aspects of research proposals—for example, research design and purpose—require scientific expertise to assess. Yet the researcher cannot be the final arbiter of his or her own proposal. The research imperative and potential conflicts of interest may militate too strongly against a balanced ethical assessment, especially when positive undertakings may be required to safeguard patient interests. Generally, research must be independently reviewed by an institutional REB. REBs integrate scientific, clinical, ethical, legal, and community representation in light of relevant circumstances to review a research proposal's scholarly and ethical value. They may authorize lower standards for consent or disclosure, where higher standards would preclude socially beneficial research and where the risk of research is low or effectively mitigated. Alternatively, REBs may compel researchers to institute stronger measures to safeguard patient well-being. REBs are a check and balance on human research, and represent an institutional commitment to scholarship that balances research's social importance with the rights of research subjects.

CLINICAL EQUIPOISE AND SCHOLARLY MERIT

If a physician should feel that a certain treatment is in a subject's best interests, is a randomized treatment protocol acceptable? The notion of clinical equipoise helps navigate this tension between the aims of research and the aims of therapy. Clinical equipoise occurs when there is genuine uncertainty regarding appropriate therapy for a disease. In clinical trials, researchers experience clinical equipoise when they perceive an even chance that the treatment regime will be as effective as the control regime. For many diseases, a control regime that meets this criterion will be the current standard of care, **not** placebo. To sketch the point simply, when clinical equipoise exists, randomization is compatible with the duty of beneficence because there is no certain knowledge to suggest that the patient would benefit more from one regime than another.

Clinical equipoise relates to the concept of scholarly merit. When clinical equipoise is not the case, that is, if there is already reasonable certainty in the professional community regarding the research question or hypothesis, the utility of the research is questionable. All research that involves human subjects, whether the project is a chart review or a trial of an invasive intervention, involves some risk to the subjects. If the research will not produce new knowledge, then subjects are exposed to risk for no good reason. Other factors impacting the utility of the research effort include the research question, which should be nontrivial; the design of the study, which must be adequate to address the question posed; and the inclusion criteria, which must isolate patients for whom the test and control treatments are equally appropriate and screen out confounding elements. These factors are issues of scholarly merit. Because their evaluation requires expertise in the field and its methodologies, REB review may require independent peer or expert input. To be ethical, research must meet a standard of scholarship.

CONSENT AND DISCLOSURE

Is clinical consent required? If so, to what standard? The first article of the Nuremberg Code, a set of principles developed at the Nuremberg "Doctors' Trial," in the aftermath of inhumane experiments on humans performed by the Nazis, articulates an absolute requirement for consent that is informed, voluntary, and capable. This standard applies to clinical trials, where there may be substantial risk to patients undertaking novel interventions. In clinical trials (and other sorts of research, e.g., population surveys) the dual role of clinician-researchers may give rise to a perception that research will benefit the patient, even if it does not; or that clinical care may be affected if the patient refuses participation. Patients must be free to decline participation at any time without prejudice to the care they can expect from their care providers. Care providers and research staff may need to operate at some distance from each other to prevent coercion. And continuing opportunities to withdraw should be provided and respected.

But what about chart reviews, or epidemiologic studies in which obtaining consent from all patients involved would be excessively onerous? In such studies, the major risk to patients is that their health information may be exposed. Identifiable health information is sensitive information, in which subjects have a continuing interest. In certain jurisdictions, the conditions under which health information, identifiable or deidentified, can be accessed for research purposes without consent may be outlined in legislation. Generally, REBs are reasonable: where the risk is minimal and well managed, and the social benefits substantial, and otherwise unattainable, consent and disclosure may be waived.

Notably, the Nuremberg Code leaves no room for research involving incompetent patients, whether they are children or incompetent adults. These individuals may yet benefit from participation in research, for example, in a clinical trial that gives them access to new treatments. The group to which these individuals belong, for instance, the subset of children to whom the research applies, may benefit from the new knowledge generated. Newer formulations of consent requirements allow the participation of incompetent individuals through consent by SDM. However, parents of potential child-subjects are generally obliged to seek their children's best interests: If a child does not stand to benefit directly from research, the legal ability of a parent to consent to participation is questionable. The law around this issue is unclear in Canada, except in Quebec. In general, research should not pose a serious risk to the subject; if children are sought as subjects, their participation must be necessary to the project; and a child's refusal to participate should be respected, whatever the child's capacity.

As with consent, the requirement of disclosure may vary with the research project. For a chart review involving hundreds of charts, with proper safeguards for patient information, it seems prohibitive that researchers should be required to contact each and every patient for disclosure. Consent and health information statutes and the guidance of the institutional REB will determine the extent of investigators' obligations. Of course, riskier undertakings, like clinical trials, will require disclosure. In court cases that have addressed the issue, the standard of disclosure has been determined to extend beyond the usual clinical standard. It has been characterized as "the most exacting duty possible, requiring full and frank disclosure of all risks, no matter how rare or remote, as well as other material information about the research." The experimental nature of any novel treatments offered should be emphasized to distinguish them from routine clinical care. Developments that alter the material risks and benefits of participation may need to be disclosed as they occur. Investigators are responsible for ensuring patient understanding.

Importantly, informed consent is a necessary, but not a sufficient, requirement for participation in research. REB reviewers and investigators must also consider factors such as scholarly merit, conflicts of interest, and the risk/benefit profile. Potential research participants **cannot** consent to otherwise unethical research, even if their consent is fully autonomous.

CONFLICTS OF INTEREST IN RESEARCH

Many entities influence and have a stake in the research enterprise. Of these interests, the commercial link between industry and the research community has attracted much attention. Industry contributes significantly to health research, undoubtedly facilitating research that otherwise would not be possible. Where the scientific and ethical standards of research are upheld, the commercial incentive may be socially beneficial. However, numerous commentators and high-profile cases of commercial conflicts of interest have brought public attention to bear on commercial involvement in research. For example, in 1996, Dr. Nancy Olivieri identified adverse effects of the drug deferiprone during a clinical trial. The pharmaceutical company and research sponsor, Apotex, insisted that she abide by confidentiality clauses attached to her research funding, jeopardizing the safety of her research participants.

The fiduciary responsibility of a physician to his or her patients is a duty of utmost loyalty. It requires that the fiduciary refrain from conflicts of interest and, where this is not possible, that the fiduciary resolve conflicts of interest in the patients' favor. Applied to the research setting, this means that physicians are obliged to disclose conflicts of interest to regulators, and to patients when performing disclosure for consent. Physicians should maintain their scientific and clinical independence, and must resolve conflicts of interests in favor of research participant welfare.

PROFESSIONALISM AND THE REGULATION OF HEALTH CARE PROFESSIONALS

Professionalism refers to the practice of medicine according to a common set of norms and standards, characterized by ethical conduct, clinical independence, and self-regulation. These norms and standards are developed and enforced by physicians themselves, through physician organizations that control practitioners' entry to the health care market.

Health care is an imperfect market. Patients are unable to know when or if they will be sick. The diagnosis, treatment, and prevention of illness require years of training. Health care decisions can impact third parties, and stricken patients may not be in a position to make autonomous decisions. The public is exposed to substantial harm in a "free" (i.e., unregulated) health care market. To protect their citizens, governments intervene in the supply and provision of health services to produce a uniform standard of care.

Provincial governments accomplish this purpose by restricting the supply of medical practitioners to specially certified and licensed individuals, governed by physician-run colleges. However, allowing physicians to determine their own standards of professional entry and practice creates an occupational monopoly through which physicians have acquired extraordinary power and privilege. This arrangement is justifiable only insofar as

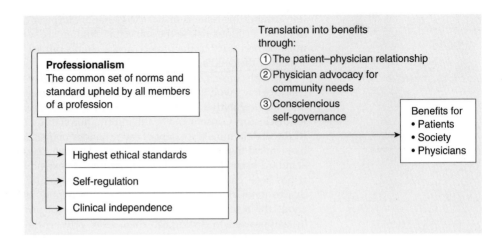

Figure 2.2 Professionalism. With abstractions from the CMA policy, **Medical Professionalism.**

it continues to serve the public interest. Physicians are therefore charged by statute, and obliged by social contract, to set and uphold common standards of conduct, collectively, and as individuals. Additionally, standards of professional conduct translate principles of patient autonomy, beneficence, nonmaleficence, justice, and patient-centered care into clinical practice. Adhering to professional norms ensures sound care, helps guarantee fidelity to the core principles of medicine, and maintains the public's trust in the profession.

Challenges to professionalism interfere with the ethical and clinically independent practice of medicine according to commonly accepted norms and standards. Personal factors, such as alcoholism, overwork, marital strife, loneliness, and financial distress, may affect an individual's ability to practice medicine. The line between the professional and the personal can be indistinct. Personal problems may affect patient care. Equally, professional responsibilities may weigh down personal life. Professionalism therefore requires achieving balance and equanimity in both clinical **and** personal matters.

Impairment occurs when personal factors interfere with the professional practice of medicine. Physicians have a duty to prevent practice-under-the-influence.

The 2005 CMA Policy, **Medical Professionalism**, identifies other challenges to professionalism, including resource restraints, commercialism (e.g., the market mentality and commercial interests), and consumerism (e.g., patient demand for unnecessary or inappropriate interventions). These challenges are environmental and systemic. They express identifiable social trends that impact the professionalism of physicians not only at the level

 MCCQE C₂LEO Essentials
Professionalism

Physicians should conduct themselves according to the common norms and values of the profession.

- Practice should be characterized by clinical independence and the highest ethical standards. Dignity, respect, integrity, and honesty are essential.
- Possess and maintain medical expertise.
- Practice without impairment by substances, ill health, or other incapacity.

As a self-regulating profession, physicians have responsibilities of loyalty to patient welfare and to the public interest.

MCCQE C₂LEO Essentials
Physicians and Industry

Relationships with pharmaceuticals
- Are regulated by an ethical code
- Must not affect independent clinical judgement
- Must not impinge on duty to one's patients

Table **2.3**	**Professional Expectations of Physician–Pharmaceutical Interactions**
Situation	**Expectation**
Drug samples	Should not result in material gain for the physician or practice
CME	Physician-organizers must control organization, content, and choice of activities Funds from commercial sources should not be directed to individual attendees (e.g., no industry funding of individual travel bursaries) Allocation of promotional displays should not be influenced by sponsorship
Industry-sponsored research	Sponsors should guarantee that results will be made public within a reasonable period Remuneration for enrolling patients is unacceptable, except to recover costs Physicians should disclose relevant relationships to industry to research subjects and to academic journals
Investment in pharmaceuticals	Should be avoided if it might inappropriately affect clinical practice
Personal gifts	Should not be accepted
Teaching aids	Are acceptable only if they do not refer to specific agents, services, or products

Selected and abridged from the CMA Policy, *Physicians and the Pharmaceutical Industry*.

of individual practitioners but collectively as well. Of these challenges, physician relations with industry have received particular attention.

Drugs consume more and more health care spending every year—spending that remunerates pharmaceutical companies. Because physicians direct and control consumer access to the prescription drug market, the pharmaceutical industry has a commercial interest in influencing physician-prescribing practices. Commercial interests further the public good when pharmaceuticals encourage the adoption of safer, more effective, or more cost-effective treatments. They set the public back when, for example, expensive drugs with no benefit over cheaper alternatives are aggressively marketed, or when physicians experience pressure to suppress negative clinical outcomes. With respect to drugs, physicians need to assess industry claims independently, on the basis of sound evidence, to maximize the social benefit of the commercial incentive. More generally, physicians should maintain their professional distance and clinical independence.

REGULATION OF MEDICAL PRACTICE

MCCQE C₂LEO Essentials
Regulation of Medical Practice

- Health care is an imperfect market. Unregulated, it would subject consumers to unacceptable risk.
- Physicians' competence and conduct is legally (and ethically) regulated to protect patients and society in general.
- The objectives of regulation are performed by self-regulating physician licensing and certification bodies.
- Certification indicates that a practitioner has met certain requirements of education, knowledge, and competency. Certification bodies include the MCC, the CFPC, and the RCPSC.
- Licensure from a provincial board or college is a legal requirement for medical practice.
- Licensure is nontransferable between provinces.
- Physician representation and advocacy are carried out by distinct medical associations (i.e., the CMA and its provincial chapters) separate from the regulatory functions of licensing and certification.
- The CMPA is a medical defence association.

CERTIFICATION AND LICENSING

Medical practice is regulated at the level of input and output. Input regulation throws up barriers to entry into the health care market, and might in turn be conceptualized as consisting of two sorts of schemes: certification and licensure. In a certification regime, certain agencies are granted exclusive powers to certify individuals as having met particular performance or educational standards. Certification provides a "quality signal" to patients, hospitals, and other organizations interested in acquiring or accessing physician services; and certified practitioners gain an advantage in the health care market. Canada's physician certification bodies include the CFPC, the RCPSC, and the MCC. These three organizations set national standards for family practice, specialty practice, and independent medical practice, respectively. The national character of these organizations means that the medical degree and certification are portable from province to province.

Under a licensing regime, unlicensed individuals are legally prohibited from providing certain services. Licensing represents an increased level of state intervention in the health care market beyond certification because unlicensed practitioners are excluded from the market altogether. Physician-run colleges or boards, established in each province by statute, govern licensing. Licensure is nontransferable from province to province, and must be sought and awarded by the college or board responsible for medical licensing in each province of practice. Additionally, provincial colleges typically require certification from the MCC, as well as certification from one of the CFPC or RCPSC. In practice, then, uncertified physicians are excluded from medical practice, although certifying bodies bear no responsibility for licensing.

SELF-REGULATION

Physician certification and licensing bodies are self-regulating. Their operations, the standards they set and enforce, and the policies for which they advocate are determined by physicians themselves. The responsibilities of certification and licensure require considerable medical expertise and organizational resources, which would need to be acquired or contracted by nonphysician regulators. Physicians fulfill these duties more effectively and efficiently by self-regulation. Self-regulation also makes use of collegiality and peer pressure to increase compliance with medical standards. However, the interests of the profession may occasionally clash with the interests of the public. To prevent conflicts of interest, professional advocacy is carried out separately by distinct medical associations—the CMA and its provincial chapters. Medical associations neither certify nor license, and membership is voluntary. Medical student and resident associations perform analogous functions for medical students and residents, respectively.

Finally, the CMPA, a legal defence fund, looks after the legal interests of individual practitioners. In return for annual membership fees, the CMPA provides members with legal representation in the event of a malpractice suit, and foots the bill for settlements or damages awarded to plaintiffs.

OUTPUT REGULATION

Output regulation concerns actual performance, after the fact. Penalties assessed against deficient care or conduct provide an incentive to maintain professional standards. Disciplinary proceedings, whereby provincial colleges leverage their powers to grant, revoke, or suspend medical licensure to penalize breaches of professional standards, are an important form of output regulation. Legal liability is another form of output regulation.

GENERAL ORGANIZATION OF HEALTH CARE IN CANADA

In the Canadian constitutional framework, the provinces have primary responsibilities for health care, executed through a range of statutes that vary from province to province. The federal government nevertheless performs an important and varied role in health care that goes beyond merely funding provincial efforts.

CONSTITUTIONAL UNDERPINNINGS

Except for marine hospitals and quarantine, which are matters of federal jurisdiction, the 1867 Constitution Act apportions responsibility for much of what we recognize as health care to the provinces. The federal government therefore has no power to mandate or

Table **2.4**	**Overview of Physician Organizations**		

Major Function(s) (Simplified)	Organization	Licensure/Certification/ Membership Required for Practice?	Comments
Licensing	Provincial College of Physicians and Surgeons	Yes	Provincial colleges determine licensing, scope of practice, standards of practice, and codes of conduct
Certification	MCC	Yes	Evaluate medical graduates according to national standards for independent medical practice
Certification and PGME	CFPC	One of certification with the CFPC or RCPSC	Certify family physicians, set criteria for family medicine residency programs, advocate for family medicine as a specialty
Certification and PGME	RCPSC		Certify specialists, set criteria for specialty residency programs
Advocacy	CMA	No	Support provincial medical associations, represent physicians nationally, develop clinical practice policies
Advocacy	Provincial Medical Association	No	Advocate for physicians, negotiate terms of work with provincial ministries of health
Advocacy and professional development	Specialty organizations	No	Publish clinical practice guidelines, provide continuing education, advocate for specialities
Legal representation, malpractice suits	CMPA	No	Provide legal representation in the event of malpractice suits, provide financial support against settlements or damages awarded to plaintiffs

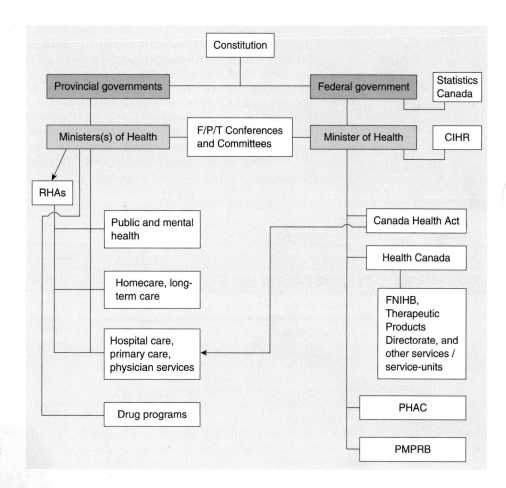

Figure 2.3 General Organization of Health Care in Canada. Organizational scheme, simplified. (Figured modified with permission from Marchildon G. *Healthcare systems in transition: Canada.* Toronto: University of Toronto Press; 2006.)

Table **2.5**	Additional Federal Powers Related to Health
Constitutional Responsibility for	**Application to Health**
Criminal law	Laws governing narcotics, food and drugs, and tobacco
Indians and reserves; the militia and military; and penitentiaries	Health care for status Indians, military personnel, veterans, RCMP members, and inmates falls under federal jurisdiction
Taxation and spending	Federal funding for the CIHR, Genome Canada, the Canada Health Services Research Foundation, and other programs that impact health care knowledge and delivery Federal-provincial transfer payments that help fund provincial health care systems
Patents of invention and discovery	The regulation of the prices of patented drugs through the PMPRB
POGG	The POGG power is invoked in situations of crisis or to address issues of "national concern" The POGG power has never been tested in respect of health care; its applications remain theoretic

interfere directly with a province's arrangements for the provision of health care to its citizens. However, the constitution grants the federal government powers which affect health care, including responsibility for patents, and for the criminal code. These powers are listed in Table 2.5.

Particularly important is the federal spending power. The national CHA framework leverages this power, through the use of conditional federal-provincial transfer payments, to achieve specific aims among and within the provinces.

THE CANADA HEALTH ACT—A "NARROW BUT DEEP" SYSTEM OF HEALTH CARE INSURANCE

The *CHA* was passed in 1984, consolidating and building on two previous acts, the 1957 federal *HIDS Act* and the 1966 federal *Medical Care Act*. The CHA establishes criteria and conditions that must be met before provinces qualify for a full federal cash contribution for health care. Provinces must establish a **publicly administered** health care insurance program that provides **universal, comprehensive, portable, and accessible** coverage.

In addition to these five conditions, Section 20 of the CHA prohibits user charges and extra billing. Whereas the CHA **permits** the federal government to withhold portions of the cash transfer if its five conditions are breached, it **requires** the federal government to deduct at least the amount of the user fee or extra billing from federal-provincial cash contributions until user fees and extra billing are eliminated.

Despite the lack of federal jurisdiction in health care, the **CHA** framework has fostered the establishment of provincial health care plans along national principles. The public

Table **2.6**	Conditions of the Canada Health Act
Condition	**Each Provincial Health Care Insurance Plan Must**
Accessibility	Not impede or preclude reasonable access to insured health services (**Note 1**)
Comprehensiveness	Cover all medically necessary hospital, physician, and surgical-dental (i.e., those that require a hospital setting) services
Portability	Cover new residents to the province within a waiting period of not more than 3 mo; cover residents leaving the province during a waiting period for new coverage; pay for insured services for residents temporarily out-of-province or out-of-country (**Note 2**)
Public administration	Be operated on a nonprofit basis by a public authority designated by the province
Universality	Insure all insurees at uniform terms and conditions

Note 1: This condition is an addition to principles outlined in previous health care legislation. It targets such practices as user charges, which impede access for those with lower incomes.

Note 2: The rates of pay for out-of-province services are defined according to rates for similar services in the province of delivery. Those for out-of-country services are defined according to rates in the home province.

Quebec's health insurance plan does not meet portability requirements. The federal government has not pursued this breech.

MCCQE C₂LEO Essentials

User Fees and Extra Billing

- **User fees** and **extra billing** refer to fees charged to insured patients for the provision of goods or services covered by the universal provincial health insurance plan.
- User fees typically refer to fees charged by hospitals or health care facilities.
- Extra billing refers to fees charged by physicians.
- User fees and extra billing are prohibited by the CHA. The costs of insured medical or hospital services should be borne by taxpayers through the publicly administered provincial health insurance program, and not by individual patients.

health care system established by the CHA has been characterized as "narrow, but deep": within the narrow range of services that fall under the notion of "comprehensiveness" (i.e., medically necessary physician, hospital, and surgical-dental services), Canadians are very well provided for. The CHA framework represents an understanding that health care is a social good best provided for by the public weal, and that all citizens deserve adequate care regardless of their circumstances. The CHA act has been criticized for defining services that fall under its ambit by provider and setting (i.e., physician and hospital services). Health care has changed much since the days of the HIDS and *Medical Care* Acts. Take-home drugs, home care, long-term care, and the services of allied health professionals have become common, and increasingly important to patient-centeredness. For example, home care, not only reduces the cost of unnecessary hospitalization but also maintains patient autonomy by allowing the patient to remain independent in the setting of his or her choice for as long as possible. And take-home drugs impose a rapidly escalating cost on patients. Yet the CHA confers no obligation that provincial insurance plans should provide for these services. For the most part, provinces have voluntarily taken it upon themselves to establish public financing for prescription drugs, long-term care, home care, and certain other services. As a side effect, public financing for these services varies widely across Canada, and may be subject to user fees and other barriers to accessibility.

The CHA does not outlaw private funding for health care. However, six provinces have statutes that outlaw private health insurance for medically necessary services covered by the public insurance scheme. The other provinces discourage private health care insurance by preventing clinicians from operating in both private and public sectors. In effect, then, private financing—that is, private insurance and out-of-pocket payments—plays little role in health care that falls under the CHA framework. However, private sources of funding coexist with public funding for home care, long-term care, and prescription drugs. Additionally, private sources provide most coverage for dental services, vision care, and CAM, services for which public insurance funding is minor.

The balance of private funding in health care has implications for accessibility. Public insurers in Canada community-rate their premiums, providing a single, flat fee for all individuals. Private insurers, on the other hand, may obey the commercial incentive to limit liability for risky or expensive patients. They may risk-rate, that is, charge higher premiums for higher-risk individuals, or exclude certain patients from coverage. Because higher health risk often coincides with lower socioeconomic status, a regressive effect may arise in sectors dominated by private financing. Those least able to afford care may need to pay proportionally more to finance their health needs. The role of private financing in health care is a topic of hot debate, especially in light of *Chaoulli v. Quebec*, a 2005 legal case in which the Supreme Court of Canada found Quebec's prohibition against private health insurance contrary to the Quebec Charter of Rights and Freedoms.

MORE DETAILS—WHO DOES WHAT?

The provinces and territories regulate health professionals, hospitals, and other aspects of health care provision. Provinces and territories administer hospital and medical services through a universal single-payer system, remunerate physicians through FFS schedules negotiated with the provincial medical association, and run some specialized mental health and public health services. Provinces, to varying degrees, also provide or fund a variety of home care and long-term care services. All provinces also administer provincial drug plans.

In the last two decades, health care reform efforts have led provinces to adopt geographic health regions that bear responsibility for hospitals, long-term care, home care, and public health (e.g., illness prevention, population health assessment, emergency planning and preparedness, among other things). These RHAs receive global budgets and distribute health resources in light of local circumstances.

The federal roles in health care stem from the powers outlined in Table 2.4. Notably, the federal department of health, Health Canada, is responsible for administering the *CHA*; and for regulating drugs, medical devices, natural health products, and biologics. The FNIHB of Health Canada is responsible for the health needs of Canada's aboriginal peoples.

The PMPRB is a quasi-judicial watchdog that reviews and regulates wholesale drug prices for patented drugs. The PHAC, established in 2004, is a federal agency that performs a wide range of public health functions, and has responsibility for national disease centers and laboratories.

Statistics Canada helps meet Canada's health information needs. The CIHR is Canada's national health research funding agency.

At the intergovernmental level, the Conference of F/P/T Ministers of Health is the premier policy-making instrument. A range of organizations can be considered intergovernmental, being created by F/P/T agreement, with various arrangements for funding and governance. Examples include the Canadian Institute for Health Information, Canadian Blood Services, and the Health Council of Canada.

CHAPTER 3

Cardiology and Cardiovascular Surgery

Yi Zhen Ting, Mohamed Firdaus B. Mohamed Mydeen, Mohamed Shahul Hameed, and Nicholas Giacomantonio

HYPERTENSION

DEFINITION

- A BP of **>140/90 mm Hg** on three separate occasions. If there is end-organ damage, diagnosis is made on the first visit.
- ~95% of Canadians will develop HTN in an average life span.

Table **3.1**	JNC Classification of HTN	
Category	**Systolic (mm Hg)**	**Diastolic (mm Hg)**
Normal	<120	<80
Pre-HTN	120−139	80−89
Stage 1 HTN	140−159	90−99
Stage 2 HTN	≥160	≥100

ASC Box

HTN

Effect of CO and SVR on BP:

$CO = HR \times SV$ $MAP = TPR \times CO$

$BP \sim CO \times TPR$ $CO = MAP / TPR$

$MAP = dBP + 1/3$ pulse pressure

APPLIED SCIENTIFIC CONCEPTS

AUTOREGULATION

↑ CO → ↑ MAP, detected by **aortic and carotid baroreceptors** → vasodilation → ↓ TPR and hence ↓ CO (to balance the initial ↑ CO)

PRESSURE NATRIURESIS

↑ MAP = ↑ **renal perfusion, ↑ GFR, and ↓ aldosterone** → ↑ Na + H_2O excretion (natriuresis)

THE RENIN-ANGIOTENSIN-ALDOSTERONE SYSTEM

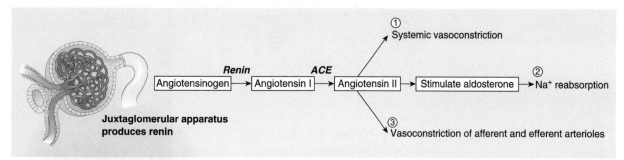

Figure 3.1 Renin-angiotensin-aldosterone system.

CAUSAL CONDITIONS

1. **1°** (essential HTN—95% of cases)
2. **2° HTN**

- Renal/vascular (↑ CO)
  - RF, polycystic kidney disease, CoA, RAS
- Endocrine (↑ SVR)
  - Hyperthyroidism, adrenal adenoma (↑ aldosterone, ↑ cortisone), **pheochromocytoma,** hyperparathyroidism

Reversible RF: obesity, poor dietary habits, high Na^+ intake, sedentary lifestyle, high EtOH and/or coffee consumption, high stress, high normal BP, illicit drug use (e.g., cocaine), herbal med (e.g., ma huang, ginseng, licorice, ginger)

APPROACH

Hx

- Age of **onset, duration**, prior Rx and response, Hx of refractory HTN? **associated Sx** (chest pain, palpitations, SOB, renal problems, headaches, diaphoresis, polyuria, hematuria, edema), Hx, or symptom of sleep apnea
- Family Hx, meds, diet, coffee intake, and EtOH
- **End-organ damage** (stroke/TIA, MI, CHF, renal disease, retinal disease), CV risk stratification
- Elicit **hypertensive emergency** (hypertensive encephalopathy, strokes, dissecting thoracic aortic aneurysm, malignant HTN, acute LV failure, acute glomerulonephritis)

Px

- BP measurement with calibrated instrument and appropriate cuff size
- **Fundi** (copper wire, cotton wool spots, AV nicking, papilledema), complete **CV exam** (clubbing, cyanosis, peripheral pulses, bruits, JVP, apex beat, parasternal heave, heart sounds and murmurs, compare U/E and L/E BP), lungs auscultation, Abdo exam for **renal mass and bruits**, edema, weight

Ix

Standard Workup

Electrolytes, BUN, CR, fasting gluc., U/A, lipid profile (fasting total cholesterol, HDL, LDL, triglycerides), EKG (to evaluate LVH Δs)

2° Causes Workup
1. Renal and vascular
   - **Renovascular** (older pt, Hx of atherosclerosis, renal artery bruit)
     - Captopril renal scan/duplex U/S, MRI, angiography
     - **Unilateral** RAS: normal Cr
     - **Bilateral** RAS: hypervolemic, ↑ Cr
   - Renal parenchymal
     - BUN, Cr, Cr clearance (also see Chapter 13)
   - CoA
     - ↓ LE pulses, radiofemoral delay, **systolic** murmur, LVH, rib notching on CXR
     - ECHO, aortogram
2. Endocrine
   - TSH, cortical, urinary VMA, PTH, aldosterone, renin, renin/aldosterone ratio

Mx

Annual F/U with high normal BP is recommended as 40% of pts with sBP 130 to 139 mm Hg or dBP 85 to 89 mm Hg develop HTN in 2 years. Home BP monitoring.

Goal ↓ BP to <140/90 mm Hg; and if pt has diabetes or renal disease, BP <130/80 mm Hg

Pharmacologic Rx
- Select med with minimal or Ø adverse effects on diabetes, asthma, and that benefits CHF or myocardial ischemia.

• Initiate pharmacologic Rx for hypertensive pt **refractory to lifestyle** Δs or pre-HTN + diabetes/renal disease.

HTN Alone

Thiazide diuretics, β-blockers, ACEIs, ARBs, long-acting CCBs as first-line Rx

• **If still Ø response** to Rx despite max tolerated dose or Rx-related adverse effect, add CCB/ARB/α-receptor blocker/centrally acting agents (methyldopa).

CLINICAL BOX

Target Organ Damage in HTN

Cerebrovascular disease

TIA

Ischemic or hemorrhagic stroke

Vascular dementia

Hypertensive retinopathy

LV dysfunction

CAD

MI

Angina

CHF

CKD

Hypertensive nephropathy

Albuminuria

Peripheral artery disease

Intermittent claudication

Table **3.2**	Antihypertensives for Pt with Other Comorbidities
Condition	**Antihypertensives**
DM	ACEI or ARB
Asthma	CCB (nondihydropyridine)
MI	ACEI, β-blocker
Angina	β-Blockers, long-acting CCB
CRF	ACEI or ARB (with caution)
CHF	ACEI, β-blocker, diuretics

CLINICAL BOX

Urinary Albumin Secretion

Identify urinary albumin secretion for **DM** and **CKD**: Rx differs without proteinuria **albumin/creatinine ratio (ACR)** >30 mg/mmol is AbN

CLINICAL BOX

Exogenous Aggravators of HTN

Prescription Drugs
• NSAIDs, including coxibs
• OCP and sex hormones
• Corticosteroids and anabolic steroids
• Vasoconstricting/sympathomimetics
• Calcineurin inhibitors (cyclosporin, tacrolimus)
• EPO and analogs
• MAOIs
• Midodrine

Other
• Salt
• Excessive EtOH use
• Sleep apnea
• Licorice root
• Stimulants including cocaine

CLINICAL BOX

Things to Consider

ACEIs and ARBs are contraindicated in pregnancy.

β-Blockers are not recommended for pts older than or 60 years without indication.

Avoid diuretic-induced hypokalemia by using K^+ sparing agent.

CLINICAL BOX

Lifestyle Therapies in HTN

Intervention	Target
Reduce foods with added Na	<100 mmol/d
Weight loss	BMI <25 kg/m²
EtOH restriction	≤Two drinks/d
Exercise	At least four times/wk, 30–60 min of moderately intense activity
Dietary patterns	Refer to Canada's food guide
Smoking cessation	Smoke free environment
Waist circumference	<102 cm for men, <88 cm for women

HYPERTENSION IN ELDERLY

ASC Box

HTN in Elderly

Factors that contribute to the ↑ prevalence of HTN in the elderly:

↓ **Compliance** of arterial wall

↓ NO dependent arterial vasodilation

↓ Numbers of functioning nephrons

↑ **Collagen**, ↑ **vascular thickening**, ↓ **elasticity**

↓ CV physiological reservoir

DEFINITION

A BP of **>140/90 mm Hg**. Isolated **systolic** HTN (sBP >140; dBP <90) is more common in the elderly population. Prevalence may reach 60% to 80% in pts aged 60 years and older.

APPLIED SCIENTIFIC CONCEPTS

- Age-related Δs in aortic vascular property
  - ↑ Age → progressive **thickening of arterial walls**—predominantly in the intimal layer → ↑ intimal to medial thickness ratio
  - ↑ **Fragmentation** and **depletion** of arterial **elastin** coupled with medial **deposition** of matrix **metalloproteins** and **collagen**
  - Collectively, this leads to thicker and stiffer arteries, predominantly **central elastic arteries.**
  - In elderly, ↑ sBP is characterized by **widened arterial pulse pressure** or Δs in vascular morphology associated with ↑ age → **small artery constriction** that ↑ the reflected component of the pulse wave
  - **Large artery stiffening** that ↑ the velocity of the reflected wave, where it moves from **diastole** to **systole** hence ↑ the sBP

CAUSAL CONDITIONS

See Hypertension

- 1° HTN
- 2° HTN
  - **Med** related (Na$^+$ retaining agents e.g., mineralocorticoids, anabolic steroids, NSAIDs, antidepressants, sympathomimetics e.g., pseudoephedrine, herbal agents)
  - **Endocrine:** thyrotoxicosis, pheochromocytoma, Cushing disease, 1° aldosteronism, hyperparathyroidism, hyper/hypothyroidism
  - **Renal:** renovascular disease (RAS), renal parenchymal disease
  - **Vascular:** aortic coarctation
  - **Sleep apnea**
- Other causes
  - **White coat HTN**
  - **Pseudohypertension** also prevalent in the elderly population due to thickening and calcification of the arteries

APPROACH

Hx

In addition to usual Hx taking for HTN:

- **Meds:** Prescribed, OTC and herbal drugs
- **Past medical history:** DM, chronic renal disease, pre-HTN, hyperlipidemia, previous CAD
- **Social Hx:** smoking, EtOH intake, dietary habits (↑ salt and ↑ fat diet)

Px

- **Vitals:** BP (compare for both arms), weight, height, BMI, waist circumference (assess for MS)
- **Head and Neck:** funduscopy for retinal Δs, thyroid exam, JVP, carotid bruit
- **Chest:** signs of CHF, palpable murmur
- **CV exam:** murmurs, Abdo aorta bruit, renal artery bruit, Abdo aorta aneurysm

Ix

See Ix for HTN.

Mx

sBP and **pulse pressure** should be regarded as major predictor of outcome.

- Rx should be initiated when sBP >160 mm Hg or >140 mm Hg when pt has other RF like **diabetes** and **smoking.**

HTN in Elderly

The elderly population is susceptible to postural and postprandial hypotension. Careful assessment and Mx of these problems must be done before initiating Rx.

CLINICAL BOX

Pharmacological Options

- HTN alone: thiazide-type diuretics
- HTN + atherosclerosis: ACEI
- HTN + post-MI: β-blockers
- HTN + DM: ACEI

- **Nonpharmacologic Rx:** lifestyle modification, achieve target BMI through **diet and exercise, Na restriction**, cessation of smoking, judicious consumption of EtOH
- **Pharmacologic Rx:** initiated if the above is inadequate
- Benefit in treating **systolic** HTN in the elderly is **two to four times greater** than in younger pt with 1° HTN.
- **Thiazide** diuretic—**First-line** choice for elderly pt. Use **lower doses** (half of what is usually used in younger population) to minimize side effects like postural hypotension due to sluggish autoregulation in the elderly population.
- Periodically monitor electrolytes; hypokalemia may negate any CV benefit.
- **Dihydropyridines** such as nifedipine may also be used as an alternative.
- Subsequent and additional Rx: see Hypertension

HYPERTENSION IN CHILDHOOD

DEFINITION

An **sBP** or **dBP** of **>95th percentile** for corrected age and gender

CAUSAL CONDITIONS

Prevalence is <1%, often from identifiable causes.

Table **3.3**	**Causal Conditions of HTN in Childhood**	
Neonates and Young Infants	**Children and Adolescents (1–10 yr)**	**Children and Adolescents (11 yr and Older)**
a. ↑ **CO** Congenital renal disease b. ↑ **SVR** Ischemic renal disease Neurogenic tumors CoA Hypercalcemia	a. ↑ **CO** Renal parenchymal disease (**most common**, up to 70% of cases) b. ↑ **SVR** Renovascular disease CoA (less common)	a. **1° HTN** b. **2° HTN** Renal disease Endocrine disorders Med related

APPROACH

Hx

In addition to routine Hx taking for HTN R/O 2° HTN:
Neonates: failure to thrive, seizure, irritability or lethargy, respiratory distress, CHF
Children: headaches, fatigue, blurred vision, epistaxis, Bell palsy; obtain birth Hx, nutritional Hx, and developmental milestone

Px

In addition to routine Px for HTN, perform BP measurement in infants and very young children with **automated devices** and check BP tables for normal values. Plot height and weight on growth chart.

Ix

In addition to routine Ix of HTN:

- **ABG**, postductal O_2 saturation
- Imaging: **CXR, ECHO, chest MRI**
- Abdo U/S may reveal tumors or structural anomalies of the kidneys or renal vasculature
- Monitoring of BP on a 24-h basis may help in diagnosing **white-coat** HTN and provides information about the risk of target end-organ damage

Mx

- **Nonpharmacologic:** weight reduction for obesity-related HTN; regular exercise and changing sedentary activity; dietary modification (**salt restriction, low fat diet**); avoidance of 2° smoke; and excess EtOH intake
- Pharmacologic

HTN in Childhood
Asymmetry in renal size suggests renal dysplasia or RAS. Renal or extrarenal masses suggest a Wilms tumor or neuroblastoma, respectively.

Table **3.4**	Antihypertensives in Childhood HTN
Antihypertensives	**Doses**
Thiazide diuretics	1 mg/kg/d PO q.d. initially; can be given upto 3 mg/kg/d with max dose of 50 mg/d, associated with less prominent complications such as hypokalemia, gluc. intolerance, adverse lipid effects
Metoprolol	1–2 mg/kg/d PO divided b.i.d. initially; may gradually ↑ to 6 mg/kg/d; **not to exceed** 200 mg/d
Enalapril[a]	0.08 mg/kg/d PO q.d. or divided b.i.d.; not to exceed 5 mg/d initially; may gradually ↑ to 0.6 mg/kg/d; **not to exceed** 40 mg/d
Amlodipine	For children 6–17 yr: 2.5–5 mg q.d.
Spironolactone	1 mg/kg/d PO q.d. or divided b.i.d. initially; may gradually ↑ to 3.3 mg/kg/d; **not to exceed** 100 mg/d
Losartan	0.7 mg/kg/d PO q.d.; **not to exceed** 50 mg/d initially; may ↑ to 1.4 mg/kg/d; **not to exceed** 100 mg/d

[a]needs dose adjustment in renal disease

Use of any antihypertensive drugs is effective in reducing BP in pediatric population. The choice is based on physicians' preference. **ACEI** is recommended for children with **DM and microalbuminuria** or **proteinuric renal disease**.

Table **3.5**	Rx for Hypertensive Emergencies in Childhood
Antihypertensives	**Doses**
Labetalol	0.2–1 mg/kg/dose up to 40 mg/dose as an IV bolus or 0.25–3 mg/kg/h IV infusion
Nicardipine	1–3 μg/kg/min IV infusion
Na nitroprusside	0.53–10 μg/kg/min IV infusion to start

PREGNANCY-ASSOCIATED HYPERTENSION

RATIONALE

Ten percent to 20% of pregnancies are associated with HTN, >5% complicated by chronic HTN, 6% have preeclampsia, and 6% of pregnant women get gestational HTN.

DEFINITIONS/CAUSAL CONDITIONS

Table **3.6**	Four Major Hypertensive Disorders in Pregnancy
Hypertensive Disorders	**Features**
Chronic HTN	• BP >140/90 • Occur before pregnancy, <20 wk of pregnancy, or persists for >12 wk postpartum
Preeclampsia–eclampsia	• Syndrome of new onset of HTN with **proteinuria after 20 wk** of gestation

Preeclampsia superimposed on underlying **HTN**	• Three different subcategories
	  a. **Preeclampsia** superimposed on **chronic HTN**
	  b. Preeclampsia superimposed on chronic HTN **and proteinuria**, both present before 20-wk gestation. Pt has severe exacerbation of BP, with sBP >160 mm Hg and dBP >110 mm Hg in last half of pregnancy
	  c. **Preeclampsia** superimposed on **gestational HTN**

Gestational HTN	• Presenting ≥20 wk of pregnancy, **Ø proteinuria**. Two subtypes
	  a. **Transient** HTN of pregnancy, resolves 12-wk postpartum
	  b. **Masked chronic** HTN, persists beyond 12-wk postpartum

ASC Box
Pregnancy-Associated HTN

- The earliest pathologic Δ that happens in preeclampsia occurs in **uteroplacental circulation**.
- In preeclampsia, **cytotrophoblast** fails to invade the myometrial portion of uterus.
- The large tortuous vascular channels does not develop, and vessels narrow leading to **placental hypoperfusion**.

APPLIED SCIENTIFIC CONCEPTS

- Δs in the **uteroplacental circulation** (impaired trophoblast invasion and placental ischemia) that occurs in **preeclampsia**
- Chronologic Δs resulting from **placental ischemia** are as follows:
  - As pregnancy progresses → **AbN uterine vasculature** → **placental hypoperfusion**
  - Late placental Δs 2° to hypoperfusion → **atherosis**, arteriole sclerotic narrowing, thrombosis, fibrinoid necrosis, **infarction of placenta**
  - Ischemic placenta → release of proinflammatory cytokines and mediators of oxidative stress in maternal bloodstream → ↑ capillary permeability as well as activation of endothelial cells and coagulation system. The **key player** in pathogenesis of preeclampsia appears to be **sVEGFR-1**, an antagonist of PGF and VEGF.

APPROACH

GOAL

1. To **differentiate preeclampsia** from other conditions that presents with HTN
2. **Determine** the **severity** of the condition
3. Preserving **fetal well-being** by performing assessment

Hx

- **Gestational age**
- Sx of preeclampsia: **visual disturbance**, new onset headache, epigastric or RUQ pain, rapidly progressing peripheral edema, rapid weight gain
- Past medical Hx: **previous episodes** of preeclampsia or eclampsia, BP from previous pregnancies, presence of chronic HTN

Px

- If ↑ risk of preeclampsia, perform **rollover test** (BP in L lateral position, and 5 min after turning to the supine position, an ↑ ≥15 mm Hg in dBP is positive)
- **Head and Neck:** Check the eyes for signs of retinal **vasospasm or retinal edema.**
- **CVS:** S_4 on auscultation, diminished distal pulses from signs of end-organ damage from chronic HTN, carotid bruit
- **Neurologic exam:** Check reflexes and look for **clonus**, as it is a sign of severe preeclampsia.
- **Abdo:** RUQ tenderness (liver swelling and capsular stretch), Abdo bruit (RAS)
- Signs of 2° chronic HTN: Cushing syndrome for glucocorticoid excess, hyperthyroidism

Ix

Fetal well-being: Perform **nonstress test or biophysical profile. U/S** to evaluate growth and amniotic fluid volume

Mx

- **Achieve a target sBP 130 to 150 mm Hg and dBP 80 to 100 mm Hg.**
- Ensure safety of mother's health.
- Ensure safe delivery of infant not requiring intensive neonatal care.

R
HTN in Pregnancy

Avoid ACEIs/ARBs—teratogens, fetal renal agenesis, fetal hydramnios

Atenolol is a category D drug (unsafe in pregnancy)—causes IUGR

Careful with nitroprusside—potential fetal cyanide poisoning

Table **3.7**	**Laboratory Tests in Pregnancy-Associated HTN**
Hct	Hemoconcentration—preeclampsia
Platelet count	Thrombocytopenia signifies severe preeclampsia
Serum CR	↑ suggests severe disease
AST, ALT	↑ signifies hepatic dysfunction, indicative of severe disease
LDH	↑ in level is a sign of hemolysis
Serum UA level	Not diagnostic, but levels ↑ in preeclampsia (marker of tubular dysfunction).
Coagulation function test	PT, aPTT, fibrinogen concentration is not routinely done
24-h urine	≥300 mg/d of **protein** supports the diagnosis of preeclampsia

Table **3.8**	**Mx of Pregnancy-Associated HTN**
HTN of **any etiology**	**Bed rest:** Although largely recommended, Ø large trials to support its implementation
Mild **gestational HTN**	1. **Antihypertensives:** Not recommended for sBP <160 mm Hg and dBP <110 mm Hg as it is not shown to improve neonatal outcome 2. **Fetal well-being:** Ask pt to observe fetal movement, obtain **biophysical profile weekly** as soon as diagnosis of HTN is made, **U/S** exam to monitor fetal growth every 3–4 wk 3. **Delivery:** Ø later than 40-wk gestation
Severe **gestational HTN**	1. **Antihypertensives** • Begin **labetalol** 20 mg IV and ↑ between 20 and 80 mg at every 10-min interval. Give up to a cumulative dose of 300 mg if needed • **Hydralazine:** Begin with 5 mg IV over 1–2 min. If BP goal is not achieved in 20 min, give 5–10 mg bolus depending on initial response. Max bolus dose is 20 mg. Associated with hypotension • **CCB:** Sustained release of nifedipine 30 mg PO and immediate release of nicardipine are options 2. **Delivery:** Indicated if pregnancy is near term
Mild **preeclampsia**	1. **Delivery:** Definitive Rx to prevent maternal and fetal complications. Ø later than 40-wk gestation 2. **Antihypertensives:** Not indicated as it does not alter the course of disease or alter perinatal morbidity or mortality 3. **Antenatal corticosteroids: Betamethasone** 12 mg IM 2 dose 24 h apart to promote fetal lung maturity. This is for women <34-wk gestation 4. **Anticonvulsant Rx: Magnesium sulphate** 4–6 g IV as loading dose over 20 min then 2 g/h continuous infusion. Initiated during labor or while administering corticosteroid or PG before planned delivery
Severe **preeclampsia**	1. **Delivery:** Indicated regardless of gestational age to minimize risk of maternal and fetal complications 2. **Antenatal corticosteroids: Betamethasone** 12 mg IM 2 dose 24 h apart to promote fetal lung maturity. This is for women having <34-wk gestation 3. **Anticonvulsant Rx: Magnesium sulfate** as in mild preeclampsia.

MALIGNANT HYPERTENSION

DEFINITION

Hypertensive emergencies are life-threatening conditions associated with ↑ in BP $\geq 180/120$ mm Hg. The following are two major syndromes:

1. **Malignant HTN:** HTN with retinal **hemorrhages, exudates,** or **papilledema;** may also have renal involvement, known as **malignant nephrosclerosis.**
2. **Hypertensive encephalopathy:** clinical presentation of **cerebral edema** caused by **breakthrough hyperperfusion** from severe and sudden ↑ of BP

APPLIED SCIENTIFIC CONCEPTS

MECHANISM OF VASCULAR INJURY

- Mild to moderate ↑ in BP → arterial and arteriolar **vasoconstriction.** This maintains tissue perfusion at a relatively constant level and prevents pressure from being transferred to smaller, more distal vessels.
- However, with ↑ severe HTN → autoregulation fails → ↑ in arteriole and capillary pressure → damage to vascular wall, disruption of endothelium (**breakthrough vasodilation**).
- Endothelial damage → leakage of plasma constituents → obliteration of vascular endothelial lumen
- Role of renin-angiotensin↑ BP → natriuresis + renal vascular injury → ↑ renin which ↑ angiotensin II → exacerbating HTN

Ischemic consequence of an excessive response to Rx could happen when autoregulation capacity is exceeded at the lower pressure end of an organ's autoregulatory curve:

Autoregulation → arterial and arteriole vasodilatation → tissue perfusion maintained during Rx of HTN

$$Q = P/R$$

⚛ ASC Box

Malignant HTN

Hypertensive encephalopathy

Signs of **cerebral edema**, caused by breakthrough vasodilation from autoregulation failure.

It is characterized by the insidious onset of **headache, nausea**, and **vomiting** followed by **nonlocalizing neurologic Sx** such as **restlessness** and **confusion**.

If not treated, this will eventually lead to seizures and coma.

Malignant HTN

Be careful of ischemic consequences of an excessive response to Rx.

A parallel ↓ in both P and R will maintain Q. But when ↓ P (due to excessive response to Rx) while R maintains the same → ↓ flow → ischemia.

CAUSAL CONDITIONS

1°

Rapid rise in BP in a pt with **chronic essential HTN** (most common), due to uncontrolled HTN or antihypertensive drug withdrawal

2°

- ↑ CO: **uremia** with fluid overload, **acute renal disease** (acute glomerulonephritis, scleroderma crisis), thyrotoxicosis, 1° hyperaldosterone
- ↑ Vascular resistance: **renovascular HTN**, pheochromocytoma, drugs (cocaine, food interactions with MAOI), cerebrovascular causes (infarction, SAH)

APPROACH

Hx

- **Presenting complaint:** Assess for specific Sx suggesting **target organ damage**: (a) **chest pain** (myocardial ischemia/MI), (b) chest pain radiating to the back (aortic dissection), (c) dyspnea (pulmonary edema, CHF), and (d) neurologic Sx (headache, nausea, vomiting, visual disturbances, seizure).
- **Past medical Hx:** duration and severity of **preexisting HTN**, previous renal and cerebrovascular disease, thyrotoxicosis, Cushing disease, SLE
- **LMP** for female pt in reproductive age-group, oral contraceptive use
- **Med:** antihypertensive Rx and **compliance**, use of sympathomimetics (including OTCs), use of illicit drugs, for example, cocaine

Px

- **Vitals:** lying and standing BP. BP on both arms (asymmetry suggests aortic dissection)
- **Head and neck:** Check for retinal hemorrhage, exudates, and papilledema which suggest an emergency.
- **CVS:** JVP, crackles, peripheral edema
- **Abdo:** Abdo mass, bruit, palpable pulsations
- **CNS:** level of consciousness, visual field, focal neurologic signs

Ix

- **Laboratories:** electrolytes, BUN, CR, U/A for evaluation of renal impairment, CBC and smear to diagnose microangiopathic anemia
- Other lab tests: toxicology, pregnancy, endocrine
- **Imaging:** CXR (for pt presenting with chest pain/dyspnea), noncontrast head CT/MRI (stroke/hemorrhage), CT (aortic dissection)

Table **3.9** Pharmacotherapy in Malignant HTN	
Antihypertensive Rx for Malignant HTN	**Mode of Action/Dose**
Na nitroprusside	An arteriolar and venous dilator, given IV **initial dose**: 0.25–0.5 μg/kg/min; **max**: 8–10 μg/kg/min. Acts within seconds, short duration of 2–5 min. Potential **cyanide toxicity**, especially with renal insufficiency
Nicardipine	An arteriolar vasodilator, given IV **initial dose**: 5 mg/h, **max**: 15 mg/h
Labetalol	An α- and ß-adrenergic blocker, given IV bolus/infusion. **Bolus**: 20 mg initially followed by 20–80 mg q10 min to a total dose of 300 mg. **Infusion**: 0.5–2 mg/min
Fenoldopam	A peripheral dopamine-1 receptor agonist, given IV **initial dose**: 0.1 μg/kg/min; titrated at q15 min, depending on BP response
Hydralazine	An arterial vasodilator, given IV bolus 10–20 mg every 20 min. If Ø effect after 20 mg, try another agent. Rx of choice in eclampsia and gestational HTN
Phentolamine	A reversible nonselective α-adrenergic antagonist. Given IV bolus 5–10 mg every 5–15 min

Mx

Therapeutic Goal

1. Initial aim is to **rapidly reduce the dBP** to ~100 to 105 mm Hg. This should be done **over 2 to 6 h**. The initial fall in BP should not exceed 25% of the current BP.
2. Avoid ischemic events (stroke/MI) that could result from overaggressive Rx: BP ↓ below the autoregulatory range.
3. Switch to appropriate oral Rx once the BP is under control. dBP should be slowly reduced to 85 to 90 mm Hg over 2 to 3 mo.

HYPOTENSION

ASC Box

Hypotension

Biochemical process derangement in prolonged, severe shock:

1. **Ion pump dysfunction** across cellular membrane
2. Intracellular **edema**
3. **Intra**cellular contents leaking into **extra**cellular space
4. Intracellular **pH derangement**

DEFINITION

A physiologic state of **overwhelming reduction in systemic tissue perfusion** leading to ↓ tissue oxygenation

APPLIED SCIENTIFIC CONCEPTS

Effects of reduced tissue perfusion are **reversible at the early stage**. Prolonged, severe hypotension on systemic tissue perfusion → ↓ O_2 delivery → cellular deprivation → cellular hypoxia.

APPROACH

Hx

Obtain Hx from relatives, **medical records**. Recent complaints/activities, allergies, Δs in **med**, drug intoxication, **premorbid illness**.

Px

Assess **ABC**. Examine swiftly and efficiently for (a) volume status; (b) meningeal signs; (c) absent breath sounds/crackles, consolidation; (d) heart arrhythmia, murmurs, rubs; (e) Abdo tenderness, bowel sounds, ascites/distension, masses, rectal bleeding; (f) swollen calf; (g) cold/hyperemic skin, rash; and (h) check for muffled heart sound, JVD, hypotension (the **Beck triad**) suggesting CT, pulses paradoxus.

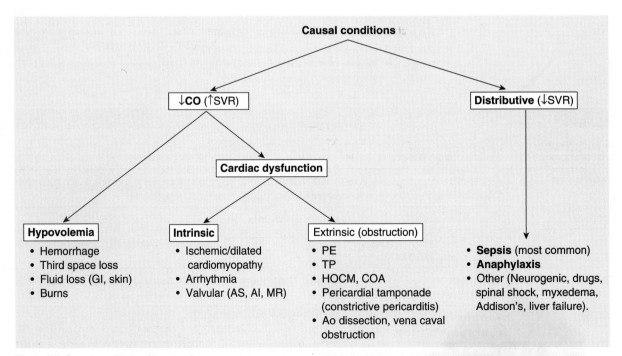

Figure 3.2 Causal conditions of hypotension.

Table **3.10**	Findings in Different States of Shock		
Findings	**Hypovolemic**	**Cardiogenic**	**Distributive**
HEENT	Dry conjunctivae and mucous membrane	Scleral icterus (MAHA from mechanical valve, CHF → nutmeg liver)	Flushy/swollen face, angioedema (swelling of lips and tongue)
JVP, carotid pulse	↓ JVP	↑ JVP, pulsus parvus et tardus (AS)	↓ JVP, delayed carotid, meningeal sign
Heart	Tachycardia	Arrhythmia, tachycardia /bradycardia, S_3 gallop, ventricular heave, murmurs, rub, distant heart sounds, pulsus paradoxus	Tachycardia
Lungs	Tachypnea, Kussmaul's breathing	Crackles (CHF), absent breath sounds, rub	Shallow breaths
Abdo	Tenderness, distension, absence of bowel sounds, pulsatile masses	Distended (hepatic congestion from CHF)	Tenderness, distension, rebound tenderness, absent bowel sounds, pulsatile masses
Skin	Cold, clammy	Cold, clammy/warm hyperemic skin	Warm, hyperemic, rashes, petechiae, urticaria, cellulitis
Neuro	Agitation, confusion, delirium, obtundation, coma	Agitation, confusion, delirium, obtundation, coma	Agitation, confusion, delirium, obtundation, coma, spinal cord injury
Rectal	Bright red blood, melena, occult blood in stool	Hemorrhoids (portalcaval venous engorgement)	↓ anal tone (spinal cord injury)
Ix	CBC, electrolytes, BUN, Cr, amylase, lipase, lactate, abdo X-ray, U/A	CBC, electrolytes, BUN, Cr, D-dimer, cardiac enzymes, ABG, toxicology screen, CXR, EKG, PCWP in ICU	CBC with differentials, electrolytes, lactate, toxicology screen, amylase, lipase, blood culture, spinal XR, EKG, ECHO, cardiac enzymes, TSH, procalcitonin
Causes	Hemorrhage, third space loss, GI fluid loss	Ischemic/dilated cardiomyopathy, arrhythmia, mechanical (valvular i.e., AS), PE, TP, tamponade	Sepsis, anaphylaxis, neurogenic, spinal shock

Ix

CBC, electrolytes, LFT, CR clearance, amylase/lipase, fibrinogen degradation product, lactate, cardiac enzymes, ABG, toxicology, CXR, ECHO, EKG, Tn, pro-BNP, U/A. Continuous monitoring is required to assess response to Rx.

Mx

Acute Mx for all shock states:

1. **Stabilize the pt:** ABC—airway, 100% O_2, two large-bore IVs, and **Trendelenburg** position (↑ venous return, cerebral perfusion)
2. **Monitors:** automatic BP, pulse oximetry, cardiac monitoring
3. **Diagnose cause** of shock based on signs and Sx in Table 3.10 and manage accordingly.
4. Consider **ICU admission** if IV vasopressors are needed or refractory hypotension.

Hypovolemic Shock

Rapid **volume repletion**

- For **hypovolemic nonhemorrhagic shock**
  - Give **crystalloids** (0.9% N/S or Ringer's lactate) 1 to 2 L IV bolus, then replace fluid accordingly to **maintain sBP >90 mm Hg** or **minimum MAP of 60**, urine output >0.5 mL/kg/h.
- For **hypovolemic hemorrhagic shock**
  - Cross match and **transfuse** in addition to giving crystalloid. **Maintain Hct 30% to 35%.** Control bleeding. Buffer Rx, added to replacement fluid when blood pH <7.10 (i.e., in cases of massive transfusions).

⚑

Hypotension

Immediate therapeutic goal—maintain sBP >90 mm Hg or minimum MAP of 60, urine output >0.5 mL/kg/h.

Distributive Shock

1. Rapid **fluid repletion**: Give 4 to 6 L N/S.
2. **If Ø response** to fluid resuscitation: Give dopamine.
3. **Septic shock**
   - **Empiric antibiotics**
     - Third-generation cephalosporins + aminoglycoside **or** imipenem alone (two to three blood cultures from different sites, before antibiotic Rx whenever possible). Antimicrobial Rx must be tailored to blood culture findings, once available.
     - Probable gram-positive sepsis: Add vancomycin or nafcillin.
     - Anaerobes suspected: clindamycin or metronidazole (Flagyl)
     - Legionella sepsis: erythromycin
     - Fungemia: amphotericine B
     - Drainage and debridement of wound as needed
   - **Recombinant activated protein C** in the ICU setting
4. **Neurogenic shock:** Load methylprednisolone 30 mg/kg over 15 min, then infuse 5.4 mg/kg/h for next 24 h.
5. **Anaphylactic shock:** See Anaphylaxis later in the chapter.

Cardiogenic Shock

As per Hx, Px, and Ix, **treat underlying cause** based on ACLS, ATLS protocol. Also see Chapter 5.

- Treat **pulmonary edema**: O_2, IV furosemide, and morphine; consider IABP
- If Ø pulmonary edema, **fluid challenge** with 250 mL N/S over 10 to 15 min. Repeat one to two times if still Ø edema. When BP of pt ↑, titrate infusion to maintain sBP >100.

Dopamine: In low doses (2 to 3 μg/kg/min), acts on renal **dopaminergic** and splanchnic vascular beds, causing vasodilatation in these beds. In midrange doses (4 to 8 μg/kg/min), acts on **β-adrenergic** receptors to ↑ HR and contractility. In high doses (>10 μg/kg/min), acts on **α-adrenergic** receptors to ↑ SVR and raise BP. Titrate as required. Maintenance doses <20 μg/kg/min usually are satisfactory for 50% of the pts treated.

CLINICAL BOX

Five Common Features of Shock

1. **Hypotension**, either sBP <90 mm Hg or a drop of >40 mm Hg in sBP
2. **Cool**, clammy **skin** (except for distributive shock → warm, dry skin)
3. **Oliguria** (<0.5 mL/kg/h)
4. △ in **mental status** (agitation → confusion → obtundation)
5. **Metabolic acidosis**

Other findings: tachycardia, orthostatic hypotension, poor skin turgor, ↓ sweat, dry mucous membrane

CLINICAL BOX

Physiologic Variables in Different States of Shock

Physiologic Variables	Preload	Pump function	Afterload	Tissue Perfusion
Clinical measurement	PCWP	CO	SVR	Mixed venous O_2 saturation
Hypovolemic	↓	↓	↑	↓
Cardiogenic	↑	↓	↑	↓
Distributive	↓ or ←→	↑	↓	↑

ANAPHYLAXIS

DEFINITION

Anaphylaxis is an **IgE-mediated**, immediate hypersensitive allergic reaction to protein substances. In Canada, anaphylaxis causes ~50 fatalities/year and 1/5,000 admissions.

CAUSAL CONDITIONS

ASC Box

Anaphylaxis

Mediators involved in anaphylaxis

- **Initial minutes:** Histamine, tryptase, PGs (PGD_2, PGF_{2a}), LTs (LTB_4, LTC_4, LTD_4, LTE_4), and platelet activating factor
- **Hours later:** Same cells release cytokines—IL-4, IL-13, and TNF

Table **3.11** Anaphylaxis Causal Conditions	
Anaphylaxis (IgE Mediated)	**Anaphylactoid Reactions (Non–IgE Mediated)**

Therapeutic agents: Antibiotics (PCN most common), vaccines, allergen immunotherapy, local anesthetics
Foods: Peanuts and tree nuts (almonds, Brazil nut, Hazel nut), grains, eggs, seafood, milk
Human proteins: Hormones, enzymes, heterologous, serum, blood and blood products
Venoms: Hymenoptera, snake, fire ant
Latex (inhaled or contact)
Idiopathic
	1. **Direct release of mediators from mast cells**
	  • Drugs: Opiates, neuromuscular blockers
	  • Hypertonic solutions
	  • Exercise
	2. **Immune complex/complement mediated:**
	  • Blood and blood products, gamma globulin, antisera, dialysis membranes
	3. **Arachidonic acid metabolism modulators**
	  • ASA/NSAIDs, COX-2 inhibitor
	4. **Multiple/unknown mechanisms**
	  • RCM, sulfites, idiopathic anaphylaxis

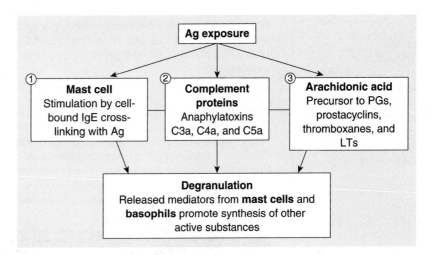

Figure 3.3 Events that trigger anaphylactic reaction.

APPROACH

Hx

Once pt is stable, ask about:

- **Ingestion** that occurred within minutes: food, beverage, candies, prescription, and OTC drugs
- Recent **environmental exposure**: contact with insects, bite, sting, plants, fluids, gas
- Recent **physical activities** such as exercise and sexual activity

Table **3.12** Manifestations of Anaphylaxis	
Physiological Δs	**Systems Involved**

• ↑ in vascular permeability
• Vasodilation → hypotension and tachycardia
• Mucus secretion
• Stimulation of autonomic nervous system
• Enhanced gut motility
• Platelet aggregation
	Skin: Pruritus, flushing, urticaria/angioedema, diaphoresis
	Neurologic: Dizziness/weakness, sense of impending doom, syncope, seizures
	Eyes: Conjunctival injection, lacrimation, periorbital edema, pruritus
	CV: Conduction disturbances, tachycardia, bradycardia, arrhythmias, hypotension, cardiac arrest
	Respiratory tract
	  • Nose/oropharynx: Sneezing, rhinorrhea, nasal congestion, metallic taste
	  • Upper airway: Hoarseness, stridor, sense of choking, laryngeal edema
	  • Lower airway: Cough, tachypnea, wheezing, dyspnea, cyanosis
	GI: Nausea/vomiting, Abdo cramping, bloating, diarrhea

Px

Most common signs and Sx: **urticaria, angioedema, flushing, pruritus**

Ix

Serum histamine and serum tryptase, allergy testing (done 4 wk after anaphylactic event)

Mx

Initial Acute Mx

Airway: Airway and cardiopulmonary status (A, B, C) rapidly assessed. Immediately intubate when stridor, worsening mental status, or respiratory arrest is present.

Epinephrine: Give epinephrine 0.3 to 0.5 mg IM (0.3 to 0.5 mL of 1:1,000 dilution) to anterolateral thigh. Can be repeated every 3 to 5 min prn.

IV access: two 14- to 16-gauge IV catheters placed in preparation for fluid resuscitation

O_2 administration: Give 100% O_2.

Removal of causal agent: Stop culprit drug.

Constant monitoring: Monitoring of cardiopulmonary status. Check vital signs, pulse oximetry, and telemetry.

Acute Mx

N/S rapid bolus: Treat hypotension with rapid infusion of 1 to 2 L IV. Repeat prn.

IVepinephrine: If poor response to IM epinephrine and IV saline, give epinephrine 0.5 to 1 mL of 1:10,000 through IV (mix 1 mL of 1:1,000 dilution into 9 mL of N/S to make 10 mL of 1:10,000). Consider giving epinephrine 1 to 6 μg/min as an IV drip, titrated to response.

Salbutamol: Treat bronchospasm with 2.5 to 5 mg in 3-mL saline through nebulizer; repeat prn.

Antihistamine (H_1 blocker): Give all pts a second-generation antihistamine (e.g., cetirizine). Diphenhydramine 25 to 50 mg IV is used only if IV meds are required.

Antihistamine (H_2 blocker): Give all pts ranitidine 50 mg IV or famotidine 20 mg IV.

Corticosteroid: Consider giving methylprednisolone 125 mg IV or dexamethasone 20 mg IV.

Prevention of future attacks: Prescribe epinephrine autoinjectors (e.g., EpiPen). Avoidance of known allergen.

Allergy referral: Pts should be referred to an allergy specialist for evaluation.

Anaphylaxis

Rapid progressions of Sx, hypotension, syncope, dysrhythmia, chest pain, stridor, respiratory distress (wheezing, ↑ work of breathing, constant dry cough), stridor (one of most common cause of death in anaphylaxis is airway obstruction).

CLINICAL BOX

Anaphylaxis is a clinical diagnosis, when it is confirmed by **any one** of the following **three** criteria:

1. **Acute onset** from minutes to few hours with either skin and mucosal involvement and **one or more** of the following:
   - **Respiratory compromise:** dyspnea, wheeze-bronchospasm, stridor, ↓ expiratory flow, hypoxemia.
   - **Reduced BP** or associated Sx of end-organ dysfunction: hypotonia, collapse, syncope, incontinence.

2. **Two or more** of the following that occur rapidly (minutes to hours) after exposure **to a likely allergen for pt**:
   - Skin and mucosal tissue: generalized hives, swollen lips-tongue-uvula, itching, flushing
   - **Resp compromise:** (as mentioned earlier)
   - *Reduced BP* or associated Sx: (as mentioned earlier)
   - Persistent *GI Sx*: crampy Abdo pain, vomiting

3. **Reduced BP** after exposure to **known antigen for pt** (minutes to hours):
   - Reduced sBP <90 mm Hg or >30% ↓ from pts baseline

CLINICAL BOX

Observation After Anaphylaxis

For mild to moderate attacks, 8 h should suffice as biphasic response occurs within 8 h. Admission for all cases of severe anaphylaxis.

CHEST PAIN (ANGINA)

RATIONALE

Chest pain is more commonly benign in the 1° care setting. Coronary heart disease primarily occurs in pts older than 40 years, also affects younger men and women (20% men and 8%

women aged 30 to 34). Physicians must recognize the presentation of CAD and assess its RFs.

APPLIED SCIENTIFIC CONCEPTS

ASC Box

Chest Pain

Causes of ↑ MOD:

- ↑ HR
- ↑ Myocardial contractility
- ↑ Myocardial work → ↑ MOD
- ↑ Afterload + ↑ preload → ↑ wall tension

MOD exceeds myocardial O_2 **supply** → stimulation of chemosensitive and mechanoreceptive receptors of unmyelinated cardiac nerve cells → angina.

VALUE OF EKG AND CARDIAC MARKERS

WHO criteria for MI diagnosis: two out of these three—(a) chest pain—cardiac specific, (b) EKG-ST Δs, T-wave inversions, and (c) ↑ cardiac enzymes

EKG
Ischemia: downsloping or horizontal ST depression

Infarction: ST elevation or T-wave inversion

Cardiac Markers
Tn I or T: Most sensitive and specific. Typical rise and fall in appropriate setting is highly indicative of diagnosis in STEMI and NSTEMI. Detectable 4 to 6 h after injury, peaks at 24 h. Serial cardiac Tn I is still the most specific cardiac marker for myocardial damage in ESRF setting.

CK-MB isoforms
Less sensitive and specific, present in skeletal muscle, tongue, diaphragm, intestine, uterus, prostate. CK-MB2/CK-MB1 ratio is measured, and is positive if ratio is 1.7. Is an early marker for acute MI, detected in serum 2 to 4 h after onset and peaks 6 to 9 h. An important marker in myocardial reinfarction.

R

Chest Pain

R/O five deadly causes of chest pain: UA, MI, aortic dissection, TP, and PE

CAUSAL CONDITIONS

1. **CV** (25% of causes, 50% in elderly pts)
Ischemic
   - Angina pectoris, coronary vasospasm, small vessel disease MI (<2% in 1° care)
Nonischemic
   - Aortic dissection: dilating, dissecting (hypertensive, cystic necrosis, Marfan syndrome)
   - **Pericarditis:** infectious, post-MI, post-CABG (Dressler syndrome), uremia, connective tissue disease
2. **GI** (20%)
   - Esophageal spasm, esophagitis, Mallory Weiss tear, peptic ulcer disease, biliary disease, and pancreatitis
3. **Neuropsychiatry** (10%)
   - Cardiac neurosis, anxiety, depression, somatoform
4. **Pulmonary/mediastinal** (5%)
   - Pulmonary embolus, tracheitis, mediastinal/pulmonary malignancy, pneumothorax, and pleuritis
5. **Musculoskeletal and cutaneous**
   - Costochondritis, chest wall pain

Hx

Table **3.13**	Hx of Angina
Spatial	**Temporal**
Location, quality, intensity (scale 1–10), radiation, associated Sx, relieving/aggravating factors	When (duration, frequency, previous episodes, status of pain at presentation) is the pain getting worse? Is it same as past coronary event (if applicable)? Is it present at rest or only on exercise? Is it getting more frequent or intense?

Table **3.14**	Five Deadly Causes of Chest Pain and Findings	
Disorder	**Typical Presentation**	**Findings in Exam and Ix**
Angina NB: UA is: New angina Pain that ↑ in frequency/more severe Pain at rest	• Substernal pressure radiating to neck, arm, and jaw • Duration <30 min • ± Dyspnea, diaphoresis, N/V, aggravated by exertion, relieved by nitroglycerine or rest **NB:** Relief by nitroglycerine not reliable indicator of angina	**EKG:** Down slopping or horizontal ST ↓ is predictive of CAD; ST ↑ highly predictive • Physiologic Δs: ↓ BP • Imaging: Wall motion abnormalities—ECHO **NB:** HR must achieve ≥85% maximal predicted HR (220-age) for exercise stress test to be diagnostic
MI	• Same as angina, but ↑ intensity of distress • >30 min • ± Dyspnea, anxiety, nausea, diaphoresis	• **EKG** Δs (ST ↑ ≥0.5 mm, T wave inversion), new LBBB, sustained VT • Positive Tn and CK-MB • **Signs:** Pulmonary edema 2° to ischemia, new/worsening MR murmur, hypotension, bradycardia, tachycardia, S_3 gallop or worsening rales
Aortic dissection	• Sudden onset tearing, sharp pain anterior or posterior midscapular	• **Signs:** Asymmetric BP/pulse, HTN/hypotension (2° to tamponade, AI/aortic rupture), pulse deficit, AI murmur (diastolic murmur), CHF (2° to AI) • **Imaging** **CXR**: Widened mediastinum, pleural effusion (but cannot r/o dissection) **CT:** False lumen. Fast, noninvasive, high sensitivity (85% for proximal; 90% for distal). Spiral and multislice ↑ sensitivity **TEE:** Can assess pericardium, AI. Sensitivity >95% for proximal and 80% for distal **MRI:** (Gold standard) sensitive and specific, >98%; but not readily available, time consuming **Aortography:** Sensitivity <90%, time consuming; can assess coronaries but not intramural hematoma
TP	• Sudden onset, unilateral, sharp, pleuritic pain	• Unilateral hyper resonance, ↓ breath sounds • **CXR**: PTX
Pulmonary embolus	• Sudden onset, pleuritic • Tachypnea, tachycardia	• **ABG**: Hypoxemia • **Imaging**: Positive V/Q scan or angiogram

Table **3.15**	Determinants of Myocardial Work and O_2 Supply	
Factors that determine MOD	**Myocardial O_2 supply**	
• HR • sBP (clinical marker of afterload) • Myocardial wall tension (preload + myocardial muscle mass) • Myocardial contractility	• O_2 carrying capacity of blood Affected by O_2 tension, Hb concentration • Degree of O_2 unloading from Hb Affected by 2,3 diphosphoglycerate levels • Coronary blood flow	

APPROACH

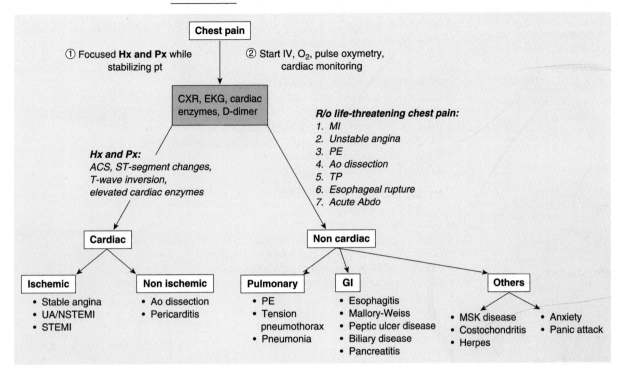

Figure 3.4 Approach to chest pain.

Mx

Ischemic Cardiac Chest Pain

Stable Angina

- **Immediate:** morphine (2 to 4 mg IV), O_2 (4 L/min, nasal prongs), nitroglycerin (0.4 mg, 1 spray repeat three times over 3- to 5-min intervals), ASA (160 to 325 mg crushed or chewed), β-blocker
- **Once stable:** statin, lifestyle Δs, stress test, angiography, ECHO

UA/NSTEMI

- **Anti-ischemic:** morphine, O_2, nitroglycerin, β-blocker
- **Antithrombotic:** ASA, clopidogrel, heparin, GpIIb/IIIa inhibitors
- **Admit to CCU if needed:** once stable—as angina
- **Decide:** early coronary intervention versus initial medical Rx

STEMI

- **Immediate assessment:** Assess ABCs, vital signs, IV access, 12-lead EKG, assess for eligibility for fibrinolytic or reperfusion Rx, cardiac biomarkers (Tn I or T and CK-MB) at presentation, 8 h, 16 h, electrolytes and coagulation studies, portable CXR.
- **Immediate Rx:** Give **morphine, oxygen, nitroglycerin and aspirin**.
- If pt candidate for fibrinolytics: must administer drug $\leq$30 min on arrival to ED **or**
- **Percutaneous coronary intervention:** Performed $\leq$90 min by skilled operator at experienced center
- **Other adjuncts:** β-blockers, ACEIs, statins
- Admission to **ICU** for observation after pt is stabilized
- **Once stable:** Statin, lifestyle Δs, future **cardiac risk stratification** using stress test, ECHO, angiography $\pm$ angioplasty/stenting or CABG

Nonischemic Cardiac Chest Pain

Aortic Dissection

- **Medical:** $\downarrow$ BP first with IV β-blockers (propanolol/esmolol/labetalol), then $\downarrow$ sBP with IV vasodilators (nitroprusside) titrate till sBP 110 mm Hg and HR 60 bpm.
- Control pain with morphine prn.

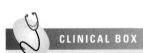

CLINICAL BOX

Mnemonic for CAD RFs

SHOULD FAST: **S**moking, **H**ypertension, **O**vulation (lack of) that is menopause, **U**nhealthy lifestyle (sedentary, high-fat diet), **L**ipid, **D**iabetes, **F**amily history, **A**ge, **S**ex, **T**wo that is second line marker (lipoprotein (a), cardiac CRP, homocysteine).

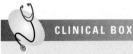

CLINICAL BOX

Early, more aggressive lipid lowering regimen provides greater benefit against death or CV events in ACS pts. For example, atorvastatin 80 mg

Antithrombotic Rx of UA/NSTEMI

Enoxaparin preferred to UFH, 20% ↓ in death/MI

CLINICAL BOX

GPIIb/IIIa Inhibitors

- Give in pt when PCI is planned, ↓ 50% in death/MI
- Consider upstream eptifibatide/tirofiban

CLINICAL BOX

Angiography in UA/NSTEMI

- Done within 24 to 48 h ↓ 25% in death/MI (with stents and GPIIb/IIIa)
- Indicated if high risk: Recurrent ischemia, + Tn, STΔ, TRS ≥3, CHF, ↓ EF, recent PCI, CABG. Angiography within 6 h superior to "cooling off" for 3 to 5 d

CLINICAL BOX

1° PCI for STEMI

- Transfer to center for 1° PCI superior to lysis

Surgery:

For proximal dissection: root replacement for **all** acute cases

For distal dissection: only for progressive chronic cases/significant branch artery involvement/aneurysm/uncontrolled HTN

Pericarditis

- **R/O infectious causes:** Hx and CXR
- **R/O noninfectious causes:** BUN, Cr, ANA, RF, common malignancies
- **Viral/idiopathic cause:** anti-inflammatory drugs (ibuprofen 800 mg t.i.d. plus colchicines 0.6 mg b.i.d.), steroids (prednisone 1 mg/kg) for refractory cases
- **Infectious effusion:** pericardial drainage plus antibiotics
- **Large effusions:** pericardiocentesis
- **Recurrent effusions:** pericardiectomy

TIMI RISK SCORE FOR UA/NSTEMI

- **Aged 65 years or** older
- Use of **ASA** in the last 7 d
- **Severe anginal Sx** (e.g., ≥ two anginal events in the last 24 h)
- Greater than or equal to **three RFs** for CAD
- Known coronary **stenosis of 50% or greater**
- Serum **cardiac markers**
- ST deviation on ECG

    For score of 3 to 7→consider:

1. IV GPIIb/IIIa agents
2. Heparin (low molecular weight or unfractionated)
3. Early cardiac Cath

CLINICAL BOX

Antithrombotic Rx in STEMI

- ASA: 23% ↓ in death
- LMWH: 25% ↓ in death/MI/recurrent ischemia
- GPIIb/IIIa inhibitors: In 1° PCI, start as early as possible: ↓ 60% in death/MI/urgent TVR. In lysis, Ø indication; ½ dose lytic + GPIIa/IIIb: ↓ recurrent MI, Ø Δ in mortality

CLINICAL BOX

Adjunctive Rx in STEMI

- β-Blockers: 15% ↓ in vascular mortality
- ACEI: ~↓ 10% mortality in 4 to 6 wk
- ARBs: appear ~ ACEI

CARDIAC ARREST

RATIONALE

- When an individual is in cardiac arrest, all physicians are expected to attempt resuscitation.
- Most common cause of cardiac arrest in the community is **VF**. However, heart rhythm at clinical presentation in most cases is unknown.
- Therefore, while performing resuscitation do not rely on heart rhythm but focus on **presumed sudden pulse-less condition** and **absence of evidence of a noncardiac condition as cause.**

CAUSAL CONDITIONS

Table **3.16**	**Cardiac Arrest: Causal Conditions**

Cardiac causes
1. **Abnormalities of coronary arteries** (85% of cases)
   a. CAD (MI, with angina/ silent)
   b. Coronary artery **spasm or embolism**
   c. **Tachyarrhythmias** (VF/VT and AF/AFL)
2. Abnormalities of cardiac **conduction**
   a. **Congenital**
   b. **Acquired**
      i. **Metabolic** ($\downarrow$ K$^+$, $\downarrow$ Mg^{2+}, $\downarrow$ Ca^{2+}, anorexia/starvation)
      ii. **Bradyarrhythmias**
          A. Sinus node dysfunction
          B. AV block (second and third degree)
          C. Antiarrhythmic drugs
      iii. **Other**
          A. Antimicrobial drugs
          B. Psychotropic drugs
          C. Vasodilator drugs
          D. Serotonin antagonists
          E. Street drugs
3. Abnormalities of **myocardium**
   a. **Hereditary** (hypertrophic/dilated cardiomyopathy and RV dysplastic syndrome)
   b. **Acquired** (associated with coronary atherosclerosis ischemic injury, HTN, DM)
      i. LVH
      ii. LV **systolic/diastolic dysfunction**
      iii. **Valvular** disease and atrial myxoma
      iv. **Myocarditis** and myocardial/aortic **rupture**

Noncardiac causes

a. Acute CT
b. PE
c. Airway obstruction and TP
d. 1° ED
e. Chest wall trauma

> *Mnemonic:*
> **CT**, **TP**, **PE**, **ED**,
> Trauma

APPROACH

OUTSIDE HOSPITAL SETTING

Check for responsiveness → activate emergency medical system **(911)** → assess **ABCs** → provide **basic life support** until paramedics arrive to give further support.

IN A HOSPITAL SETTING

Check for responsiveness → activate emergency medical system **(code blue/code 999)** → establish **ABCs** → set up monitors, IVs, meds → treat condition as per **ACLS** protocol according to cardiac rhythm and clinical picture.

Hx

1. If the arrest happened outside a hospital setting, ask if there was any event **witness**.
2. Ask about events preceding the arrest.
3. Ask about the **past medical Hx** of the pt that could have led to the arrest.
4. Check if the pt has an **AD** for cardiac resuscitation.

Ix

EKG, CXR, serum electrolytes, blood gas, toxic screen

Cardiac Arrest
The Hs and Ts for reversible causes of cardiac arrest:

Hypoxia, **H**ypo/hyperkalemia, **H**ypo/hyperglycemia, **H**ypovolemia, **H**ypothermia, **H**ydrogen ions (acidosis)

Tension pneumothorax, **T**amponade, **T**oxins, **T**hromboembolism (PE)/ **T**hrombosis (MI)

Mx
Perform lifesaving procedures immediately.

1. **Pericardiocentesis** for CT
2. **Tracheostomy** for airway obstruction
3. **Volume resuscitation** for acute blood loss
4. Release of air for TP
5. Give **antidote** for toxic ingestion

   While performing resuscitation, think about reversible causes.
   If resuscitation is successful:

1. **Stabilize** pt.
2. Admit to **ICU** for recovery.
3. **Establish cause of cardiac arrest** and prevent recurrence:
   • **Cardiac cause:** Refer to cardiology for long-term ICD implantation, optimization of med, pacemaker insertion, and surgery depending on the etiology of the arrest.
   • **Electrolyte imbalances:** Correct underlying cause and monitor blood work.

   If resuscitation is unsuccessful:

• **Communicate news of death** to family members and try to address questions that they might have.
• Discuss the possibility of an **autopsy** if indicated.

C₂LEO

Beneficence: special ethical responsibility of the physician to act in the **best interest of the pt.**
Autonomy: The capacity to make **informed, uncoerced decision.** In the medical context, it is the obligation to respect pts as individuals and **honor pts' preferences** in Rx.
Informed consent: For every Rx recommended, **pt must understand risk, benefits, and alternatives, including Ø intervention.**

ADs
1. **Oral AD:** Incapacitated pt's oral directive whether to give or withdraw Rx. It is more valid than a written directive if the pt was informed, directive is specific, and the decision of the pt is repeated over time.
2. **Written AD:** Can be in the form of a living will or appointing an enduring power of attorney

Living will: Pt directs physician to withdraw/withhold life-sustaining Rx when pt develops terminal disease or enters a persistent vegetative state.

Enduring power of attorney: Pt designates someone else to make medical decisions in the event when the pt loses the capacity to do so.

 C₂LEO Box

Informed Consent
Legally, informed consent requires:

1. Discussion of pertinent information
2. Pt's agreement of care
3. Freedom from coercion

   Exceptions to informed consent:

1. Pt is **not competent** in making decision
2. Implied consent, in an **emergency situation**
3. **Therapeutic privilege**—when disclosure would harm pt or undermine informed decision-making capacity
4. **Pt waives the right** of informed consent

SYNCOPE

DEFINITION

An **abrupt** and **transient LOC** followed by a **rapid** and usually **complete recovery**. Physicians are required to distinguish syncope from seizures, and benign syncope from syncope caused by serious underlying illness.

APPLIED SCIENTIFIC CONCEPTS

RELATIONSHIP BETWEEN BP, CO, AND SVR

$SVR = MAP - CVP$
$CO = X$ mm Hg/L/min
MAP = dBP + 1/3 pulse pressure

RELATIONSHIP BETWEEN CO, SV, AND HR

$CO = HR \times SV$

RELATIONSHIP BETWEEN SV, CONTRACTILITY, PRELOAD, AND AFTERLOAD

SV is determined by three main factors: preload, afterload, and contractility

Preload: ventricular volume at end of diastole; ↑ preload leads to ↑ SV **Starling's law of the heart** → energy of contraction of the muscle is proportional to the initial length of the muscle fiber.

Afterload is the resistance to ventricular ejection. This is caused by the resistance to flow in the systemic circulation and is the **SVR**.

Vascular capacitance refers to degree of active constriction of vessels (mainly veins) which affects return of blood to the heart.

Therefore, ↑ in intravascular volume → ↑ in vascular capacitance → ↑ in preload.

CAUSAL CONDITIONS

CV (~80%)

Cardiac arrhythmia
• Bradyarrhythmias, tachyarrhythmias, carotid sinus syndrome
Reduced CO
• Outflow obstruction (AS, HOCM, myxoma), inflow obstruction (due to venous return), MI
Reflex/underfill
• Vasovagal (micturition, deglutition, cough, defecation), orthostatic/postural hypotension, situational

CEREBROVASCULAR (~15%)

Carotid artery disease, TIAs, vertebrobasilar, high intracranial pressure

PSYCHIATRIC

Panic disorder, hysteria, and hyperventilation

METABOLIC

Hypoxia, **hypoglycemia**, EtOH, drugs

APPROACH

Hx

• Were **convulsions**, bowel/bladder incontinence or postictal state present? → **seizure**
• **Preceding event:** urination, defecation, swallowing, coughing, exertion of arm muscle, manipulation of neck → **situational syncope**
• Painful/emotional **stimulus** precede event? → **vasovagal syncope**
• Hx of CAD/arrhythmia, light-headedness around time of syncope, palpitations, chest pain/SOB/angina → **cardiac cause** of syncope
• Hx of diabetes, TIA, autonomic disorders → **neurogenic** syncope

---

ASC Box

Syncope
Autoregulation of Cerebral Blood Flow

• ↑ Production of vasodilators → ↓ cerebral arteriolar resistance→ reestablish cerebral blood flow
• Constriction of systemic vasculature of skin, splanchnic bed, muscles → diverting blood to brain
• ↑ Sympathetic output → ↑ contractility and ↑ peripheral resistance → ↑ **arterial pressure**

Syncope
Cardiac arrhythmias are important and dangerous cause of syncope. EKG is the most valuable Ix.

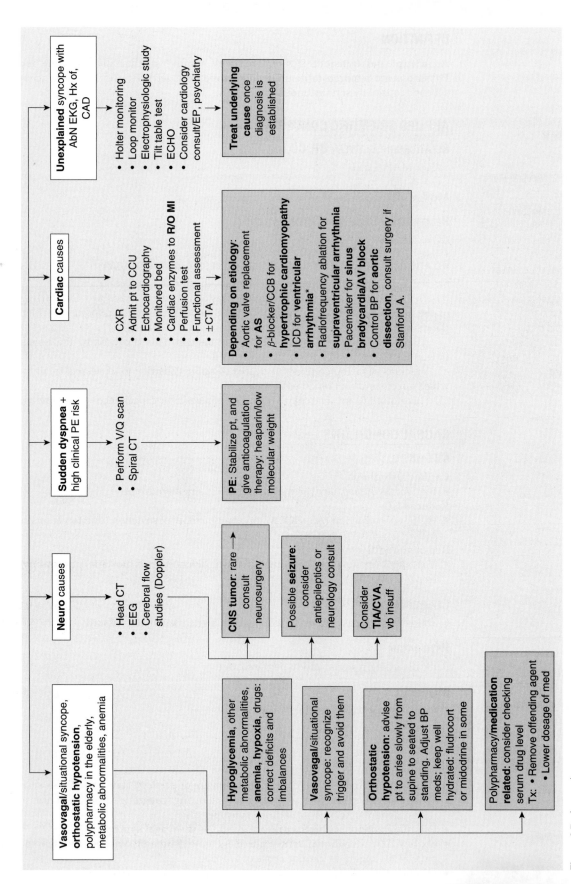

Figure 3.5 Approach to syncope.

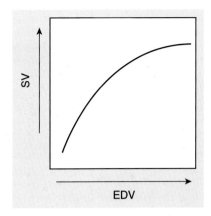

Figure 3.6 Relationship between CO and preload.

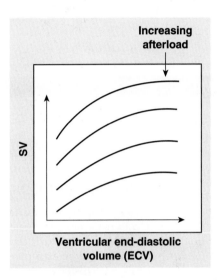

Figure 3.7 Relationship between SV and afterload.

- Feeling lightheaded upon standing, pt on antihypertensives (nitrates, diuretics, α-blockers) → **orthostatic hypotension**
- Hx of psychiatric disorder (e.g., panic attack, anxiety, hysteria, mania) → **psychogenic**
- Meds: insulin, psychoactive meds, narcotics, benzodiazepines, illicit drugs → **med related**
- Past Hx of syncope, family Hx, Hx of presyncope, syncope, and postsyncopal events
- *Syncope versus presyncope*: Pt is usually unable to recall details around the time of attack in syncope (LOC), whereas in presyncope pt would describe the events before fainting (light-headedness, dizziness).

Px

- **Vital signs:** Check BP in supine, sitting, erect position to detect any postural drop; respiratory rate for signs of hyperventilation.
- **Palpation:** Check for AbN pulse. Check parasternal area for heaves
- **Auscultation:** for murmurs, extra heart sounds, clicks
- **Neurologic exam:** Check CNs, sensation, reflexes for any lateralizing signs, mental status.
- **Injuries:** Check for injuries sustained during seizures.
- **Physiologic maneuvers:** Carotid massage (in select pts), Valsalva maneuver

Ix

CBC, electrolytes, TSH, H/H, **EKG**, ECHO, tilt table testing, **EP study** (guided by Hx) neuroimaging, EEG (if focal neuro signs or if seizure is suspected)

Mx

>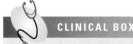
>
> **CLINICAL BOX**
>
> **Causes of Syncope**
>
> **S**eizure
>
> **V**asovagal
>
> **N**eurocardiogenic
>
> **C**ardiac
>
> **O**ccasional (situational)
>
> **P**sychogenic
>
> **E**verything else

> **CLINICAL BOX**
>
> **Hx of Syncope**
>
> **P**receding events
>
> **P**rodrome/warning
>
> **P**osition
>
> **P**reexisting condition
>
> **A**ge of onset
>
> **A**ssociated Sx
>
> **R**ecreational drugs
>
> **R**ecovery
>
> **R**ecordings (by witness, duration of the episode, injuries, number of episodes)

GENERALIZED EDEMA

RATIONALE

Pts frequently complain of swelling. Swelling often represents expansion of the interstitial fluid volume. It may be a benign condition, but at times may be caused by serious disease.

APPLIED SCIENTIFIC CONCEPTS

- **EABV:** adequacy of the arterial BV to "fill" the capacity of the arterial vasculature
- **1° Salt retention:** direct retention of Na^+ and hence H_2O in the kidneys from ↓ excretion or ↑ absorption of Na^+; occurs in **RF**, mineralocorticoid excess, and NSAID ingestion
- **2° Salt retention:** example—nephrotic syndrome ↓ intravascular oncotic pressure → ↓ EABV → activation of renal angiotensin system→ **2° renal salt retention**

> **ASC Box**
>
> **Generalized Edema**
>
> Body compartments and approximate relationship to body weight:
>
> **40%** of total body **weight** = fat, mineral, protein
>
> **20%** of total body **weight** = plasma, transcellular fluid, interstitial fluid (extracellular fluid accounts for 40% of total body H_2O)
>
> **40%** of total body **weight** = intracellular fluid (intracellular fluid 60% of total body H_2O)

STARLING'S LAW

$$\text{Net filtration} = LpS \times (\Delta \text{ hydraulic pressure} - \Delta \text{ oncotic pressure})$$

$$= LpS \times [(P_{cap} - P_{if}) - s(\pi_{cap} - \pi_{if})]$$

where

Lp = unit permeability of capillary wall

S = surface area

P_{cap} and P_{if} = capillary and interstitial fluid hydraulic pressures

π_{cap} and π_{if} = capillary and interstitial fluid oncotic pressures

s = reflection coefficient of proteins across capillary wall (0 = completely permeable; 1 = completely impermeable)

Net filtration = hydropressure (pressure pushing out from vessels) − oncotic pressure (resistance to pressure pushing out)

Examples

1. In **heart failure**: hydro pressure ($\uparrow\uparrow$) − oncotic pressure ($\emptyset\ \Delta$) = $\uparrow\uparrow$ net filtration
2. In **cirrhosis**: hydro pressure ($\emptyset\ \Delta$) − oncotic pressure ($\downarrow\downarrow$) = $\uparrow\uparrow$ net filtration, that is, less resistance to the pressure pushing out due to low albumin, therefore more net filtration.

CAUSAL CONDITIONS

$\uparrow$ Hydrostatic pressure

- CHF
- Cirrhosis

Obstruction of lymph flow

- CHF

Inappropriate renal Na and H_2O retention

- RF
- Nephrotic syndrome

$\downarrow$ Oncotic pressure

- Nephrotic syndrome
- Cirrhosis
- Malnutrition

$\uparrow$ Vascular permeability to proteins

- Angioneurotic edema (usually allergic)

APPROACH

Hx

- **Previous Hx** of any disorder (coronary disease, HTN, EtOH abuse, hepatic disease, renal disease)
- **Med** (med that can cause cardiac, hepatic, or renal disease)
- Where is the edema located?

Px and Ix

See Figure 3.8.

Mx

1. **Diuretics**
   - For **CHF**, Na$^+$ retention, and nephritic syndrome: **furosemide** (20–80 mg/d)
   - For **hepatic cirrhosis**: **Spironolactone** (starting 100 mg/d divided doses) and **furosemide** 40 mg in the morning
2. **Therapeutic paracentesis** for diuretic resistant or tense ascites causing **Abdo discomfort** or **dyspnea**
3. **Others**
   - **Venous insufficiency:** leg elevation and well-fitted, high-**compression** knee **stockings**
   - **Lymphedema: massage Rx** and **compression garment** on affected area

General Edema

Peripheral edema and ascites usually causes discomfort and aesthetic concerns. Flash pulmonary edema, caused by ARDS or CHF on the other hand, could become life threatening.

CLINICAL BOX

Contrast "Forward" (LV) to "Backward" (RV) Failure

L heart failure (forward failure)	R heart failure (backward failure)
• LV failed to pump out total volume of blood from the RV	• Failed RV output: less than input from the systemic circulation
• Cause: MI (most common), HTN, valvular stenosis, cardiomyopathy	• Cause: L heart failure, COPD, pulmonary HTN, congenital heart defects
• Clinical features: fatigue, weakness, dizziness, orthopnea, dyspnea on exertion	• Clinical features: $\uparrow$ JVP, pitting edema and hepatosplenomegaly

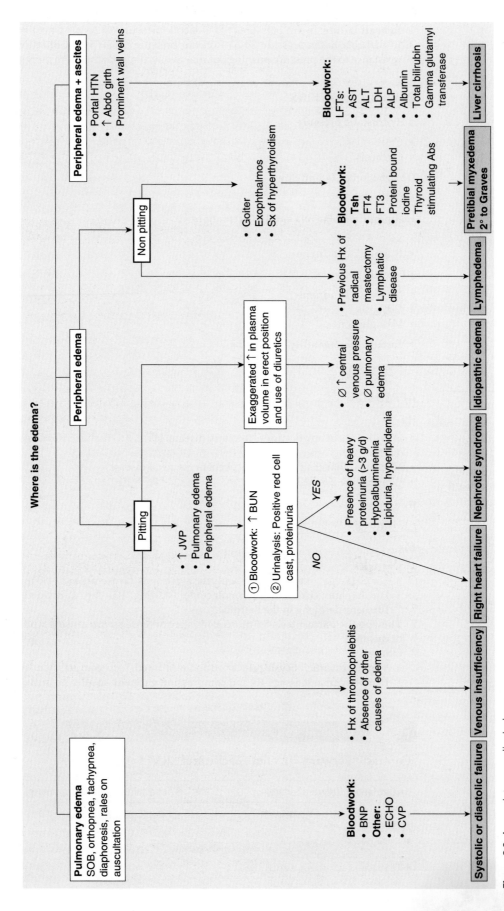

Figure 3.8 Approach to generalized edema.

Conditions that Favor Interstitial Edema

- ↑ Capillary **hydrostatic** pressure
- ↑ Capillary **permeability**
- ↓ Capillary **oncotic** pressure

Classes of Diuretics

- **Osmotic agents:** mannitol (**osmotic diuresis** at **proximal tubule**)
- **Loop agents:** furosemide, bumetanide (**reduction of Na⁺ reabsorption** [leads to K⁺ loss at distal tubule]; reduction of medullary hypertonicity at thick **ascending loop of Henle**)
- **Thiazides:** hydrochlorothiazides, chlorthalidone, metolazone, clopamide, mefruside (**reduction of Na⁺ reabsorption** [leads to K⁺ loss at distal tubule] at **cortical diluting segment** of nephron)
- **K sparing diuretics:** spironolactone, triamterene, amiloride (**inhibition of Na⁺ exchange with K⁺, H⁺** [K⁺ retention]; aldosterone antagonism; aldosterone independent at **distal tubule**)

ABNORMAL PULSE

RATIONALE

The characteristics of arterial pulse should be assessed as an integral part of the Px. Carotid, radial, femoral, posterior tibialis, and dorsalis pedis pulses should be examined **bilaterally**. Δs in **amplitude, contour, and upstroke** should be determined. Compare R and L radial pulses as well as brachial and femoral pulses.

APPLIED SCIENTIFIC CONCEPTS

At very low speed, blood flow is laminar. When there is ↑ in velocity from either narrowing of blood vessels ($\downarrow l$) or ↑ flow rate, at some point the transition is made to turbulent flow.

$$\text{FLOW} = \frac{\Delta P \times \pi \times r^4}{8 \times \eta \times l}$$

(Δp = pressure difference between two ends ; r = radius of the tube ; η = viscosity of fluid ; l = length of tube)

CAUSAL CONDITIONS

Table **3.17**	**Causal Conditions of AbN Pulses**
Unequal or delayed pulses	a. **Obstructive arterial disease** (i.e., atherosclerosis) b. **Aortic disease** Dissection (>20 mm Hg Δ between arms), aneurysm, coarctation (brachiofemoral delay), supra/valvular AS (pulses **tardus et parvus**; delayed and weak) c. **Takayasu arteritis** (systemic Sx: fever, weight loss, myalgia, erythema nodosum, intermittent HTN): Asymmetric BP (>20−30 Δ) and pulses, aortic and subclavian bruits, absent pulses (rare), retinal and vitreous hemorrhage, cotton wool spots
Rhythm irregular/too fast/too slow	a. **Tachycardia** (>100/min) Sinus Fever, sepsis, hyperthyroid Volume depletion: Hypotension, shock, cardiac failure Anemia, hypoxemia, drugs b. **Bradycardia** (<45/min) Normal heart: During sleep, athletes, some elderly Intrinsic to heart: Infiltrative disease, collagen disease, open heart surgery Extrinsic: Vagal stimulation, drugs, hypothyroid, hypothermia, AbN K levels c. **Arrhythmia** (see **Palpitation**)

TYPES OF PULSES

Pulsus alternans
- Weak and strong pulses with fixed cycle length
- Present in: systolic dysfunction/low EF

Pulsus bisferiens
- Biphasic pulse
- Present in: AS plus AI, severe AI, and HOCM

Dicrotic pulse
- Double peak, with weaker second beat
- Present in: ↓ arterial pressure/PVR, very low EF, post AVR

Anacrotic pulse/Pulsus parvus et tardus
- Slow rising, typically with an ascending notch
- Present in AS

Corrigan pulse (H$_2$O hammer/collapsing)
- Rapid pulse then sudden collapse
- Present in AR

Pulsus paradoxus
- Exaggerated inspiratory ↑ in arterial pulse
- Present in CT, asthma, hypovolemic shock

AbN Pulses

Pulsus paradoxus with Beck triad (JVD, muffled heart sound, hypotension) is indicative of pericardial tamponade.

APPROACH

Hx

- **Previous Hx of CV disease**: congenital heart disease (PDA, CoA, AS, long QT syndrome), previous episode of MI, previous heart surgery, valvular disease, PVD, Hx of arrhythmia, pericardial/myocardial disease
- **Toxic ingestion**: med overdose, smoking (PVD), substance abuse
- **Exposure**: to extremes of temperature

Px

- Palpate radial pulse bilaterally for **radio–radio delay**
- Measure **BP in both arms and legs** using appropriately sized cuffs if CoA is suspected

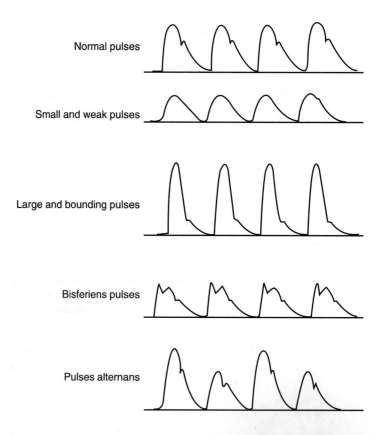

Figure 3.9 AbN volume pulses.

- Examine **popliteal pulses** if lower leg arterial disease is suspected
- Auscultate the heart for any **murmur**, extra heart sounds (S_3, S_4, clicks)

Mx

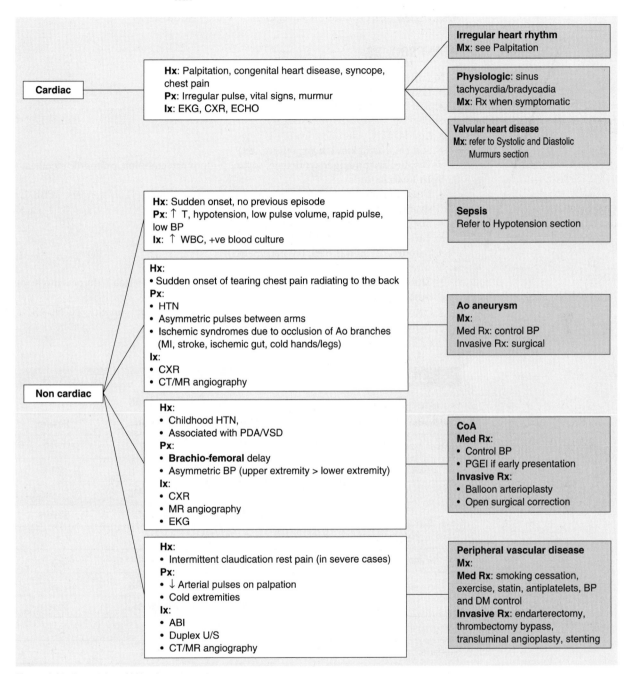

Figure 3.10 Approach to AbN pulses.

CLINICAL BOX

ABI

ABIs as high as **1.10** are normal; AbN values are those **<1.0**. Most pts with claudication have ABIs ranging from **0.3 to 0.9**. Rest pain or severe occlusive disease typically occurs with an ABI **<0.50**. Indexes **<0.20** are associated with ischemic or gangrenous extremities. ABI **>1.30** is usually associated with calcified vessels.

ABNORMAL HEART SOUNDS

RATIONALE

Pathological heart sounds are clues to underlying heart disease.

HEART SOUNDS

1. S_1
   - Loud (MS, hyperthyroidism, short PR interval)
   - Soft (mitral valve regurgitation, long PR interval, COPD)
2. S_2
   - Loud (HTN, sclerotic aorta)
   - Soft (hypotension, L heart failure, AS)
   - Ø split (Eisenmenger syndrome, severe pulmonary embolus, pulmonic stenosis)
3. **Split heart sounds**
   - Delayed pulmonary valve closure (pulmonary embolus/HTN/stenosis, RBBB, L to R shunt)
   - Fixed split (ASD)
   - Early aortic closure (MR, VSD)
   - Paradoxical split (LBBB, RV pacemaker)
4. **S_3 and S_4**
   - Third heart sound (dilated ventricle with volume overload, hyperkinetic heart, mitral/TR, L/R heart failure)
   - Fourth heart sound (hypertrophic and ischemic cardiomyopathy, HTN, AS, acute ischemia causing a stiff ventricle)

Table **3.18**   **Classification of Valve Stenosis and Regurgitation**

	AS		
Indicator	**Mild**	**Moderate**	**Severe**
Mean gradient (mm Hg)	≤25	25–40	≥40
Valve area (cm²)	≥1.5	1.0–1.5	≤1.0
	MS		
	Mild	**Moderate**	**Severe**
Mean gradient (mm Hg)	≤5	5–10	≥10
Valve area (cm²)	≥1.5	1.0–1.5	≤1.0
	AR		
	Mild	**Moderate**	**Severe**
Angiographic grade	1+	2+	3–4+
Doppler vena contracta width (cm)	≤0.3	0.3–0.6	≥0.6
Regurgitant fraction (%) (Cath/ECHO)	<30	30–49	≥50, LV size ↑
	MR		
	Mild	**Moderate**	**Severe**
Angiographic grade	1+	2+	3–4+
Doppler vena contracta width (cm)	≤0.3	0.3–0.69	≥0.70
Regurgitant fraction (%) (Cath/ECHO)	≤30	30–49	≥50, LA and LV size ↑

Table **3.19**	Six Grades of Intensity of Murmur
Grade I	Very faint, heard only when listener has "tuned in"
Grade II	Also faint, but can be identified after placing stethoscope on chest
Grade III	Moderately loud
Grade IV	Loud with palpable thrill
Grade V	Very loud, with thrill; may be heard when stethoscope is partly off the chest
Grade VI	Very loud, with thrill; heard without stethoscope

AbN Heart Sound

A pericardial rub, heard on auscultation usually as a two to three component sound is a sign of pericarditis—which warrants attention. The rub is loudest during systole, grating, scratching, or rasping in nature and is body position dependent, leaning forward ↑ its intensity.

5. **Extra heart sounds and clicks**
   • Ejection sounds (early systolic)—AS and PS
   • Opening sounds (early diastolic)—MS, TS
   • Clicks (mid-systolic)—mitral valve prolapse
   • Pericardial rub—pericarditis

   Up to 60% of pts have a mid-systolic murmur and 90% of them would have a normal ECHO. Murmur is considered innocent when there is **absence** of other AbN findings (i.e., AbN S_2, signs of heart failure).

Table **3.20**	Indications for Surgery of Some Common Cardiac Conditions	
Condition	**Indication for Surgery**	
ASD	L to R shunt >2:1	
VSD	L to R shunt >2:1	
PDA	Always	
CoA	Always	
PS	Pressure gradient >50 mm Hg	
AS	Angina Effort syncope L heart failure Pressure gradient >50 mm Hg EKG shows LVH with strain	
AR/AI	Angina L heart failure EKG shows LVH with strain	
MS	Symptomatic (dyspnea and effort intolerance) Pulmonary HTN Tight MS	
MR	Significant and progressing Sx	

SYSTOLIC AND DIASTOLIC MURMURS

RATIONALE

Without cardiac findings and normal splitting of second heart sounds, systolic murmurs are often innocent. Diastolic murmurs are almost always pathologic.

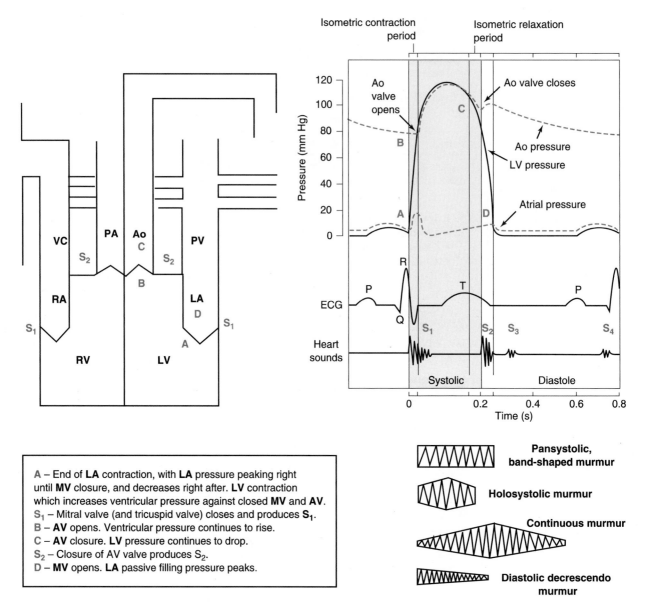

A – End of **LA** contraction, with **LA** pressure peaking right until **MV** closure, and decreases right after. **LV** contraction which increases ventricular pressure against closed **MV** and **AV**.
S_1 – Mitral valve (and tricuspid valve) closes and produces S_1.
B – **AV** opens. Ventricular pressure continues to rise.
C – **AV** closure. **LV** pressure continues to drop.
S_2 – Closure of AV valve produces S_2.
D – **MV** opens. **LA** passive filling pressure peaks.

Figure 3.11 Heart sounds.

CAUSAL CONDITIONS

SYSTOLIC MURMUR

Holosystolic murmurs
• MR, TR, VSD
Mid-systolic ejection murmurs
• AS, aortic valve sclerosis, PS
• ↑ Semilunar blood flow, innocent mid-systolic murmurs **Late-systolic murmurs:**
• Mitral valve prolapse, tricuspid valve prolapse, papillary muscle dysfunction

DIASTOLIC MURMUR

Early diastolic murmurs
• AR, PR
Mid-diastolic murmurs
• MS, TS
• Atrial myxoma
Late-diastolic murmurs
• Complete heart block

Murmur
A systolic murmur with a triad of angina, syncope, and dyspnea or impaired exercise tolerance is highly suspicious of AS.

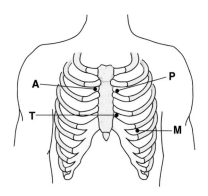

Figure 3.12 Site of auscultation.

APPROACH

Hx

- Hx of **previous heart conditions**: **congenital cardiac lesions**, childhood murmur, previous heart surgery, Hx of heart failure, **MI**, previous myocarditis/endocarditis, any known **cardiomyopathy** (HOCM)
- Previous infections: Hx of **rheumatic fever**, sexually transmitted disease (aortitis 2° to syphilis), **bacterial endocarditis** (from IV drug use)
- **Collagen disease**: SLE, scleroderma
- **Genetic disorder**: Marfan syndrome (MVP), Down syndrome (ASD, VSD)
- Rheumatology: RA, AS
- Malignancy: **carcinoid syndrome** (diarrhea, flushing, R heart failure)

Px

Seven components of murmur:

1. **Timing** (early, middle, late)
2. **Shape** (intensity over time: crescendo, decrescendo, crescendo–decrescendo, and plateau)
3. **Location**
4. **Radiation**
5. **Intensity** (loudness)
6. **Pitch** (low, medium, high: use bell for low pitch and diaphragm for high pitch)
7. **Quality** (blowing, harsh, rumbling, musical)

Ix

EKG: Determine sinus rhythm. Detect ventricular failure.

CXR: Determine placement of the heart and signs of cardiac failure (pulmonary congestion).

ECHO: able to define the anatomy of the heart and great vessels and to detect valve damage and estimate severity of disease; **color Doppler flow** on the **TTE**—has higher accuracy, quantitative

Cardiac Cath: Useful for anatomic diagnosis and also provides
- Pressure gradient across stenotic valves
- Degree of regurgitation
- Magnitude of shunting

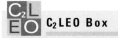 **C₂LEO Box**

Physicians' Legal Liability for Negligence (Civil Liability in Quebec)
Physicians are **legally liable to their pts for causing harm** through a failure to meet the standard of care that is applicable under the particular circumstances under consideration. A physician may be found legally liable to pt if a diastolic or systolic murmur, when associated with other cardiac findings was considered innocent and not investigated or referred for further assessment.

Table **3.21**	**Mx of Murmur**			
	Etiology	**Sx, Px**	**Ix**	**Mx**
MS	**Rheumatic heart disease** Calcification of leaflets Bacterial endocarditis	Malar flush, AF, CHF **Opening snap** after A_2, **mid-diastolic rumbling** murmur after opening snap at apex loud P_2, **low-pitched**, tapping apex beat, thrill LLD position ↑ murmur	Transmitral gradient measured by **doppler ECHO** **Swan-Ganz** Cath: PCWP	**Medical:** β-blocker and **diuretics** **Anticoagulation** if AF present **Surgical:** balloon valvoplasty
MR	**Myxomatous degeneration of the mitral valve** IHD Infective endocarditis Collagen vascular diseases Rheumatic heart disease Trauma Dilatation of the LV	SOB, pulmonary edema, fatigue, orthopnea, PND Heard best at apex, radiates to the **axilla, high-pitched, holosystolic,** P mitrale, laterally displaced PMI, LV heave	**EKG:** LA enlargement and LVH, ± AF in chronic MR **CXR:** enlargement of the LA and the LV **ECHO**: TTE with color Doppler flow showing backflow from LV to LA	**Hypo**tensive: IABP **Normo**tensive: nitroprusside, ACEI, and hydralazine **Anticoagulation** if AF present **Surgery**: repair vs. replacement
MVP	**Myxomatous degeneration** Genetic variants of fibrillin, elastin, collagen I and II 7% prevalence, F:M is 3:1.	Usually **asymptomatic**, **late systolic** murmur, midsystolic **click** Can progress to **MR**	**EKG:** arrhythmia, APCs, PVCs **ECHO:** shows AbN valve anatomy, regurgitant flow	**Endocarditis prophylaxis** (amoxicillin) for dental procedures Prolapse **Rx Ø needed**, unless symptomatic
AS	**Acute rheumatic fever** Bicuspid aortic valve Calcification of aortic valve	SOB, CHF, syncope, angina **Midsystolic** crescendo-decrescendo, second **IC,** radiating to the neck **Pulses parvus et tardus,** sustained apical beat, paradoxical S_2 split, pulsus alternans ↑ murmur with squatting, ↓ with standing (opposite to HOCM)	**EKG:** LVH **CXR:** cardiomegaly **Cardiac Cath with Doppler ECHO:** measure of blood velocity **ECHO:** valve P gradient $= 4$ $(\text{velocity})^2$ mm Hg	Use afterload reducers with **precaution** (diuretics, β-blockers) **Infective endocarditis prophylaxis** **Surgery:** valve replacement
AR	**Idiopathic aortic root dilatation** HTN Bicuspid aortic valve Rheumatic fever Marfan syndrome Aortic dissection Syphilis	CHF and angina **Three murmurs:** **High-pitched, blowing decrescendo diastolic murmur** at LLSB **Midsystolic** murmur at the base **Austin-Flint** —low pitched, mid-diastolic murmur	**EKG:** Could be N, L axis deviation, prominent Q wave in I, AVF, V_3 to V_6 **ECHO:** Regurgitant flow and LV size **Cardiac Cath:** LV function, aortic valve leaflet anatomy, especially needed for valve replacement candidate	**Afterload reducers:** digoxin, ACEI, nifedipine, hydralazine, and diuretics

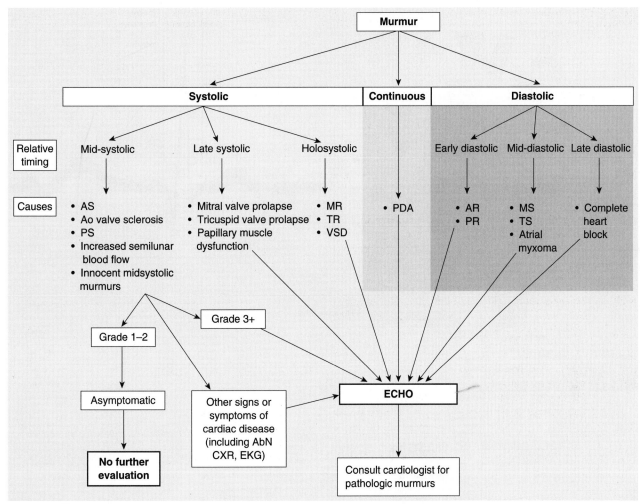

Figure 3.13 Approach to murmurs.

PALPITATION

DEFINITION

Unpleasant awareness of the forceful, rapid, or irregular beating of the heart

APPLIED SCIENTIFIC CONCEPTS

1. Depolarization of **SA node** (electrical activity spontaneously generated) → 2. **Atrial** depolarization → 3. Depolarization of **AV node** (there is a delay in the conduction, causing PR segment), the **bundle of His**, bundle branches → 4. Depolarization of **Purkinje fibers** and myocardial cells

CAUSAL CONDITIONS

1. Cardiac (50%)
   - **Arrhythmia:** SVT, PVC
   - **Heart defects:** valvular disease, cardiomyopathy, shunts, myxoma
2. **Psychiatric (33%)**
   - Panic attack, AD, stress, depression
3. **Endocrine**
   - Thyrotoxicosis, hypo/hyperglycemia, pheochromocytoma

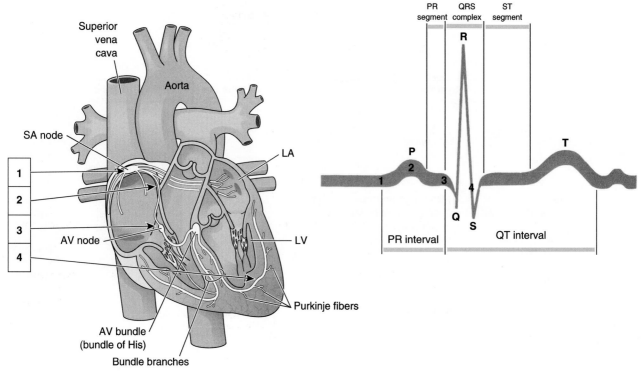

Figure 3.14 Cardiac electrophysiology.

ASC box

Palpitation

Role of autonomic system in development of arrhythmias:

1. **Sympathetic** stimulation of β_1 adrenergic receptors → ↑ SA node automaticity and ↑ rate of pacemaker depolarization → ↑ HR for example, exercise, emotional stress
2. **Parasympathetic** stimulation through vagus nerve → ↓ pacemaker current → ↓ pacemaker firing rate → ↓ HR
3. Arrhythmias like SVT and ventricular tachyarrhythmia can occur during catecholamine excess such as during exercise or at times of stress.

> **Palpitation**
> In VF, there is Ø organized pumping of the ventricles. Death is inevitable within seconds to minutes unless there is immediate intervention.

4. **Others:** ↑ in CO
   - ↑ **Demand:** anemia, pregnancy, fever, thyrotoxicosis, exercise, Paget disease
   - **Meds:** sympathomimetics, vasodilators, β-blocker stopped, cocaine, amphetamines, caffeine, nicotine

APPROACH

Hx

Age of onset, type of palpitation (**regular vs. irregular**), Hx of cardiac disease, onset and offset of palpitation, associated Sx (syncope, chest pain, and dyspnea), psychiatric illness, med (including OTC), drugs, and caffeine intake

Px

Look for presence of **murmur**, extra heart sounds (S₃, S₄, clicks, snap), assess **JVP**, and listen for basilar crackles.

Ix

EKG with rhythm strip.

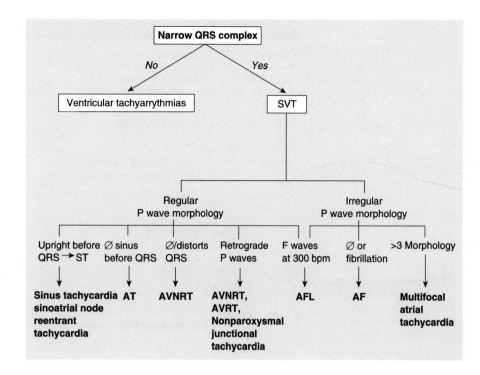

Figure 3.15 SV arrhythmias.

Laboratory work: Consider Hb to R/O anemia, TSH to R/O thyroid disorder, metabolic panel to R/O electrolyte imbalance.

Ambulatory monitoring: done only when Hx, physical and EKG do not establish a definitive diagnosis

Mx

Noncardiac

Sx indicating **psychiatric** etiology:

• Refer to psychiatric, relaxation technique, and cognitive behavioral Rx, see Chapter 19.

2° Metabolic Derangement
• Correct underlying deficits/excess

2° to Med, Caffeine
• Stop offending agent
• Optimize med dosage

Cardiac
• Diagnose and treat rhythm

AF
Irregularly irregular pulse is indicative of AF. Rate control is as effective as rhythm control with regards to mortality (AFFIRM). But in severe heart failure, rhythm control might be needed as reattained atrial "kick" provides ~10% to 15% ↑ in CO.

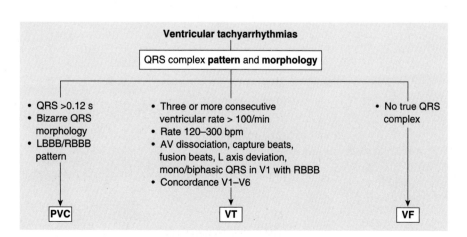

Figure 3.16 Ventricular tachyarrhythmias.

Table **3.22**	Mx of Palpitation	
Rhythm	**Acute Rx**	**Long-Term Rx**
Unstable	**Cardioversion** per ACLS	Not applicable
ST	Treat underlying cause	Not applicable
AT	**β-blocker or CCB**	β-blockers or CCB ± antiarrhythmics radiofrequency ablation
AVNRT or AVRT	Vagal maneuvers, **adenosine**, CCB, and β-blockers (**avoid** IV verapamil and digoxin if suspect accessory pathway)	Radiofrequency ablation CCB or β-blockers ± antiarrhythmics
AF	**β-blockers, CCB, digoxin**	Pt **with** underlying structural **heart disease**: antiarrhythmic Rx + anticoagulation Pt **without heart disease** and asymptomatic: rate control (β-blockers, CCB) + anticoagulation
AFL	**β-blockers, CCB, digoxin**	Radiofrequency **ablation** β-blockers or CCB ± antiarrhythmics
MAT	**CCB**	Treat underlying disease process AVN ablation + PPM
VT	**Unstable** pt: DC cardioversion **Stable** pt: DC cardioversion and antiarrhythmics	AICD
VF	**Cardioversion** as per ACLS	AICD

CLINICAL BOX

Four variables are independent predictors of cardiac etiology.

- Event **d**uration of >5 min
- Hx of **h**eart disease
- Description of an **i**rregular heart beat
- **M**ale sex

CLINICAL BOX

Rx of SVT: ABCDE

Adenosine

β-Blocker

Calcium channel blocker

Digitalis

Excitation (vagal stimulus)

CLINICAL BOX

AF

- Cardioversion: If duration >48 h, cardioversion has 2% to 5% chance of precipitating CVA, therefore must either visualize LA with TEE to R/O thrombus.
- Rhythm control: Recent trial data suggest rhythm control offers Ø mortality benefit to rate control + anticoagulation in pt with recurrent AF.

CHAPTER 4

Dermatology

Andrea Cheung, Dr. Nisha Mistry, and Dr. Harvey Lui

SKIN RASH: MACULES

DEFINITION

Table **4.1**	Primary Lesions
Macule	<1 cm flat discolored lesion
Patch	>1 cm flat discolored lesion
Papule	<1 cm palpable raised superficial lesion
Plaque	>1 cm confluence of papules
Nodule	<1 cm lesion with significant depth
Tumor	>1 cm lesion with significant depth
Cyst	>1 cm fluid-containing lesion
Telangiectasia	Dilated superficial blood vessels
Pustule	<1 cm elevated lesion containing pus
Vesicle	<1 cm elevated lesion containing serous fluid
Bulla	>1 cm elevated lesion containing serous fluid
Wheal	Transient blanchable papule or plaque

CAUSAL CONDITIONS

ERYTHEMATOUS MACULES

Possible Causes
- Drug eruption
- Infectious exanthems
- Secondary syphilis (palms and soles)
- Rheumatic fever (erythema marginatum)

Location
Trunk and proximal extremities

Lesion
Blanchable and diffuse

Table **4.2**	**Secondary Lesions**
Excoriation	Scratch mark on the skin
Lichenification	Area of diffuse thickening with increase in skin markings due to rubbing or scratching
Scales	Increased stratum corneum cells that are shedding
Crusts	Dried exudates of blood, serum, or pus
Fissure	Linear breaks in the skin
Erosion	Disruption of the epidermis
Ulceration	Irregular excavations extending into the dermis or deeper
Atrophy	Thinning or depression of the skin
Scar	Connective tissue formations that replace lost tissue
Hypopigmentation	Decreased skin pigment
Hyperpigmentation	Increased skin pigment
Depigmentation	Complete absence of skin pigment

PHOTO-DISTRIBUTED MACULES
Drug Photosensitivity Reactions

Table **4.3**	**Phototoxic vs. Photoallergic Drug Reactions**	
	Phototoxic Drug Reaction	**Photoallergic Drug Reaction**
Common agents	NSAIDs, quinolones, tetracyclines, amiodarone, phenothiazines	Soaps, fragrances Caused by interaction of photoallergen and UVA
Location	Face, "V" of upper chest, dorsa of hands and forearms	
Prevalence	More common	Less common
Clinical presentation	Presents as an exaggerated sunburn: erythema, edema, vesicles/bullae	Pruritic eruption indistinguishable from allergic contact dermatitis
Dose dependency	Dose related	Triggered at any dose

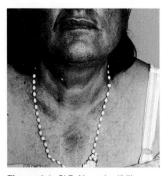

Figure 4.1 SLE. Note the "V" photodistribution of the upper chest.

(From Goodheart HP. *Goodheart's photoguide of common skin disorders*, 2nd ed. Philadelphia: Lippincott Williams & Wilkins; 2003.)

Collagen/Vascular

SLE lesions
• Erythema in malar distribution (**butterfly rash**) or
• Diffuse erythema in photodistribution

Dermatomyositis lesions
• Violaceous, periorbital **heliotrope rash** with edema
• Erythema of face, neck, and upper trunk (**shawl sign**)
• Violaceous papules over knuckles (**Gottron papules**)

HYPOPIGMENTED MACULES
Tinea Versicolor (Pityriasis Versicolor)
• Associated with overgrowth of *M. furfur*

Lesions
• Mottled distribution of round/oval hyper- or hypopigmented macules with fine scaling
• Most commonly found on the trunk

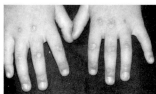

Figure 4.2 Dermatomyositis. Gottron papules are violaceous, flat-topped papules located over the joints of the fingers.

(From Goodheart HP. *Goodheart's photoguide of common skin disorders*, 2nd ed. Philadelphia: Lippincott Williams & Wilkins; 2003.)

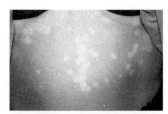

Figure 4.3 Tinea versicolor. Oval hypopigmented macules which are accentuated in the summer with tanning and can resemble vitiligo.

(From Goodheart HP. *Goodheart's photoguide of common skin disorders*, 2nd ed. Philadelphia: Lippincott Williams & Wilkins; 2003.)

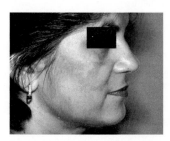

Figure 4.4 Melasma of the cheeks.

(From Goodheart HP. *Goodheart's photoguide of common skin disorders*, 2nd ed. Philadelphia: Lippincott Williams & Wilkins; 2003.)

DIAGNOSIS
- Hyphae and spores seen on KOH prep ("**spaghetti and meatballs**")

TREATMENT
- Selenium sulfide lotion
- Oral ketoconazole

Vitiligo
An autoimmune reaction against melanocytes; associated with other autoimmune diseases including pernicious anemia, Hashimoto's thyroiditis, and diabetes mellitus type 1

Lesions
- Acquired depigmented macules or patches with sharp margins
- May be isolated or generalized
- Typically around the eyes, mouth, on digits, extensor surfaces, low back, and genitalia

DIAGNOSIS
- Wood's lamp to distinguish hypopigmentation from depigmentation
- Absence of melanocytes on histology and microscopy
- Lab tests if thyroid disease, diabetes, or pernicious anemia suspected

TREATMENT
- Sun protection (including sunscreens)
- Camouflage preparations
- Repigmentation with narrow band UVB and topical corticosteroids or topical immuno-modulators
- Depigmentation for extensive disease using topical depigmenting agents on normally pigmented skin

HYPERPIGMENTED MACULES
Postinflammatory Hyperpigmentation
Common causes
- Following acne, psoriasis, lichen planus, atopic dermatitis, or any type of trauma

Lesions
- Usually limited to site of inflammation
- Indistinct borders
- Occurs especially in darker skin types

TREATMENT
- Observation (almost all cases will resolve spontaneously)
- Topical hydroquinone

Melasma
Affects females ≫ males

Common causes
- Sun exposure
- Triggered by pregnancy and hormone use

Lesions
- Acquired well-demarcated geographic patterned macules and patches with irregular margins
- Most commonly on the central face (cheeks, forehead, nose, upper lip)

TREATMENT
- May regress spontaneously
- Skin-lightening agents: hydroquinone, azelaic acid, tretinoin
- Chemical peels
- Sun protection

Fixed Drug Eruption
- An adverse drug reaction

Lesions
- Sharply marginated, round/oval, erythematous macules evolving to plaques, bullae, and erosions; recurrent episodes may leave prominent hyperpigmented macules
- This drug eruption is "fixed" because it recurs at the same location(s) each time the drug is taken

DIAGNOSIS
- Clinical; drug challenge/withdrawal

SKIN RASH: PAPULES

DEFINITION

See Skin Rash: Macules

CAUSAL CONDITIONS

Table **4.4**	Papules: Causal Conditions	
Type	**Cause/Location**	**Differential Diagnosis**
Isolated papules	Tumors	Dermatofibroma, BCC, hemangioma, melanoma, nevus, SCC, pyogenic granuloma
	Infections	Fungal infections, wart
	Keratoses	Actinic keratosis, keratoacanthoma, seborrheic keratosis, milia
Papular eruptions	Acneiform	Rosacea, acne vulgaris, perioral dermatitis
	Dermatitis	Seborrheic dermatitis, contact dermatitis, dyshidrotic dermatitis, atopic dermatitis
	Other dermatologic	Psoriasis, pityriasis rosea, miliaria, lichen planus
	Infections	Folliculitis, molluscum contagiosum, syphilis, infections, viral exanthem, warts, bacillary angiomatosis
	Systemic conditions	Dermatomyositis, SLE, lymphoma, neurofibromatosis, sarcoidosis, urticaria, vasculitis, xanthomas
	Arthropod bites	Scabies, pediculosis, insect bites
	Drug eruptions	Antibiotics, other drugs
Plaques	Infections	Candidiasis, cellulitis, fungal, tinea, Lyme disease, syphilis
	Systemic conditions	Acanthosis nigricans, neutrophilic dermatoses, granuloma annulare, SLE, lymphoma, scleroderma, myxedema, necrobiosis lipoidica, sarcoidosis, vasculitis
	Other dermatologic	Atopic dermatitis, eczema, ichthyosis, lichen planus, lichen sclerosus, pityriasis rosea, psoriasis, seborrheic dermatitis
Vesicles and bullae	Infections	Congenital syphilis, fungal, herpes simplex/zoster, impetigo, Staphylococcal scalded skin, varicella
	Immune/allergic/drugs	Dermatitis herpetiformis, atopic dermatitis, contact dermatitis, pemphigus/pemphigoid, SLE, vasculitis, Stevens-Johnson syndrome, toxic epidermal necrolysis, erythema multiforme
	Other	Diabetes, burns, scabies, insect bite reactions
Pustules	Face	Acne vulgaris, rosacea, perioral dermatitis, tinea barbae, staphylococcal folliculitis, impetigo
	Trunk	Bacterial/fungal infections of sweat glands or follicles, arthropod bites
	With fever	Varicella, syphilis, gonococcus, drugs, psoriasis

APPROACH

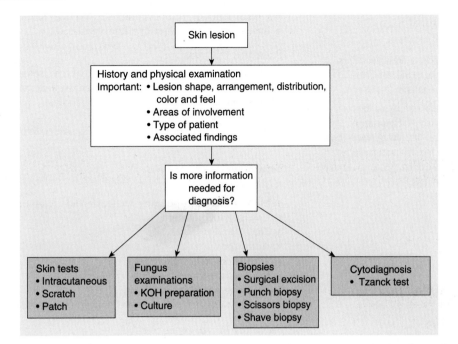

Figure 4.5 Approach to skin lesions.

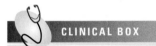
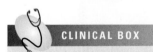
ACNE VULGARIS

Combination of comedones, papules, pustules, and in severe cases nodules and cysts

Treatment

Mild Acne

- Topical antibiotics (clindamycin/erythromycin)
- Benzoyl peroxide
- Topical retinoids (tretinoin/adapalene/tazarotene)

Moderate Acne

- Addition of oral antibiotics (minocycline/doxycycline/tetracycline)
- OCP/antiandrogens in females

Severe Acne

- Oral isotretinoin

ROSACEA

Most commonly seen in fair-skinned individuals between the age of 30 and 50

Variants

Stage 1—erythema and telangiectases

Stage 2—papulopustular rosacea; nodules may be present if severe

Stage 3—hyperplastic and phymatous rosacea (e.g., rhinophyma)—coarse facial features plus soft tissue hyperplasia

Triggers
- Hot beverages
- Spicy foods
- Alcohol
- Sun
- Heat

Clinical Signs of Psoriasis

Koebner phenomenon: Physical trauma to the skin causes a lesion to form.

Auspitz sign: Scale removal results in the appearance of minute droplets of blood. (Note that this is not routinely tested for these days because of infectious risks.)

Treatment
- Topical metronidazole gel or cream
- Oral antibiotics (minocycline/doxycycline/tetracycline)
- Laser for telangiectasia or rhinophyma

PSORIASIS VULGARIS
- Elbows, knees, scalp, nails, intergluteal fold, soles, and feet are predilection sites. Lesions themselves consist of chronic recurrent well-demarcated red scaling papules and plaques.
- Nail changes (pitting, oil drops, onycholysis, subungual hyperkeratosis) are also commonly seen.
- It is important to note that psoriasis is associated with psoriatic arthritis in 10% to 20% of cases.

Treatment
Body Lesions
- Medium- to high-potency corticosteroid cream or ointment
- Calcipotriol ointment
- Tar
- Anthralin
- Tazarotene gel or cream
- Intralesional triamcinolone
- Phototherapy (UVB, PUVA)
- Systemic drugs (methotrexate, acitretin, cyclosporin, biologics)

Facial and Intertriginous Lesions
- Low-potency corticosteroid cream or ointment
- Tacrolimus ointment/pimecrolimus cream

Scalp Lesions
- Tar shampoo
- Topical corticosteroid lotion/solution/foam
- Calcipotriol solution
- Tazarotene gel

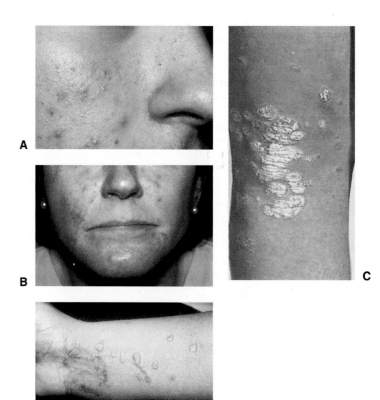

Figure 4.6 Papular skin lesions. Acne vulgaris (**A**), rosacea (**B**), psoriasis (**C**), and lichen planus (**D**). (Images A, B, D from Goodheart HP. *Goodheart's photoguide of common skin disorders*, 2nd ed. Philadelphia: Lippincott Williams & Wilkins; 2003. Image C reprinted with permission from Bickley LS. *Bate's guide to physical examination and history taking*, 8th ed. Philadelphia: Lippincott Williams & Wilkins; 2003.)

> **CLINICAL BOX**
>
> **Lichen Planus and Hepatitis**
>
> 20% of patients with lichen planus may have Hepatitis C; therefore, all patients with risk factors should undergo a hepatitis screen.

LICHEN PLANUS

Chronic pruritic purple, polygonal, planar (flat-topped) mainly seen on wrists and legs; white reticulated lesions of mucosal surfaces (lips and buccal mucosa)

Treatment
- Lichen planus is usually very difficult to treat
- Rule out a drug-induced lichenoid reaction which can be indistinguishable from idiopathic lichen planus
- Low-potency topical corticosteroids cream

PERIORAL DERMATITIS

1 to 2 mm erythematous papulopustules distributed periorally with sparing of the vermilion border; occasional periorbital distribution; may be caused by topical steroid abuse

Treatment
- Topical metronidazole
- Topical erythromycin
- Systemic antibiotics (minocycline/doxycycline/tetracycline)

SKIN TUMORS/ULCERS

> **CLINICAL BOX**
>
> **Hemangiomas**
>
> 70% of hemangiomas regress by age 7.

DEFINITION

- A tumor is a skin lesion with significant depth measuring >1 cm.
- An ulcer is an excavation extending into the dermis or deeper.

CAUSAL CONDITIONS

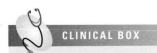

> **CLINICAL BOX**
>
> **Dimple Sign**
>
> The classic finding of a dermatofibroma.

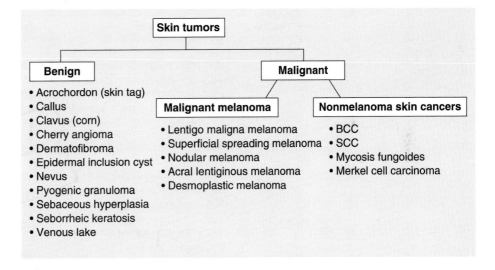

Figure 4.7 Skin tumors: causal conditions

```
                    Skin tumors
                   /           \
              Benign           Malignant
                               /        \
  • Acrochordon (skin tag)  Malignant melanoma   Nonmelanoma skin cancers
  • Callus
  • Clavus (corn)           • Lentigo maligna melanoma    • BCC
  • Cherry angioma          • Superficial spreading melanoma  • SCC
  • Dermatofibroma          • Nodular melanoma    • Mycosis fungoides
  • Epidermal inclusion cyst • Acral lentiginous melanoma  • Merkel cell carcinoma
  • Nevus                   • Desmoplastic melanoma
  • Pyogenic granuloma
  • Sebaceous hyperplasia
  • Seborrheic keratosis
  • Venous lake
```

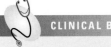

> **CLINICAL BOX**
>
> **Gardner Syndrome**
>
> A rare familial condition associated with colon cancer where multiple epidermal inclusion cysts are found.

APPROACH

BENIGN SKIN TUMORS

Nevus

Melanocytic nevi, or moles, are small pigmented macules, papules or nodules arising from the proliferation of melanocytic nevus cells.

Subtypes of Melanocytic Nevi
- Junctional nevus
- Compound nevus
- Dermal nevus
- Congenital nevus
- Dysplastic/atypical nevus
- Halo nevus
- Blue nevus

Figure 4.8 Melanocytic nevi. Compound nevus **(A)**, halo nevus **(B)**, and dysplastic/atypical nevus **(C)**. Note the raised center and indistinct border giving a "fried-egg" appearance. (Images from Goodheart HP. *Goodheart's photoguide of common skin disorders*, 2nd ed. Philadelphia: Lippincott Williams & Wilkins; 2003.)

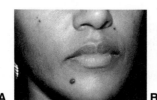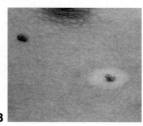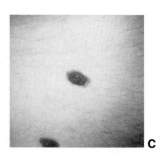

A   B   C

MALIGNANT TUMORS

Nonmelanoma Skin Cancers and Malignant Melanoma

Table **4.5**	Nonmelanoma vs. Malignant Melanoma	
	Nonmelanoma Skin Cancers	**Malignant Melanoma**
Risk factors	1. UV light exposure (especially UVB) 2. Ionizing radiation exposure (e.g., uranium miners, childhood cancer survivors) 3. Chronic immunosuppression 4. Smoking 5. Phototherapy with psoralens 6. Chronic ulcers/scars 7. Arsenic ingestion 8. Actinic keratoses	1. Skin type I/II (fair skin, red hair, blue eyes) 2. Dysplastic nevus syndrome 3. Congenital nevi 4. Multiple common or atypical nevi 5. Personal history of melanoma 6. FHx of atypical nevi or melanoma 7. Excessive sun exposure, especially sunburns during childhood 8. Immunosuppression 9. Genetic markers (CDKN2A mutation)
Metastases	BCC: extremely rare SCC: 5%–10%	Common
Clinical features	BCC: pearly papule or nodule with peripheral telangiectasias (multiple other presentations also possible) SCC: sharply demarcated scaling or hyperkeratotic papule, plaque, or nodule	**A**symmetry **B**order irregularities **C**olor variegation **D**iameter >6 mm **E**volution
Treatment	**BCC** Surgical excision Mohs' microscopic surgery Electrodessication and curettage Radiation therapy Topical imiquimod cream Topical 5-fluorouracil cream Photodynamic therapy **SCC** Surgical excision Photodynamic therapy for superficial SCCs (*in situ* only) Topical imiquimod to treat Bowen disease (SCC *in situ*) Cryotherapy or imiquimod to treat actinic keratosis (precursor to SCC)	Surgical excision • *in situ*: 0.5 cm margins • <2 mm thick: 1 cm margins • ≥2 mm thick: 2 cm margins Lymph node dissection Adjuvant therapy with interferon α-2b Palliative therapy (chemotherapy and radiation therapy)
Prevention	Sun avoidance and sun protection Avoidance or protection from carcinogenic chemicals (e.g., arsenic) Regular skin self-examination	Sun avoidance and sun protection Screening in patients with FHx, dysplastic and multiple nevi Regular skin self-examination

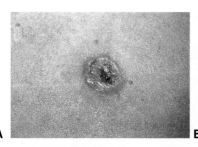
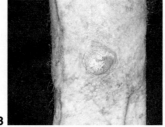
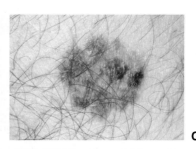

A   B   C

Figure 4.9 Malignant tumors: nodular BCC **(A)** note the pearly rolled border characteristic of BCC, SCC **(B)**, and superficial spreading melanoma **(C)**.

(Image A: Courtesy of the American Cancer Society, Inc. Atlanta, GA, Image B & C: From Goodheart HP. *Goodheart's photoguide of common skin disorders*, 2nd ed. Philadelphia: Lippincott Williams & Wilkins; 2003.)

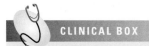

CLINICAL BOX

Side Effects of Interferon α-2b

- Myelosuppression
- Liver toxicity
- Thyroid dysfunction

Lymphoma

- Mycosis fungoides: T-cell lymphoma with primary involvement of the skin
- Mycosis fungoides presents as thin scaly red plaques that often have highly irregular shapes
- Mycosis fungoides with extensive infiltration presents as **leonine facies**

Treatment

- Topical corticosteroids
- Nitrogen Mustards
- Narrowbend UVB or PUVA
- Total body electron-beam therapy

PRURITUS

DEFINITION

- The sensation provoking a desire to scratch
- The most common symptom in dermatology
- Can be associated with primary skin disease or an underlying systemic disorder

CAUSAL CONDITIONS

ATOPIC DERMATITIS

A hypersensitivity reaction characterized by severe pruritus and dry skin; associated with a personal or FHx of atopy.

Aggravating Factors
- Inhalants (dust mites/pollens)
- Foods (controversial)
- Winter
- Wool clothing
- Emotional stress

Lesions
- Erythematous patches/papules/plaques with edema
- May be linear with scales, crusts, and excoriations from scratching or secondary infections
- Lichenification (thickening with accentuated skin markings)
- Fissures and Dennie-Morgan folds (infraorbital eyelid fold)

Stages
Infantile stage: Extensor surfaces, face, scalp

Childhood stage: Flexural surface, lichenification present

Adult stage: Hand eczema and xerosis

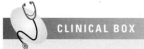

CLINICAL BOX

Type 1 Hypersensitivity

Urticaria is a type 1 (IgE mediated) hypersensitivity reaction.

Table **4.6**	**Pruritus: Causal Conditions**
With Skin Lesions	
Primary skin disease	Dermatitis herpetiformis
	Bullous pemphigoid
	Mycosis fungoides
	Psoriasis
	Lichen planus
	Mastocytosis
Parasitosis	Scabies
	Pediculosis
Allergy	Atopic dermatitis/eczema
	Urticaria
	Allergic dermatitis
Bites	Arthropods
Psychiatric	Neurotic excoriations
	Parasitophobia
Without Skin Lesions	
Drugs/food	OCP
	Steroids
	Phenytoin
Obstructive biliary disease	PBC
	Cholestasis of pregnancy
	Cholestasis from drugs
Hematologic	Polycythemia vera
	Lymphoma
Uremia	Renal failure
Malignancy	Adenocarcinomas
	SCCs
	Gastric carcinoids
Endocrine	Thyrotoxicosis
	Hypothyroidism
	Diabetes mellitus
Other	Xerosis (e.g., winter itch)

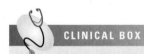

CLINICAL BOX

Pruritus and PBC

Pruritus is the presenting symptom in 50% of patients with PBC.

OBSTRUCTIVE BILIARY DISEASE

Common Causes
- PBC
- Renal disease
- Cholestasis of pregnancy
- Cholestasis from drugs

Lesions
- Excoriations from scratching; commonly starts on the palms and the soles and then becomes generalized
- Jaundice

Treatments
- Bile acid resins (cholestyramine, colestipol)
- Opioid antagonists (naloxone)

ENDOCRINE DISORDERS

Thyrotoxicosis
- Intractable itching in 4% to 11% of patients; believed to be due to increased blood flow

Hypothyroidism
- Pruritus caused by xerosis

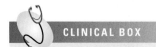

Diabetes Mellitus
- Pruritus caused by anhidrosis from diabetic neuropathy/autonomic dysfunction
- Pruritus vulvae/ani secondary to candidiasis, dermatophyte, and bacterial infections

APPROACH

HISTORY, PHYSICAL EXAM, AND INVESTIGATIONS
- Identify underlying dermatosis or systemic disease

INVESTIGATIONS
For generalized pruritus without primary skin lesions

- CBC and differential
- LFTs: Bilirubin, transaminases and alkaline phosphatase
- Renal function tests: BUN, creatinine, urinalysis
- Thyroid function test: TSH
- Fasting blood sugar
- Stool and serology for parasites
- Others: Chest x-ray

MANAGEMENT
- Avoidance of scratching to break the itch-scratch cycle
- Avoid using excessively hot water for showers/baths
- Use of appropriate topical +/− systemic +/− other therapies
- Treat underlying disorder

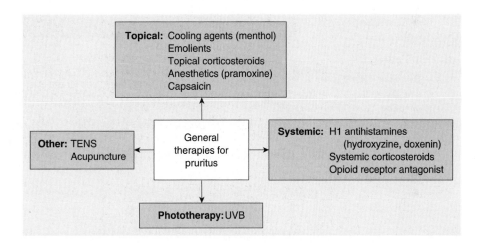

Figure 4.10 Therapies for pruritus.

URTICARIA/ANAPHYLAXIS

DEFINITION

Acute urticaria = urticaria where recurrence lasts <6 wk
Chronic urticaria = urticaria with recurrence lasting >6 wk

CAUSAL CONDITIONS

APPROACH

HISTORY AND PHYSICAL EXAMINATION

Table **4.7**	Urticaria: Causal Conditions					
Urticaria						
IgE-Dependent	**Direct Mast Cell Release**	**Complement Mediated**	**Arachidonic Acid Metabolism**	**Physical**	**Other**	
Drugs (antibiotics, e.g., penicillin; hormones, e.g., insulin; local anaesthetics)	Opiates Muscle relaxants Radio-contrast agents	Serum sickness Transfusion reactions Infections Urticarial vasculitis	ASA NSAIDs	Dermatographism Cold Cholinergic Solar Delayed pressure	Mastocytosis	
Physical contact (animal saliva, plant resins, latex, metals, lotions, soap)						
Insect sting (bees, wasps, hornets)						
Aeroallergens (plant resins, animal dander, essential oils)						
Food/additives (chocolate, shellfish, nuts, yeast)						
Parasitic infections (ascaris, strongyloides, filarial, schistosomal)						

CLINICAL BOX

Urticaria: Pediatrics

More than 80% of urticaria seen in the pediatric population is caused by **infection**.

CLINICAL BOX

Type 1-4 Hypersensitivity Reactions

Type I: Immediate hypersensitivity (IgE mediated), for example, urticaria

Type II: Cytotoxic reactions (IgG and IgM mediated), for example, Goodpasture syndrome

Type III: Immune complex reactions (soluble immune complex and complement mediated), for example, serum sickness

Type IV: Delayed-type reactions (lymphocyte mediated), for example, contact sensitivity

Serum Sickness

A reaction to IVIG or antibiotics occurring 5 to 21 days after the exposure

Minor form presents with
1. Fever
2. Urticaria
3. Arthralgia

Major form = Minor form criteria plus
4. Angioedema
5. Arthritis
6. Lymphadenopathy

Mastocytosis

Caused by an abnormal accumulation of mast cells in the skin and at different systemic sites that release histamine following exposure to various drugs.

Presentation

- Brown macules and papules that urticate when stroked

MANAGEMENT

- Avoidance of triggers (alcohol, anesthetic muscle relaxants, opioids)
- Antihistamine use
  - First generation → hydroxyzine, diphenhydramine
  - Second generation → loratadine, fexofenadine

CLINICAL BOX

Antihistamines

First-generation antihistamines are the most potent and have the quickest onset of action.

Second-generation antihistamines are nonsedating and longer acting.

ANGIOEDEMA

CLINICAL BOX

Angioedema and Urticaria

Angioedema may occur in approximately half of those affected by urticaria.

Angioedema by itself may be related to the use of ACEIs.

DEFINITION

Angioedema may affect the tongue, larynx, and pharynx, thereby causing significant mortality by airway obstruction.

APPROACH

Treatment of anaphylaxis/angioedema involving tongue/larynx/pharynx

1. Secure the ABCs
2. IM epinephrine (1:1000) 0.3 to 0.5 mL
3. Administration of systemic corticosteroids and β-agonists

HAIR DISORDERS

CLINICAL BOX

Hair Changes

Hair changes can provide clues to an underlying disease process.

DEFINITION

Alopecia: Hair loss
Cicatricial alopecia: Hair loss associated with fibrosis and scar tissue (scarring alopecia)

CAUSAL CONDITIONS

Table 4.8 Alopecia Causal Conditions

Cicatricial alopecia		Noncicatricial alopecia	
Infection	Severe folliculitis Dissecting cellulitis	Infection	Tinea capitis Secondary syphilis
Skin conditions	Bullous diseases Lichen planopilaris Discoid lupus erythematosus	Autoimmune conditions	Alopecia areata Alopecia totalis Alopecia universalis
Chemical alopecia	Hair dyes Hair relaxers	Stressors	Telogen effluvium Anagen effluvium Traumatic alopecia Trichotillomania
Tumors	Primary tumor of the scalp Metastatic tumor to the scalp	Hormonal/genetic	Androgenetic alopecia

CLINICAL BOX

Depigmentation

Depigmentation of the hair shaft can be caused by protein or copper deficiency.

CLINICAL BOX

Androgenetic Alopecia

Most common cause of noncicatricial alopecia in both men and women

CLINICAL BOX

Exclamation Point Hairs

Short, broken-off hairs known as **exclamation point hairs** are a hallmark feature of alopecia areata.

APPROACH

INVESTIGATIONS

Baseline

- CBC
- Ferritin
- TSH
- Microscopic examination and fungal culture, if fungus suspected

Other

- Scalp biopsy
- ANA
- Androgens

MANAGEMENT

Androgenetic Alopecia (Pattern Hair Loss)

Cause

The action of androgens on scalp hair follicles and genetic predisposition

Treatment

Topical minoxidil (men and women)

Oral finasteride (men only)

Hairpieces

Hair transplantation

Telogen Effluvium

Cause

Increased daily hair loss triggered by any physical or mental stressor to the body (e.g., illness, childbirth, medications)

Treatment

Full regrowth expected with no treatment

Alopecia Areata

Cause

An autoimmune disease causing localized round or oval patches of hair loss; when all scalp hair is lost it is called **alopecia totalis** and when all body hair is lost the term **alopecia universalis** is used.

Treatment

Steroids (topical/intralesional/systemic)

Minoxidil

Topical anthralin

Topical contact sensitizers

NAIL DISORDERS

DEFINITION

Onycholysis: Separation of the nail plate from the nail bed

Onychogryphosis: Severe thickening of the nail plate with deformed shape

Onychomycosis: Chronic fungal infection where the nail plate becomes friable; onycholysis and subungual hyperkeratosis will be present

CAUSAL CONDITIONS

Table **4.9**	**Causal Conditions of Nail Disorders**

Shape Change	
Description	**Causal Conditions**
Hourglass nail/finger clubbing	CVD
	Lung disease
	GI disorders
	Chronic methemoglobinemia
Hollow/spoon-shaped/koilonychia	Iron deficiency
	Malnutrition
	Diabetes
	Old age
Hypoplastic	Fetal alcohol syndrome
	Nail-patella syndrome
Onycholysis	Psoriasis
	Thyroid disease
	Trauma
	Fungal infections
Onychogryphosis	Chronic inflammation
	Tinea
	Psoriasis
Onychomycosis	Fungal infection
	T. rubrum
	T. mentagrophytes

Surface Change	
Description	**Causal Condition**
Transverse grooves/Beau's lines	Serious acute systemic disease
Transverse white lines/transverse leukonychia	Hypoalbuminemia
	Chemotherapeutic agents
	Poisons
Pitting	Psoriasis
	Alopecia areata
	Eczema
	Paronychia
	Inflammatory damage

Color Change				
Yellow	**Black**	**Brown**	**Splinter Hemorrhages**	**Blue-Green**
1. Tinea	1. Hematoma	1. Nicotine	1. Trauma (most common)	1. Pseudomonas
2. Jaundice	2. Melanoma	2. Psoriasis	2. Bacterial endocarditis	2. Drug-induced (e.g., AZT)
3. Tetracycline		3. Poisons (e.g., excessive fluoride ingestion)	3. Blood dyscrasias	
4. Hypoplasia/dysplasia of lymphatics		4. Melanonychia striata		
		5. Melanoma		

APPROACH

PARONYCHIA

Red, painful lesion around the nail fold

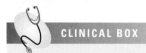

CLINICAL BOX

Subungual Hematoma vs. Melanoma

Only a biopsy can give a definitive diagnosis

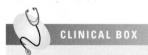

CLINICAL BOX

Herpetic Whitlow

Commonly seen in health care professionals before the institution of Universal Precautions.

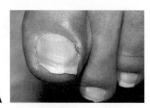

A

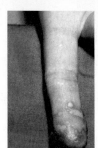

B

Figure 4.11 Local nail problems. Acute paronychia **(A)** and herpetic whitlow **(B)**.

(From Goodheart HP. *Goodheart's photoguide of common skin disorders*, 2nd ed. Philadelphia: Lippincott Williams & Wilkins; 2003.)

Cause

Most commonly a *S. aureus* infection if acute; when seen in thumb suckers/nail biters/nail pickers and those who do a lot of "wet" work it is generally chronic and associated with *C. albicans*

Treatment

Glucocorticoids

Minimize irritants and water exposure

Treat the secondary infection

HERPETIC WHITLOW

Painful grouped vesicles on an erythematous base located on the distal finger

Cause

Infection with HSV

Treatment

Self-limiting disease

Antiviral (e.g., acyclovir) may be beneficial

ONYCHOCRYPTOSIS/INGROWN NAILS

Inflammation and soft tissue hypertrophy $+/-$ secondary infection occurring when the lateral edge of the nail plate impinges on the nail fold

Cause

Onychomycosis

Incorrect technique of nail cutting

Repetitive trauma

Poor foot hygiene; poorly fitting shoes

Treatment

Barrier placement between nail plate and nail fold

Excision of the portion of nail plate pressing on the nail fold

$+/-$ Antibiotics

CHAPTER 5

Emergency Medicine

Meghan Brison, Julian J. Owen, Dr. John Crossley,
and Dr. Christopher Hall

ANAPHYLAXIS

CLINICAL BOX

Anaphylaxis Statistics

- 50 fatalities per year in Canada
- True incidence is unknown due to under-reporting and differences in defining "anaphylaxis"

ASC Box

Cytokines Contributing to the Late-Phase Response

IL-4—↑ IgE secretion

IL-5—recruitment and activation of leukocytes

TNF-α—contributes to systemic anaphylactic shock

RATIONALE

- Anaphylaxis is a rapidly progressive, life-threatening allergic reaction.
- In children, foods are the most common allergens.
- Anaphylaxis is a clinical Dx based on Hx and P/E.
- Patient Tx demands rapid recognition of the condition, aggressive airway and CV support, and prompt administration of meds.

APPLIED SCIENTIFIC CONCEPTS

- There is a spectrum to allergic/hypersensitivity reactions with local dermatologic manifestations at one end and anaphylactic shock at the other.
- Anaphylaxis is an IgE-mediated, immediate onset, hypersensitivity reaction to a protein Ag. It requires a prior "sensitizing" exposure to the Ag.
- Anaphylactoid reactions are clinically identical to anaphylaxis but are not IgE mediated. Reactions can occur upon initial exposure to the Ag. (see Fig. 5.1)

CAUSAL CONDITIONS

Table 5.1	Common Anaphylaxis-Inducing Ags
Foods	Peanuts/nuts, seafood, eggs, cow's milk
Hymenoptera envenomation	Bees, wasps, fire ants
Drugs/therapeutic agents	β-Lactam Abx, NSAIDs, antineoplastic meds, ACEIs, vaccines, local anesthetics
Human products	Blood products, insulin
Iatrogenic	**Latex, radiocontrast material**

CLINICAL BOX

Anaphylaxis Differential Dx

- Other types of shock: hypovolemic, septic, cardiogenic
- Other causes of acute Resp failure: asthma, PE, epiglottitis
- Flush syndromes: carcinoid, menopausal Sx, pheochromocytoma
- "Restaurant" syndromes: MSG or sulfite sensitivity
- Excess endogenous production of histamine
- Nonorganic disease: panic attack, Münchhausen
- Other: vasovagal syncope, hereditary angioedema, ACEI angioedema

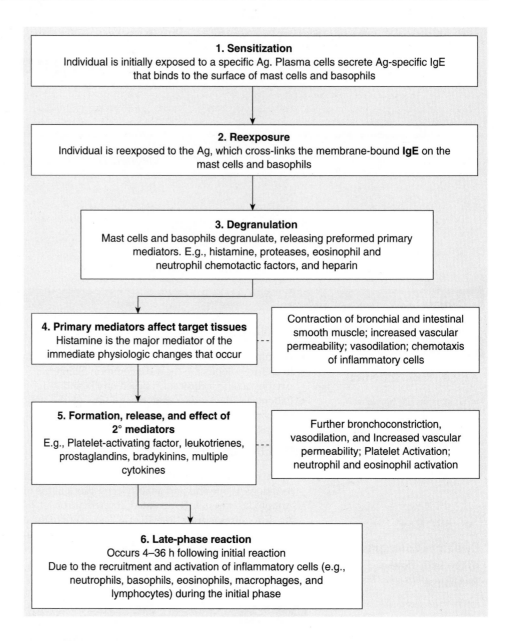

Figure 5.1 Anaphylaxis: cellular mechanisms, immune mediators, and physiologic Δs.

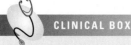

Types of Anaphylaxis

Biphasic Anaphylaxis
Recurrence of Sx 4 to 32 h (mean 10 h) after the initial episode. Occurs in up to 20% of patients and is due to the release of 2° mediators and the late-phase response.

Protracted Anaphylaxis
Refractory Resp distress or hypotension despite appropriate medical Rx.

APPROACH/KEY OBJECTIVES

- Anaphylactic shock is a form of distributive shock, and therefore requires aggressive fluid resuscitation to prevent CV collapse.
- Patients may initially present with mild Sx but will rapidly deteriorate without medical Rx.
- Most patients will present with Sx within 1 h of exposure to the offending Ag. However, some people may have a delayed response or will present hours later with a biphasic anaphylactic response.
- Anaphylaxis is a clinical Dx and there are no diagnostic tests of value in the emergent setting. Classically, anaphylaxis is evidence of allergic reaction with either hypotension and/or Resp distress.

PERTINENT HX

Diagnostic Predictors

- Known allergies and previous Hx of anaphylactic reactions
- Hx of asthma or other atopic conditions (e.g., eczema)
- Recent/current exposure to any suspected causative Ags

Table **5.2**	**Common Presenting Signs and Sx in Anaphylaxis**
CNS	Anxiety, headache, ↓ level of consciousness
Resp	Oropharyngeal swelling, chest tightness, dyspnea, wheezing, stridor, inability to speak, hypoxia, apnea
CV	Hypotension, palpitations, weak/absent pulses, tachycardia, cardiac arrest
GI	Dysphagia, abdominal pain or cramping, nausea, vomiting, diarrhea
Dermatologic	Pruritus, rash, urticaria, angioedema

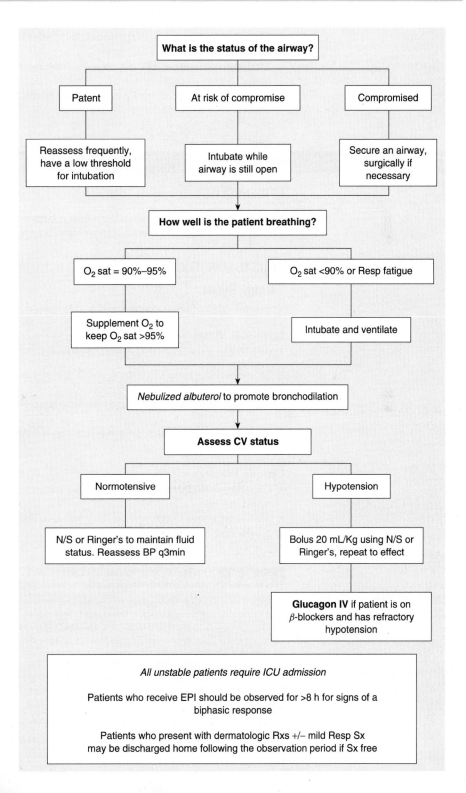

Figure 5.2 Acute Tx of anaphylaxis.

CLINICAL BOX

What Saves Lives? EPI, EPI, EPI

Adults: 0.3 to 0.5 mg IM

Children: 0.01 mg/kg IM

IV EPI: 0.1 mg, dilute 0.1 mL
1:1,000 in 10 mL N/S

Give 1 to 2 mL/min

Prognostic Predictors
- Prehospital use of EPI, antihistamines, or steroids following exposure
- Current meds—β-blockers and antihypertensives will blunt the effect of EPI and other resuscitative meds
- Chronic CV or pulmonary disease—such patients may deteriorate much more rapidly than others

   All patients presenting with signs or Sx of anaphylaxis get:

- Measures to stop any continuing Ag exposure
- Two large bore IVs
- Supplemental O_2
- Cardiac and O_2 sat monitoring
- **EPI IM or IV**—to ↓ vascular permeability, relax bronchial smooth muscle, and ↑ cardiac and peripheral vascular resistance
- **Methylprednisolone 125 mg IV**—to limit the production of leukotrienes in the late phase
- **Diphenhydramine 50 mg IV + ranitidine 50 mg IV**—to block the action of histamine at the H1 and H2 receptors

BURNS

EPIDEMIOLOGY

- Burns are common and range from minor cutaneous lesions to life-threatening injuries.
- They are a significant source of morbidity in survivors.

CAUSAL CONDITIONS

THERMAL BURNS

Types: fire (flash, flame), contact, and scalds (grease, steam, liquids spill, liquids immersion)

ELECTRICAL BURNS

Types: low voltage, high voltage, and lightning

- DC—short duration of contact, but ↑ risk of trauma because victim often thrown from source
- AC—exposure can be prolonged because source repetitively stimulates muscle contraction
- First-, second-, and third-degree burns result from interaction of current with resistance of tissues

Unique Features
- Cardiac—arrhythmia occurs in 15% of injuries, rhythms are usually benign, but can result in Vfib
- MSK—because of high resistance of muscle/ligament/bone, greatest amount of injury results here. Compartment syndromes may result +/− rhabdomyolysis

Table **5.3**	**Unique Features of Electrical Burns**
Cardiac	Arrhythmia occurs in 15% of injuries, rhythms are usually benign, but can result in Vfib
MSK	High resistance of muscle/ligament/bone; therefore, greatest injury results here. Compartment syndromes may result +/− rhabdomyolysis
Renal	High concentration of CK combined with fluid losses may result in ATN. Tx involves ++ fluid administration +/− urine alkalinization
CNS	LOC, paralysis, Resp depression, amnesia can be transient effects
Eye	May result in keraunoparalysis and fixed, dilated pupils Other eye injuries such as cataracts are frequent after lightning injury

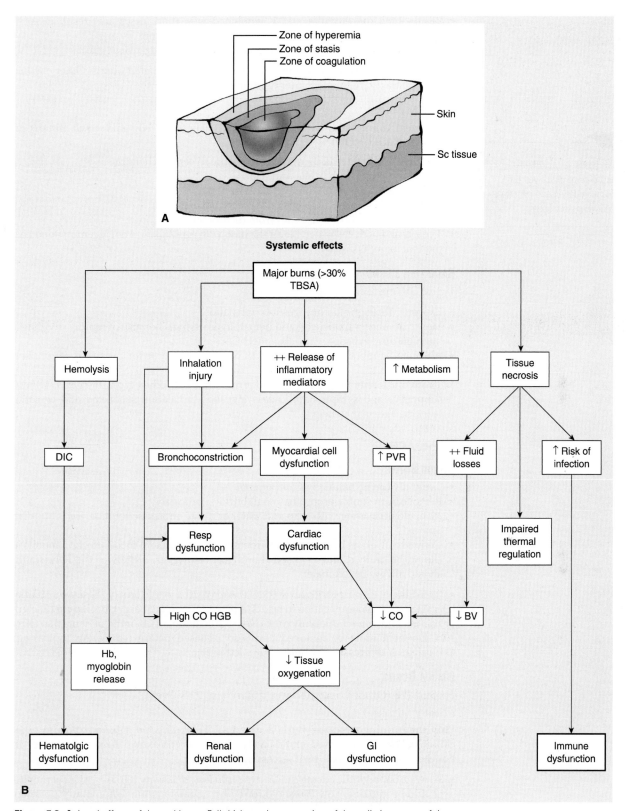

Figure 5.3 A: Local effects of thermal burns. Full thickness burns consists of three distinct zones of tissue.

Zone of coagulation: white, charred central portion. Consists of necrotic tissue.

Zone of stasis: red, may blanch with pressure initially, but fragile blood supply gives way to AVN.

Zone of hyperemia: red, blanches with pressure and has intact blood supply. Healing takes place in first wk.

Image excerpted from the Smeltzer et al., *Brunner and Suddarth's Textbook of Medical-Surgical Nursing*, 9th ed., Philadelphia: Lippincott Williams & Wilkins, 2000.

B: Systemic effects of thermal burns.

Image modified from the Smeltzer et al., *Brunner and Suddarth's Textbook of Medical-Surgical Nursing*, 9th ed., Philadelphia: Lippincott Williams & Wilkins, 2000.

- Renal—high concentration of CK combined with fluid losses may result in ATN. Tx involves ++ fluid administration +/− urine alkalinization
- CNS—LOC, paralysis, Resp depression, amnesia can be transient effects

Lightning may result in keraunoparalysis and fixed, dilated pupils. Other eye injuries such as cataracts are frequent after lightning injury.

CHEMICAL BURNS

Alkali burns ≫ acid burns because alkali dissolves protein and collagen and penetrates deeper than acid burns

Types: acid (nitric acid, sulfuric acid, HCl, oxalic acid, HF) and alkali (lime/cement, ammonia, NaOH, KOH)

- Systemic effects have occurred with exposure to certain chemicals:
  1. Hypocalcemia with oxalic acid, HF
  2. Nephrotoxicity with tannic acid, phosphorus
  3. CNS depression + hypotension with phenol exposure
  4. Liver failure, ATN, and death from dichromate poisoning
- Tx early and with ++ water. Neutralization with acid/alkali is not recommended because thermal injury is greater.

RADIATION BURNS

Types: UV, medical/therapeutic

- Exposure through skin or ingestion/inhalation
- Most common Sx involve GI and hematologic systems because of rapidly dividing cells, but high-dose exposure may also affect CNS
- Absolute lymphocyte count within 48 h is best indicator for prognosis of whole body exposure
- Tx involves removing clothing and irrigation as in other types of burns. Otherwise, supportive and symptomatic unless ingestion/inhalation suspected and chelating or blocking agents may help

APPROACH

MINOR BURNS

- Generally can be handled as outpatients
- Remove burn source promptly to halt burning process
- Meticulous cleaning with soap and water or dilute antiseptic solution. Td immunization prn
- Controversy exists over blister debridement, but in general those affecting mobile joints should be drained and cleansed thoroughly. However, blisters of the hands and feet should always be left intact.

Traditional empiric Rx involves Rx with topical Abx in the form of 1% silver **sulfadiazine** (Dermazine) (avoid application to face or if patient has sulfa allergy), **bacitracin** (Baciguent), or **bacitracin/neomycin/polymyxin B** (Neosporin ointment). Remind patients that all excess Abx ointment must be removed and skin cleansed before reapplying topical agents. Occlusive, clean dressings should be applied regularly.

MAJOR BURNS

Hx and P/E (Often Combined as Primary and 2° Survey)

Primary Survey

Stop the burning process—Burn degree and TBSA affected ↑ with exposure time. All clothing should be removed immediately. Rinse burn areas with large amounts of water. For chemical burns, brush away excess before rinsing.

- **Airway:** Supraglottic edema can lead to rapid loss of airway. 100% O_2 + O_2 sat monitoring should be initiated. Low threshold for ETT if stigmata of inhalation injury present (side panel).
- **Breathing:** Bronchoconstriction and inhalation injury are managed with PP ventilation to overcome ↑ stiffness. Tx of coexistent CO or cyanide toxicity must be considered.
- **Circulation:** 2x large bore IVs, inserted in unburned skin (preferably U/E) for rapid volume expansion. Estimate using Parkland for first 24 h (see clinical box Parkland Formula).

Inhalation Injury Rx

- 100% O_2 to ↓ half-life of CO Hgb in blood
- Consider use of hyperbaric O_2 and/or oscillator ventilator

Signs of Inhalation Injury

- Hx of enclosed fire/flame injury
- Burns to neck or face
- Singed eyebrows and nasal vibrissae
- Stridor, inspiratory grunting
- Hoarseness, difficulty speaking
- Cough, soot-tinged sputum

- ↓ LOC
- High RR, low Po_2 saturation, accessory muscle use
- Crackles, wheezes, rhonchi on auscultation
- Circumferential burn to chest
- Cardiac instability +/− ischemia

Secondary Survey: "**ABCDEFGHI**"

Caution: list given below is not the order in which resuscitation efforts are performed

- **A**nalgesia—++ high-dose narcotics, titrated for extreme agitation and pain
- **B**urn depth/TBSA area/body weight—depth and TBSA are needed for calculation of approximate fluid requirements (Fig. 5.4 and Table 5.3)
- **C**atheter (urinary)—most reliable and least invasive method for assessing appropriate fluid resuscitation
- **D**ressings and wound care—initially, clean all burn areas with water and cover with clean dressings. Avoid applying wet dressings to a patient with extensive burns because of the risk of hypothermia. Prophylactic Abx are not indicated, but topical agents may be used such as **bacitracin** (Baciguent) or **silver sulfadiazine** (Dermazine)
- **E**scharotomy—may need to incise burn tissue (eschar) for circumferential burns causing distal ischemia. Consider use of Doppler U/S to assess peripheral pulses
- **F**luids/fasciotomy—Parkland used to estimate fluid requirements. Fasciotomy may be needed for compartment syndromes (usually the result of electrical burns)
- **G**astric tube—burns >20% TBSA often have an ileus that may last 4 to 5 days postinjury. NG/NJ tubes indicated for administration of drugs and maintaining nutritional status (major burns = ↑↑ metabolic rate and ↑ need for supplements)
- **H**istory—salient PMHx including comorbidities, allergies. Consider abuse paediatric population if Hx or pattern of injury is suggestive
- **I**mmunization (Td)—prn

Lab Investigations
- CBC, Lytes, BUN, Cr, gluc., INR, PTT
- ABG, CO-Hgb (if suspect CO poisoning)
- ECG, CK-MB, CK, and MB (if suspect electrical injury). U/A with urine MB prn
- T&X if anticipating early debridement
- β-HCG if fertile female

Imaging
- CXR +/− bronchoscopy (if suspect inhalation injury)
- CT of the head used liberally if altered LOC

Neglect/Abuse in Pediatric Patients

Burns are frequently a sign of caregiver abuse in children. Often the pattern and Hx may suggest abuse:
- Burns to the back of hands/feet, buttocks, perineum, and legs
- Burns with a well-demarcated edge may represent an immersion-type burn
- Other signs of abuse including old and new fractures, bruises, cigarette burns

Parkland Formula

Fluid required (ml of RL) = 4 × kg body wt × TBSA

- ½ given in first 8 h from time of injury, ½ given in next 16 h
- TBSA used is for second- and third-degree burns only. Electrical, fourth-degree burns require greater amounts
- Parkland formula only provides estimate of total fluid needs. Most accurate measurement of adequate fluid resuscitation is a return of normal U/O: 0.5 mL/kg in adult, 1.0 mL/kg in child, and up to 2.0 mL/kg in infants

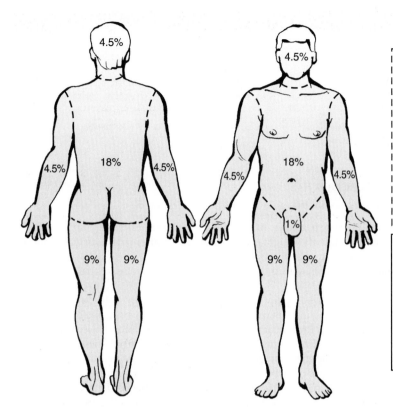

Estimating TBSA

- "Rule of 9's" commonly used. Body surfaces are broken into multiples of 9 (see diagram)
- Patient's hand approximates 1% of TBSA
- Rule of thumb: contribution of head in children > adults and contribution of legs in children < adults

Head
18% (infants) ⟶ 14% (child) ⟶ 9% (adult)

Each leg
14% (infant) ⟶ 16% (child) ⟶ 18% (adult)

Patients requiring specialized care

- Second and third degree burns > 10% BSA
- Second and third degree burns on face, hands, and perineum
- Circumferential or splash burns
- Electrical burns (including lightning)
- Chemical burns;
- Pediatric burns suspicious for neglect or abuse

Figure 5.4 Estimating TBSA. Image excerpted from the *Emergency Series*.

Table **5.4**	**Estimating Burn Depth**			
	First Degree (Superficial)	**Second Degree (Superficial or Deep Partial)**	**Third Degree**	**Fourth Degree**
Appearance	Red	Red or blanched white, fluid-filled blisters	White, leathery, or black and charred	Similar to third degree
Layers involved	Epidermis	Epidermis, superficial (papillary) dermis +/− deep (reticular) dermis	Epidermis, both layers of dermis	Epidermis, dermis, and subcutaneous tissue including fascia, muscle, bone
Sensory	Very painful, tender to touch; two-point discrimination intact	Very painful, tender to touch; two-point discrimination intact or diminished	Numb, two-point discrimination lost	Numb, two-point discrimination lost
Healing	Complete, within several days	Usually without scarring, within 2 wk, or may see hypertrophic scar formation, contracture across joints	Skin grafting necessary	Extensive debridement, reconstruction of specialized tissues, and skin grafting necessary

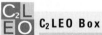 **C₂LEO Box**

In patients with serious burns, determination of capacity is often difficult. In such cases, obtaining consent from SDMs is undertaken after the patient is initially stabilized. Physicians have a duty to provide necessary emergency care even when consent cannot be obtained.

Communicate realistic prognosis to serious burn victims or their SDMs. In situations where mortality approaches 100%, continuing care should be a decision made by SDMs or in consultation with hospital ethics boards.

POISONING

EPIDEMIOLOGY

- 5% to 10% of ED visits
- >5% ICU admissions
- >50% are younger than 6 yr (typically unintentional in pediatric population)

CAUSAL CONDITIONS

Table **5.5**	**Typical Poisons**		
Common Agents			
Household products (30%)	Cleaning substances (detergents, soaps, and shampoos) Cough and cold remedies Cosmetics Plants and other environmental substances		
Metals		Iron, lead	
Potentially Lethal			
Drugs Causing Excitation States		**Drugs Causing Depressive States**	
Anticholinergic	Antihistamines, TCAs, phenothiazines, atropine	Cholinergic	Insecticides, nerve agents, nicotine, pilocarpine, urecholine
Sympathomimetic	Cocaine, amphetamines, MDMA (ecstasy), ephedrine, theophylline	Opiate/sedative	Heroin, morphine, benzodiazepines, barbiturates, meprobamate, EtOH
Hallucinogens	LSD, mescaline, phencyclidine, psilocybin	CVS	β-Blockers, CCBs
Serotonin	MAOI, SSRI, meperidine, TCA, L-tryptophan	Cellular	CO, H_2S, cyanide
TCAs	Amitriptyline, doxepin	Simple asphyxiants	CO_2, inert gases
Drugs inducing metabolic acidosis (BP usually low)	Ethanol, methanol, ethylene glycol, ASA, NSAID, tylenol		

APPROACH TO THE POISONED PATIENT

Hx

- Notoriously unreliable; obtain collateral from witnesses, family members, police/EMS for completion
- Questions to ask:
  1. What was taken? How much? By what route? Time since exposure? Coingestions?
  2. Details about the environment the patient was found in (presence of pill bottles, suicide note, smells/odours, needles)
  3. Intentional versus accidental, previous suicidal attempts
- Other things to consider:
  1. How caustic is the agent?
  2. How potentially severe is the exposure?
  3. Is this patient a "toxic time bomb"? (Consider delayed presentations of toxicity)
- Standard PMHx, particularly comorbid conditions, psychiatric conditions, meds taken (and what patient has access to) and allergies, because all these may influence resuscitation efforts

P/E

- Attention to ABCs crucial
- Vital signs = **Most important** in the toxic patient. Look for Δs in HR, BP, RR, O₂ sat, temperature, and CBS
- Focus on CVS, Resp, and CNS exams

Table **5.6**   **Common Toxidromes**

	Toxidrome	Vital Signs	Appearance	Pupils	Mental Status	Other
Excitation states	Anticholinergic "hot as a hare, dry as a bone, red as a beet, blind as a bat, and mad as a hatter"	• ↑ Temperature • Possible ↑ HR	• Dry mucous membranes • Erythematous	• Mydriasis	• Disoriented, agitated • Reaching blindly for objects • Large ODs can lead to depressive state (sedation, coma)	• ↓ bs and ↓ GI motility • Urinary retention
	Sympathomimetic "fight or flight"	• ↑ HR • ↑ BP • ↑ Temperature	• Wet mucous membranes • Diaphoretic • Erythematous • ↑ Psychomotor activity	• Mydriasis	• Agitated, "reved up"	
	Serotonin "wet dog shakes"	• ↑ Temperature	• Whole body tremor • May be diaphoretic; shivering; fever; diarrhea	• Not characteristic	• Altered or normal mental status	• ↑ Reflexes • ↑ Tone
Depressive states	Cholinergic "secreting from every orifice"/ "wet from head to toe"	• ↓ HR • May see ↓ BP • May see ↓ RR and Resp failure	• Diaphoretic • Lacrimation • Salivation • Fasciculations	• Miosis common, may see mydriasis	• Altered or normal mental status	• Nausea + vomiting • Defecation • Urination • Bronchorrhea
	Opiod or sedative/hyponotics "depressed all over"	• ↓ RR • ↓ HR • ↓ BP • ↓ Temperature	• Range from stuporous/drunk to coma	• Miosis, possible nystagmus	• ↓ LOC	

Osm can be calculated by FPD or BPE. It is imperative that FPD be used if you suspect EtOH ingestion—there will be a false negative for OG because these substances will boil away

CLINICAL BOX

OG and AG

OG

Serum Osm = calculated by lab by FPD

Calculated Osm = (2 × Na) +BUN + gluc.

N = 280 to 290 mOsM per L

OG = calculated − actual Osm

N is < 10 mOsM per L

AG

AG = Na − (Cl + HCO₃)

Normal is 8 to 12, some centers use 10 to 14

• Check for breath odours, which may point to small list of poisons
• Putting it all together: Does the P/E fit any of the common toxidromes?

LABWORK/INVESTIGATIONS

• Routine: CBC, Lytes, gluc., ASA + acetaminophen + EtOH levels, blood gas, serum Osm (see subsequent text), ECG
• Additional tests to consider: INR/PT, LFTs, RFTs, specific drug levels, β-HCG if fertile female, urine tox screen (often unhelpful from a Tx perspective, but can identify other drug exposures)

OG

• With acute ingestions, presence of unmeasured osmoles may indicate a potentially lethal OD.
• Common causes of elevated OG = EtOH ingestions (isopropyl alcohol, ethylene glycol, methanol, ethanol) and others such as alcoholic ketoacidosis and lactic acidosis.
• Life-threatening ODs can be seen without a change in the OG. Results must be interpreted with caution and within the clinical picture.

AG

• Typical trend is to see ↑ OG initially with the ingestion of EtOHs, followed by ↑ AG as the EtOHs are metabolized and result in a metabolic acidosis.
• If specific drug levels have been obtained, it is important to match the amount of drug in the blood with the elevation in OG.

Imaging

• Consider AXR (indications = "**CHIPES**")
• Consider CXR on an individual basis

Table **5.7**	Interpretation of the AG		
Elevated AG Acidosis "MUDPILES"		**Normal AG Acidosis "HYPERCHLOREMIC"**	**Narrow AG "HARDUPS"**
Methanol **U**remia **D**iabetic ketoacidosis/alcoholic ketoacidosis **P**araldehyde **I**soniazid, iron **L**actate **E**thylene glycol **S**alicylates		Usually due to ++ saline administration because of high Cl content	**H**yperventilation **A**cetazolamide, acids, Addison disease **R**enal tubular acidosis **D**iarrhea **U**reterosigmoidostomy **P**ancreatic fistula **S**aline

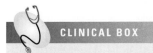

CLINICAL BOX

"CHIPES"

Calcium, **Ch**loral hydrate, **CC**l4

Heavy metals

Iron

Potassium

Enteric-coated

Salicylates

Tx

Supportive Care

- Attention to ABCs crucial: all potentially toxic patients should receive cardiac monitoring + oximetry. IV access should be established
- Frequent reassessments for clinical improvement or deterioration
- +/− repeat bloodwork

Gastric Decontamination

General principle: ↓ absorption or ↑ excretion of ingested poisons. Generally only effective if time since exposure ≤2 h or if delayed toxicity expected. There is limited data to support most methods of gastric decontamination. AC may have some benefit in specific instances (see Table 5.8).

Enhanced Elimination

HD or hemoperfusion as well as alkalinization of urine or diuresis are used to enhance elimination.

Specific Antidotes (if Available)

- Poison control is helpful in virtually all toxic exposures
- Form 1—indicated if intentional ingestion suggested by Hx

Table **5.8**	Methods of Gastric Decontamination	
Method	**Principle**	**Indications/CIs**
SOI	Induced vomiting to prevent gastric absorption	Must avoid if drug is caustic; no longer used in ED setting, but may still have some application in prehospital pediatric OD
OGL	Large OG tube is flushed with N/S or water followed by aspiration of the fluid + tox/pills to ↓ gastric absorption	May be considered if bezoar in stomach or delayed absorption of substance + threat of severe toxicity
NA	Aspiration of stomach contents through NG to ↓ gastric absorption	NG not large enough to remove pills or pill fragments
WBI	PEG solution used to flush bowel to ↓ absorption/↑ excretion	Patient must be conscious and cooperative for procedure; contraindicated if suspect significant ileus or high risk of perforation
AC or MDAC	Charcoal binds to drug and prevents systemic absorption	Not useful for EtOHs, caustics, most metals; patient must be able to protect airway or there is a risk for aspiration and ↑ morbidity
Cathartics	↓ Bowel transit time to ↑ excretion	Not indicated in ED

COMMON TOXICOLOGY PROBLEMS

Table **5.9**	Rx of Common Ingestants		
	Pathophysiology	**Clinical Presentation and Diagnostics**	**Rx**
Methanol	Metabolism to formic acid and elimination of folate stores leads to toxicity. Metabolism occurs by EtOH dehydrogenase in the liver	• Delayed presentation common (can be 6–24 h); EtOH ingestion delays presentation further • OG, AG may be normal or elevated • ↓ LOC, ataxia, stupor, lethargy, coma • Visual complaints common: blurry vision, ↓ acuity, "snowstorm" perception • CNS effects: ↓ LOC, Parkinsonism in late stages	• EtOH has greater affinity for EtOH dehydrogenase and saturates it, preventing breakdown of methanol into its toxic metabolites • Fomepizole has even greater affinity and less S/Es than EtOH • $NaHCO_3$ used for acidemia • HD for severe toxic ingestions; must ↑ EtOH or fomepizole if used • Consider folate supplementation
Salicylates	• Early: Resp alkalosis due to stimulation of CNS chemoreceptors • Late: metabolic acidosis • Severe toxic dose >300 mg/kg, toxic dose considered to be >150 mg/kg	• Symptom onset 3–8 h after ingestion • Dehydration common • Adults: mixed acid–base with Resp alkalosis and metabolic acidosis • Children: metabolic acidosis only; indistinguishable from Reye syndrome • Salicylate levels helpful to determine severity	• WBI or AC for large ingestions; AC may be helpful >2 h after ("It's never to late to aspirate with salicylate") • ++ Fluids +/− dextrose +/− K • $NaHCO_3$ to ↓ tissue distribution and ↑ urine elimination • HD for severe toxic ingestions
Acetaminophen	• Metabolized almost exclusively in the liver; 5% forms toxic metabolite • Toxic metabolite is conjugated by glutathione and excreted; in OD glutathione stores are depleted and hepatocytes are susceptible to the effects of the toxic metabolite, leading to a picture of hepatotoxicity • Toxic dose reported as 150 mg/kg or >7.5 g ingested	• Initial Sx of anorexia, nausea +/− vomiting, and diaphoresis subside in 24–48 h; patient may then become asymptomatic • This is the "calm before the storm" and patients may later present as hepatic failure if ingestion is severe enough	• Toxicity determined by Rumack-Matthew nomogram; must draw acetaminophen levels at 4 h post-ingestion and to determine probable or possible hepatic toxicity • NAC is specific antidote and is 100% effective in preventing toxicity if given within 8 h of severe ingestion • Liver transplantation may be only choice if hepatic failure imminent
TCAs	• Tertiary amines block norepinephrine and serotonin reuptake, and their metabolites, 2° amines predominantly affect norepinephrine reuptake • Also have anticholinergic and antihistaminic effects	• Symptom onset within 6 h • Dx made on clinical grounds; no specific levels • May see dizziness, confusion, agitation, and variable anticholinergic effects; presentation is often nonspecific • ECG findings characteristic: may see prolonged QRS, PR, or QT +/− right axis deviation of terminal 40 mV of QRS (seen as R wave in lead aVR and S wave in lead I)	• Rx is supportive • AC if ingestion <2 h • Benzodiazepines for seizures • $NaHCO_3$ for ECG changes • ++ Fluids +/− pressors for hypotension

HYPERTHERMIA

DEFINITION

Hyperthermia is defined as an elevation in core temperature 2° due to thermoregulatory failure. This is in contrast to fever, which is a cytokine-mediated elevation in core temperature. It is important that this distinction is made. Hyperthermia can be a medical emergency.

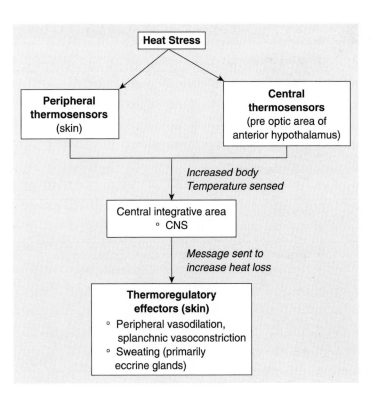

Figure 5.5 Mechanisms of heat regulation following heat stress.

CAUSAL CONDITIONS

ASC Box

Heat Regulation

A balance between heat load (from environment or 2° to ↑ metabolic heat) and heat dissipation. Hyperthermia is caused by conditions that ↑ heat load (from the environment or from ↑ metabolic heat) or diminish heat dissipation.

Table **5.10**	Causal Conditions of Hyperthermia			
	↑ Heat Load		Diminished Heat Dissipation	Sepsis
From Environment	**Metabolic Heat**			
Exertional (heavy exercise in high ambient temperature)	Thyroid storm, pheochromocytoma		Patient specific factors (obesity, anhidrosis, extremes of age, schizophrenia, alcoholism, hypothalamic/cerebral stroke, status epilepticus)	Encephalitis, brain abscess, meningitis, Td
Nonexertional or classic (persistent environmental exposure or impaired thermoregulation)	MH NMS		Drugs/tox ingestions (diuretic use, anticholingerics, sympathomimetics, salicylate toxicity, serotonin syndrome, cocaine)	

APPROACH

Severity is important: heat illness occurs along a spectrum. Hyperthermia is defined as any temperature >38°C.

Table **5.11**	Focused P/E	
System	**What to Look for**	**What Investigations Might Help**
Cardiac	• ↑ HR, ↑ BP (initially); BP may be ↓ 2° to dehydration • Arrhythmias • Ischemic Δs • High output failure	• ECG • Lytes + Ca
Resp.	• ↑ RR • Pulmonary edema • Pulmonary hemorrhage (2° to DIC)	• CXR
Neurologic	• Seizures or coma suggestive of cerebral edema • Hypertonia suggestive of NMS, MH	• CT head • CK
GI	• Hepatic failure (2° to severe dehydration/vasoconstriction) • Pancreatitis (2° to severe dehydration/vasoconstriction)	• ALT, AST +/− full LFTs • gluc. • Lactate +/− ABG • Amylase, lipase
Renal	• RF (2° to severe dehydration or rhabdomyolysis)	• U/A • BUN, Cr, CK • Urine myoglobin
Hematologic	• DIC	• CBC (look for consumptive thrombocytopenia) • INR/PTT +/− D-dimer and fibrinogen

Table **5.12**	Severity of Heat Illness		
Minor Heat Illness	**Heat Exhaustion**	**Heat Stroke**	

1. Heat cramps
  • Isolated cramps of most-worked muscle groups
  • Sweating + isotonic fluid replacement
2. Heat edema
  • Commonly nonacclimatized or elderly persons
  • Must R/O cardiac, hepatic, venous, or lymphatic disease
3. Heat syncope
  • Commonly occurs in elderly
  • Must R/O cardiac, neurologic disease
4. Prickly heat/heat rash/miliaria rubra/lichen tropicus
  • Pruritic vesicles on erythematous base, confined to clothed areas
	• Temperature 37.5°C– 40.5°C
	• Mental function intact
	• Malaise, fatigue, headache
	• ↑ HR, + orthostatics, clinical dehydration
		• Temperature classically >40.5°C
		• CNS dysfunction (coma, seizures, death)
		• Liver transaminases ↑
		• "Classical" heatstroke occurs usually in an elderly patient due to ↓ heat dissipation
		• "Exertional" heatstroke tends to occur in younger individuals due to exercise in high ambient temperatures +/− high humidity	

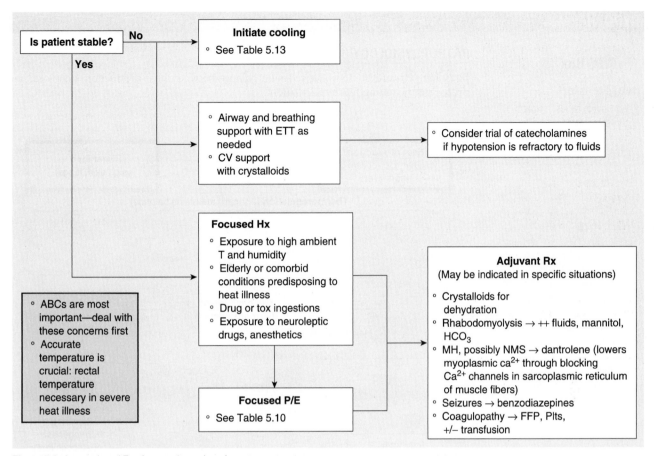

Figure 5.6 Approach and Tx of severe hyperthermia.

Table **5.13**	**Comparing Cooling Techniques**[a]		
	Methods	**Advantages**	**Disadvantages**
Ideal	• Evaporative cooling or body cooling unit • Ice water immersion	• Rapid, whole body cooling • Avoids shivering thermogenesis, which may generate heat during cooling process • Ice water immersion particularly effective in hypotensive patient → promotes vasoconstriction	• Specialized equipment needed (fans, water at 40°C, etc.) • Ice water immersion may complicate resuscitation efforts
Adjuncts	• Ice packs applied to groin and axillae • Cooling blankets • Peritoneal lavage • Gastric + rectal lavage • CPB	• Inexpensive, generally available in most Eds	• Little evidence to support peritoneal, gastric, and rectal lavage • Specialized equipment and personnel needed for CPB

[a]All cooling efforts must be **stopped** at 39°C to avoid "overshoot" hypothermia.

HYPOTHERMIA

Heat Transfer

- Conduction—loss of heat through direct contact; for example, submersion in cold water (Most common form of heat loss in accidental hypothermia)
- Convection—loss of heat through indirect contact via molecular motion; for example, wind blowing
- Radiation—loss of heat through indirect contact via infrared electromagnetic radiation; for example, radiation of heat to cold objects in the same room
- Evaporation—loss of heat through insensible fluid dissipation from skin or lungs; for example, sweating

PATHOPHYSIOLOGY

Body temperature homeostasis relies on balance between heat production, heat loss, and properly functioning thermoregulation.

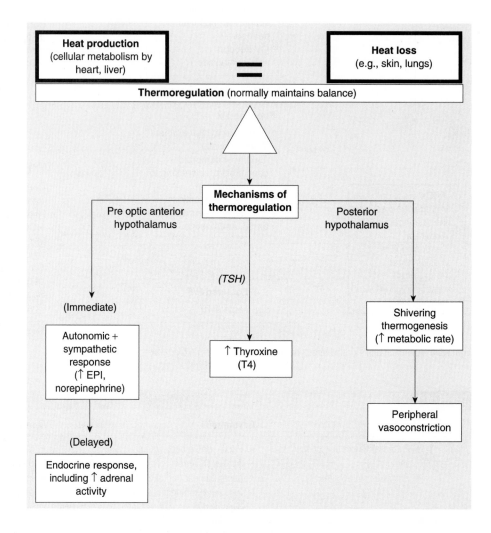

Figure 5.7 Pathophysiology of thermoregulation.

Table **5.14**	Causal Conditions of Hypothermia	
↓ **Heat Production**	**Impaired Thermoregulation**	↑ **Heat Loss**
• Endocrine (hypopituitarism, hypothyroidism, adrenal insufficiency) • Insufficient fuel (hypoglycemia, malnutrition) • Neuromuscular inactivity (age, impaired shivering)	Central a. Metabolic (cirrhosis, uremia) b. Drug/OD (barbiturates, phenothiazines, tricyclics, insulin) c. CNS (stroke, trauma, SAH, Parkinsonism, hypothalamic dysfunction, MS) Peripheral (spinal cord transection, neuropathy, DM, neuromuscular disease)	• Accidental/immersion hypothermia (exposure to cold air, water) • Vasodilatation (drugs, EtOH, tox, sepsis) • Skin disorders (burns, exfoliative dermatitis) • Iatrogenic (cold infusion)

APPROACH

Hx

Concomitant EtOH/other tox, Hx of previous illness, namely thyroid disease, CV/Resp disease, neuromuscular or CNS disease, endocrinologic etiologies such as adrenal insufficiency, and hypopituitarism

P/E

- Temperature determination is crucial: rectal temperature is most accurate; oral temperature typically 0.5 less and affected by food/fluids, breathing patterns, smoking; and axillary temperature typically 1.0 less, and least accurate.
- Focus on CNS, CVS, and Resp exams

LABWORK/INVESTIGATIONS

CBC, Lytes, gluc., INR/PTT, ABG, amylase, ECG, CXR

Tx

See algorithm mentioned in the subsequent text.

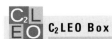

C₂LEO Box

Physicians are legally obligated to meet the standard of care, which includes continuing the resuscitation of the hypothermic patient until all reasonable efforts have been made.

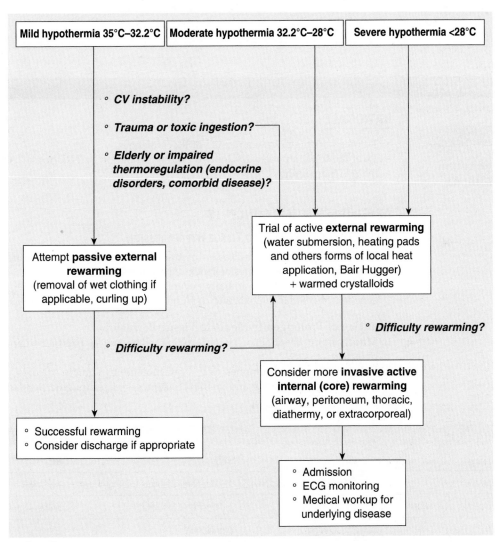

Figure 5.8 Approach to hypothermia.

Table **5.15**	Comparing Rewarming Techniques		
	Methods	**Advantages**	**Disadvantages**
Passive external	• Insulating material used to cover patient only	• Inexpensive	• Must be able to generate sufficient heat to allow spontaneous rewarming
Active external	• Bath immersion at 40°C • Hot water bottles • Heating pads • Forced-air warming systems (Bair Hugger)	• More rapid warming (required in CV instability, moderate or severe hypothermia, and thermoregulatory failure) • Minimizes energy expenditure	• Difficult resuscitation and monitoring if immersion bath used • Local heat application may cause thermal injury
Active internal (core)	• Warmed crystalloids • Heated, humidified O_2 at 41°C • PD • Heated irrigation (gastric, thoracic, pericardial) • Diathermy (with ultrasonic or microwaves) • Extracorporeal (venovenous, HD, continuous AV, and CPB)	• More rapid warming (required in CV instability, severe hypothermia, and thermoregulatory failure) • ↓ Hypothermic pulmonary damage associated with heated, humidified O_2 • Extracorporeal techniques are advantageous with concomitant ingestion of dialyzable substance	• Can be very invasive • Electrolyte disturbances with dialysis (hypokalemia) or gastric irrigation • Some techniques (CPB) require specialized personnel/equipment • Very rapid rewarming may cause DIC, pulmonary edema, ATN

TRAUMA/ACCIDENTS

CLINICAL BOX

Top Causes of Trauma Fatalities in Canada

1. MVC
2. Falls
3. Firearms

RATIONALE

• Trauma patients present a myriad of Rx challenges.
• Tx of the trauma patient is founded on the evaluation and Rx of the "**ABCDEs**" as per the ATLS guidelines.

APPLIED SCIENTIFIC CONCEPTS

SHOCK: TISSUE HYPOXIA 2° TO TISSUE HYPOPERFUSION

• Shock is a common complication of trauma. Although there are different types, the definition and consequences of shock remain the same.
• The effects of shock are initially reversible. However, prolonged O_2 deprivation → generalized cellular hypoxia and dysfunction of the biochemical cellular processes.

Sequelae of Prolonged Inadequate Tissue Perfusion

1. Mitochondrial dysfunction → anaerobic metabolism → production and accumulation of lactate
2. Release of stress hormones (e.g., catecholamines, glucocorticoids, glucagons) → glycogenolysis, lipolysis, and insulin resistance → ↑ serum gluc. and lactate

Table **5.16**	Four Major Categories of Shock and Associated Physiologic Δs		
	CO	**SVR**	**BP**
Hemorrhagic/hypovolemic	↑ [a] (↑ HR, ↑ contractility)	↑ (Peripheral vasoconstriction)	Narrowed pulse pressure
Distributive (e.g., septic, anaphylactic)	↓ (↓ Preload)	↓ (Peripheral vasodilation)	Widened pulse pressure
Cardiogenic	↓ (↓ Contractility)	↑ or Normal	↓
Obstructive (e.g., tamponade, PE, tension pneumothorax)	↓	↑ (Primarily due to venocongestion)	↓

[a] BP and HR are poor indicators of hemorrhagic and distributive shock as they depend on the patient's underlying health and physiologic reserve. CO will initially ↑ but, as hemorrhage continues, the patient will eventually decompensate leading to ↓ CO and BP.

General Presentation of Circulatory Shock

- Patient appears unwell
- Tachycardia
- Tachypnea/hypoxemia
- Elevated serum lactate
- Severely ↓ U/O
- Arterial hypotension despite fluid bolus

Holds for all types of shock, regardless of cause

3. Initiation of inflammatory events → activation of neutrophils, which bind to the vascular endothelium and release toxic free radicals + proteolytic enzymes → cell membrane, DNA, and organ damage

Eventually:

- Ion pumps in cell membrane malfunction → cells become edematous → intracellular contents leak into ECF and intracellular pH regulation becomes inadequate
- Once cells are no longer able to maintain homeostasis they undergo necrosis
- Generalized cell death → organ dysfunction and subsequent failure
- Death ensues in the face of global organ system failure

WOUND HEALING

- Emergency Tx of wounds emphasizes the restoration of tissue function, strength, and cosmesis, while minimizing blood loss and risk of infection.
- The skin is made up of four layers: epidermis, dermis, superficial fascia, and deep fascia.

CAUSAL CONDITIONS

- Blunt and penetrating traumas
- Motor vehicle accidents

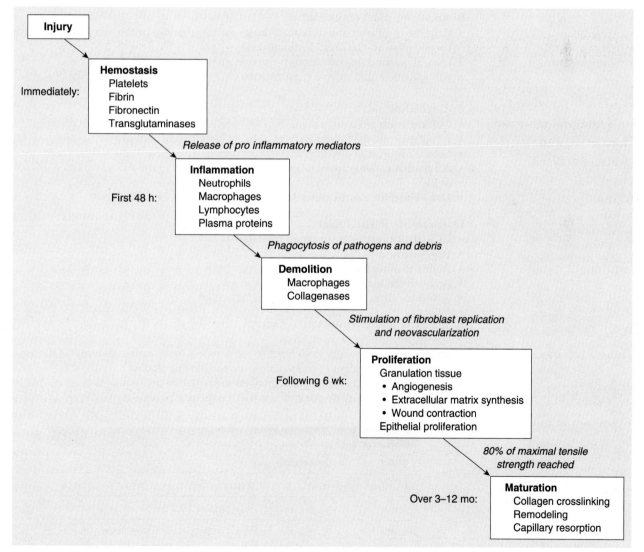

Figure 5.9 Sequence of wound healing. Wound healing is not a linear process. Rather all of the cellular Δs are occurring simultaneously to facilitate rapid tissue repair. Image is modified from *Pathology,* 3rd ed.

- Closed bony and soft tissue trauma
- Occupational; sport; domestic
- Lacerations and wounds from other causes

APPROACH

"SAMPLE" Hx:

S—Signs and symptoms of injury/illness
A—Allergies
M—Medications
P—Past Medical History, pregnancy
L—Last oral intake, including EtOH/drugs (present in 30% of cases)
E—Events surrounding the accident/trauma

PRIMARY SURVEY IN THE TRAUMA PATIENT —THE "ABCDEs"

A: Airway with C-Spine Control

- Maintain C-spine control until spinal injury can be ruled out
- Assess the airway to ensure that it is patent and free of FBs, fluids, and so on.
- Examine for facial/tracheal injuries that may → airway compromise/obstruction
- Jaw-thrust maneuvers, oro- and nasopharyngeal airways to improve the airway
- Definitive airways are needed in any patient with a GCS <8 or if risk of the patient losing his/her airway

B: Breathing and Ventilation

- Examine chest wall and auscultate lungs for compromise of the ventilatory structures (pneumothorax, flail chest, hemothorax)
- Place all patients on continuous pulse oximetry
- **All** patients should receive supplemental O_2, regardless of ventilatory capacity

C: Circulation

- Quickly assess circulatory status by LOC, peripheral pulses, BP, and skin color
- Hypotension in the trauma patient is due to hemorrhage until proven otherwise
- Look for sources of bleeding; manage any external bleeding through direct pressure
- **All** trauma patients get two large bore IVs, preferably in the AC fossa, and a 2-L bolus of RL
- Draw blood for trauma panel at time of IV cannulation (see side panel)

D: Disability (Neurologic)

- GCS (see Traumatic Head Injury for details)
- Pupils—size and reactivity
- Ability to move hands and feet
- Assess rectal tone
- Assess for signs of impending cerebral herniation

E: Exposure and Environmental Control

- Completely expose all body areas
- Rapidly examine patient from head-to-toe to assess for any gross deformity, substantial bleeding, or other signs of immediately life-threatening trauma
- Cover patient quickly with warm blankets to prevent hypothermia
- An external warming device and warm IV fluids may be necessary

Mechanical ventilation may be necessary, but beware of converting a simple pneumothorax to a tension pneumothorax.

CLINICAL BOX

Critical Adjuncts to Primary Survey

- Regular vitals
- Pulse oximetry
- ECG + telemetry
- IV fluids—2 L of RL
- Urinary catheter
- Gastric catheter
- Temperature control

CLINICAL BOX

"6 Places to Bleed"

1. Head
2. Chest
3. Abdo
4. Pelvis (3 L)
5. Legs (1 L each)
6. Street (i.e., environment)

CLINICAL BOX

Trauma Lab Panel

- CBC
- G&S or cross-match
- INR, PTT
- Lytes
- BUN, Cr
- β-HCG in female

Consider:

- ABG
- Lipase, amylase
- LFTs
- Drug panel

Table **5.17**	**Hemodynamic Status**
Status	**Description**
Unstable	Vitals continue to deteriorate despite 2 L of IV fluid resuscitation
Stable	Vitals (including U/O) are stable, but are not necessarily normal
Normal	Normal vitals and shows no signs of inadequate tissue perfusion

CLINICAL BOX

Diagnostic Studies

- AP CXR
- AP pelvis
- C-spine series
- DPL or FAST
- Additional XR of suspected injuries
- CT head/Abdo as appropriate

CLINICAL BOX

Indications for DPL

- Unstable patient, typically those with blunt abdominal trauma
- FAST is unavailable or is equivocal

Table **5.18**	2° Survey in the Trauma Patient—the "Head to Toe Exam"
Begins once resuscitation measures are underway and vitals are stabilizing	
Head	Assess for lacerations, contusions and fractures of the scalp, face, and skull. Test the CNs
EENT	Assess visual acuity, pupils (size, reactivity), EOM, Battle's sign, tympanic membrane (intact, CSF or blood present), and facial fractures
Chest	Palpate chest wall, beginning at clavicles and extending down the length of the rib cage Look for subcutaneous emphysema, tracheal deviation, and flail segments
CVS	Assess heart sounds, JVP, and bilateral BP Consider cardiac tamponade and aortic transaction
Abdo	Inspect, auscultate, palpate, and percuss Assess for intra-abdominal injury and pelvic stability
Spine	Assess when logrolling patient off spine board. "Walk" fingers down the spine assessing for deformities. Test sensation in the major dermatomes
Rectum and genitalia	Urethral bleeding, injury to the genitalia, rectal tone and bleeding, high-riding prostate
Extremities	Palpate all long bones and move all joints
	Assess peripheral pulses

DISPOSITION FOLLOWING INITIAL STABILIZATION

- Disposition depends on the patients' hemodynamic stability, the severity of the injuries, and the need for specialist services (typically surgical specialties).
- Patients not requiring immediate surgical Tx may be admitted to the ICU for close observation.
- Other: observation in ED, admit to ward, direct to OR, transfer to a trauma center

INDICATIONS FOR TRANSFER TO A TRAUMA CENTRE AND/OR ADVANCED CARE

- The stable patient who requires specialized investigations (e.g., CT) or access to a specialty service (e.g., surgery)
- Consider in the unstable patient who requires definitive Rx not available at the current hospital (e.g., worsening neurologic state refractory to all stabilization efforts)
- Note: Prehospital services routinely transfer patients who are <30 min from scene to trauma center directly, bypassing local hospitals

POTENTIAL COMPLICATIONS OF TRAUMA TX AND RESUSCITATION

- Decubitus ulcers—may occur after only a short period of immobilization on a hard spinal board or in a C-spine collar. To minimize risk, patients are routinely taken off spinal board ASAP if thoracic and lumbar spines can be cleared clinically. C-spine collar often remains in place until C spine cleared radiographically.
- DVT and PE —particularly in orthopedic and spinal cord traumas. Prophylaxis in at-risk patients consists of daily subcutaneous enoxaparin or LMWH.
- Transfusion complications—infection (HBV, bacterial pathogens); immunologic (↓ cell-mediated immunity, proinflammatory effects); metabolic (hypothermia, acidosis, coagulopathy, hyperkalemia, hypocalcemia, and citrate toxicity); and mistransfusion (ABO incompatibility).

INJURY PREVENTION

- Trauma is largely a "disease of the young" and is the leading cause of death in persons aged 1 to 44 yr

- >85% of traumatic injuries are unintentional and many are preventable.
- Major prevention strategies include campaigning and legislation around:
  - Seatbelt use
  - Driving—EtOH consumption implicated in ~40% of fatal MVAs
  - Bicycle helmet use → up to 88% ↓ in risk of head and severe brain injuries
  - Gun locks

ABDOMINAL INJURIES

CLINICAL BOX

Estimating TBV

Infant = 90 mL/kg

Child = 80 mL/kg

Adult = 70 mL/kg

RATIONALE

- Abdominal trauma divides into two broad categories: blunt and penetrating
- Severe abdominal injuries may initially exhibit few clinical signs.
- The mechanism of injury and an understanding of abdominal organ anatomy should guide one's level of suspicion for injury and subsequent investigations.

APPLIED SCIENTIFIC CONCEPTS

- Abdominal injuries can result in a large amount of occult blood loss.
- The physiologic Δs associated with hemorrhage reflect the body's attempt to maintain CO, tissue perfusion, and oxygenation despite ↓ blood volume and O_2 carrying capacity.
- Caution needs to be taken with children and young patients, those with large CV reserve, and the elderly or those on adrenergic-blocking meds as they have ↓ CV reserve.
- **Mental status is the most specific "vital sign,"** as declining mentation reflects cerebral hypoperfusion and hypoxia.

Table **5.19**	Classification of Hemorrhage and Associated Physiologic Δs			
	Class I	**Class II**	**Class III**	**Class IV**
Blood loss (% of TBV)	<15%	15%−30%	30%−40%	>40%
HR	<100	>100	>120	>140
BP	Normal	Normal	↓	↓↓
Pulse pressure	Normal	↓	↓↓	↓↓↓
RR	Normal	20−30	30−40	>35
U/O (mL/h)	>30	20−30	5−15	Scant
Mental status	Slightly anxious	Mildly anxious	Anxious, confused	Confused, lethargic

(Adapted from the American College of Surgeons ATLS Guidelines.)

CLINICAL BOX

Total Allowable Blood Loss

$$TBV \times \frac{(Hbi - Hbf)}{Hbi}$$

Where Hbi = initial hemoglobin and Hbf = threshold hemoglobin for transfusion

Example: for a 70-kg healthy adult

$$(70)(70) \times \frac{(145 - 80)}{145} = 2.2L$$

Therefore, after ~2 L of blood loss, the patient will require PRBC transfusion.

Table **5.20**	Indications for Transfusion of PRBCs in Trauma
Absolute	**Relative**
Hb < 80 g/L in any patient	• Hb < 100 g/L in a patient with known CV disease • Suspected or known massive hemorrhage • Persistent hypotension following 2 L of IV crystalloids • Evidence of end-organ dysfunction 2° to hypoxia

Table **5.21**	Common Mechanisms and Associated Abdominal Injuries	
	Mechanism of Injury	**Commonly Injured Organs**
Penetrating trauma	Stab wounds; missile/gun shot wounds	Spleen, liver, pancreas, duodenum, small intestine, colon
Blunt trauma	Motor vehicle/bicycle/all-terrain vehicle crash; auto vs. pedestrian injury; fall from height; child abuse	Spleen, liver, GU tract, pelvis

In general, blunt trauma is associated with higher mortality rates.

CLINICAL BOX

FAST

Assesses for free fluid in four areas—the four "**P**s": **P**erisplenic, **P**erihepatic, **P**elvic, and **P**ericardial

CLINICAL BOX

Values for Positive DPL

Gunshot = 5,000 RBC/mL

Blunt = 100,000 RBC/mL

Stabbing = 10,000 RBC/μL

CLINICAL BOX

Causes of Hypotension in the Abdominal Trauma Patient

- Acute blood loss/hemorrhagic shock
- Spinal shock
- Toxic ingestion
- Pregnancy
- Acute and chronic Resp or cardiac disease

CLINICAL BOX

Fluid Regimen in the Trauma Patient

All trauma patients should receive 2 L of crystalloid, and PRBCs as indicated thereafter

CAUSAL CONDITIONS

- In blunt trauma, compressive forces disrupt tissues and rupture hollow viscera.
- Any penetrating trauma to the lower chest, flank, back, and pelvis must be considered to have caused an abdominal injury until proven otherwise.
- Rapid decelerations can cause relatively mobile organs to move abruptly about their tethers (e.g., the small bowel at the ligament of Treitz) resulting in injury.

APPROACH

- Almost all injuries to the abdominal viscera produce nonspecific signs and Sx, many of which take hours to days to develop.
- A tense and distended Abdo suggests ↑ intra-abdominal pressure and may indicate abdominal compartment syndrome.
- DPL: Infusion and drainage of 1 L of saline into the Abdo and analysis of the number of RBCs present. Used for determination of intra-abdominal bleeding. Like FAST, DPL does not localize the injury and cannot identify retroperitoneal injury.

INDICATIONS FOR EMERGENT SURGICAL CONSULTATION AND LAPAROTOMY

- Hemodynamically unstable patient with abdominal, back or flank trauma
- Obvious GI evisceration
- P/E findings consistent with peritonitis
- Transabdominal gunshot wound
- Penetrating wound that extends through the fascia ± a positive DPL
- Free air present on either plain XR or CT
- Abdominal organ injury as seen on CT that requires surgical repair

APPROACH

CONSERVATIVE VERSUS SURGICAL TX

- A hemodynamically stable patient with a positive DPL, FAST, or CT and no indications for emergent laparotomy is a candidate for conservative Rx.
- Most patients with blunt hepatic and splenic injuries are managed nonoperatively, with individuals younger than 55 yr most likely to benefit.
- Patients with ongoing bleeding, particularly splenic, may require angiography ± vessel embolization.

Table **5.22**	Diagnostic Investigations in the Evaluation of Abdominal Trauma				
	P/E	**FAST**	**DPL**	**CT**	**Exploratory Laparotomy**
Rapid	Yes	Yes	Yes	No	No
Sensitive	No	Yes	Yes	Yes	Yes
Specific	No	No	No	Yes	Yes
Repeatable	Yes	Yes	Yes	Yes	Yes
Invasive	No	No	Yes	No	Yes

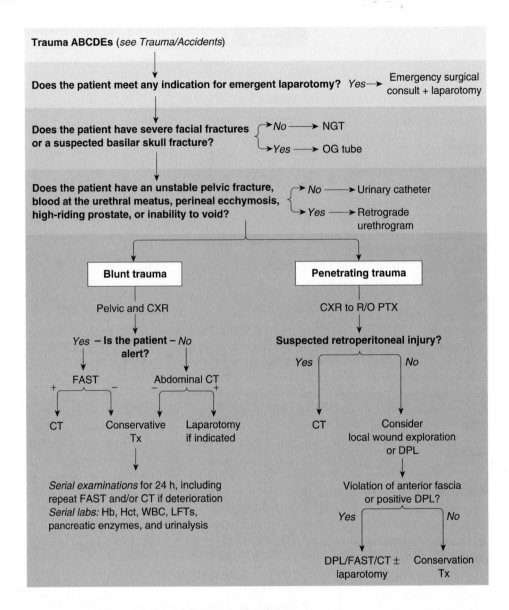

Figure 5.10 Initial Tx of the abdominal trauma patient.

BITES, ANIMAL/INSECTS

EPIDEMIOLOGY

- 1% total ED visits
- Most occur in children
- Can lead to significant morbidity or even death.

CAUSAL CONDITIONS

1. Dog bites
2. Cat bites
3. Human bites
4. Insect bites/stings—often cause local inflammatory reaction. Systemic illness is uncommon
   - Mosquitoes can transmit infectious disease (malaria, yellow fever, dengue, encephalitis, and filariasis)
   - Tick-borne illness
   - Blackflies, deerflies, and horseflies may cause systemic allergic reactions
5. Snake bites (see Figs. 5.11 and 5.12)

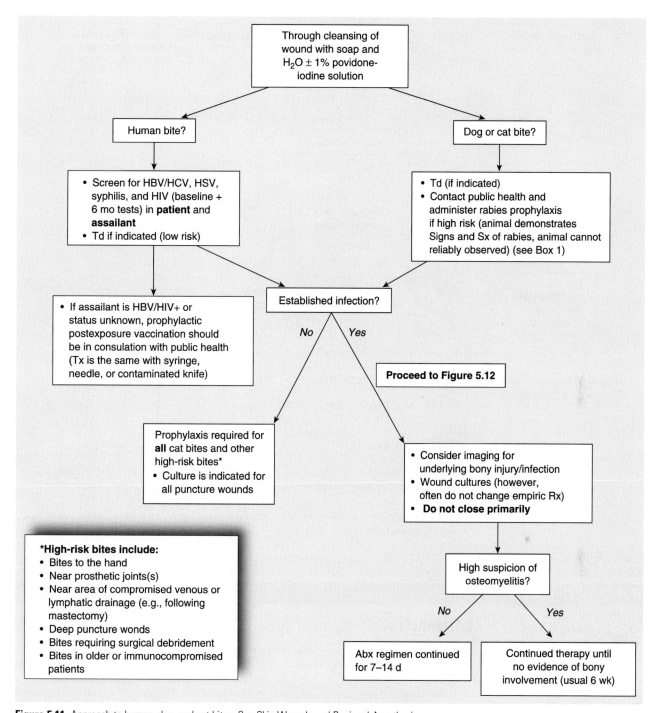

Figure 5.11 Approach to human, dog, and cat bites. See Skin Wounds and Regional Anesthesia.

RABIES PROPHYLAXIS

- High suspicion with bites or scratches from bat, bobcat, coyote, fox, raccoon, skunk, or wolf, especially if unprovoked attack
- Indicated if animal/human has confirmed rabies or status of animal is unknown and cannot be observed for 10-d period
- Must contact public health for vaccine and Ig
- Rabies Ig (20 IU/kg): $\frac{1}{2}$ infused to wound, $\frac{1}{2}$ in separate IM dose (e.g., deltoid or buttock)
- Rabies vaccine (1 mL, IM): to be given in opposite deltoid on days 0, 3, 7, 14, 28

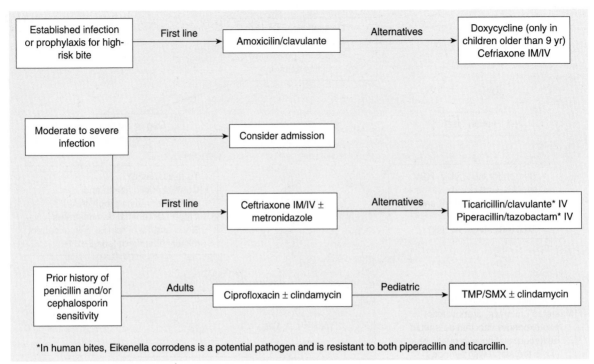

*In human bites, Eikenella corrodens is a potential pathogen and is resistant to both piperacillin and ticarcillin.

Figure 5.12 Appropriate Abx choice for human, dog, and cat bites. (Based on the 2005 Edition of Anti-infective Guidelines for Community-acquired Infections)

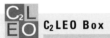 **C₂ LEO Box**

Fight bites, unlike animal bites, may result in litigation and appropriate documentation, including photographs, should be obtained. Physicians are obligated to testify and act as medical experts in such cases.

As well, screening for HBV/HCV, HIV, and syphilis is evaluated on a case basis. In Canada, patients can refuse HIV testing.

BONE/JOINT INJURY

Pelvis and femur fractures are life-threatening injuries.

RATIONALE

- In the trauma patient, major fractures can be associated with other significant injuries.
- Most fractures are rarely immediately life threatening and their Tx is initially a low priority.
- In the pediatric population, unexplained fractures should raise the question of potential child abuse.

APPROACH

- Emergency Tx of fractures involves ruling out open fractures, assessment of neurovascular status distal to the injury, analgesia, imaging of the injury, limb splinting, and reduction as appropriate.
- Once there is no immediate threat to life, open fractures should be managed urgently (irrigation, splinting, Td, IV Abx) due to ↑ risk of osteomyelitis.
- The overall aim of fracture Rx is to return normal alignment and length to the bone and then provide support to the reduced fracture.
- Soft tissue injuries are best managed by the assessment and Rx of any associated bone or joint injuries.
- Once healing is occurring appropriately, early return to function and rehabilitation should be encouraged.

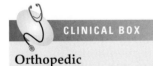

CLINICAL BOX

Orthopedic Emergencies

- Knee/hip dislocation
- Ankle reduction
- Reduction of the fractured cold, pulseless limb

Table **5.23**	Tx Based on Type of Bone/Joint Injury
Tx Approach	**Indication**
Supportive sling	• Postreduction of shoulder or radial head dislocation • Clavicle, shoulder girdle, and humeral neck fractures • Nondisplaced radial head fractures
Closed reduction and cast immobilization	• Closed, stable fractures that are able to be reduced without operative intervention and do not have significant overlying soft tissue injuries • Fractures must not meet any requirements for ORIF
Closed reduction and continuous traction	• A temporizing measure used while patient awaits definitive fixation (external or internal) • Often used because the patient is not medically stable enough to tolerate surgery • Permits Rx of associated soft tissue injury at the fracture site • E.g., crush/comminuted long bone and pelvic fractures
Internal skeletal fixation (percutaneous pinning)	• Displaced proximal humerus and supracondylar fractures, postreduction • Distal radius fractures, postreduction
ORIF	• Open, unstable, or intra-articular/periarticular fractures • Failure to obtain closed reduction of fracture

CHEST INJURIES

Thoracic Trauma Emergencies

- Airway obstruction
- Flail chest
- Large hemothorax
- Cardiac tamponade
- Pneumothorax
- Open
- Tension

These are life-threatening conditions that may result in hypoxia, hypercarbia, and acidosis.

RATIONALE

- Patients who have suffered a thoracic trauma frequently present with Resp distress and/or shock.

CAUSAL CONDITIONS

- Penetrating trauma: stab wounds; missile/gunshot wounds; iatrogenic
- Blunt trauma: steering wheel blow to sternum; falls; explosions; crush

APPROACH

- Thoracic injuries have the potential to compromise all of the patient's ABCs (see Trauma/Accidents).
- Therefore, suspicion of a specific thoracic injury demands immediate, appropriate investigation (see Fig. 5.25).

CLINICAL BOX

Beck's Triad: Cardiac Tamponade

1. Elevated JVP
2. ↓ BP
3. Muffled heart sounds

Table **5.24**	Common Injuries Associated with Thoracic Trauma
Lungs	Tracheobronchial tree injury Pulmonary contusion Hemothorax Pneumothorax (open, closed, tension)
MSK	Clavicle; sternum; rib fracture Flail chest
Esophagus	Esophageal rupture
Great vessel	Aortic rupture Aortic dissection
Heart	Pericardial trauma (pericarditis, acute/delayed tamponade) Myocardial trauma (contusion, coronary vessel injury)
Diaphragm	Diaphragmatic injury

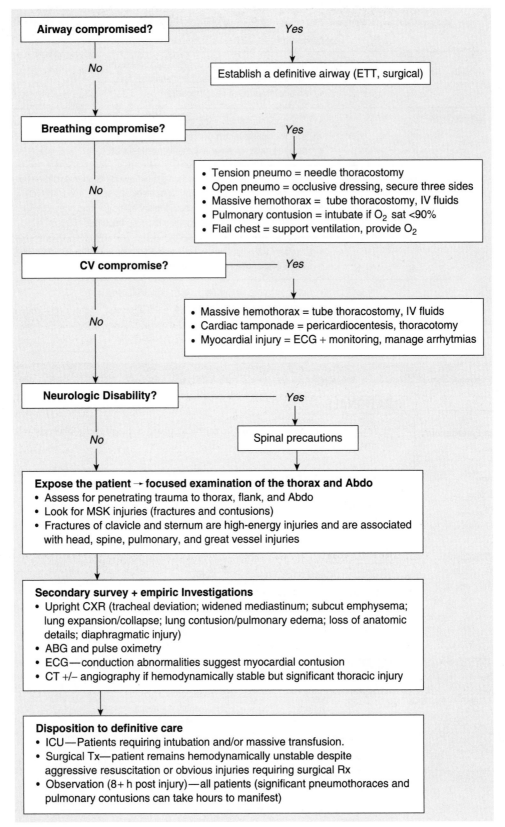

Figure 5.13 Initial Tx of the thoracic trauma patient.

Table **5.25**	Clinical Presentation of Obstructive versus Hypovolemic Shock	
Signs and Sx	**Obstructive (e.g., Cardiac Tamponade)**	**Hypovolemic (e.g., Severe Hemothorax)**
Breath sounds	Normal	↓ (On affected side)
Heart sounds	Muffled	Normal
BP	↓	↓
JVP	Elevated	↓ or flat

Hx

- Determine the mechanism of injury—blunt versus penetrating—and the force sustained.
- Obtain a Hx of pain associated with the thoracic trauma. Delayed onset of pain suggests flail chest and/or worsening pneumothorax/hemothorax.

CLINICAL BOX

CXR Signs of Aortic Disruption

- Widened mediastinum (>8 cm)
- Indistinct aortic knob
- Depressed left main bronchus
- Tracheal deviation (right)
- NG tube deviation
- Widened right paratracheal stripe (>5 mm)
- Apical capping
- Loss of space between the pulmonary artery and aorta

CLINICAL BOX

Indications for Immediate ED Thoracotomy

Indications

- Acute hemodynamic instability or cardiac arrest in the ED **and**
- Penetrating thoracic injury ± signs of electrical cardiac activity
- Blunt thoracic injury + electrical cardiac activity
- Great vessel injury
- Cardiac tamponade
- Suspected air embolus
- Known esophageal, tracheal, or bronchial injury

Not Indicated If:

- Patient with blunt trauma and no sign of electrical cardiac activity
- No qualified surgeon present

CLINICAL BOX

Presentation of Acute Aortic Rupture

- Chest or midscapular pain
- Dyspnea
- Hoarseness
- Dysphagia

May be asymptomatic

DROWNING/NEAR DROWNING

RATIONALE

- Near drowning/submersion victim = survival following submersion in a liquid and subsequent distress requiring medical attention
- Drowning = death 2° to a submersion event
- Additionally, the temperature of the water plays a pivotal role in patient Tx and outcome

CLINICAL BOX

Drowning

- Drowning injuries carry a ~12% case fatality rate
- Second cause of injury-related mortality in children
- Males account for 80% of victims older than 12 mo
- Estimated that for each case of fatal drowning there are up to six near-drowning cases

The vast majority of children younger than 4 yr drown in the domestic setting, e.g., bath-tubs, large buckets of water, and artificial pools.

CAUSAL CONDITIONS

CAUSES OF SUBMERSION INJURY

- Inability to swim or an individual's overestimation of personal capability
- Risk-taking behaviour
- Boating accidents, particularly if not wearing a life jacket
- Substance abuse (associated with up to 50% of adult drowning deaths)
- Inadequate adult supervision
- Concomitant illness—trauma, seizure, CVA, cardiac event
- Hyperventilation
- Hypothermia

APPROACH

- Unexpected submersion → panic, breath-holding, and an attempt to reach the water surface. Hypoxia develops and the patient begins to swallow water → eventual aspiration when no longer able to breath-hold.
- Initial studies comparing fresh versus saltwater near-drowning emphasized differences in Lytes, hemolysis, and shifts within the fluid compartments.
- However, the physiological differences associated with fresh versus saltwater near-drowning are theoretic as >11 mL/kg of water must be aspirated before they occur and most drowning victims aspirate <4 mL/kg.

INITIAL TX OF THE SUBMERSION INJURY PATIENT

Hx

- Elicit a Hx of the events surrounding the submersion and if resuscitative measures were started.
- Determine the quality of the liquid in which the patient was submerged—mud, sewage, and particulates significantly ↑ the risk of developing ARDS and pulmonary infections.
- Try to discover the relative temperature of the liquid into which the patient was submerged.

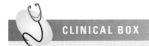

CLINICAL BOX

Aspiration

The quantity of the water aspirated determines the pulmonary sequelae more so than the composition.

CLINICAL BOX

Diving Reflex

Present in infants and children. Results in apnea and bradycardia on stimulation of cold water on the face → shunting of blood to the brain and heart. May prolong the tolerable submersion time.

Table **5.26**	**Relevant Pathophysiology of Submersion Injury**	
Temperature	Hypothermia	↓ Cerebral metabolism; ↓ LOC; faster exhaustion; cardiac dysrhythmias
Resp	Disruption of surfactant with aspiration of 1–3 mL/kg Noncardiogenic pulmonary edema ARDS; Resp acidosis	Alveolar collapse; atelectasis
CVS	Severe hypoxia and metabolic derangements	CVS collapse; cardiac dysrhythmias
Metabolic	Hypoxia and CO_2 trapping	Resp acidosis; metabolic acidosis
CNS	Hypoxia, acidosis, and hypothermia Hypothermia → ↓ cerebral metabolism. ? neuroprotective	Hypoxia and acidosis → neuronal death

Trauma ABCDEs (see Trauma/Accidents)

In particular, in the submersion injury patient:

- C-spine control if submersion injury was associated with trauma
- Assess patient's core temperature (i.e., rectal temperature)
- Assess for signs of Resp injury, including the presence of ARDS
- Assess for CVS collapse and dysrhythmias (e.g., bradycardia, AF)
- Assess for signs of cerebral edema (e.g., lethargy, ↓ LOC, pupils)

Initial Tx

Outcome in a patient who has absent vital signs is highly dependent on how quickly CPR is initiated.

Upon arrival in the ED:

- Initiate continuous cardiac monitoring and pulse oximetry
- Intubate if $PaCO_2$ >50 mm Hg or PaO_2 <60 mm Hg
- Insertion of rectal temperature probe if patient is lethargic or unstable
  - Initiate rewarming if T <36°C
  - Continue rewarming until core temperature is between 32°C to 35°C as cerebral death cannot be diagnosed in hypothermic patients
- Insert Foley catheter and monitor U/O (as an indication of renal function)
- Naloxone and gluc. are appropriate if Hx suggests confounding factors
- There is no evidence for giving empiric corticosteroids or Abx.

Investigations
- ABG—to assess acid–base status
- Lytes, BUN, Cr, U/A—~50% have renal dysfunction due to lactic acidosis and hypoperfusion; may develop rhabdomyolysis
- INR, PTT—patients may develop a coagulopathy associated with hypothermia
- ECG—to monitor for dysrhythmia
- CXR—may initially underestimate the severity of the pulmonary injury
- C-spine XR if traumatic injury
- Investigations to R/O contributors/causes of submersion (e.g., intoxication, hypoglycemia, cardiac arrest, CVA)

Disposition
- All symptomatic patients require hospitalization.
- Patients who are asymptomatic may be observed for a 6- to 8-h period. If O_2 sat on room air, CXR and ABG results remain normal, patients may be safely discharged home into the care of a competent adult. Instructions to return in the event of any Resp distress must be given.

FACIAL INJURIES

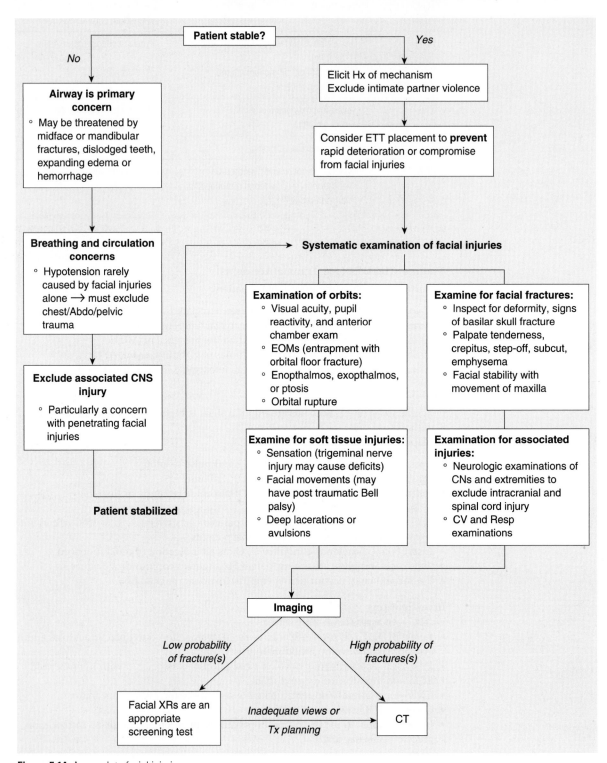

Figure 5.14 Approach to facial injuries.

HAND AND WRIST

RATIONALE

- Injury to the hand is a common chief complaint in the emergency room.
- Rx success and eventual outcome depends on the severity of the initial injury, how quickly repair is performed, the skill of the treating physician, and subsequent rehabilitation efforts.

CAUSAL CONDITIONS

- Tendon injury
- Nerve injury
- Bone and/or joint injury

APPLIED SCIENTIFIC CONCEPTS

Table **5.27**	Muscles of the Hand and Wrist—Innervation and Function	
	Muscles	**Function**
Ulnar		
Forearm	FCU	Wrist flexion
	FDP—D4, D5	Flexion at the DIP joints
Hand	*Hypothenar muscles*:	
	ODP	Facilitates opposition of D5 with D1
	ADM	Abduction of D5 at MCP joint
	FDMB	Flexion of D5
	Dorsal and palmar interossei	Abduction and adduction of digits
	Adductor pollicis	Adduction and opposition of the thumb
	Palmaris brevis	—
	Lumbricals—third and fourth	Permit flexion at MCP joints when PIP and DIP joints are extended
Median		
Forearm	FCR	Flexion and radial deviation of the wrist
	PL	Flexion of the wrist
	Pronator teres	Pronation of the forearm
	FDS FDP—D2, D3FPL	Flexion at the PIP joints
	Pronator quadratus	Flexion at the DIP joints
		Flexion of the thumb
		Pronation of the hand
Hand	*Thenar muscles*:	
	APB	Abduction of the thumb
	FPB	Flexion of the thumb
	OP	Opposition of the thumb
	Lumbricals—first and second	Same as third and fourth lumbricals
Radial		
Forearm	Brachioradialis	Flexion at the elbow
	ECRL and ECRB	Extension and abduction about the wrist
	Extensor digitorum	Extension of digits, wrist, and elbow
	EPB	Extension of the proximal phalanx of D1
	EPL	Extension of the distal phalanx of D1
	EI	Extension of D2
	EDM	Extension of D5
	ECU	Extension and adduction about the wrist
	APL	Abduction of the thumb

ASC Box

Hand Muscles

- Extrinsic muscles: the muscle bellies originate outside of the hand (in the forearm) but their tendons insert within the hand.
- Intrinsic muscles: muscle origins and insertions are within the hand.

APPROACH

Hx

- Patient ID—age, hand dominance, occupation, hobbies
- Type of injury (laceration, crush, fall, bite)
- Environment in which injury occurred (clean vs. contaminated; home vs. work)
- Position of the hand/wrist at the time of the trauma
- Any loss of sensation or mobility since accident, any hand/wrist pain
- Any Rx provided to date, Td prophylaxis

INVESTIGATION

- Any patient who has suffered a significant hand or wrist trauma should have hand ± wrist XRs with three views (PA, lateral, and oblique).
- A good rule of thumb is that any injury with associated swelling should be radiographically investigated.
- If there are lacerations/punctures, the wounds should be explored under local anesthesia to determine depth, injury to any adjacent structures, and presence of any remaining FBs.

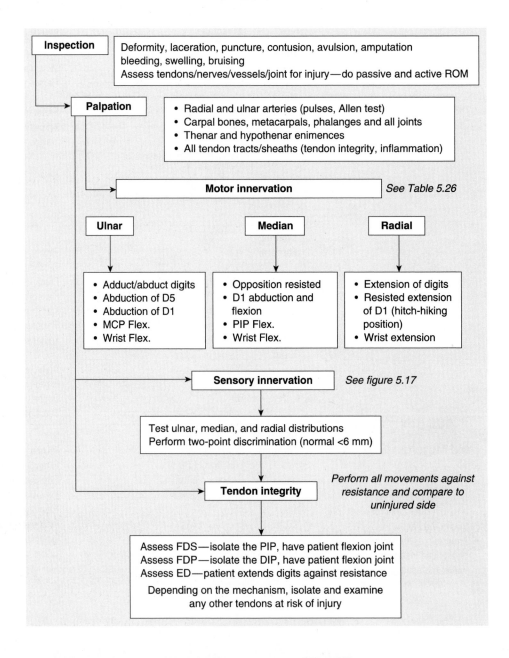

Figure 5.15 Initial assessment of hand and wrist injury.

Table **5.28**	Indications for Surgical Consultation in Hand/Wrist Injury
Immediate:	Vascular injury with signs of tissue ischemia
	Substantial amputation (beyond DIP, amputated part present)
	Highly contaminated wounds (requiring surgical debridement)
	Unstable/irreducible/open/intra-articular/periarticular fractures
	Severe crush injuries
	Compartment syndrome
	Joint dislocation (e.g., MCP)
Delayed[a] (within 24–48 h):	Tendon laceration
	Nerve laceration
	Unstable ligamentous injury
	Reduced dislocations and fractures

[a]All patients awaiting delayed consultation must be placed in a splint.

INITIAL TX

- All patients who sustain a significant injury to the hand should receive follow-up with a plastic surgeon. This includes all patients with fractures of the hand and/or carpal bones
- Conservative Tx (e.g., NSAIDs, analgesics)—closed distal phalanx fracture; stable proximal and middle phalanx fractures (can be "buddy taped" for the first few days postinjury); soft tissue injuries
- Splints—dislocations postreduction; stable injuries that are not amenable to surgical intervention, patients who are poor surgical candidates
- Occupational therapy/physiotherapy—any patient who has an injury to the dominant hand that results in a functional limitation; all patients who require prolonged splinting or surgical Tx

"Position of Safety" Splinting

- Patients with hand injuries should be splinted in the "position of safety."
- The "position of function" is used in forearm and wrist injuries.

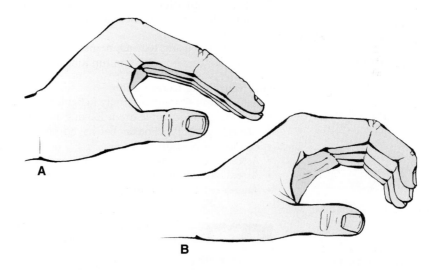

Figure 5.16 Position of safety versus position of function. **A:** Position of safety = wrist in 20° to 30° extension, MCPs in 90° flexion, IP joints in full extension. **B:** Position of function = wrist in 20° to 30° extension, MCP and IP joints have full ROM (patient should be able to make the "OK" sign and have an adequate grasp)

HEAD TRAUMA, BRAIN DEATH, AND ORGAN TRANSPLANTATION

RATIONALE

- Most head trauma is mild and associated with a good long-term prognosis.
- Appropriate use and interpretation of head CT imaging is necessary to detect serious TBI.
- Prevention of 2° brain injury in the TBI patient improves outcomes.

ASC Box

$CPP = MAP - ICP$

$CBF = CPP/CVR$

CPP = cerebral perfusion

MAP = mean arterial pressure

CBF = cerebral blood flow

CVR = cerebrovascular resistance

Avoid

1. Hypotension/shock
2. Hypoxia
3. Fever
4. Seizures
5. Hypo-/hyperglycemia

Be Alert! A LOC may have been the **cause** of the trauma. Always consider other causes of impaired consciousness.

CLINICAL BOX

Etiology of TBI

1. Falls (45%)
2. MVC (36%)
3. Assaults (9%)

CLINICAL BOX

Classification of Head Injury

- Mild: GCS 13 to 15
- Moderate: GCS 9 to 12
- Severe: GCS <9

APPLIED SCIENTIFIC CONCEPTS

- ICP reflects the balance of pressures exerted by CSF blood and the brain on the walls of the cranium.
- Monroe-Kellie doctrine: Compensation for ↑ volume of one component of the cranial vault (i.e., blood, CSF, or brain matter) necessitates an equal ↓ in the volume of another.
- Normal ICP = 8 to 10 mm Hg and pathologic ICP is ≥ 20 mm Hg
- A major complication in head injuries and leading cause of 2° brain injury is ↑ ICP, often due to an intracranial hematoma.
- Additionally, anything that compromises or exacerbates cerebral metabolism may result in 2° brain injury.

CAUSAL CONDITIONS

1. Skull fracture/penetrating injury
2. Hemorrhage/hematoma
3. Cerebral contusion
4. Edema

APPROACH

Determined by severity of head injury

MILD

- Focused neurologic exam (e.g., level of alertness and orientation, pupils, CNs, reflexes)
- CT as per the Canadian CT Head Rules (not applicable if age younger than 16 yr, use of coumadin, or obvious open skull fracture)

MODERATE

- Full neurologic exam (see subsequent text)
- CT head

SEVERE

Tx of ABCs and Vitals

- Intubate if GCS <8, patient is unable to protect his/her airway, or neurologic deterioration is anticipated.
- Ventilate prn using 100% O_2 to maintain O_2 sat >90%.
- Place two large-bore IVs and run Ringers or N/S to prevent hypotension.

Full Neurologic Examination

- Assess pupil size and reactivity to light.
- Perform a fundoscopic exam looking for papilledema and hemorrhages, especially if suspecting ↑ ICP or Shaken Baby syndrome.
- Perform a CN exam.
- Assess rectal tone and reflexes (DTRs and Babinski).
- Assess motor function in all four limbs and sensation in all major dermatomes.
- Reassess vitals and neurologic status every 15 min!

Table **5.29**	**Glasgow Coma Scale**[a]		
	Movement	**Verbal**	**Eye Opening**
1	No movement	No response	No eye opening
2	Decerebrate posturing	Incomprehensible	Opens to pain
3	Decorticate posturing	Inappropriate words	Opens to voice
4	Withdraws from pain	Confused	Spontaneous
5	Localizes to pain	Oriented	—
6	Obeys command	—	—

[a]Best score = 15/15; worst score = 3/15.

Investigations

CT Head

Table **5.30**	**Presentation of TBI on Head CT**					
	Immediate Findings		**Early Findings**			**Evolving Findings**	
	IVH	**SAH**	**Epidural Hematoma**	**Intracerebral Contusion and Hemorrhage**	**Acute Subdural Hematoma**	**Cerebral Edema**	**Diffuse Axonal Injury**
Mechanisms of Injury	Caused by shearing of vessels within the brain parenchyma	May be 2° to trauma or due to rupture of an aneurysm	Due to meningeal artery injury, typically the middle meningeal artery	Caused by shearing of vessels within the brain parenchyma	Injury of the bridging veins running from the surface of the brain to the superior sagittal sinus	Vasogenic, cytotoxic, or hydrocephalic in nature	Shearing of axons due to deceleration or rotational forces about the brain
Location	Lateral ventricles and third ventricle	Blood collects in the space between the arachnoid and the pia	Blood collects between the skull and the dura mater	Most commonly located in the frontal and temporal lobes	Blood collects between the dura and arachnoid layers	May be localized to area of injury or may be diffuse	In the deep white matter and midbrain
Appearance on CT	Focal areas of blood within the ventricles	Area of high density that is spread thinly over the convexity of the brain	Usually biconvex (the "lens" sign)	Diffuse area of high density in the brain parenchyma, adjacent to the bony prominences	Usually crescent shaped. Acute = high density	Shift of midline structures, particularly if focal edema	The CT may initially be normal. Evolves to show loss of gray-white interface and/or multiple small hemorrhages

 C₂LEO Box

Informed consent is needed for all investigations and Rx. Suffering a TBI does not automatically render a patient "incapable" and it is important to fully assess and document the patient's competency to consent to Rx.

Canadian CT Head Rules

CT of any patient with a mild TBI (GCS = 13 to 15) plus:

- High risk factors
  - GCS <15 2 h after injury
  - Suspected open or depressed skull fracture
  - Any sign of basilar skull fracture
  - Two or more episodes of vomiting
  - Older than 65 yr
- Medium risk factors
  - Amnesia before impact of ≥30 min
  - Dangerous mechanism (pedestrian struck by motor vehicle, occupant ejected from vehicle, fall from ≥3 ft or ≥5 stairs)

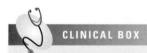

CLINICAL BOX

Presentation of ↑ ICP

- Headache
- Nausea, vomiting
- ↓ Level of consciousness
- Papilledema

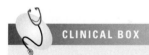

CLINICAL BOX

Shaken Baby Syndrome

Owing to the violent shaking of infant's body or head → acceleration–deceleration injury and cervical whiplash

Suspect with subdural hematomas + retinal hemorrhages

CLINICAL BOX

Skull Fractures

Skull fractures significantly ↑ the probability of an intracranial lesion

Signs of Basilar Skull Fracture

- Battle's sign: postauricular ecchymosis
- Raccoon eyes
- CSF rhinorrhea or otorrhea
- Hemotympanum or laceration of the external auditory canal

Determination of Brain Death

To be able to declare a patient neurologically dead, one must be an independently practicing physician with skill and experience in severe brain injury and neurologic death (typically performed by NSx, anesthesia, or critical care practitioners).

Minimum Criteria for Neurologic Death

- Absence of clinical neurologic function in the presence of a known, irreversible proximate cause. Requires definite clinical or neuroimaging evidence.
  or
- Patient is in a deep, unresponsive coma with an absence of both spontaneous movement and movement originating in the CNS (e.g., CN function, motor responses to pain, seizures, decorticate, and decerebrate posturing). Spinal reflexes may persist!

Confounding Factors

- Unresuscitated shock
- Hypothermia—a core temperature <34°C in adults
- Severe metabolic disorder—may be causing a potentially reversible coma
- Peripheral nerve/muscle dysfunction/neuromuscular blockade—may account for the lack of response to painful stimuli
- Clinically significant drug intoxications—EtOH, barbiturates, sedatives, and so on

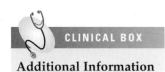

Confounding factors should always be considered and, if present, reversed before determination of neurologic death can be made.

CLINICAL BOX

Diagnostic Tests in Determining Brain Death

- Apnea test—preoxygenate the patient; discontinue mechanical ventilation but deliver 100% O_2 through ETT. Observe for ventilatory effort. Test is complete when: ABGs show pH $\leq$ 7.28, $PaCO_2$ $\geq$60 mm Hg, and a $PaCO_2$ $\geq$20 mm Hg from baseline
- Assess brainstem reflexes—gag and cough, pupillary constriction, corneal reflex, and vestibulo-ocular reflex should all be absent
- Ancillary tests—four-vessel cerebral angiogram or radionucleotide CBF imaging can be done for confirmation

PRINCIPLES OF ORGAN DONATION

- If a patient is a candidate for organ donation, practitioners who are members of the organ donation team are not permitted to participate in the determination of brain death.
- When a death has occurred or is considered imminent, the organ donation team within the hospital/facility should be notified immediately.
- An assessment of the patients' suitability to be an organ donor must be performed, and includes investigation for potentially transferable infections and malignancies.
- Importantly, the final decision to donate organs or tissues is made by the patient, or the SDM if the patient was unable to express his/her wishes.
- Decisions must be made free of coercion and in open consultation with the treating physician and/or organ donation team member.

CLINICAL BOX

Additional Information on Organ Donation

www.ccdt.ca

www.giftoflife.on.ca

PERIPHERAL NERVE INJURY

RATIONALE

- Peripheral nerve injuries commonly occur in combination with other traumatic injuries and may go unrecognized.
- Assessment requires knowledge of the distribution of the peripheral nerves and types of nerve injury.

APPLIED SCIENTIFIC CONCEPTS

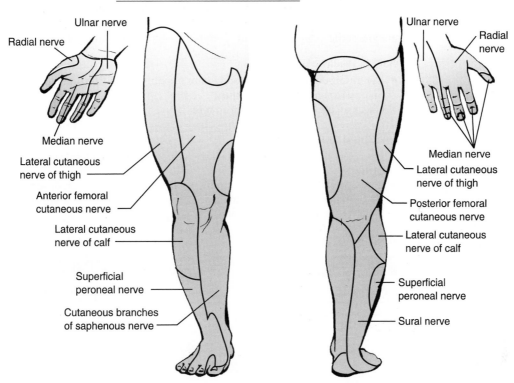

Figure 5.17 Sensory distribution of peripheral nerves: anterior and posterior. See Chapter 5, section on Spinal Trauma for the major dermatomes. Image modified from *Bates' Guide to Physical Examination and History Taking*, 8th ed.

CAUSAL CONDITIONS

Table **5.31**	**Causes and Types of Peripheral Nerve Injury**		
Etiology	**Contusion**	**Compression/Stretch**	**Laceration**
Common mechanisms	Sport-related "burner"/"stinger"	Fractures and dislocations	Penetrating trauma and open fractures
Nerve injury	Neurapraxia	Axonotmesis	Neurotmesis
Neural damage	Disruption of impulse transmission; demyelinization of the axon sheath	Injury to the nerve fibers; Wallerian degeneration of axons; neural sheath remains intact	Severing of the nerve, including the neural sheath
Clinical presentation	Transient paralysis; may have minimal sensory loss	Complete loss of nerve function (sensory, motor, and autonomic)	Complete loss of nerve function (sensory, motor, and autonomic)

⚛ ASC Box

Seddon's Classification

Grade 1—neurapraxia

Grade 2—axonotmesis

Grade 3—neurotmesis

APPROACH

PERTINENT HX

- Mechanism of injury suggests possible site of injury (e.g., spinal vs. peripheral).
- Gradual onset of sensory/motor Sx suggests chronic neurodegeneration, neuromuscular junction disease, or myopathy.

GENERAL INSPECTION

- Inspect for dislocations, fractures, penetrating traumas, compartment syndrome, and other causes of peripheral nerve injury.

Assess for compartment syndrome

LOCALIZE THE LESION

- Map the sensory and motor Sx. Do deficits follow a peripheral nerve or dermatomal/myotomal pattern?
- Symmetric Sx make traumatic peripheral nerve injury unlikely.

ASSESS INJURY SEVERITY

- Determine degree of sensory and motor impairment. Do the findings suggest neurapraxia or a more significant nerve injury?
- Check all appropriate pulses, cap refill

INVESTIGATIONS

- If suspect orthopedic or spinal injury, perform appropriate investigations (e.g., XR, CT, MRI).
- If an open wound, carefully examine for laceration/transaction of surrounding nerves.
- If closed injury, carefully document degree of sensory and motor impairment and regions affected. No immediate specialized investigations.

RX

Table **5.32**	**Rx and Mechanism of Recovery for Nerve Injuries**	
Injury	**Rx**	**Mechanism of Recovery**
Neurapraxia	Watchful waiting; serial follow-up until full return of nerve function	Remyelinization occurs, typically within 1 mo
Axonotmesis	Watchful waiting; 2° surgical repair can be performed months postinjury if axonal regrowth fails to occur	Axon regrows 1 mm/d; Function recovers in order of innervation
Neurotmesis	If obvious laceration, primary surgical repair with approximation of neural sheath ends; Otherwise 2° surgical repair	Spontaneous healing is impossible; Surgical repair is necessary and healing is always imperfect

CLINICAL BOX

Special Investigations:

- EMG: done at least 2 wk postinjury in order to detect the presence of Wallerian degeneration
- Nerve conduction studies: used to test the function of large sensory and motor nerves

CLINICAL BOX

Differential Dx of TBI

Metabolic	DM, uremia, nutritional deficiencies
Infectious	HIV, syphillis, lyme disease
Nervous	Spinal cord lesion, plexopathy, Guillain-Barre, carpal tunnel, nerve entrapment, ataxia
Toxic	Lead, pesticides, CO

SKIN WOUNDS/REGIONAL ANESTHESIA

CAUSAL CONDITIONS

- Lacerations
- Avulsions
- Puncture wounds
  - Bite wounds (human, domestic/nondomestic animal
  - Other (knife, needles, missiles)
- Crush injuries (avulsions, bites, and crush injuries are usually "untidy" widespread tissue damage, severe or prolonged contamination)

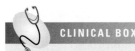

Scarring

It is important to tell patients that **all** wounds through the dermis will scar. Certain factors can affect wound healing and optimize scar formation.

Host factors that influence wound healing include immunosuppressive conditions (DM, HIV), drug use (chronic steroids), smoking, keloid formation, and ability to keep wound clean and dry.

Wounds requiring special attention:

- Heavily contaminated with soil, dirt, and fecal material
- Crush injuries with significant tissue loss/necrosis
- Immunocompromised host
- Injuries to tendon, nerve, and blood vessels
- Underlying fractures, joints
- Animal bites from humans, cats, and dogs

APPROACH TO PATIENT WITH SKIN WOUND

See also Bites, Animal/Insects

Hx

- Mechanism of injury, timing (most wounds can be closed <12 h from injury, facial lacerations up to 24 h safely without infection)
- Elicit Td status
- Human bites: HIV, HBV/HCV status of individuals
- Animal bites: type of animal, provoked versus unprovoked attack, rabies status (if known)

P/E

- Note proximity of tendons, blood vessels, nerves, or underlying joints
- Look for FBs
- Note the presence of more than one wound
- Search for signs of infection: local skin Δs such as erythema, warmth, excessive pain, purulent drainage, or systemic features such as fever/chills

INVESTIGATIONS

- Consider XR to search for radiopaque FBs or possible underlying bone lesions (fracture, joint penetration, osteomyelitis in delayed or late presentation of deep wound)
- Consider wound culturing if there is systemic infection present (high fever, chills, cellulitis locally, +/− pus drainage from wound)

RX

6 Cs of Wound Closure

1. **Cold** (anesthesia). Topical (LET, EMLA) or infiltrated (lidocaine, bupivacaine) anesthetic used for virtually all wound closures. Decrease pain associated with local anesthetic by using 25- to 27-gauge needle with slow rate of infiltration, and entering the wound margins versus intact skin outside of wound
2. **Clean.** Wound itself should be cleaned with N/S or tap water. The key to preventing infection is "irrigation, irrigation, irrigation!" Skin around the wound should be cleaned with chlorhexidine or equivalent. Do not put in wound because of damage to tissue edges (may cause necrosis and impaired wound healing)
3. **Cut.** If indicated, debride heavily contaminated and/or necrotic tissue from wound
4. **Closure**
5. **Cover.** Apply sterile dressing +/− topical Abx prn
6. **Care.** Inform patients of local and systemic signs of infection, how to care for their sutures/staples/glue/skin tape, and instructions on follow-up for when sutures and so on should be removed

Types of Wound Closure

Primary Closure

Wound is closed immediately. It is used for uncomplicated skin lacerations in which the risk of infection is very low. Typically these are uncontaminated, simple lacerations that present within 12 h to the ED (or up to 24 h for facial/scalp lacerations). Wounds that should not be closed primarily include puncture wounds, hand bites, extensive crush injuries, and those requiring extensive debridement.

2° Closure

Wound is left open and allowed to heal by granulation and contraction. It is preferred if there is significant risk of infection, or the wound cannot be adequately explored or irrigated. The wound is left open to allow for possible drainage of purulent material. It may be used only in small wounds where cosmesis is not a significant factor, as this method tends to leave a large scar.

Delayed Primary Closure

Wound is left open, typically for 3 to 5 d, followed by closure. It is reserved for wounds that pose a significant risk of infection, but which require closure for cosmesis, or those

EPI Use

- Allows for hemostasis, but may ↑ the risk of infection
- Traditionally never used in areas with terminal blood supply (i.e., lacerations to "fingers, toes, penis, ears, and nose")

Maximum doses of common anesthetic agents:

- **Lidocaine** 5 mg/kg
- **Lidocaine + EPI** 7 mg/kg
- **Bupivacaine** 2 mg/kg
- **Bupivacaine + EPI** 3 mg/kg

Suture Material

Absorbable: surgical or chromic gut, polyglactin (Vicryl), polyglycolic acid (Dexon)

Nonabsorbable: silk and monofilament synthetic alternatives such as nylon (Ethilon) or polypropylene (Prolene)

Anatomic Location and Suture Size

Scalp	4–0
Face	5–0 to 6–0
Hands, feet	5–0
Trunk, back	3–0 to 4–0
Arms, legs	4–0 to 5–0

Suture Closure Techniques

1. Simple interrupted
2. Continuous
3. Horizontal mattress
4. Vertical mattress
5. Deep dermal

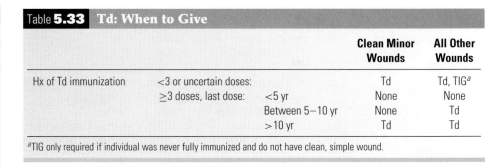

Table 5.33 Td: When to Give

			Clean Minor Wounds	All Other Wounds
Hx of Td immunization	<3 or uncertain doses:		Td	Td, TIG[a]
	≥3 doses, last dose:	<5 yr	None	None
		Between 5–10 yr	None	Td
		>10 yr	Td	Td

[a]TIG only required if individual was never fully immunized and do not have clean, simple wound.

with a significant amount of tension. Typically they are cleaned thoroughly, debrided prn, and an antimicrobial mesh (e.g., Bactigras) is placed over the wound for 3 to 5 days to see if purulent material is present. If none is present, the wound may be closed as above.

Methods of Wound Closure

- Suture—traditional method of closure with very good approximation and cosmetic results. There are multiple suture techniques and materials to approximate a wide variety of wounds (e.g., high vs. low tension, superficial vs. deep).
- Staples—often used in low-tension wounds in noncosmetic locations such as the scalp, or to achieve quick hemostasis or closure in trauma situation.
- Glue—useful only if wound is well-approximated. Has antimicrobial properties; easy to use.
- Skin tape—least effective for high-tension wounds, but rapid application and good closure of simple, nongaping wounds.

RX AFTER WOUND CLOSURE

Consider immunization against:

1. Td
2. Rabies (see Bites, Animal/Insects)
3. Prophylactic Abx for:
   - Deep puncture wounds of the hands or feet
   - Delay in irrigation and debridement
   - Heavily contaminated wounds and those contaminated with pus, saliva, or vaginal secretions
   - Immunocompromised host or presence of prosthetic joints
   - High-risk animal bites and all cat bites (see next section)

TAKE HOME POINTS

1. All skin wounds through the dermis will leave a scar! It is important to notify the patient and try to minimize scar formation.
2. Infection is the main complication of skin wounds and can be prevented in most cases.
3. Td status should be obtained and documented for any skin wound you encounter in the ED.
4. Rabies should be a consideration in all animal bites; Abx should be given to high-risk wounds.

Ten (easy) steps to prevent infection

1. Irrigation!
2. Irrigation!
3. Irrigation!
4. Chlorhexidine around edges
5. Sterile technique
6. Debridement (if indicated)
7. Removal of FBs
8. Wound approximation
9. Abx prophylaxis (if indicated)
10. Follow-up care

SPINAL TRAUMA

EPIDEMIOLOGY

- Most common cause of SCI is MVAs, falls, sports-related injuries, or weapons/assault
- M:F = 4:1
- Peak age for SCI is 35 yr

CAUSAL CONDITIONS

1. Trauma (fracture dislocation of vertebral column, penetration injury)
2. Acute disc rupture
3. Ruptured arteriovenous malformation
4. Spontaneous epidural hematoma

TYPES OF INJURY

- Complete—loss of sensory and motor function below spinal level. Complete paralysis of Resp muscles below level must be considered. Prognosis = poor if no motor or sensory function recovered after 24 to 48 h (spinal shock)
- Incomplete—some preservation of sensory or motor function below the lesion site. Resp muscles below lesion also affected variable.

  Generally, three types of incomplete SCI:

1. Anterior cord—no motor, no pain/temperature sensation, but preserved vibration/proprioception/touch functions. Mechanism: hyperflexion, anterior spinal artery compromise, or disc herniation
2. Central cord—motor deficit > sensory loss (variable), with arms > legs affected. Mechanism: hyperextension (patients with spinal stenosis 2° RA, OA, AS)
3. Brown-Sequard—ipsilateral motor deficit with loss of vibration/proprioception/touch sensation and contralateral loss of pain/temperature sensation. Mechanism: hemisection of cord (penetrating trauma, blunt injury)

APPROACH

In prehospital care, all trauma patients should be immobilized (spinal board + hard collar).

HX AND P/E (OFTEN COMBINED)

- ABCs are most important
- Vital signs—look for signs of shock: hypovolemic shock (↑HR with ↓BP) or neurogenic shock (↓ HR with ↓ BP)
- Hx—include mechanism of injury (flexion, extension, rotation, axial loading, penetrating), function, LOC
- Spinal level
  - Determine level of lesion, complete versus incomplete and perform full neurologic exam (see Figure 5.18 and Table 5.34)
  - Document early and reassess for improvement/deterioration
  - Examination of motor power in arms and legs, sensation, superficial reflexes, and DTRs
  - Make sure to check for sacral sparing or other subtle signs of incomplete SCI
- Exposure—log roll with C-, T-, L-precautions prn. Check rectum for tone, masses, and blood

CLINICAL BOX

Prognosis of incomplete SCI:
Central cord > Brown-Sequard > anterior cord

CLINICAL BOX

Spinal Injury Prevention

Primary prevention is the key: targeting high-risk groups is most effective, such as hockey players (checking from behind), swimmers (hazards of shallow water diving), and skiers (loss of control)

2° (prehospital care) includes immobilization with hard collar and spine board in all suspected injuries; attention to airway; routine trauma procedures

CLINICAL BOX

Immobilization Technique

- Immobilization takes place with hard collar + head supports + long board
- Four people needed to maintain immobilization while logrolling:
  1. For in-line immobilization of H&N
  2. Torso (including pelvis and hips)
  3. Pelvis and legs
  4. Leader directing logroll + removal/splinting of long board

C3,4,5 keep your patient alive

CLINICAL BOX

Special Airway Considerations

- C-spine precautions, C-spine precautions, C-spine precautions!
- Low threshold for intubation. Consider threats to airway as in all other causes of trauma (head injury, facial fracture, inhalation injury, intoxication)
- In-line stabilization + jaw thrust for intubation

SPECIAL BREATHING CONSIDERATIONS

- Cephalad injury ≫ caudal injury for Resp complications. Complete injury has worst effect than incomplete injury, as there is some preservation of ventilation in the latter.
- Injury to C1-3—often complete Resp failure. Frequently causes death at the scene 2° to apnea. Requires mechanical ventilation indefinitely.
- Injury to C3-5—variable Resp paralysis with lesions closer to C3 resulting in greater potential for failure.
- Injury to C5-8—spontaneous breathing intact. Patients may require ventilatory support postinjury, but recover fully.
- Intercostal muscle paralysis leads to paradoxical breathing (inward during inspiration).
- Abdominal muscle paralysis leads to ↑ abdominal compliance and ↓ expansion of lower rib cage by diaphragm.
- Quadriplegic patients have blunted response to dyspnea and display abnormally small ↑ in ventilatory drive in setting of hypercapnia.

IMAGING

- Trauma trio often needed: C-spine, CXR, and pelvic XR. Consider adding T, L spines (see side panel for indications). Upright films contraindicated in potential spine injury.

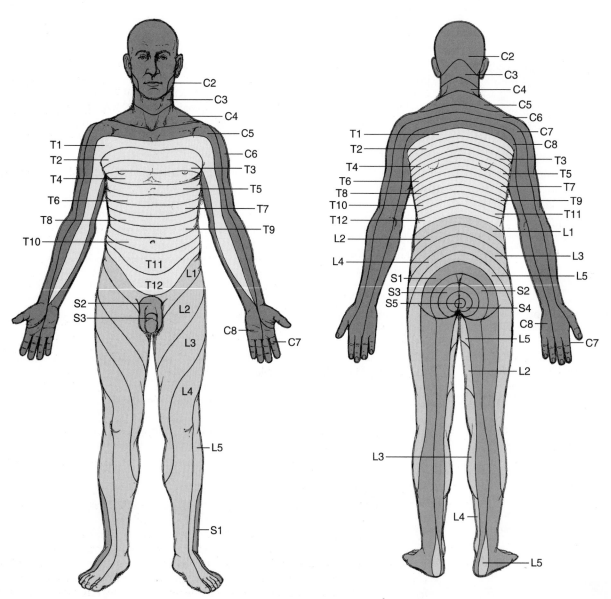

Figure 5.18 Determination of spinal level. Image excerpted from *The Clinical Practice of Emergency Medicine*, 3rd ed.

Table **5.34**	Determination of Spinal Level		
Level	**Sensory**	**Motor**	**Reflex (Type[a])**
C2,3,4	Cape distribution around neck	Intact diaphragm breathing	None
C5	Lateral aspect of arm, just below deltoid	Abduction of shoulder	Biceps (D)
C6	Thumb	Flexion at elbow	Brachioradialis (D)
C7	Volar tip, middle finger	Extension at elbow	Triceps (D)
C8	Volar tip, little finger	Finger flexion	—
T1	—	Finger abduction	—
T2-10	Intercostal space below rib T2-10	Intercostal muscles	Abdominal (S) for T8-12
L1	Lateral aspect hip	Hip flexion	None
L2	Medial inner thigh		
L3	Lateral aspect knee	Knee extension	Patellar tendon (D)
L4	Medial calf	Dorsiflexion of foot	
L5	Webspace between first and secondtoes	Dorsiflexion great toe	Hamstring
S1	Lateral aspect of foot	Planter flexion of foot	Ankle jerk (D), Babinski (S)
S2,3,4	Perianal		Anal (S)

[a] D, deep tendon reflex; S, superficial tendon reflex.

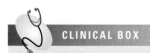

CLINICAL BOX

When to consider T, L-spine injury: "**SPPINE**"

Step-off

Palpable tenderness, **P**araspinal bruising

Injury to C-spine

Neurologic deficit

Elderly

- In the awake, alert, and low risk patient, the CCR has been developed to determine the need for C-spine radiography.
- CT may be needed to better image spine fractures.
- Consider CT head if suspect ICB.
- Consider FAST or CT Abdo (low threshold because sensory deficits may mask intra-abdominal injury).

Tx

- Airway—ETT for compromised airway
- Breathing—use of chest tubes prn
- Circulation—shock may require ++ fluids +/− vasopressors in the case of spinal shock
- Foley to monitor U/O or decompress bladder if the spinal injury/shock present
- Pain meds—narcotics and NSAIDs commonly used to control pain and ↓ inflammation
- Use of steroids controversial (see subsequent text)
- Consult NSx for definitive Tx

Corticosteroids in Spinal Trauma
- Issue: Edema that may develop in acute spinal cord trauma is thought to contribute to neurologic deficits. Steroids thought to prevent this swelling through anti-inflammatory properties.
- Evidence: Three randomized, double-blind, prospective, multicenter trials by NASCIS group. MPSS effects on neurologic outcome of SCI patients was evaluated. All three trials found no significant difference between those who received steroids and those who did not. *Post hoc* subgroup analyses of the data from NASCIS trials II and III found a significant benefit of MPSS within 8 h of injury and guidelines were produced based on these data. A follow-up study with questionable methodology did demonstrate a positive effect of MPSS administered within the first 8 h in spinal cord injuries.
- Recommendation by CAEP: There is insufficient evidence to support the use of high-dose MPSS in SCI. Currently, there is only level III evidence and the use of MPSS in SCI remains only a Rx "option" and should be undertaken • only in consultation with a neurosurgical service.

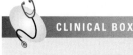

CLINICAL BOX

Organizations to help patients/families:

Canadian Paraplegic Association (http://www.canparaplegic .org/en/)

National Spinal Cord Injury Association (http://www.spinalcord .org/)

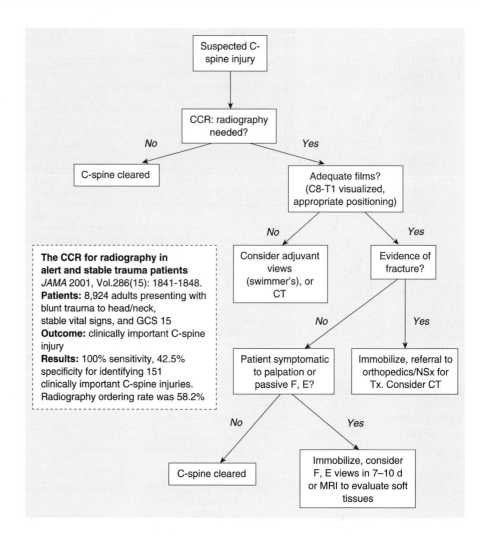

Figure 5.19 Clearing the C-spine. **Clinical note:** It is important to remove patient from spine board as soon as possible to prevent complications such as decubitus ulcers, aspiration, and airway compromise.

URINARY TRACT INJURIES

EPIDEMIOLOGY

- Up to 10% of trauma patients have associated injuries to kidney or collecting system
- Upper tract = kidney and ureters
- Lower tract = bladder, posterior and anterior urethra

Table **5.35**	**Mechanism and P/E Features of Urinary Tract Injuries**			
	Upper Tract Injuries		**Lower Tract Injuries**	
	Kidneys	**Ureters**	**Bladder**	**Urethra**
Mechanism	• High energy, blunt forces to back or flank • Fall from height • Deceleration injury • Penetrating trauma		• Bladder and posterior urethral injuries are commonly associated with pelvic fractures (rami or pubic symphyseal disruption); they may also occur in the setting of penetrating trauma and should be suspected with any abdominal trauma • Anterior urethral injuries are associated with external forces (straddle injury, bicycle riding, monkey bars); consider sexual abuse	
P/E	• Hematuria, ecchymoses, tenderness, or masses, open wounds in anatomic proximity to kidney and ureters, or associated lumbar, lower thoracic, or lower rib fractures		• Pelvic fractures, hematuria (gross), suprapubic tenderness, abdominal distension, open wounds near bladder	• Blood at urethral meatus, penile or scrotal hematoma, high-riding prostate, lacerations or contusions to testicles or vaginal introitus • Elicit Hx about voiding difficulty or incontinence, and ED

Important: deal with life-threatening injuries first—GU injuries often discovered later when patient is stable

CLINICAL BOX

Contraindications to catheter insertion

- Blood at meatus
- Hematomas/lacerations on external genitalia
- High-riding prostate
- Hx of difficulty voiding

The above signs may be associated with a partial urethral tear.

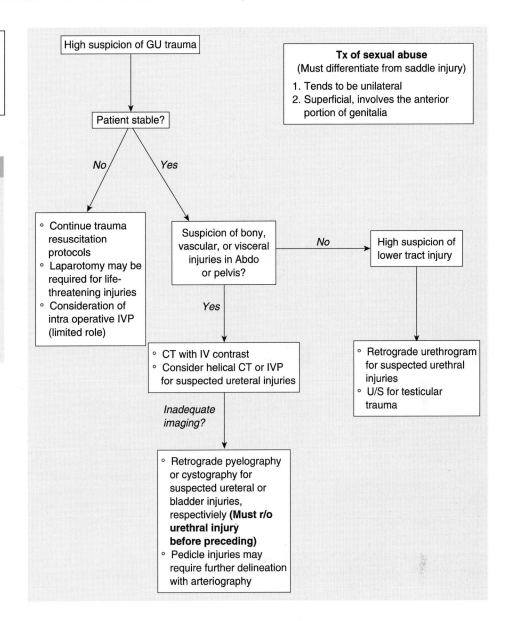

High suspicion of GU trauma

Patient stable?

No → **Continue trauma resuscitation protocols** · **Laparotomy may be required for life-threatening injuries** · **Consideration of intra operative IVP (limited role)**

Yes → **Suspicion of bony, vascular, or visceral injuries in Abdo or pelvis?**

No → **High suspicion of lower tract injury**

Yes → **CT with IV contrast** · **Consider helical CT or IVP for suspected ureteral injuries**

Inadequate imaging?

→ **Retrograde pyelography or cystography for suspected ureteral or bladder injuries, respectively (Must r/o urethral injury before preceding)** · **Pedicle injuries may require further delineation with arteriography**

High suspicion of lower tract injury → **Retrograde urethrogram for suspected urethral injuries** · **U/S for testicular trauma**

Tx of sexual abuse
(Must differentiate from saddle injury)
1. Tends to be unilateral
2. Superficial, involves the anterior portion of genitalia

Figure 5.20 Approach to imaging the urinary tract in trauma Features of sexual abuse (must differentiate from saddle injury)
1. Tends to be unilateral
2. Superficial involves the anterior portion of genitalia

Table **5.36**	Tx of Urethral Injuries				
Anterior, Contusion	**Anterior, Partial Tear**	**Anterior, Complete Tear**	**Posterior, Partial Tear**	**Posterior, Complete Tear**
• Conservative; +/− urethral catheter	• Urethral catheter with Abx • Alternatively, can use suprapubic cystotomy	• Surgical repair	• Urethral or suprapubic drainage	• Surgery + suprapubic drainage

VASCULAR INJURY

RATIONALE

- Vascular injuries are increasingly common.
- One needs to have a high index of suspicion for vascular injury, particularly in the setting of orthopedic trauma.

CAUSAL CONDITIONS

- Laceration
- Contusion/spasm
- Compression
- FB

APPROACH

- There is a high mortality associated with trauma to the major vessels and most patients do not reach definitive care. Therefore, most vascular injuries seen in hospital are peripheral vascular traumas.
- It is vital to quickly identify and treat vascular injuries as they carry significant short- and long-term consequences (hemorrhagic shock, distal limb ischemia, thromboembolic events, true and false aneurysms, and fistulae formation).
- Some vascular injuries may be subclinical on initial assessment. Therefore, serial exam in the at-risk patient is necessary.
- Arterial injuries can be divided into two large clinical categories: occlusive or hemorrhagic. Importantly, injuries that involve arterial transection have both occlusive and hemorrhagic features.

The two common vascular emergencies in the trauma patient are arterial injury and compartment syndrome.

CLINICAL BOX

Warm Ischemia

Six hours after sustaining a vascular injury, 10% of patients will have irreversible neuromuscular injury. After 12 h, the incidence is 90%.

Table **5.37**	Occlusive versus Hemorrhagic Arterial Injuries	
	Occlusive Injury	**Hemorrhagic Injury**
Hx	• Penetrating wound within 1 cm of a neurovascular bundle • Obvious arterial transection • Peripheral neuropathy • Hx of stasis, previous limb trauma, intermittent claudication, or other RF for arterial thrombosis or embolism	• Orthopedic injuries, particularly knee dislocation and fractures
P/E		
Vitals	Normal, unless other concomitant injuries or arterial transection	Hemodynamically unstable
Hematoma	May be present	Present, pulsatile if arterial source
Pulse deficit	Present, quantify with an API	May be present if arterial transection
Distal ischemia	Present if lesion is fully occlusive	May be present if arterial compromise

ARTERIAL INJURY

Hx

See Historical Features listed in Table 5.37.

P/E
- Hemodynamically unstable
- Pulsatile bleeding/hematoma or any of the 6 P's of arterial insufficiency carries a >90% incidence of arterial injury
- Capillary refill >3 s in the presence of other physical findings of arterial injury
- Isolated peripheral nerve injury (as 50% of peripheral vascular injuries have an associated nerve injury)

COMPARTMENT SYNDROME

Hx
- Crush or long bone injury; unrecognized/uncontrolled bleeding into a fascial compartment; repair + reperfusion of vascular injury; coagulopathy; burns; orthopedic surgery; binding casts/dressings

CLINICAL BOX

6 Ps of Arterial Insufficiency

In order of severity:

Pain

Pallor

Polar (cold)

Pulseless

Paresthesias

Paralysis

Vascular Injury Dx Test

- CBC, if hemorrhage
- Plain XR (fractures, FB)
- U/S +/− duplex
- Handheld Doppler
- API
- Angiography
- Surgical exploration

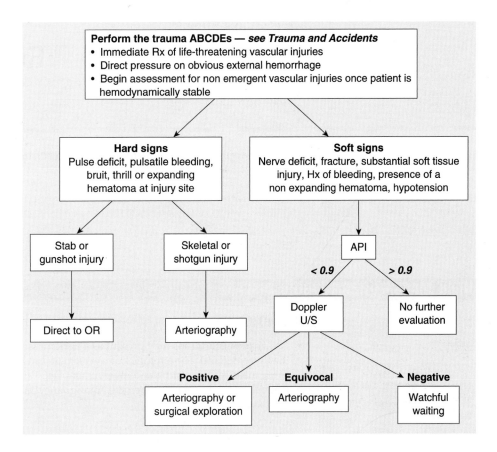

Figure 5.21 Initial assessment for vascular injury.

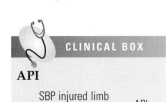

API

$$\frac{\text{SBP injured limb}}{\text{SBP unaffected limb}} = \text{API}$$

- Measure by placing BP cuff proximal to injury and by placing Doppler distally to determine sBP
- API <0.90 requires further investigation (angiography)

Risks of Tourniquets and Clamps

- Vessel clamping can → crushing of nearby nerves
- Tourniquets → ↑ compartment pressure; ↑ risk of venous thrombi 2° to stasis

P/E
- Pain out of proportion to injuries or findings on P/E
- Pain on passive stretch or active flexion of the compartment in question
- Paresthesias in the distal peripheral nerves that cross the compartment
- Patients may not exhibit the 6 P's of arterial insufficiency
- Compartment pressure >30 mm Hg or within 30 mm Hg of patients' dBP

Tx of Arterial Bleeding
1. Apply direct pressure to the site of bleeding. Minimize the use of tourniquets and avoid the use of clamps
2. If suspect bleeding from a noncompressible site but no signs of poor perfusion, consider limiting the amount of IV fluid given (to prevent dislodging thrombus, hemodilution, and coagulopathy)
3. Serial Hb; G&S/cross-match
4. Definitive Tx involves surgical reanastomosis + flushing of the distal circulation with heparin (systemic anticoagulation is discouraged)
5. Preoperative mannitol and broad-spectrum Abx are used to prevent compartment syndrome and infection respectively
6. Serial compartment pressures following reperfusion to recognize early compartment syndrome

Disposition
- Vascular surgery should be consulted as soon as a vascular injury requiring surgical Tx is identified.
- If vascular surgery is not present in the current medical facility and there exists a high index of suspicion for vascular injury, do not delay patient transfer to perform diagnostic investigations.
- Patients with Sx of vascular injury/compromise and those at risk of limb ischemia or compartment syndrome should be admitted for observation.

CHAPTER 6

Endocrinology

Daphne Yau, Dr. Jeremy Gilbert, and Dr. René Wong

NECK MASS/GOITER/THYROID DISEASE

DEFINITION

- A variety of conditions may present as a neck mass; **these may or may not be related to the thyroid gland**. The etiologies of a neck mass can be grouped according to the location of the mass, and thyroid gland involvement (see Table 6.1).
- Regardless of thyroid involvement, **malignancy must be ruled out** when assessing a neck mass.

APPLIED SCIENTIFIC CONCEPTS

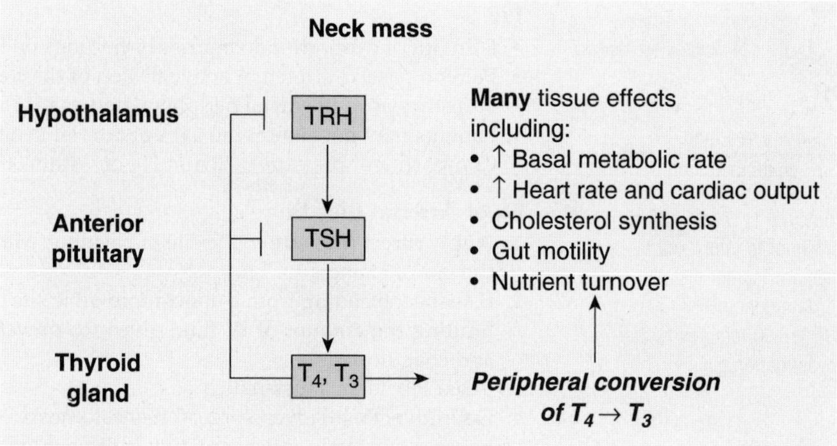

Figure 6.1 The hypothalamic-pituitary-thyroid axis. Thyroid hormone secretion is a prototypical example of the classic hypothalamic-anterior pituitary-peripheral gland axis. **T_4 is the major secretory product and T_3 is the more bioactive form. Conversion of T_4 to T_3 occurs at the pituitary thyroid and other tissues. T_4 and T_3 exert feedback inhibition on TRH and TSH secretion.**

ASC Box
Thyroid Hormone Synthesis
Iodine is **essential** for thyroid hormone synthesis:

- Dietary iodine is converted to iodide and taken up by the thyroid gland.
- Thyroid peroxidase uses the iodide to iodinate the protein thyroglobulin within follicular cells to produce T_3 and T_4.

CAUSAL CONDITIONS

See Table 6.1

APPROACH

DIAGNOSIS

General

- The key to evaluating a neck mass is to **determine if the thyroid gland is involved, and to exclude malignancy** for both thyroid and nonthyroid causes (Table 6.1, Fig. 6.2).
- Age can be used to narrow the differential diagnosis. For instance, benign neoplasms, such as hemangiomas and lymphangiomas, are much more common in infants and children.

Table **6.1**	**Differential Diagnosis of Neck Mass**
Mechanism	**Differential Diagnosis**
Midline (chin to sternal notch)	
Thyroid	Thyroid cancer
Within thyroid	
Associated with hyperthyroidism	Graves disease, toxic multinodular goitre, toxic adenoma, subacute thyroiditis, iodine-induced
Associated with Hypothyroidism	Hashimoto thyroiditis, postablative, postpartum thyroiditis, iodine deficiency, acute thyroiditis
Nonthyroid	Thyroglossal cyst, dermoid cyst
Lateral	
Cystic	Branchial cysts
Noncystic	Benign lymphadenopathy: reactive, inflammatory
	Malignancy: lymphoma, rhabdomyosarcoma, neuroblastoma, cancers of the thyroid or salivary glands, nasopharyngeal cancer
	Benign neoplasm: hemangioma[a], lymphangioma[a], cystic hygroma[a].
Congenital	Benign or malignant neoplasm: teratoma, neuroblastoma

[a] **Seen predominantly in infants and children**

Malignancy

- Certain historical elements, as well as particular signs and symptoms, ↑ the likelihood of malignancy. For thyroid malignancy, these are listed in Clinical box Thyroid Malignancy. Suspicious nodules should be evaluated by FNAB as it has a high sensitivity for detecting thyroid cancer (Clinical box Thyroid Imaging).
- For other types of cancer, the clinical findings depend on the particular malignancy, but may include lymphadenopathy, symptoms due to compression or infiltration of adjacent structure, and systemic symptoms such as fever, chills, and night sweats (see Chapter 15).

Thyroid Disease

- The presence of thyroid disease may be apparent from the clinical findings (Clinical boxes Hyperthyroidism: Signs and Symptoms and Hypothyroidism: Signs and Symptoms). A **goiter** is an enlarged thyroid. Goiter can be classified as diffuse (involves the whole gland) or nodular; associated with autonomous hormone secretion (i.e., toxic); and benign or malignant. Thyroid disease may be present in the absence of a goiter.

 CLINICAL BOX

Thyroid Malignancy

Risk factors
- Personal or family history of thyroid cancer
- History of multiple endocrine neoplasia
- Age: <20 or >60 yr
- Male
- Head and/or neck radiation in childhood or adolescence

Suspicious features
Nodule
- Suspicious features on ultrasound
- Rapid growth
- Hard or firm consistency
- Fixation to adjacent tissues
- Absence of pain or tenderness. **Note however that the presence of pain does not preclude malignancy.**

Other
- Vocal cord paralysis
- Regional, especially cervical, adenopathy

CLINICAL BOX

Hyperthyroidism: Signs and Symptoms

General: nervousness, ↑ sweating/heat intolerance, fatigue, weight loss/gain, weakness, leg swelling, tremor

Skin and hair: skin changes

Eye: upper eyelid retraction, lid lag

H&N: goiter ± autonomous hormone secretion

CVS: palpitations, tachycardia, atrial fibrillation, bruit

Respiratory: dyspnea

GI: hyperdefecation, splenomegaly

GU: ↓ menstrual flow, gynecomastia

Specific to Graves disease

Infiltrative ophthalmopathy

Infiltrative dermopathy

Thyroid bruit

Thyroid acropathy

Vitiligo

Premature hair graying

Note: Thyrotoxicosis is another term describing the manifestations of excess thyroid hormone.

Consider thyroid storm with a sudden change in mental status, fever and tachycardia out of proportion to fever, and GI, cardiac, or CNS symptoms of thyrotoxicosis.

CLINICAL BOX

Hypothyroidism: Signs and Symptoms

General: weakness, lethargy, fatigue, cold intolerance, ↓ sweating, weight gain, anorexia, sleepiness, slow movements

H&N: slow speech, hoarseness, goiter

Skin and hair: dry/coarse/cold skin, coarse hair, hair loss

Eye: periorbital puffiness

CVS: bradycardia, diastolic hypertension

GI: constipation

GU: menstrual problems, sexual dysfunction

CNS: impaired memory, paresthesias, impaired learning

Myxedema coma is a complication of hypothyroidism associated with profound lethargy or coma, hypothermia, bradycardia, and hypotension.

- **Thyroiditis**, inflammation of the thyroid gland, can present with hyperthyroid or hypothyroid symptoms. Any type of thyroiditis may present initially as hyperthyroidism, followed by hypothyroidism and possibly restoration of euthyroid status (see Table 6.2). Acute thyroiditis can present with symptoms and signs of infection, in association with a tender thyroid on palpation.
- **Hashimoto or autoimmune thyroiditis** is the **most common cause of hypothyroidism in North America**. Its prevalence ↑ with age. **Graves disease** is the **most common cause of spontaneous hyperthyroidism in individuals younger than 40 yr of age**. Both are more common in females.
- Many causes of **hyperthyroidism** and **hypothyroidism** exist, a selection of which are listed in Table 6.1.
  - Hyperthyroidism may also arise from production of a thyroid stimulator (e.g., TSH, hCG) in certain disease states, extrathyroid sources of thyroid hormone, and mutations in the thyroid hormone receptor.
  - Hypothyroidism may result from surgery, chemicals (including foods and therapeutic agents), congenital conditions, and disorders of the hypothalamus or pituitary gland.
- If clinical evidence of thyroid involvement is present, thyroid function status should be ascertained, starting with serum TSH levels. If abnormal, T_4 and T_3 levels, and the presence of TAb should be determined (Table 6.2). Imaging investigations such as thyroid scan and high resolution ultrasonography can be used to help clarify the diagnosis (Clinical box Thyroid Imaging).
- These results in the context of the clinical findings will likely pinpoint the cause of the disorder.

Consider screening for hypothyroidism in women anticipating pregnancy or who are pregnant – asymptomatic maternal hypothyroidism can have adverse effects on the developing fetus.

MANAGEMENT

- Treatment of hyperthyroidism and thyroiditis depends on the etiology (Table 6.2), whereas thyroid hormone replacement with **levothyroxine** is the primary type of therapy for hypothyroidism.
- Treatment options for hyperthyroidism include **antithyroid medications (e.g., thionamides), radioiodine therapy** and **surgery** (Clinical box Treatment of Hyperthyroidism).
- A neck mass due to nonthyroid causes should be managed appropriately.

Initiate antithyroid therapy in pregnant patients with symptomatic hyperthyroidism to minimize thyrotoxicosis-induced complications.

| Table **6.2** | Diagnosis (top) and Management (bottom) of Hyperthyroidism and Thyroiditis |

Condition	TSH	T_3, T_4	TAb	RAI Uptake	Notes
Hyperthyroidism					
Graves disease	↓	↑	+	↑	
Toxic adenoma	↓	↑	−	↑	Single nodule
Toxic multinodular goiter	↓	↑	−	↑	Multiple nodules
Iodine-induced/Jod-Basedow effect	↓	↑	−	↓	
Thyroiditis					
Autoimmune (Hashimoto)	↑	↓	+	↓	
Acute	↓	↑	±TAb	None	Extreme pain, evidence of infection, ↑ ESR
Subacute, classic/silent/postpartum	↑	↓	±TAb	None	±Extreme tenderness

Condition	Management
Hyperthyroidism	
Graves disease	Antithyroid medications
Toxic adenoma	RAI therapy; surgery if large, symptomatic nodule
Toxic multinodular goiter	RAI therapy; surgical resection to alleviate or preempt obstructive symptoms
Subacute thyroiditis	See text in the cell below for management of subacute thyroiditis
Iodine-induced/Jod-Basedow effect	Discontinue or reduce iodine load
Thyroiditis	
Autoimmune (Hashimoto)	Levothyroxine therapy; surgery to alleviate symptoms or cosmetic symptoms
Acute	Treat cause of infection; drainage Mild: NSAIDs; severe: glucocorticoids
Subacute, classic	Hypothyroid phase: levothyroxine replacement until TSH levels normalize
Subacute, silent or postpartum	Symptomatic treatment. Hypothyroid phase: levothyroxine replacement until TSH levels normalize

CLINICAL BOX

Thyroid Imaging

Thyroid scan

- Technetium-99 m pertechnetate is concentrated by the thyroid gland and detected by a gamma camera
- Reveals information about the gland's size, shape and location of functional activity
- Uptake can be quantified when performed in conjunction with an uptake assay, usually RAI-123

High resolution ultrasonography

- Differentiates between solid and cystic nodules
- Detects nodule characteristics suspicious for malignancy (e.g., irregular margins, small calcifications)
- Used to guide FNAB

CLINICAL BOX

Treatment of Hyperthyroidism

Antithyroid drugs

(+) Least invasive, with lower risk of permanent hypothyroidism

(−) Lower permanent remission rate (∼33% to 50%)

(−) Propylthiouracil preferred in pregnancy—less risk of fetal goitrous hypothyroidism than methimazole because crosses placenta less readily

(−) Common side effects: rash, pruritis, fever, arthralgias

(−) Rare but potentially fatal adverse reactions: agranulocytosis, hepatitis

RAI

(+) Faster ↓ in thyroid hormone levels

(−) Permanent hypothyroidism likely

(−) Slight risk of thyroid storm after treatment

(−) May precipitate new or ↑ ophthalmopathy

(−) Pregnancy and breastfeeding must be avoided 6 to 12 mo afterward

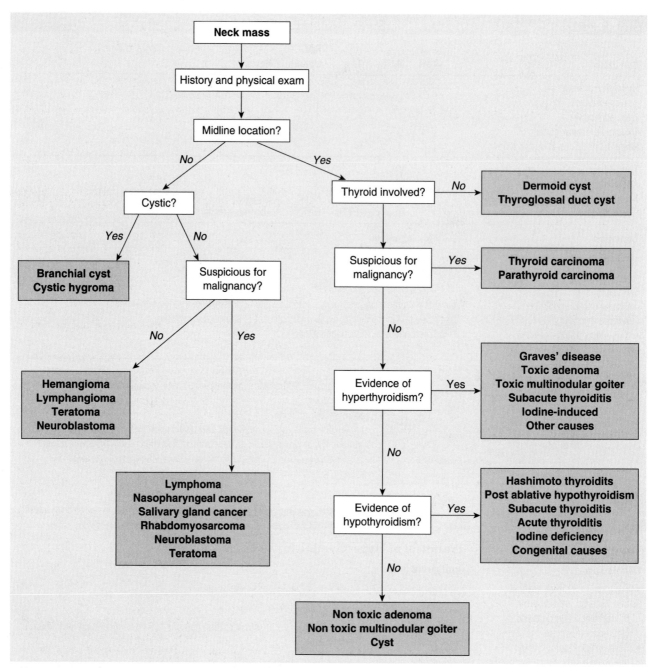

Figure 6.2 Approach to investigating a neck mass.

HYPERGLYCEMIA

DEFINITION

- DM refers to a group of common, heterogeneous disorders sharing the defining feature of hyperglycemia. Perturbations are seen in carbohydrate, lipid and protein metabolism, to the detriment of multiple organ systems. Type 2 DM accounts for 85% to 90% of DM cases.
- While acute metabolic complications can be life-threatening, chronic hyperglycemia also results in significant morbidity and mortality due to macrovascular and microvascular complications. The latter can be significantly reduced by intensive (i.e., near normal) glycemic control. Such control appears to have beneficial effects on macrovascular complications as well.

ASC Box

Glucose Homeostasis

Insulin and glucagon are the key hormones that maintain glucose homeostasis. In response to nutrient ingestion, particularly glucose, the pancreatic β-cell secretes **insulin** in response to a rise in blood glucose. Insulin stimulates glucose uptake into insulin-sensitive tissues, such as skeletal muscle, and inhibits hepatic glucose production causing glucose levels to return to normal. Therefore, defects in the β-cell and/or peripheral insulin-sensitive tissues can cause diabetes.

Glucagon is secreted in response to falling plasma glucose concentrations, and stimulates glycogenolysis, gluconeogenesis, lipolysis and ketogenesis.

APPLIED SCIENTIFIC CONCEPTS

- In **type 1 DM**, an **absolute** insulin deficiency exists due to destruction of the pancreatic β-cells.
- In **type 2 DM**, there is a **relative** insulin deficiency—circulating levels are insufficient to overcome the degree of peripheral insulin resistance. Insulin resistance results from reduced glucose uptake into tissues and reduced inhibition of hepatic glucose production
- Other causes of hyperglycemia are listed in Table 6.3

CAUSAL CONDITIONS

Table **6.3**	**Differential Diagnosis of Hyperglycemia**
Form of DM	**Examples**
Type 1 Autoimmune Idiopathic	
Type 2	
Other types	
Genetic defects in β-cell function or insulin resistance	Insulin receptor gene mutations, maturity-onset diabetes of the young
Other genetic syndromes	Down syndrome, Klinefelter syndrome, Turner syndrome, Huntington disease, Friedreich ataxia, porphyria
Diseases of the exocrine pancreas	Chronic pancreatitis
Endocrine disease	Cushing disease, acromegaly, pheochromocytoma
Drug- or chemical-induced	Glucocorticoids, thiazides, thyroid hormone, phenytoin, β-adrenergic agonists
Infections	Congenital Rubella, Cytomegalovirus, Coxsackie virus
Other uncommon immune-mediated forms	**Stiff-man** syndrome, anti-insulin receptor antibodies
GDM	

Risk Factors for type 2 DM

- High-risk ethnic group (i.e., African, Hispanic, Asian, Aboriginal, Pacific Islander)
- First degree relative with type 2 DM
- BMI >25 **or** central obesity with normal BMI
- Habitual physical inactivity
- Previously identified impaired glucose tolerance or impaired fasting glucose
- Hypertension
- Dyslipidemia (TG >2.82 mmol/L, HDL <0.9 mmol/L)
- History of GDM
- Delivery of an infant >4.0 kg
- Condition associated with insulin resistance (e.g., PCOS)

APPROACH

DIAGNOSIS

- Given the high proportion of undiagnosed cases of type 2 DM, screening using FPG is recommended every 3 yr beginning at age 45; and at younger ages and/or more frequently if risk factors are present (Clinical box Risk Factors for Type 2 DM)
- To diagnose DM, **one of the three criteria listed in Fig. 6.3 must be met on two separate occasions.** The need for a second, confirmation measurement arises from intraindividual variation in glucose levels.
- If untreated, GDM, diabetes occurring during pregnancy, has potentially severe consequences for both mother and fetus. Screening for GDM at 24 to 28 wk in women >25 yr is recommended. If the patient is at high risk (obesity, previous GDM, first-degree relative with DM), she should be screened at the initial obstetric visit.
- Individuals with prediabetes (Clinical box Prediabetes) are at ↑ risk of developing type 2 DM. Lifestyle interventions have been demonstrated to reduce the risk of progression to DM.

MANAGEMENT

- Lifestyle interventions, including education, diet modification, physical activity, and behavioral modifications, are integral to optimal diabetes management. Successful implementation of these strategies often requires a multidisciplinary approach to management.
- To gauge glycemic control, patients should monitor their own blood glucose levels; individual patient characteristics will determine when and how frequently.

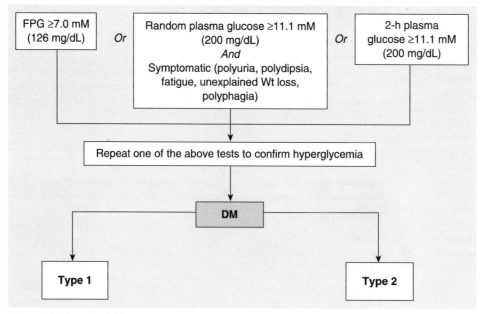

Figure 6.3 Diagnosing DM.

CLINICAL BOX

Prediabetes

- Individuals whose glucose levels do not meet the criteria for diabetes but are nonetheless elevated are considered to have **prediabetes**:
  - **Impaired FPG: 6.1 to 6.9 mmol/L**
  - **Impaired glucose tolerance: 7.8-11.0 mmol/L**

DKA presents with hyperglycemia, hyperketonemia, and metabolic acidosis.

Consider HHS in severe hyperglycemia associated with altered mental status and dehydration.

- HbA1c reflects average blood glucose levels for the previous 2 to 3 mo, and should also be measured every 3 mo to assess glycemic control.
- **Recommended nonpregnant glycemic targets** are as follows:
  - HbA1 C $\leq$7% (<6% if safely achievable)
  - FPG = 4 to 7 mmol/L
  - 2 h PPG = 5 to 10 mmol/L
- Glycemic targets during pregnancy: FPG = 3.8 to 5.2 mmol/L, 2 h PPG = 5.0 to 6.6 mmol/L
- The choice of pharmacologic agents depends on individual patient characteristics (i.e., severity of hyperglycemia, degree of insulin resistance vs. impaired insulin secretion) and preferences (see Table 6.4).
- Insulin preparations are combined to mimic endogenous insulin secretion. A common regimen uses long-acting insulin to control FPG, and rapid-acting preparations with meals to control PPG.

ACUTE COMPLICATIONS

- Acute complications include **DKA, HHS and hypoglycemia**. Hypoglycemia occurs due to insulin excess, while DKA and HHS result from insulin insufficiency. In DKA, insufficiency occurs in the setting of excess counter-regulatory hormones (ASC box Fasting Glucose Homeostasis).
- Diagnosis of these conditions, and treatment of severe hypoglycemia is outlined in Fig. 6.4. For diagnosis and treatment of hypoglycemia, see Hypoglycemia.
- Patients with DKA or HHS should be rehydrated with normal saline, and given insulin bolus and infusion until ketosis has cleared. Electrolytes, particularly K^+, should be replaced as needed. Glucose, electrolytes, osmolality, arterial blood gases, and volume status should be monitored until the patient's condition has stabilized.
- The cause of the metabolic decompensation can often be determined from the history.

CHRONIC COMPLICATIONS

- Chronic complications encompass microvascular (retinopathy, nephropathy, neuropathy) and macrovascular (atherosclerosis, CAD, cerebrovascular disease, peripheral vascular disease) complications. Screening for chronic complications should be performed **at the time of diagnosis in type 2 DM, and for type 1 DM as outlined in Table 6.5.**

Table **6.4**	Pharmacologic Therapy for Diabetes	
Group	**Examples**	**Mechanism**
Insulin secretagogues		
Sulphonylureas	Glyburide, gliclazide, glimepiride	Stimulate insulin secretion
Meglitinides	Nateglinide, repaglinide	Stimulate insulin secretion
Insulin sensitizers		
Biguinides	Metformin	↑ Muscle and liver insulin sensitivity; ↓ hepatic glucose production
Thiazolidinediones	Pioglitazone, rosigliazone	↑ Muscle and adipose tissue insulin sensitivity
Other		
α-Glucosidase inhibitors	Acarbose	Delays intestinal carbohydrate absorption by inhibiting brush border α-glucosidase
Insulin preparations		See ASC box Glucose Homeostasis
Rapid-acting	Insulin lispro, insulin aspart, regular insulin	
Intermediate-acting	NPH insulin	
Long-acting	Insulin glargine, insulin detemir	

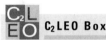

C₂LEO Box

Statutory Reporting Obligations

- Patients with sufficiently severe retinopathy may pose a potential hazard to themselves or others while driving.
- These patients should be advised to stop driving, and must be reported to the Ministry of Transportation (mandated under the **Highway Traffic Act**).
- Similar requirements exist for operation of an airplane or railway equipment.

- Neuropathies can be classified as diffuse (symmetric), focal (asymmetric), or autonomic.
  - Distal symmetric polyneuropathy, a diffuse neuropathy, is the most common form of diabetic neuropathy.
- Focal neuropathies include limb neuropathies (median nerve most commonly affected) and cranial neuropathies involving cranial nerves III or VI. An oculomotor neuropathy typically presents with **ptosis, diplopia, and pupillary sparing**.
- Autonomic neuropathies may present with abnormalities in heart rate and vascular dynamics leading to exercise intolerance, orthostatic hypotension or silent myocardial infarction; gastroparesis, alternating diarrhea and constipation, urinary retention, impotence.
- Primary and secondary prevention strategies for chronic complications include intensive glycemic, BP, and lipid control; lifestyle modification such as smoking cessation and the use of angiotensin-converting enzyme-inhibitors and antiplatelet therapy. Foot care should involve daily foot inspections, appropriate footwear and foot hygiene, as well as early detection and prompt, aggressive treatment of foot injuries and infections.
- The appropriate specialists should be consulted for the screening and/or management of chronic complications as necessitated by the patient's condition. Retinopathy screening, for instance, should be performed by an ophthalmologist.

Table **6.5**	Diagnosis of the Chronic Complications of Diabetes
Complication	**Screening Recommendations**
Microvascular	
Retinopathy	Annual dilated fundoscopic exam by ophthalmologist for nonproliferative and proliferative diabetic retinopathy Type 1 DM: start at 5 yr after diagnosis.
Nephropathy	Annual screening for microalbuminuria: albumin excretion rate = 30–300 mg/24 h on 2/3 samples Type 1 DM: start at 3 yr duration or with the onset of puberty.
Neuropathy	Annual screening for loss of sensitivity at big toes to 10 g monofilament or vibration Type 1 DM: start screening after 5 yr duration or with the onset of puberty.
Macrovascular	Presence of hypertension, dyslipidemia, and/or evidence of atherosclerosis, CAD, cerebrovascular or peripheral vascular disease (see Chapter 6).

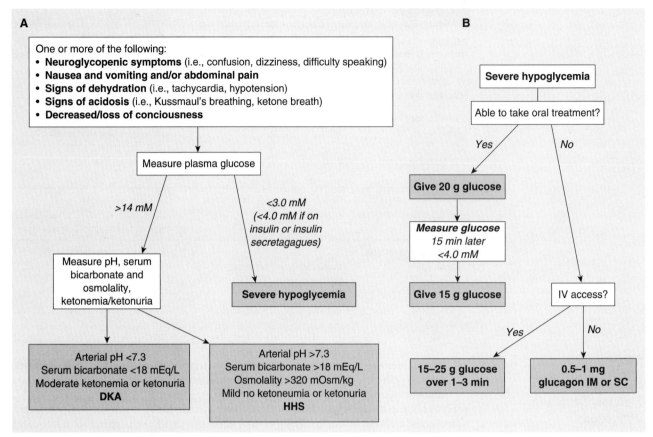

Figure 6.4 Acute complications of DM. **A:** Diagnosis of acute complications. **B:** Treatment of severe hypoglycemia.

HYPOGLYCEMIA

DEFINITION

- The requirement of the body, particularly the brain, for glucose as an energy source renders **hypoglycemia** or low blood glucose an often urgent, potentially life-threatening condition.
- Numerous regulatory factors normally prevent the occurrence of hypoglycemia (ASC box Fasting Glucose Homeostasis).
- Causes differ between adult and younger populations, and can be classified according to whether the I:G is elevated or low.

> ### ASC Box
> #### Fasting Glucose Homeostasis
> Several mechanisms maintain glucose homeostasis in response to falling plasma glucose concentrations:
>
> 1. Insulin suppression
> 2. Glucagon release
> 3. Epinephrine release
> 4. GH and cortisol release (after several hours)
>
> Glucagon, epinephrine, GH and cortisol are known as **counter-regulatory** (i.e., glucose-raising) factors. Glucagon promotes a rise in plasma glucose by simulating glycogenolysis and gluconeogenesis. After an overnight fast, the liver is the predominant source of endogenous glucose production.

CAUSAL CONDITIONS

Table **6.6**	Differential Diagnosis of Hypoglycemia
Mechanism	**Differential Diagnosis**
High I:G Adults	• Drugs: exogenous insulin, sulphonylureas, others (e.g., pentamidine, quinine) • Insulinoma, islet hypertrophy • Autoimmune: insulin or insulin receptor autoantibodies • Related to food intake: alimentary hyperinsulinism, idiopathic
Infants/children	• Maternal DM • Congenital hyperinsulinism (mutations in insulin secretory pathway) • Insulinoma
Low I:G Adults	• Critical illness: severe hepatic failure, cardiac disease, sepsis, anorexia nervosa, starvation/severe malnutrition • Extrapancreatic mesenchymal neoplasms (IGF-2 overproduction): hepatocellular, adrenocortical, carcinoid, leukemia, lymphoma • Hormone deficiencies (cortisol, GH): AI, hypopituitarism • Drugs: ethanol, salicylate intoxication
Infants/children	• Preterm or small for gestational age • Hormone deficiencies: Hypopituitarism, adrenal hypoplasia, congenital adrenal hyperplasia • Ketotic hypoglycemia of childhood • Enzymatic defects in carbohydrate, protein or lipid metabolism

Hypoglycemia presents differently in infants, and can include apnea, cyanotic spells, hypothermia, hypotonia and poor feeding. Infants and children are less tolerant to fasting than adults.

APPROACH

DIAGNOSIS

- Diagnosis of hypoglycemia should **not** rely solely on either clinical findings or plasma glucose measurements.
- Diagnosis should include **demonstration of Whipple triad and a supervised 72-h diagnostic fast during which circulating glucose, insulin and C-peptide levels are measured at appropriate intervals.** Serum should be screened for sulphonylureas.
  - Insulin levels should be interpreted in the context of prevailing glucose concentrations.
  - C-peptide serves as a marker for endogenous insulin secretion.
- Whipple triad provides compelling evidence of hypoglycemia: (i) a low plasma glucose concentration (<3.0 mmol/L), (ii) signs and symptoms consistent with hypoglycemia (Clinical box Hypoglycemia: Signs and Symptoms), and (iii) relief of those symptoms when the plasma glucose concentration is raised.

CLINICAL BOX

Hypoglycemia: Signs and Symptoms

Adrenergic: due to the perception of physiologic changes caused by autonomic nervous system activity
- Palpitations
- Tremor
- Anxiety
- Sweating
- Hunger
- Paresthesias
- Pallor
- Diaphoresis

Neuroglycopenic: directly due to CNS neuronal glucose deprivation
- Behavioral changes
- Confusion
- Fatigue or weakness
- Warmth
- Visual changes
- Seizure
- Loss of consciousness
- Death if prolonged or severe

- As a first step, the I:G can be calculated from simultaneously measured insulin and glucose levels (Fig. 6.5).
- The most common cause of hypoglycemia is drug-induced, especially due to insulin, sulphonylurea, or alcohol use. In neonates, the most frequent cause associated with hyperinsulinism is maternal diabetes mellitus.

AI

Hypoglycemia should be treated promptly; individuals with severe hypoglycemia may be unable to treat themselves and require assistance.

- AI is the inability to produce adrenal steroid hormones.
  - AI may arise from failure of the adrenal glands (primary AI) or the hypothalamic-pituitary axis (secondary AI). All adrenal steroids—glucocorticoids, mineralocorticoids and adrenal androgens—are usually deficient in primary AI. However, mineralocorticoid secretion is often intact in secondary AI, resulting in differences in clinical presentation.
  - The causes of primary AI include autoimmune, infectious and infiltrative disease, adrenal metastasis, adrenal hemorrhage/thrombosis, and adrenoleukodystrophies. The most common cause of secondary AI is long-term, high dose glucocorticoid administration.
- In contrast, acute AI or adrenal crisis is an inability of the adrenal cortex to ↑ steroid release during significant stress, potentially in the setting of chronic AI, or a sudden inability to secrete adrenal steroids. **Acute AI is a potentially life-threatening medical emergency**.
  - Common causes in developed countries include autoimmune disease, long-term glucocorticoid therapy, infectious disease, or pituitary or hypothalamic disorders; abrupt cessation of long-term, high-dose glucocorticoid therapy; and adrenal hemorrhage. The latter may arise from a number of conditions including a complication of anticoagulant therapy, disseminated intravascular coagulation, or sepsis.
- The clinical presentation of AI depends on the rate of onset, severity and duration of the deficiency, as well as whether the AI is primary or secondary (see preceding text).
  - Symptoms include fatigue, weakness, anorexia, and weight loss. GI symptoms of nausea, vomiting, and diarrhea are frequently seen. Patients may also report salt craving and/or arthralgias.
  - On exam, hypotension is usually present; hyperpigmentation also occurs if the AI is primary but not secondary. The hyperpigmentation commonly occurs in sun-exposed areas, pressure points, mucous membranes, axillae, nipples, palmar creases and new (vs. old) scars.
  - Electrolyte disturbances are commonly hyponatremia and hyperkalemia. However, hyperkalemia is not usually present in secondary AI due to maintenance of aldosterone secretion. Patients may also possess hypoglycemia and/or hypercalcemia.
- Key manifestations of acute AI include hypotension, hyponatremia, and hyperkalemia. Abdominal pain, anorexia with nausea and vomiting may be present. Acute AI may also be associated with hypoglycemia (see Chapter 13).
- Although static blood measurements may suggest AI, dynamic testing is required to definitely diagnose AI. A commonly used test is the cortisol response to ACTH stimulation. Plasma cortisol levels are measured at 0 and 30 min after administration of cosyntropin, the first 24 amino acids of endogenously secreted ACTH. A normal response is defined as a peak plasma cortisol level >500 nmol/L. Other dynamic tests can also be used to diagnose AI, and a prolonged ACTH stimulation test can be performed to distinguish between primary and secondary AI.

MANAGEMENT

Consider acute AI when unexplained hypoglycemia presents in the context of hypotension, hyponatremia ± hyperkalemia.

- An acute episode of hypoglycemia usually requires urgent treatment. Plasma glucose levels should be supported while investigating underlying causes.
- Underlying causes should be treated.
- In DM, the complication-reducing benefits of intensive glycemic control must be weighed against the risk of hypoglycemia and hypoglycemia unawareness (Clinical box Hypoglycemia Unawareness).
- Treatment for AI consists of glucocorticoid replacement (e.g., hydrocortisone, 20 mg/d titrated to the lowest dose the patient can tolerate; prednisone and dexamethasone are other options) and for primary AI, mineralocorticoid therapy as well (fludrocortisone, 0.1 mg/d titrated by symptoms, BP, electrolyte levels and plasma renin activity).

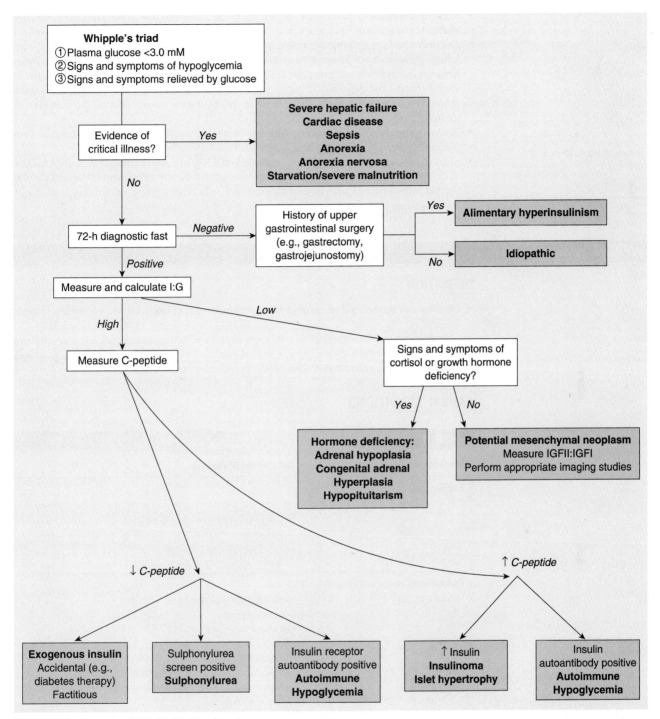

Figure 6.5 An approach to investigating hypoglycemia.

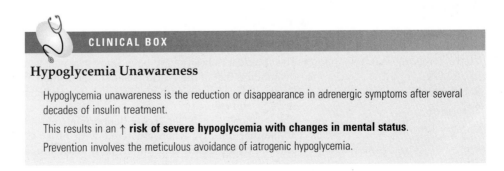

CLINICAL BOX

Hypoglycemia Unawareness

Hypoglycemia unawareness is the reduction or disappearance in adrenergic symptoms after several decades of insulin treatment.

This results in an ↑ **risk of severe hypoglycemia with changes in mental status**.

Prevention involves the meticulous avoidance of iatrogenic hypoglycemia.

- Administration of IV fluids (0.9% saline or 5% dextrose in 0.9% saline) should be initiated immediately if acute AI is suspected. Treatment with supraphysiologic or stress doses of glucocorticoids (e.g., 2 mg dexamethasone or 100 mg hydrocortisone; IV every 6 h) should follow. However, an attempt to obtain blood test results (cortisol, ACTH, electrolytes, glucose) should be made prior to administering stress dose steroids, pending the patient's condition and the degree of clinical suspicion. Supportive measures should be taken as required. Once the patient has stabilized, precipitating causes should be sought and treated.
- Severe hypoglycemia (requiring the assistance of another individual): Treatment is outlined in the section on hyperglycemia (Fig. 6.4B).
- Mild to moderate hypoglycemia: Ingestion of 15 g of carbohydrate (10 g for children <5 yr or <20 kg), preferably as glucose or sucrose tablets or solution. Plasma glucose should be retested 15 min later, and retreated with another 15 g of carbohydrate if glucose <4.0 mmol/L.

WEIGHT GAIN/OBESITY

DEFINITION

- **Obesity** can be defined as an abnormal accumulation of body fat in proportion to body size.
- Obesity is a major health concern—it is associated with a number of serious comorbidities, such as hypertension, dyslipidemia, and derangements in glucose homeostasis, as well as ↑ mortality (Clinical box Common Comorbidities of Obesity).

CAUSAL CONDITIONS

Table **6.7**	**Differential Diagnosis of Obesity**
Mechanism	**Differential Diagnosis**
Exogenous	
↑ Energy intake	
Dietary	Overeating, frequent eating, high-fat diet
Social, behavioral	Socioeconomic, cultural, psychological
Iatrogenic	Drugs, hormones, hypothalamic surgery
↓ Energy expenditure	Sedentary lifestyle, smoking cessation
Endogenous	
Neuroendocrine	Growth factor deficiency
	Cushing syndrome
	Hypothyroidism
	PCOS
	Hypogonadism
Genetic	Dysmorphic syndrome (e.g., Prader-Willi Syndrome)
	Defects in genes modulating obesity (e.g., neuropeptide Y, POMC)
	Family history of obesity

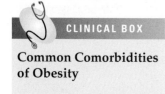

CLINICAL BOX

Common Comorbidities of Obesity

Hypertension

Dyslipidemia

CVS disease

DM/impaired FPG

Sleep apnea

Ovulatory dysfunction

APPROACH

DIAGNOSIS

- The criteria for obesity vary between expert panels; however the most widely accepted definition is that of the World Health Organization, which defines obesity as a **BMI >30 kg/m²**. BMI correlates with body fat, but the relationship is independently influenced by sex, age, and ethnicity.
- The location of body fat accumulation is an important feature of obesity. **Central or abdominal obesity, when clustered with other CVS risk factors including hypertension, dyslipidemia and abnormal glucose homeostasis, is known as the MetSyn.**

Clinical box Definition of Central Obesity provides the definitions of central obesity, and Table 6.8 defines the criteria for MetSyn. Individuals with MetSyn are at ↑ risk of CVS morbidity and mortality, as well as developing DM.

• The diagnostic goals in obesity are to determine if there are secondary causes for the obesity; identify the presence of comorbidities (Table 6.7, Clinical box Comorbidities of Obesity); and ascertain the dietary and activity habits of the patient to highlight avenues for lifestyle modification (Fig. 6.6). The history of obesity is important as sudden or rapid onset accompanied by other symptoms and/or comorbidities is highly suspicious for pathologic or drug causes, as opposed to a lifelong history of being heavy with a stable adult weight.

CLINICAL BOX

Definition of Central Obesity*

		Waist Circumference (cm)
All ethnicities except those listed below	**Male**	≥94
	Female	≥80
Chinese, Japanese, South Asians**	**Male**	≥90
	Female	≥80

*International Diabetes Federation definition
**South Asians: based on a Chinese, Malay, Asian-Indian population

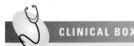

CLINICAL BOX

Drug Therapy for Obesity

Sympathomimetics (approved for short-term use only)

Diethylpropion

Phentermine

Sibutramine

Benzphetamine

Phendimetrazine

Lipase inhibitors (approved for long-term use)

Orlistat

MANAGEMENT

• Obesity is usually a chronic condition requiring a multidisciplinary approach to management.

• Treatment should begin with lifestyle interventions, including dietary improvements and ↑ physical activity, as well as behavioral modifications facilitating these changes. Dietary improvements include a reduction in caloric intake, and potentially changes in nutrient composition (e.g., ↓ fat, ↑ protein and fiber to promote health and satiety). Regarding physical activity, emphasis should be placed on incorporating ↑ activity into daily routines. Patients, particularly those with sedentary lifestyles, should be instructed on how to ↑ their level of activity safely.

• Drug therapy should be tried in patients who have failed lifestyle interventions or who possess comorbidities and a BMI >27 (Clinical box Drug Therapy for Obesity). Gastric bypass surgery is indicated as a last resort, and is recommended in individuals with progressive obesity, a BMI >40, or a BMI >35 with comorbidities.

• Screening and follow-up of comorbidities, including elements of the MetSyn, should be performed regularly, and managed by the appropriate specialists if necessary.

Table **6.8**	**International Diabetes Federation Worldwide Consensus Definition of the MetSyn**		
Central obesity[a,b] and two or more of the following			
HTg		≥1.7 mmol/L	**Or** treatment for this lipid abnormality
Low HDL	**Male**	<1.03 mmol/L	**Or** treatment for this lipid abnormality
	Female	<1.29 mmol/L	
Hypertension		Systolic BP ≥130 or Diastolic BP ≥85 mm Hg	**Or** treatment for this condition
Elevated FPG		≥5.6 mmol/L	**Or** previously diagnosed DM

[a]Waist circumference does not need to be measured if BMI >30 kg/m^2 as central obesity can be assumed.
[b]Definition of central obesity varies depending on ethnicity

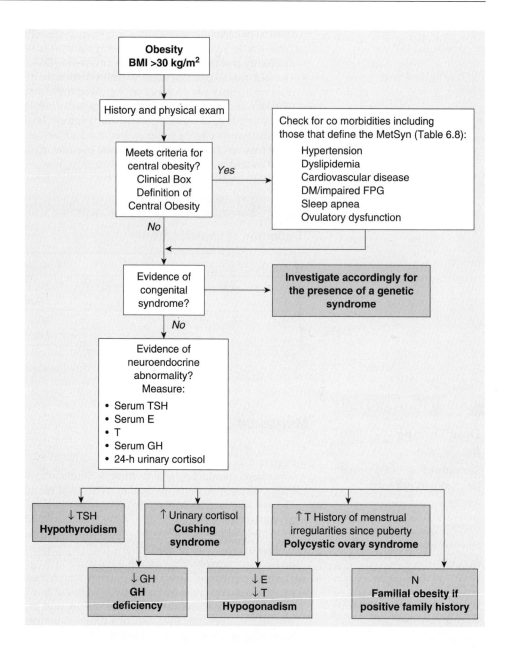

Figure 6.6 Approach to diagnosing the cause of obesity.

LIPIDS ABNORMAL, SERUM

DEFINITION

- **Dyslipidemia** refers to a group of disorders in which abnormal lipoprotein metabolism is reflected in altered levels of plasma lipids. Primary and secondary causes exist, and both may contribute to the development of dyslipidemia in an individual.
- **Hypercholesterolemia** specifically is **a major risk factor for CVS disease**.
- Screening for lipid abnormalities identifies those at ↑ risk for CAD so that early treatment can be initiated to reduce morbidity and mortality.

APPLIED SCIENTIFIC CONCEPTS

- Hypercholesterolemia, particularly **elevated LDL**, and **low HDL** are **major risk factors for atherosclerosis development**. Atherosclerosis of the coronary arteries results in CAD, commonly myocardial infarction and angina pectoris (ASC box Atherosclerosis, Chapter 3).

- Elevated plasma LDL levels can arise through an ↑ in VLDL or a ↓ in LDL catabolism.
  - ↑ VLDL arises from ↑ fatty acid delivery to the liver. This ↑ delivery can result from an ↑ in dietary fat or mobilization of fat stores.
  - ↓ LDL catabolism can arise from several factors, including an ↑ in dietary fat content. This down-regulates LDL receptor expression
- Low HDL is a major atherosclerosis risk factor because of the role of HDL in reverse cholesterol transport. Through this mechanism HDL is secreted by the liver and removes cholesterol from peripheral tissues as it circulates throughout the body, exerting a positive effect on lipid balance in the body.

CAUSAL CONDITIONS

Table **6.9**	**Differential Diagnosis of Dyslipidemia**
Mechanism	**Differential Diagnosis**
Elevated LDL	
Primary	Familial combined hyperlipidemia, familial hypercholesterolemia
	Nonfamilial/polygenic
	Endocrine, renal disease, liver disease
Secondary	Drugs (e.g., thiazides)
	Obesity, cigarette smoking
HTg	
Primary	Familial HTg
Secondary	Obesity, diabetes, renal disease
	Drugs (estrogen, tamoxifen, β-blockers, glucocorticoids, cyclosporine, ethanol)
Low HDL	
Primary	Hypoalphalipoproteinemia, LCAT deficiency, Tangier disease
	Drugs (β-blockers, benzodiazepines, anabolic steroids)
Secondary	Obesity, inactivity, cigarette smoking

APPROACH

SCREENING

- **Men >35 yr and women >45 yr should be screened every 5 yr** because the prevalence of hypercholesterolemia ↑ with age. **Screening should begin at 20 yr for either sex if risk factors for CAD are present** (Clinical box Risk Factors of CAD).
- Non-fasting serum measurements of total cholesterol or HDL can be used to identify those at ↑ risk. However, fasting LDL measurements should be used to identify therapeutic targets (see Table 6.10).

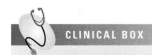

CLINICAL BOX

Risk Factors of CAD

DM

Hypertension

Cigarette smoking (current or within the previous year)

Abdominal obesity (see **Weight Gain/Obesity** for criteria)

Family history of premature CAD

Clinical evidence of hyperlipidemia (e.g., xanthomata, xanthelasma, corneal arcus)

Exertional chest discomfort, dyspnea, erectile dysfunction

Evidence of atherosclerosis

Chronic kidney disease or systemic lupus erythematous

Table **6.10**	**Treatment Targets According to CAD Risk**	
Risk Level	**Framingham 10-yr CAD Risk**[a]	**Threshold for Therapy Initiation**
High CAD or CAD risk equivalents[b]	≥20 %	Primary: LDL ≥2.0 mmol/L Secondary: TC/HDL ≥4.0 mmol/L
Moderate 2+ Risk factors	10%–19%	LDL ≥3.5 mmol/L HDL ≥5.0 mmol/L
Low 0–1 Risk factors	<10%	LDL ≥5.0 mmol/L HDL ≥6.0 mmol/L

[a]10-yr risk of cardiac death or nonfatal myocardial infarction (hard CAD risk).

[b]Clinical manifestations of noncoronary forms of atherosclerosis (peripheral arterial disease, abdominal aortic aneurysm, carotid artery disease); DM; two or more risk factors with gt;10% hard CAD risk (risk of cardiac death or nonfatal myocardial infarction).

MANAGEMENT

- Secondary causes of lipid abnormalities should be identified and treated. However, the lipid abnormality will still need to be addressed through lifestyle modification (diet, exercise) and potentially drug therapy.
- The **threshold cholesterol levels for initiation of treatment depend on the nature and number of risk factors an individual possesses** (Clinical box Risk Factors of CAD, Table 6.10). Algorithms, such as the FRS, exist which calculate parameters such as 10-yr CAD risk or change in life expectancy, based on an individual's constellation of risk factors. However, such algorithms do not account for all factors. The FRS, for instance, does not account for the influence of either diabetes or ethnicity on risk. Most individuals with diabetes have a high risk of CAD regardless of their FRS particular, and certain ethnicities such as South Asians are at ↑ risk.
- Therapeutic lifestyle changes are essential regardless of the precise lipid abnormality.
- Medication should be started immediately in those at high risk. In all other individuals, lifestyle changes alone can be tried first, with the addition of medication if lipid targets are not achieved. HMG-CoA reductase inhibitors are the mainstay of pharmacologic treatment to lower cholesterol levels. To reach target levels, however, a combination of drugs may be required (see Table 6.11).
- HTg is correlated with ↑ CAD risk. It should be managed in the context of other lipid abnormalities. Isolated HTg >11.3 mmol/L should be treated to prevent acute pancreatitis. Fibrates and niacin are first-line pharmacologic treatments.

Table **6.11**	Drugs Used in the Treatment of Lipid Abnormalities		
Class	**Effect on Plasma Lipids**	**Mechanism**	**Adverse Effects**
HMG-CoA Example: **simvastatin**	↓ LDL	Inhibits cholesterol synthesis Upregulates LDL receptors	Myopathy, hepatic dysfunction
Fibrates Example: **gemfibrozil**	↓ Tg through VLDL	Inhibits VLDL production	Nausea, abdominal discomfort, gallstone, myopathy
Niacin	↓ LDL through VLDL	Inhibits VLDL production	Flushing, hyperglycemia, pruritus, gout, elevated liver function enzymes
Bile acid-binding resins Example: **cholestyramine**	↓ LDL	Depletes bile acids Upregulates LDL receptors	Constipation, abdominal discomfort, may bind other drugs
Inhibitors of intestinal sterol absorption Example: **ezetimibe**	↓ LDL	Prevents dietary cholesterol absorption	Reversible impairment in hepatic function

POLYURIA

DEFINITION

- **Polyuria** is an ↑ in the **volume** of urine voided. This must be distinguished from urinary frequency in which the urine flow rate is not ↑.
- Polyuria can be due to either water or osmotic diuresis (ASC box Osmotic versus Water Diuresis).

ASC Box
Osmotic versus Water Diuresis

Osmotic Diuresis
Excretion of unusually large volumes of urine due to an abnormally elevated concentration of osmotically active substances in the nephron. Renal water reabsorption is **reduced.**

Water Diuresis
Excretion of large volumes of dilute urine due to intake of hypotonic fluid or an inability to properly concentrate urine. Renal water reabsorption is **normal.**

CAUSAL CONDITIONS

Table **6.12** Differential Diagnosis of Polyuria	
Mechanism	**Differential Diagnosis**
Polyuria	
Water diuresis	
Excessive intake	Polydipsia
Excessive loss	DI (central and nephrogenic)
Osmotic diuresis	Glucosuria in DM
Glucose-induced	Uricosuria in chronic renal disease
Urea-induced	
Other (e.g., due to salts, organic anions)	
Urinary frequency	

APPROACH

DIAGNOSIS

- Measuring **urine flow rate differentiates between urinary frequency and polyuria,** while U_{osm} **distinguishes osmotic from water diuresis** (Fig. 6.7).
- DM should be investigated if osmotic diuresis is due to glucosuria (see Hyperglycemia).
- If DM has been previously diagnosed, acute complications such as DKA or HHS, or inadequate glycemic control, should be pursued.
- Suspected **DI** can be confirmed with a water deprivation test (Miller-Moses Test, Clinical box Water Deprivation Test (Miller-Moses Test)). The test can also distinguish between central and nephrogenic DI.

CLINICAL BOX

Water Deprivation Test (Miller-Moses Test)

All water intake is withheld; U_{osm} and body weight are measured hourly.

When two consecutive U_{osm} measurements differ by $\leq$10% or $\geq$2% body weight has been lost, ADH is administered.

Findings in healthy individuals:
- After water deprivation: U_{osm} is two to four times greater than P_{osm}
- Response to ADH: U_{osm} ↑ by <9%

Findings in complete central DI:
- After water deprivation: **minimal ADH levels**
- Response to ADH: U_{osm} ↑ **by >50%**

Findings in nephrogenic DI:
- After water deprivation: **normal to elevated ADH levels**
- Response to ADH: failure of urine to be concentrated despite ↑ P_{osm}

MANAGEMENT

- Patients should be treated for the underlying cause of frequency.
- See Hyperglycemia for the management of DM and DKA. See Chapter 12 for chronic renal failure.
- In DI, fluid intake should be ↑ to prevent or counteract dehydration. The fluid should be hyperosmotic to the serum of the patient and given IV if necessary. Hospitalization with electrolyte monitoring may be required.

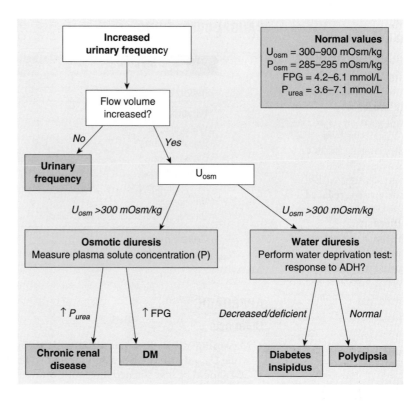

Figure 6.7 An approach to the diagnosis of urinary frequency.

- Medical treatment of DI involves the use of ADH, vasopressin analogues, and/or other drugs that either promote ADH release (e.g., carbamazepine, clofibrate), ↑ the renal ADH response (e.g., chlorpropamide) or ↑ water absorption (e.g., hydrochlorothiazide, ibuprofen, indomethacin).

SEXUAL MATURATION

DEFINITION

- Sexual development whether delayed or premature, may be due to a variety of causes, including conditions requiring medical attention (see Table 6.13).
- Moreover, sexual development is integral to adolescent perception of self-image and well-being, and its disruption may cause significant distress.

CAUSAL CONDITIONS

Table 6.13   A Classification Scheme of Abnormal Sexual Maturation

Mechanism	Differential Diagnosis
Delayed puberty	
Associated with growth failure	Constitutional, endocrine disorders, systemic diseases
Central causes	Syndromes, malformations, isolated gonadotropin deficiency, panhypopituitarism
Congenital	
Acquired	Infection, trauma, neoplasia, malnutrition, chronic systemic disease
Primary gonadal disorders	
Congenital	Chromosomal abnormality, defects in gonadal differentiation or hormonal synthesis
Acquired	Infection, trauma, neoplasia
Interruption/lack of completion	Testicular feminization, absent/hypoplastic uterus/vagina
Precocious puberty	
Central	Constitutional, CNS defect
Pseudo-precocious puberty	Autonomous ovarian/testicular function, gonadotropin-secreting tumor, adrenal pathology, hypothyroidism

CLINICAL BOX

Secondary Sex Characteristics

Female

Breast development/thelarche

Menarche

Male

Testicular and penile enlargement

Facial hair

Voice deepening

Both sexes

Pubic and axillary hair/adrenarche

Rapid height growth

APPROACH

CLASSIFICATIONS

- Delayed puberty: absence of any signs of spontaneous secondary sexual development by 14 yr of age for boys or 13 yr for girls
- Precocious puberty: any secondary sex characteristics occurring before 9 yr of age in boys, 7 yr in girls (before 6 yr if of African descent)

DIAGNOSIS

- The mechanism of delayed or precocious sexual development may arise centrally within the CNS, or distally at the gonads (Table 6.13, Fig. 6.8). A variety of congenital and acquired causes may be responsible in either case. With central precocious puberty, puberty development is normal but accelerated. Furthermore, delayed puberty may be due to an overall failure of growth.
- A thorough history that documents any symptoms of puberty, and includes a full developmental history from pregnancy through to the present should be taken. A full account of the patient's development should be elicited, including any disorders of pregnancy or abnormalities during labour and delivery, and any medical illnesses should be noted.
- A complete physical exam should be performed. Height and weight should be measured, and velocities for each parameter should be noted. The stage of secondary sexual development should be determined, with the recommendation that a non-related chaperone is present while the exam is performed. The key is to rule out an organic CNS cause.
- Investigations should include a hormone workup: gonadotropins (LH; FSH), testosterone and estrogen. Measurement of the LH and FSH responses to GnRH stimulation may be useful in distinguishing central or true precocious puberty from precocious pseudopuberty. TSH and PRL should be measured if warranted by the clinical features (i.e., features of hypothyroidism or hyperprolactinemia). Imaging studies and karyotyping should be performed as appropriate (e.g., radiographs for bone age, contrast MRI for suspected CNS lesions).
- Owing to the sensitive nature of sexual development, only the necessary examinations and investigations should be performed.

MANAGEMENT

- Identified underlying causes should be treated.
- Psychosocial support should be offered as needed. Either delayed or precocious puberty can cause significant psychological and emotional distress. Depression and suicidal ideation associated with delayed puberty have been documented; and in precocious puberty, others may have expectations that are inappropriate for the child's actual level of psychosocial and emotional developmental.
- In the case of permanent hypogonadism or constitutional delay, testosterone can be given to boys and estrogen to girls, to stimulate pubertal development.

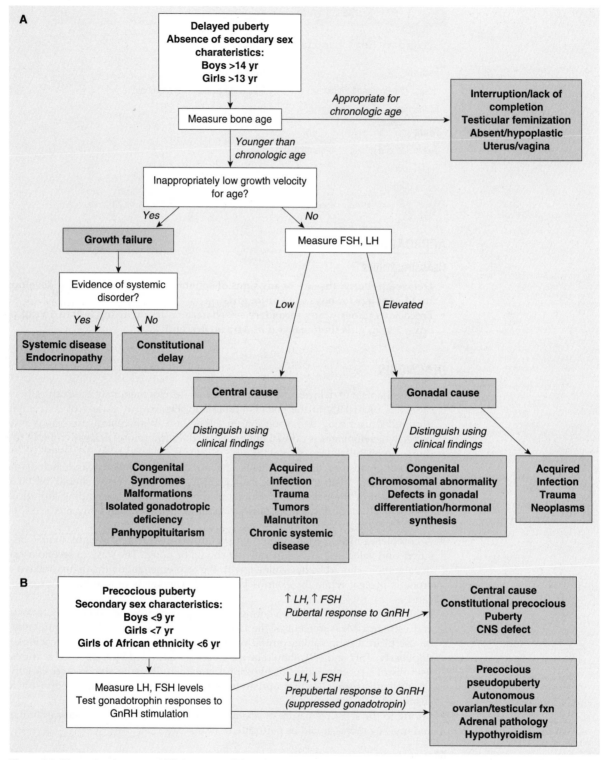

Figure 6.8 Diagnosing the cause of (**A**) delayed and (**B**) precocious puberty.

GYNECOMASTIA

DEFINITION

- **Gynecomastia** is the enlargement of the male breast due to estrogen-induced proliferation of glandular tissue.

Figure 6.9 Pathophysiological mechanisms of gynecomastia. An ↑ estrogen to androgen ratio can occur through (*1*) an ↑ in estrogen precursor formation, (*2*) an ↑ in estrogen secretion, (*3*) a reduction in testosterone secretion, or (*4*) an inhibition of testosterone action. hCG can lead to the development of gynecomastia by stimulating estrogen secretion. See Table 6.14 for specific examples.

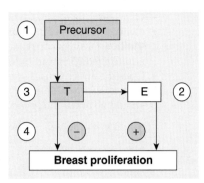

- Although gynecomastia can be physiologic, **ruling out a pathological cause such as malignancy, is critical**. Malignancy is particularly imperative to diagnose because the prognosis is worse compared to women.

APPLIED SCIENTIFIC CONCEPTS

- Estrogen is an **absolute requirement** for development of the female breast. Breast tissue possesses both **estrogen** and **androgen receptors; activation of the former stimulates proliferation, while the latter inhibits it.** Furthermore, **progesterone** is responsible for lobule development.
- Similarly, the pathophysiological mechanism of gynecomastia is **an ↑ estrogen to androgen ratio—the ratio is key as opposed to the absolute level of estrogen.** The ↑ ratio can be mediated through several mechanisms (Fig. 6.9).

CAUSAL CONDITIONS

Table **6.14**	**Differential Diagnosis of Gynecomastia**
Mechanism	**Differential Diagnosis**
Physiologic gynecomastia	Gynecomastia of the newborn Pubertal gynecomastia Gynecomastia of aging
Pathologic gynecomastia Deficient testosterone production or action Primary gonadal (testicular) failure Secondary gonadal (hypothalamus/pituitary) failure androgen insensitivity syndrome ↑ Estrogen or estrogen precursors ↑ Testicular estrogen secretion ↑ Substrate for extraglandular estrogen formation ↑ Activity of extraglandular aromatase Drugs Estrogen, estrogen mimetics Drugs enhancing endogenous estrogen production Inhibitors of testosterone synthesis or action Unknown mechanism	**Genetic**: Klinefelter syndrome, enzymatic defects in testosterone synthesis **Acquired**: infection/viral orchitis, trauma, renal failure Testicular tumors, hCG-producing tumors, true interssex Adrenal carcinomas, liver disease, hyperthyroidism Prostate cancer treatments (e.g., diethylstilbesterol), anabolic steroids hcg, clomiphene citrate Antifungals (imidazoles), antineoplastic agents, antiandrogens, spironolactone Captopril, amiodarone, methyldopa, methotrexate, isoniazid, tricyclic antidepressants, street drugs (amphetamines, heroin), alcohol
Idiopathic gynecomastia	

APPROACH

Diagnosis

- **Differentiating breast cancer from true gynecomastia (i.e., nonmalignant glandular breast tissue) is critical** (Fig. 6.10, Chapter 15).

- Gynecomastia must also be distinguished from adipose tissue or lipomastia
- Gynecomastia is **abnormal except for the three physiological conditions listed in Table 6.14**. Gynecomastia is common in adolescence (estimated 38% to 64%), and in adults aged 65 yr and older, particularly with weight gain.
- Once the above causes have been ruled out, a hormone workup should be performed as well as appropriate imaging studies if a neoplasm is suspected (Fig. 6.10). However, it should be noted that gynecomastia is most commonly idiopathic.

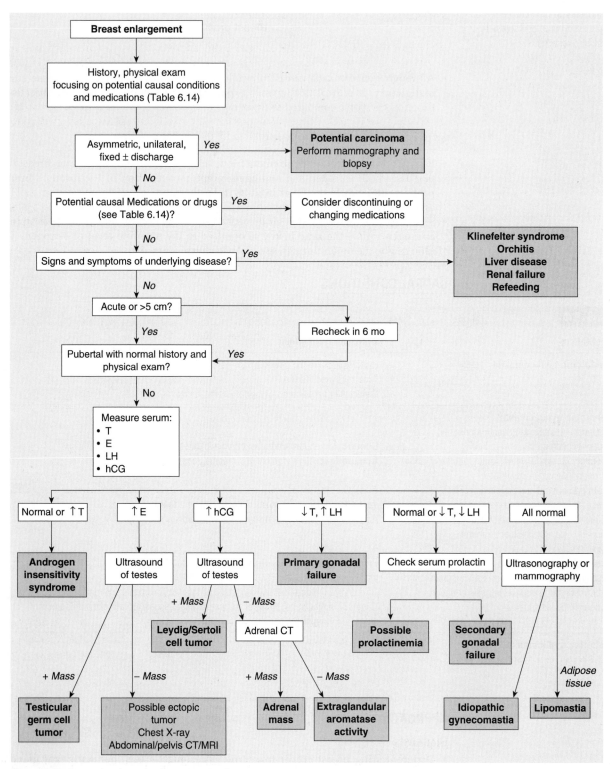

Figure 6.10 Approach to investigating gynecomastia.

MANAGEMENT

- Treat underlying causes.
- Modalities for managing gynecomastia include medications, such as **antiestrogens or aromatase inhibitors**, and surgery. Persistent and/or symptomatic gynecomastia may require surgical management.

GALACTORRHEA

ASC Box

Control of PRL Secretion

- PRL stimulates milk production or lactation in the pregnant state
- DA tonically inhibits PRL secretion as shown below
- Modulators of PRL secretion include:

+	−
Estrogen	DA
DA antagonists	DA agonists
TRH	PRL
Breast feeding	
Sleep	
Stress	

DEFINITION

- **Galactorrhea** refers to a specific type of breast discharge—that of milk or milk-like substances. Although more common in women, particular between 20 and 35 yr of age, it can occur in men.
- Although breast secretions are normal in over 50% of women of reproductive age, they nonetheless deserve evaluation to rule out pathology. Importantly, discharge may be indicative of **malignancy**; and **spontaneous, persistent galactorrhea** may reflect an underlying disease process (see Table 6.15, Fig. 6.11).

CAUSAL CONDITIONS

Table **6.15**	Differential Diagnosis of Galactorrhea
Mechanism	**Differential Diagnosis**
True galactorrhea	
Idiopathic	
Hyperprolactinemia	
Physiologic	Pregnancy, breast stimulation
Autonomous PRL production	
Pituitary tumors	Microadenomas, macroadenomas
Ectopic PRL Production	Bronchogenic carcinoma, renal cell carcinoma
↑ PRL secretion, ↓ Clearance	
Systemic disease	Hypothyroidism, chronic renal failure, liver disease
Neurogenic	Thorocotomy, burns, herpes zoster, chest wall trauma
Estrogen	OCs
Failure to inhibit PRL release	
Hypothalamic lesions	Hypothalamic tumors, histiocytosis x, empty sella syndrome
Pituitary stalk lesions	Head trauma, mass effect of sellar tumors
Drugs	Methyldopa, phenothiazines (typical antipsychotics), opiates
Abnormal breast discharge	Breast carcinoma

APPROACH

DIAGNOSIS

- Galactorrhea is mostly commonly **idiopathic.** Among known causes, the most common is **hyperprolactinemia** which, in turn, has numerous etiologies.
- **The key is to rule out breast cancer** (Fig. 6.11). The history and physical exam should therefore ascertain the nature of the discharge (color, unilateral/bilateral, spontaneous/stimulated, duration), and the presence of masses, skin changes, and adenopathy (Chapter 15).
- One should also be alert to the signs and symptoms of **hyperprolactinemia** and intracranial masses in a patient with galactorrhea (Clinical boxes Hyperprolactinemia: Signs and Symptoms, Tumor Mass Effects).

MANAGEMENT

- Underlying conditions should be managed accordingly. However, the galactorrhea may nonetheless require treatment.

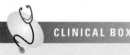

CLINICAL BOX

Hyperprolactinemia: Signs and Symptoms

Galactorrhea

Amenorrhea, oligomenorrhea

Infertility

↓ Libido

Impotence

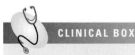

Tumor Mass Effects

Visual Disturbances
- Visual field defects
- Scotomas
- Visual acuity loss
- Cranial nerve palsies
- Headache
- Hypopituitarism
- Hypothalamic dysfunction affecting regulation of temperature, sleep, appetite, thirst, behavior, autonomic nervous system function

DA Agonists

Bromocriptine: preferred choice for the treatment of anovulatory infertility as more safety data exists on its use in pregnancy

Cabergoline: more effective and better tolerated than bromocriptine; recent concern about a possible link between medications such as cabergoline and cardiac valve fibrosis in individuals treated for Parkinson disease

Quinagolide: long-term safety data not established

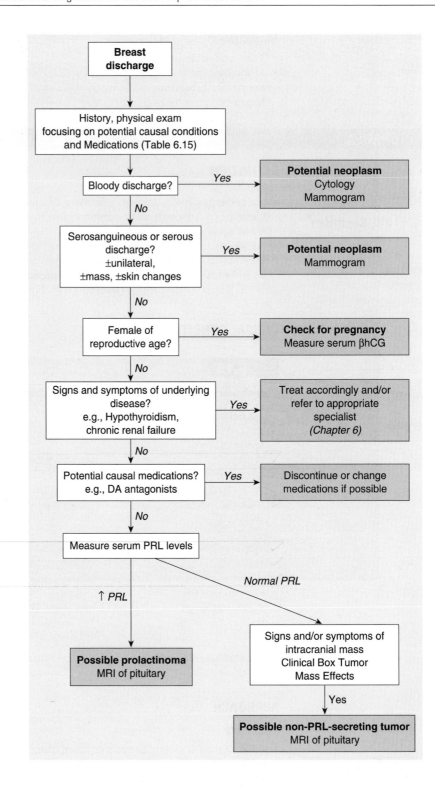

Figure 6.11 Approach to the diagnosis of galactorrhea.

Pituitary masses should be monitored for compressive effects such as visual field loss which requires surgical intervention.

- The following are indications for treatment of galactorrhea:
  - Bothersome or disabling galactorrhea
  - Reproductive or sexual dysfunction: amenorrhea, infertility, ↓ libido
  - Neuro-ophthalmic abnormalities: visual field defects, cranial nerve palsies
- Treatment is not necessary in the case of isolated galactorrhea in a patient with normal serum PRL levels as long as the patient is unconcerned, has no wish to conceive, and there is no evidence of either hypogonadism or ↓ bone density.
- The **DA agonists** are the treatments of choice for galactorrhea (Clinical box DA Agonists).
- Surgery can be considered for prolactinomas if medical therapy is unsuccessful.

HIRSUTISM/VIRILIZATION

Androgen Excess: Signs and Symptoms

Defeminization
- Menstrual irregularities
- Infertility

Virilization
- Hirsutism
- Acne
- Androgenic alopecia
- Voice deepening
- Loss of female body contours
- Clitoromegaly

DEFINITION

- **Hirsutism is defined as male-pattern growth of terminal hair in females**. Other clinical evidence of **hyperandrogenism** may accompany hirsutism, including **virilization** or the induction of masculine secondary sex characteristics, and ↑ **the likelihood of underlying pathology** (Clinical box Androgen Excess:Signs and Symptoms).
- Hirsutism should be distinguished from **hypertrichosis**, a generalized ↑ in the growth of vellous hair (short, fine, nonpigmented) in a nonsexual pattern.

APPLIED SCIENTIFIC CONCEPTS

- In patients with hirsutism, excess androgens can be produced by the ovaries, adrenal glands, or both.
- In **PCOS**, multiple abnormalities in steroid hormone metabolism exist. Ovarian production of estrogen and androgens is ↑; and conversion of the precursor androstenedione by peripheral tissues contributes to the ↑ in estrogen. ↑ LH production contributes to elevated ovarian hormones. Adrenal production of DHEAS, another androgen and estrogen precursor, is substantially ↑.

CAUSAL CONDITIONS

Table **6.16** Differential Diagnosis of ↑ Body Hair	
Mechanism	**Differential Diagnosis**
Hirsutism Androgen excess	
Ovarian source	PCOS, Idiopathic, ovarian Tumor
Adrenal source	Adrenal hyperplasia, Cushing syndrome, adrenal tumor, glucocorticoid resistance
Drugs	Danazol, norgestrel-ethinyl estradiol
Other	Hyperprolactinemia
Hypertrichosis	Idiopathic Drugs (e.g., phenytoin, minoxidil, cyclosporine) Systemic illness/conditions (e.g., hypothyroidism, malnutrition, malignancy, dermatomyositis, hyperprolactinemia)

APPROACH

DIAGNOSIS

- **Hirsutism is the most common presenting symptom of hyperandrogenism.**
- **PCOS is the most common cause of hirsutism.** However, other endocrine and drug causes of androgen excess should be excluded. PCOS is a diagnosis of exclusion based on findings of ovulatory dysfunction (anovulation or oligo-ovulation) starting at menarche and androgen excess unaccounted for by other causes (see Table 6.16).
- After excluding drug causes, steroid hormone levels should be measured (Fig. 6.12). Imaging studies are indicated if a tumor is suspected.

MANAGEMENT

- Management goals of hyperandrogenism involve the treatment of any identifiable cause and suppression of the abnormal androgen secretion.
- Treatment of hirsutism involves the use of **OCs, antiandrogens and/or mechanical forms of hair removal (see Table 6.17)**. Response to medication is generally seen by 6 to 12 mo. Medication does not completely reverse the terminalization of hair. Therefore mechanical hair removal is recommended regardless of whether medication is used.
- For anovulation in PCOS, an insulin sensitizer may be added which will act in concert with the OC.

Table **6.17**	**Medical Management of Hirsutism**
Treatment	**Comments**
OCs	First-line treatment for hirsutism Should contain ethinyl estradiol to suppress LH production
Antiandrogens	For moderate to severe hirsutism or to ensure optimal response in milder cases as their mechanism of action is different from OCs Best used with OCs to prevent pregnancy Examples: spironolactone, cyproterone, finesteride, flutamide

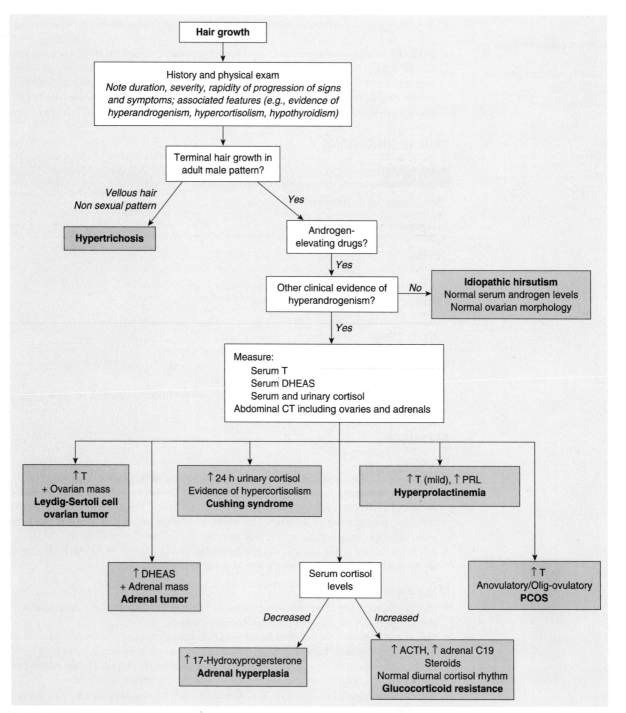

Figure 6.12 An approach to investigating hirsutism.

HYPERCALCEMIA

DEFINITION

- Ca^{2+} plays a vital role in key processes such as neuromuscular excitability, cardiac rhythm, hormone stimulus-secretion coupling, clotting, and growth. Therefore, the manifestations of hypercalcemia are diverse and can be life-threatening, particularly in the case of a hypercalcemic crisis (Clinical box Hypercalcemia: Some Key Signs and Symptoms).
- Investigations should seek to determine the underlying pathology responsible for the **hypercalcemia** because its treatment is cause dependent.

APPLIED SCIENTIFIC CONCEPTS

- The hormones **PTH, vitamin D_3 (calcitriol; 1,25-dihydroxycholecalciferol)** and calcitonin acting at the kidneys, bone, and intestine regulate serum levels of Ca^{2+} and PO_4 (see Table 6.18). Calcitonin plays a minor role in humans. Vitamin D_2 is also involved in Ca^{2+} homeostasis.
- The majority (70%) of renal Ca^{2+} reabsorption occurs at the proximal tubule; however, PTH stimulates reabsorption at the ascending loop of Henle and distal tubules. **Thiazide diuretics** enhance renal **reabsorption** of Ca^{2+} while **furosemide** enhances its **excretion**.

Table **6.18** Hormonal Control of Ca^{2+} and PO_4 Homeostasis						
	Renal Reabsorption		Bone Resorption		Intestinal Absorption	
Hormone	Ca^{2+}	PO_4	Ca^{2+}	PO_4	Ca^{2+}	PO_4
PTH	↑	↓	↑	↑	↑[a]	—
Vitamin D3	—	↑	↑	↑	↑	↑
Calcitonin	—	↓	↓	↓	—	—

[a]Indirect through vitamin D_3. PTH promotes the formation of vitamin D_3.

CAUSAL CONDITIONS

Table **6.19** Differential Diagnosis of Hypercalcemia	
Mechanism	**Differential Diagnosis**
↑ **Intestinal absorption** ↑ Intake Vitamin D-mediated	Milk alkali syndrome Granulomatous disease (e.g., tuberculosis, sarcoidosis, fungal diseases)
↑ **Bone resorption**	Malignancy Primary or tertiary hyperparathyroidism (see Hypocalcemia for secondary) Hyperthyroidism Immobilization Paget disease
↓ **Renal excretion**	Familial hypocalciuric hypercalcemia Thiazides
Miscellaneous	Advanced chronic liver disease Dehydration Hypophosphatasia Parenteral nutrition Primary infantile hyperparathyroidism

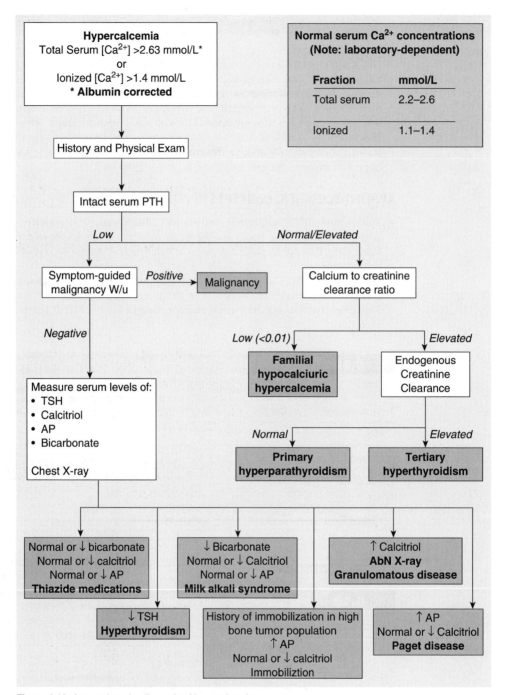

Figure 6.13 Approach to the diagnosis of hypercalcemia.

APPROACH

DIAGNOSIS

- Most cases are **asymptomatic.** Signs and symptoms may become apparent **when serum [Ca^{2+}] >3 mmol/L and one should be alert to the signs and symptoms of a hypercalcemic crisis (>3.5 mmol/L)** (Clinical box Hypercalcemia: Some Key Signs and Symptoms).
- Malignancy-associated hypercalcemia and primary hyperparathyroidism account for ~90% of cases. The former is the most common cause among hospitalized patients, while the latter is the most common outpatient cause.
- Serum Ca^{2+} exists in several forms: ionized (50%), protein-bound, particularly to albumin (45%), and complexed to anions (5%).

Hypercalcemia: Some Key Signs and Symptoms

The manifestations of hypercalcemia are variable and can involve multiple organs systems:

- Kidneys: renal failure, nephrolithiasis, nephrocalcinosis, nephrogenic DI (polydipsia, polyuria)
- Bone: osteopenia, bone pain/fractures
- Neuromuscular: muscle weakness, fatigue, ↓ level of consciousness, depressed affect
- GI: nausea, vomiting, abdominal pain, constipation
- CVS: shortened QT interval, bradycardia

Importantly, hypercalcemia, particularly a hypercalcemia crisis may also present with **nonspecific symptoms**:

- Nausea
- Vomiting
- Fatigue
- Muscle weakness
- Dehydration
- Confusion
- ↓ level of consciousness

A hypercalcemic crisis may present with nonspecific manifestations and requires urgent treatment.

Hypercalcemia occurs in advanced malignancy and is rapidly progressive.

- The **ionized Ca^{2+} concentration** is the biologically relevant fraction and therefore clinically relevant. However, its accuracy can be influenced by blood collection and handling techniques.
- **Total serum Ca^{2+}** should be corrected for albumin according to the formulae in Clinical box Serum Ca^{2+}
- Serum intact PTH levels should be measured as the initial step (Fig. 6.13).
- In patients with new onset hypercalcemia, serum intact PTH, PO_4, albumin, creatinine, alkaline phosphatase and magnesium should be measured.
- If serum intact PTH <20 pg/mL (i.e., suppressed), clinical findings should be used to dictate further laboratory investigations.

Serum Ca^{2+}

Total serum levels should be corrected for changes in serum albumin using the following formula:

$$[Ca^{2+}] \text{ corrected} = (\text{Measured } Ca^{2+}) + (40 - \text{albumin}) \times 0.02 \text{ mmol/L}$$

MANAGEMENT

- Treatment of hypercalcemia should be directed toward the underlying cause.
- One should be alert to the volume status of the patient. Should they exhibit signs of dehydration, **the initial therapy should be rehydration**.
- Patients with **any** degree of hypercalcemia with polyuria, polydipsia, dehydration, or altered mental status should be hospitalized, as should **all** patients with serum levels >3.2 mmol/L regardless of clinical presentation.

Table **6.20**	Treatment of Hypercalcemia	
Condition		**Management**
↑ **Resorption**	Malignancy	Oncology referral
	Hyperparathyroidism	**Primary:** Treat as required depending on patient characteristics (i.e., surgical vs. nonsurgical).
		Tertiary: Medication, diet and lifestyle modification to slow progression of renal disease. Nephrology referral.
	Hyperthyroidism	Thyroid workup to determine cause; treat accordingly **(Neck Mass)**. Endocrinology referral.
	Immobilization	Encourage weight bearing. Bisphosphonates to slow turnover.
	Paget disease	Bone scan and radiography to document extent of disease
↓ **Excretion**	Familial hypocalciuric hypercalcemia	No treatment required if asymptomatic and hypercalcemia mild
	Thiazides	Discontinue medication if possible
↑ **Intestinal absorption**	Milk alkali syndrome	Switch to low Ca^{2+} and low alkali intake
	Granulomatous diseases	Counsel to maintain low Ca^{2+} and vitamin D intake, limit sun exposure. Loop diuretics to accelerate Ca^{2+} excretion or glucocorticoids if hypercalcemia severe. Treat underlying disease.

HYPERPHOSPHATEMIA

DEFINITION

- **PO_4** is a key constituent in intracellular signaling and metabolism, also serving as an integral component of bone and a urinary buffer for hydrogen ions.

- The kidney excretes 90% of ingested PO$_4$. This is the **primary mechanism** for maintaining PO$_4$ homeostasis. PTH acts at the proximal tubule to **inhibit** reabsorption (Table 6.18, ASC box Renal PO$_4$ Handling and Hypophosphatemia).
- Determining if the **hyperphosphatemia** is acute or chronic, and differentiating between the major mechanisms of hyperphosphatemia are important because these factors will affect management (Table 6.21, Fig. 6.14).

CAUSAL CONDITIONS

Table **6.21**	Differential Diagnosis of Hyperphosphatemia
Mechanism	**Examples**
Artefactual	Hemolysis
↓ Excretion Renal failure	Renal failure, hypoparathyroidism, acromegaly, tumoral calcinosis
↑ PO$_4$ load Endogenous Exogenous	Tumor lysis syndrome, rhabdomyolysis, hemolysis (e.g., autoimmune) Rectal enema, PO$_4$-containing purgatives (e.g., for colonoscopy preparation), GI bleeding, transfusion-associated hemolysis, potassium repletion with potassium PO$_4$ preparations

APPROACH

DIAGNOSIS

- Hyperphosphatemia is usually identified **incidentally** or **due to the induction of hypocalcemia by the underlying condition** because there are no specific symptoms and signs of hyperphosphatemia **per se** (see Hypocalcemia).

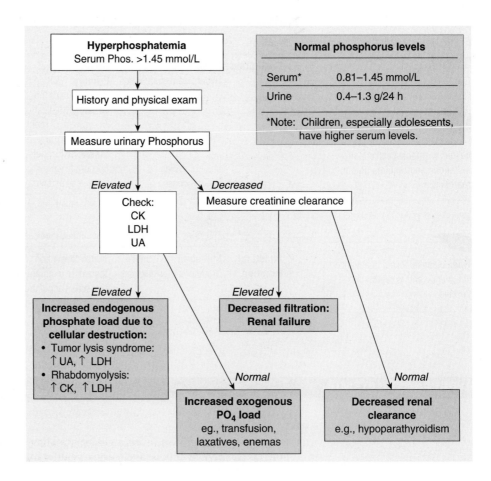

Figure 6.14 Approach to investigating hyperphosphatemia.

Acute, severe hyperphosphatemia presents primarily due to induction of hypocalcemia and should be treated aggressively.

- Reduced excretion arising in chronic renal failure is the most common cause of hyperphosphatemia. The incidence of hyperphosphatemia may be as high as 70% in populations with renal insufficiency.
- Laboratory results report phosphorus values; in the body, the element exists predominantly as PO_4 and as part of phosphorylated proteins.

MANAGEMENT

- Treatment should be directed toward the underlying disease process. Exogenous PO_4 sources should be identified and removed if possible. If renal function is intact, hyperphosphatemia often self-corrects. Saline infusion can be used to enhance PO_4 clearance by inducing natriuresis.
- Acute situations associated with hypocalcemia may require medical attention. If severe, especially in the context of renal insufficiency, hyperphosphatemia may require dialysis.
- With chronic hyperphosphatemia, such as in renal insufficiency, a low PO_4 diet and use of PO_4 binders such as sevelamer hydrochloride are often recommended.

HYPOCALCEMIA

DEFINITION

- Ca^{2+} plays a key component in numerous physiological processes (see Hypercalcemia).
- The manifestations of **hypocalcemia**, such as heightened neuromuscular excitability and arrhythmias, may be significant and require treatment, if not immediate hospitalization.
- See Table 6.18 for a description of the hormonal control of Ca^{2+} metabolism.

CAUSAL CONDITIONS

Table **6.22** Differential Diagnosis of Hypocalcemia	
Mechanism	**Differential Diagnosis**
Loss from the circulation	Hyperphosphatemia Pancreatitis Hungry bone syndrome Drugs: EDTA, citrate, foscarnet Rhabdomyolysis
↓ **Vitamin D production or action**	Renal failure Osteoblastic metastases Rickets Malabsorption Neonatal
↓ **PTH production or action**	Hypoparathyroidism: postoperative, autoimmune Congenital Pseudohypoparathyroidism Hypomagnesemia

APPROACH

DIAGNOSIS

- Signs and symptoms are **proportional to the level of hypocalcemia** and **its rate of decline** (Clinical box Hypocalcemia: Signs and Symptoms). Trousseau and Chvostek signs may also demonstrate the presence of hypocalcemia (Clinical box Clinical Tests for Hypocalcemia).
- Chronic hypocalcemia is often **asymptomatic and requires treatment to avoid complications.** It is most often due to deficiency of or resistance to PTH or vitamin D_3.

CLINICAL BOX

Hypocalcemia: Signs and Symptoms

Acute

Tetany, latent tetany

Mild

Circumoral numbness

Paresthesiae

Muscle cramps

Severe

Carpopedal spasm

Prolonged QT interval, cardiac arrhythmias

Vascular calcification

Seizures

Papilledema

Hypotension

Chronic

Cataracts

Dental changes

Skin changes

Extrapyramidal symptoms

Bone pain, fractures

Autonomic

Diaphoresis

Bronchospasm

Biliary colic

CLINICAL BOX

Clinical Tests for Hypocalcemia

Trousseau sign: carpal spasm induction by inflation of a sphygmomanometer 20 mm Hg above systolic BP for 2 to 3 min

Chvostek sign: facial muscle contraction elicited by tapping of the ipsilateral facial nerve anterior to the ear

Note: Contraction of the mouth is seen in 10% to 30% of **normal** subjects.

- The **ionized Ca²⁺ concentration** is the biologically relevant fraction and therefore clinically relevant. However, its accuracy can be influenced by blood collection and handling techniques.
- **Total serum Ca²⁺**, if used, should be corrected for albumin according to the formula below since changes in plasma protein alter the total serum Ca^{2+} concentration.

$$[Ca^{2+}]corrected = (Measured\ Ca^{2+}) + (40 - albumin) \times 0.02\ mmol/L$$

Symptoms of hypocalcemia are predominantly neuromuscular and respiratory; serum PO_4 must be checked before replacing Ca^{2+} IV.

MANAGEMENT

- Hypocalcemia requires hospitalization and immediate treatment if:
  - Symptomatic
  - QT interval is prolonged
  - $[Ca^{2+}]$ionized <0.8 mmol/L or $[Ca^{2+}]$total <1.8 mmol/L even if asymptomatic
- Treatment of acute hypocalcemia can be started before diagnosis by administering IV infusion of Ca^{2+} gluconate (10%, 1 to 2 g) over 10 to 20 min. Give Ca^{2+} IV while the infusion is being prepared.
- After normalization of Ca^{2+} levels, management should be directed toward the underlying cause of the hypocalcemia.

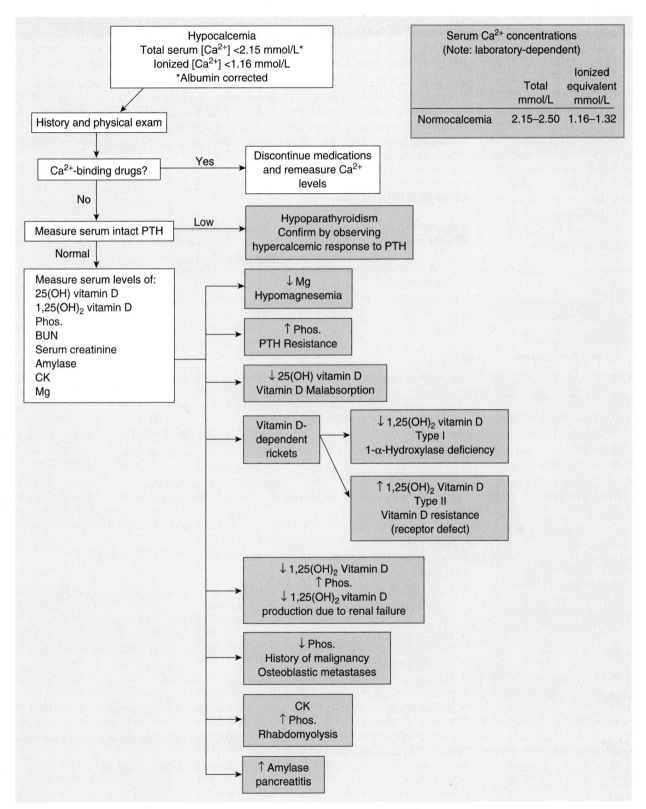

Serum Ca²⁺ concentrations (Note: laboratory-dependent)		
	Total mmol/L	Ionized equivalent mmol/L
Normocalcemia	2.15–2.50	1.16–1.32

Figure 6.15 Approach to diagnosing hypocalcemia.

HYPOPHOSPHATEMIA

ASC Box

Renal PO$_4$ Handling and Hypophosphatemia

Renal reabsorption is major mechanism controlling serum PO$_4$ levels. Reabsorption is inhibited by PTH. Factors ↓ serum PO$_4$:

- ↑ PTH
- Intracellular shift (insulin stimulation of ↑ cellular PO$_4$ uptake and utilization)

CLINICAL BOX

Hypophosphatemia: Signs and Symptoms

Acute

General: lethargy, confusion, coma

Neuromuscular: muscle weakness, paresthesias, paralysis, seizures, rhabdomyolysis

Respiratory: respiratory failure

CVS: arrhythmias, cardiomyopathy, congestive heart failure

Hematologic: hemolysis, platelet dysfunction with bleeding, leukocyte dysfunction

Note: Serious sequelae (e.g., confusion, paralysis, rhabdomyolysis, seizures, coma) occur with severe hypophosphatemia (< 0.25 to 0.32 mmol/L).

Chronic

Bone: rickets, osteomalacia

Kidney: altered renal function

Hypophosphatemia is usually asymptomatic until severe (<0.32 mmol/L).

DEFINITION

- **PO$_4$** is a key constituent of intracellular signaling and metabolism, also serving as an integral component of bone and a urinary buffer for hydrogen ions.
- **Hypophosphatemia can result in clinically significant disturbances in cellular function and multiple organ systems**, usually resulting from depletion of intracellular ATP.
- Differentiating clinically between the major mechanisms of hypophosphatemia is important for treatment (see Table 6.23).

CAUSAL CONDITIONS

Table **6.23** Differential Diagnosis of Hypophosphatemia	
Mechanism	**Differential Diagnosis**
↑ **renal excretion**	Hyperparathyroidism Osmotic diuresis Fanconi syndrome Inherited disorders (e.g., x-linked hypophosphatemia, autosomal dominant hypophosphatemic rickets) Medications: diuretics, calcitonin
↓ **Intake/absorption**	PO$_4$-binding antacids, starvation, malabsorption syndromes, chronic alcoholism (also promotes renal excretion)
Excessive skeletal mineralization	Osteoblastic metastases, hungry bone syndrome (after parathyroidectomy), healing osteomalacia/rickets
Intracellular shift	Correction of metabolic alkalosis, Resp alkalosis Refeeding after starvation Exogenous insulin administration

APPROACH

Diagnosis

- Mild hypophosphatemia is usually **asymptomatic. Hypophosphatemia usually becomes symptomatic when <0.32 mmol/L.** Symptoms are often nonspecific, diffuse, and can be life-threatening (Clinical box Hypophosphatemia: Signs and Symptoms).
- Hypophosphatemia is more common in hospitalized patients and chronic alcoholics. Among hospitalized patients, intracellular shift is the most common mechanism and usually occurs acutely.
- Laboratory results report phosphorus values; in the body, the element exists predominantly as PO$_4$ and as part of phosphorylated proteins.
- **Serum phosphorus concentrations do not necessarily correlate with intracellular PO$_4$ stores**—levels may be normal even in the presence of PO$_4$ deficiency. Although intracellular PO$_4$ depletion does not cause hypophosphatemia *per se*, depletion **predisposes** toward hypophosphatemia.
- An approach to investigating hypophosphatemia is given in Fig. 6.16.

MANAGEMENT

- Treatment should be directed toward the underlying disease process.
- Deciding whether to correct hypophosphatemia should be based on the severity of the phosphate deficit, whether the patient is symptomatic, and their overall clinical status.
- Correction of mild to moderate hypophosphatemia (>0.32 mmol/L) should be through oral replacement. **Dietary sources can be used but with caution because sources**

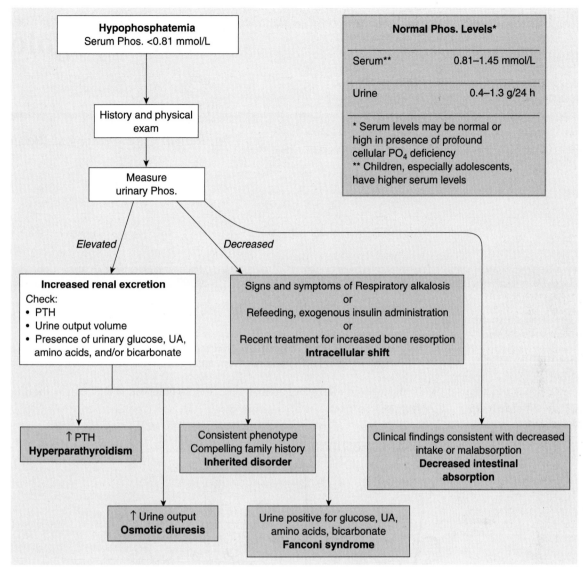

Figure 6.16 Approach to investigating hypophosphatemia.

with high carbohydrate content may precipitate intracellular shift and worsen the hypophosphatemia.
• Severe hypophosphatemia (<0.32 mmol/L) requires parenteral replacement. However, IV salts should be used with caution due to the risk of hypocalcemia and hyperphosphatemia, the latter particularly in patients with renal insufficiency.

CHAPTER 7

Otolaryngology

Jay Zhu, Raiyan Chowdhury, and Richard Liu

EAR PAIN

CLINICAL BOX

Most Common Causes of Otalgia

Primary: otitis media and externa
Secondary: dental pathology and pharyngeal infections

RATIONALE

- Otalgia: nonspecific ear pain and extremely common
  - Primary otalgia: Pain originates within the ear.
  - Referred otalgia: Pain originates from an organ that shares sensory innervation with the ear.
- Owing to the myriad of organs that share sensory innervation with the ear, the differential diagnosis is vast.

CAUSAL CONDITIONS

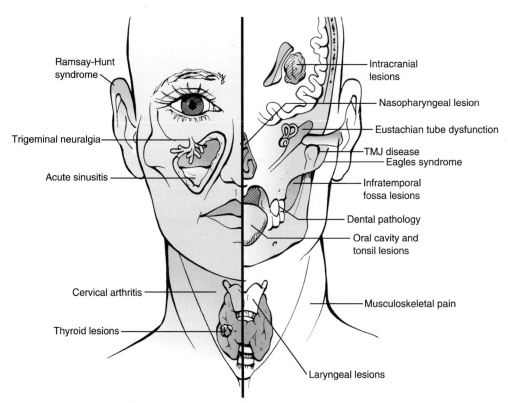

Figure 7.1 Causal conditions of ear pain.

⚛ **ASC Box**

Eustachian Tube Obstruction

- Otitis media is the most common pediatric cause of otalgia.
- Arises from Eustachian tube obstruction secondary to edema from URTI, allergies or an adequate opening
- Leads to negative middle ear pressure, causing influx of pathogens from nasopharynx
- Most common: *Strep. pneumoniae, H. flu, M. catarrhalis*, and viruses

Table **7.1**	Causal Conditions of Ear Pain	
External Ear	**Middle and Inner Ear**	**Referred Pain**
Infections • Otitis externa • Herpes simplex and zoster • Auricular cellulites • Perichondritis • External canal abscess Trauma • Lacerations • Frostbite • Burns • Hematoma Tympanic membrane • Bullous myringitis Other • Foreign body • Cerumen impaction • Neoplasm	Infection/inflammation • AOM • Otitis media with effusion • Mastoiditis • Myringitis Neoplasm Other • Wegener granulomatous	Infection/inflammation • Odontogenic infections • Sinusitis • Peritonsillar abscess • Pharyngitis • Parotitis • Thyroiditis Trauma Neoplasm Other • Neuralgia • Cervical spine disease • TMJ dysfunction • Wisdom teeth • Migraine

History of heavy tobacco and alcohol use without another evident cause of otalgia, refer to otolaryngologist to evaluate upper aerodigestive tract to rule out head and neck cancer. **Carefully examine all oropharyngeal mucosal surfaces for leukoplakia, ulcers and asymmetric masses.**

Mastoiditis is a potentially life-threatening complication of AOM. It manifests as erythema and swelling over the mastoid region, which is located immediately posterior to the external ear. If suspected, intravenous Abx and urgently refer to an otolaryngologist for surgical debridement.

APPROACH

HISTORY

- The presence of accompanying otologic symptoms, such as hearing loss, tinnitus, vertigo, and aural discharge, suggests a local cause.
- The coexistence of a dental infection or pharyngeal pain suggests a referred cause.

PHYSICAL EXAM

- An edematous external auditory canal, **with increased pain when pushing on the tragus or pulling on the pinna**, suggests otitis externa.
- An erythematous and bulging tympanic membrane suggests an AOM.
- Erythema **and fluctuance** over the mastoid region suggests mastoiditis.
- Inspect the oral cavity and oropharynx for signs of infection, dental pathology, and neoplasm.
- Inspect nasal cavity for purulent discharge, suggesting acute sinusitis.

TINNITUS

RATIONALE

- Tinnitus is the perception of sound in the absence of external auditory stimuli.
- In rare circumstances, it is due to serious organic pathology.
- **Subjective**: Only the patient can hear the noise.
- **Objective**: Sound can also be heard by the examiner.
  - This form of tinnitus is rare and occurs when the sound is produced by a para-auditory structure.

CAUSAL CONDITIONS

Table **7.2**	**Causal Conditions of Tinnitus**					
Auditory					**Para-Auditory**	**Psychogenic**
External/Middle Ear	**Cochlear-Vestibular**	**Cochlear Nerve**	**Brain Stem/Cortex**		**Pulse Synchronicity**	

• External otitis
• Wax
• Foreign body
• Otitis media
• Otosclerosis
• Trauma
	• Presbycusis
	• Drugs (ASA, aminogly-cosides, loop diuretics)
	• Otosclerosis
	• Ménière disease
	• Noise, trauma, infections, idiopathic
		• Tumor compression
		• Acoustic neuroma
		• CPA
			• Vascular ischemia
			• Chiari malformation
			• Infections (meningitis)
			• Endocrine/metabolic
			• (Paget, thyroid)
					• Pulse synchronous
					  • Vascular (arterial bruits, hyperdynamic states, aneurysm, venous hum)
					  • Glomus tumor
					• Nonpulse synchronous
					  • TMJ dysfunction, palatal myoclonus, whiplash
						• Anxiety
						• Depression

ASC Box

CNS Is Generator of Tinnitus

Perception of tinnitus is likely related to the loss of input (such as by damage or injury to the cochlea) to neurons in the central auditory pathways resulting in abnormal firing.

APPROACH

- History
  - Determine quality and laterality of the tinnitus.
  - Determine presence of past ear diseases, prolonged noise exposure, and hearing function.
  - Pulsatile tinnitus is most commonly due to a vascular pathology, such as a vascular tumor or a tortuous carotid artery.
  - Identify possible aggravating factors.
  - Excess noise exposure is the most common cause of transient tinnitus.
  - Common medications: ASA, NSAIDs, aminoglycosides, and diuretics
- Physical exam
  - Perform an otoscopy to evaluate for a middle ear infection or cerumen impaction.
  - Auscultate the head and neck region, including the carotid artery, to identify a possible cause of objective tinnitus.
- Workup
  - Routine evaluation of tinnitus includes an audiogram.

CPA tumors can present as unilateral tinnitus, order an MRI scan with gadolinium contrast to rule it out.

MANAGEMENT

- Simple procedures such as cerumen removal, myringotomy for a middle ear effusion, or cessation of ototoxic medications can help patients substantially.
- Management of the symptom is met with inconsistent success. Hearing aids or white noise generators (maskers) can reduce tinnitus.
- Modalities such as biofeedback, acupuncture, and medications have not been consistently proven to be effective.
- Educate the patient and provide reassurance to the benign nature of this condition.
- Tinnitus support groups may help the patient cope with the psychological stress.

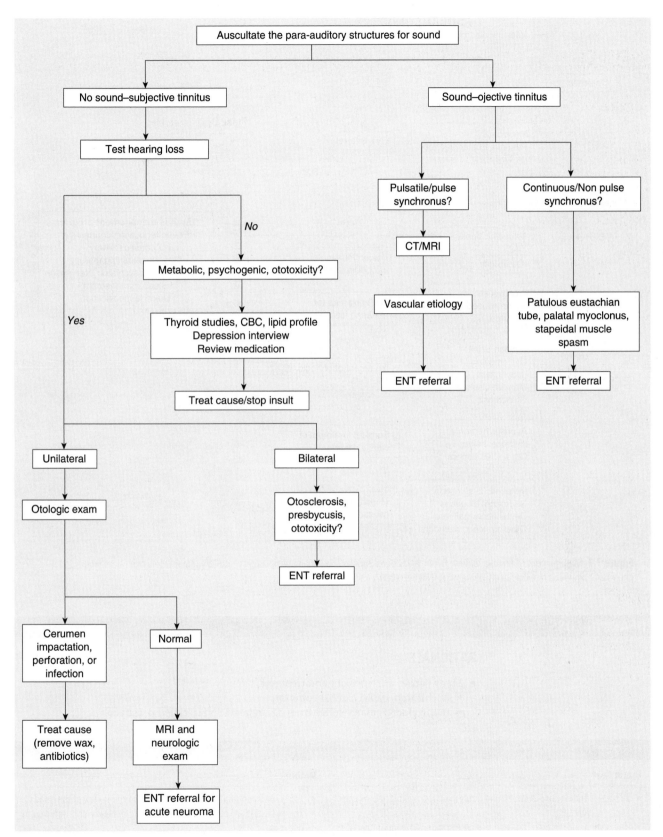

Figure 7.2 Tinnitus.

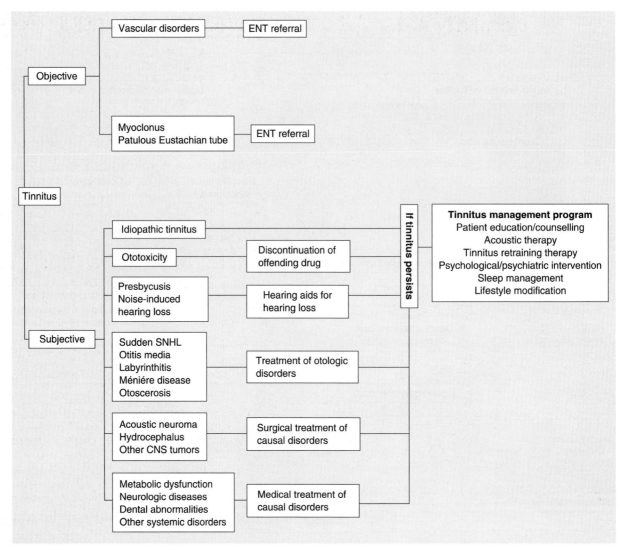

Figure 7.3 Management of tinnitus. Bailey, Byron, and Jonas Johnson. Head and neck surgery—otolaryngology, fourth edition, Figure 151.1, page 2242, Philadelphia: Lippincott Williams & Wilkins, 2006.

HEARING LOSS

RATIONALE

- Many causes are transient and treatable.
  - In children, AOM is most common.
  - In the elderly, many suffer from age-related SNHL called **presbycusis**.

Table **7.3**	Tuning Forks Test to Differentiate Conductive and SNHL
Rinne Test	**Weber**
• A 512-Hz tuning fork is struck and firmly pressed against the mastoid process. This tests BC. • The tuning fork is then replaced beside the external auditory canal to examine AC. • If AC is noted to be louder than BC, the subject has normal hearing or SNHL. Conversely, if a patient reports that BC > AC, he or she has CHL.	• A 512-Hz tuning fork is struck and held on the vertex of the head • The patient is asked if the sound is heard centrally or lateralizes to one side. • Sound lateralizes toward an ear with a CHL, and away from the side with SNHL.

Table **7.4**   **Hearing Tests to Differentiate Conductive and SNHL**

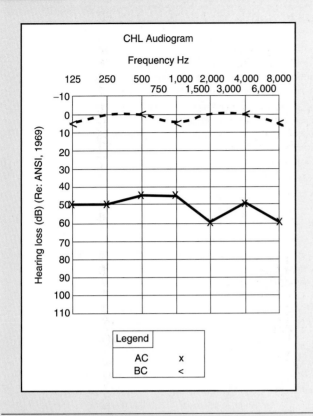

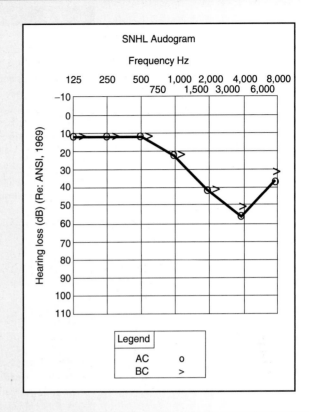

- BC thresholds (<) are normal, and therefore, sensorineural hearing is perfectly intact.
- AC thresholds (x) are significantly increased.
- The difference between AC and BC is called an **air-bone gap**.
- Air-bone gap >15 dB signifies CHL.

- The BC (>) thresholds are raised, indicating an sensorineural hearing impairment. There is no air-bone gap, and therefore, no CHL exists.

ASC Box

Hearing
- Sound waves travel through the external auditory canal to strike the tympanic membrane and vibrate the ossicles, known as the **malleus, incus, and stapes**. The energy is then transmitted to the oval window, which enters into the cochlea. The cochlea is the end organ of hearing and is divided into three fluid-filled compartments.
- The organ of Corti contains auditory hair cells and is located in the middle compartment of the cochlea. Vibrations of the stapes footplate against the oval window induces a fluid wave, which displaces these hairs cells and in turn, triggers neural activity in the cochlea. The culmination of neural signals from all hair cells are transmitted through cranial nerve VIII to the primary auditory cortex located in the temporal lobe of the brain.

- **CHL** results from interference of sound wave transmission from the outside to the cochlea. It represents a defect in the external or middle ear.
- **SNHL** is most commonly due to a defect of the cochlea, whereby processing of mechanical energy into neurologic data or its transmission to the brain is abnormal.

CAUSAL CONDITIONS

Table **7.5**	Causal Conditions of CHL (Most Common)
External Ear	**Middle Ear**

• Obstruction
  • **Cerumen impaction**
  • Foreign body
  • Exostoses
  • Tumor
• Developmental
  • Microtia
  • Canal atresia
• Inflammation/infection
  • **Otitis externa**
	• Ossicles
	  • **Otosclerosis**
	  • Ossicular discontinuity
	• Inflammation/infection
	  • **AOM**
	  • **Otitis media with effusion**
	• Mass
	  • Cholesteatoma
	  • Glomus tympanicum
	• Developmental
	  • Atresia
	  • Malformation
	• Tympanic membrane
	  • **Tympanic membrane perforation**
	  • Tympanosclerosis

Table **7.6**	Causal Conditions of SNHL	
Cochlea	**Central**	**Congenital**

• **Presbycusis**
• **Noise-induced**
• Ototoxic medications
  • Aminoglycosides
  • Chemotherapy agents
  • Loop diuretics
• Ménière's disease
• Trauma
  • Temporal bone trauma
  • Perilymphatic fistula
  • Barotrauma
	• CPA tumors (vestibular schwannoma)
	• Auditory neuropathy
	• Multiple sclerosis
		Hereditary
		  • Nonsyndromic (70%)
		  • Syndromic (30%)
		High risk birth
		  • TORCH infection
		  • Perinatal anoxia
		  • Birth trauma
		  • Low birth weight
		  • Kernicterus

APPROACH

- Common inciting factors of hearing loss: excessive noise exposure, trauma, and ototoxic medications
- In children, review the birth history for congenital hearing loss: perinatal hypoxia and infections.
  - **AOM:** otalgia, fever, and hearing loss. Infants can present with nonspecific symptoms, such as ear-tugging behavior and systemic complaints, including poor sleep, irritability, and decreased appetite.
- Presbycusis: elderly patients with progressive hearing loss with difficulty understanding speech in the setting of loud background noises

MANAGEMENT

- Bacterial AOM: *Streptococcus pneumoniae, Haemophilus influenza,* and *Moraxella catarrhalis.*
- Abx are not routinely required for uncomplicated cases of AOM.
  - If indicated, first-line Abx choice is amoxicillin.
  - Second-line treatment includes a higher dose of amoxicillin, amoxicillin-clavulanate, and second-generation cephalosporins.
- Patients with persistent or recurrent infections may be candidates for myringotomy and tube insertion.
- Prevention: ear noise protection and avoidance of ototoxic medications
  - In children, reducing the risk of AOM include avoidance of bottle feeding, sick contacts, passive smoking, and crowded living conditions, such as daycares.

VERTIGO

RATIONALE

- Dizziness is a common complaint to describe a nonspecific symptom.
- Vertigo is defined as an illusion of movement, most commonly spinning or turning of self or the environment.
  - It can be caused by abnormalities in the peripheral vestibular system or the CNS.

CAUSAL CONDITIONS

Table 7.7   Classification of Dizziness

Dizziness				
True Vertigo (50%)		**Nonvertiginous Dizziness**		
Peripheral (40%)	**Central (10%)**	**Disequilibrium (15%)**	**Presyncope (10%)**	**Psychiatric (15%)**
BPPV	CPA tumor	Peripheral neuropathy	Cardiac arrhythmias	Depression
Vestibular neuronitis	CVA	Visual impairment	Anemia	Anxiety
Ménière's disease	Multiple sclerosis		Orthostatic hypotension	Panic attack
Ototoxicity	Drugs (anticonvulsants, alcohol)			

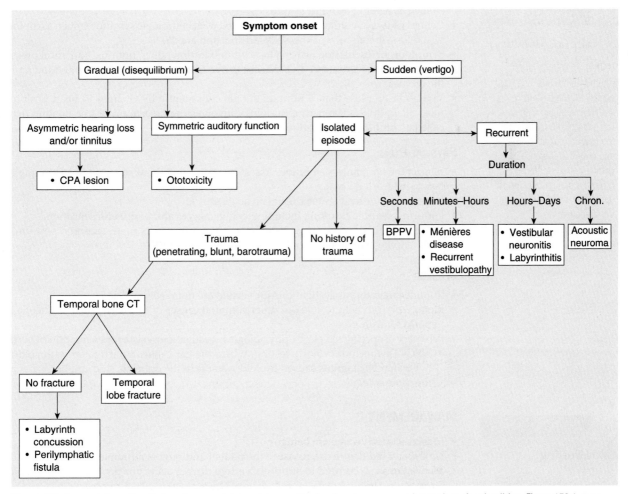

Figure 7.4 Approach to vertigo. Bailey, Byron, and Jonas Johnson. Head and neck surgery–otolaryngology, fourth edition, Figure 156.1, page 2297, Philadelphia: Lippincott Williams & Wilkins, 2006.

Table **7.8**	Peripheral versus Central Vertigo	
	Peripheral	**Central**
Nystagmus	Horizontal, never vertical Never reverses direction	Vertical or horizontal Can reverse direction with change of direction of gaze
Neurologic signs and symptoms	Absent	Common
Otologic signs and symptoms	Common	Absent
Time course	Abrupt onset/offset, never continuous due to central compensation	Tends to be continuous

Central vertigo warrants an urgent neurologic consult. See Table 7.7.

APPROACH

HISTORY

- Define whether the patient is experiencing vertigo, disequilibrium, or presyncope:
  - True vertigo is a sensation of spinning of the self or environment.
  - Dizziness without a subjective feeling of rotation is not vertigo and should be approached differently.
- Peripheral vertigo is episodic and never continuous for a matter of weeks, due to central compensation. It is often provoked by sudden changes in head position.
  - Peripheral etiologies of vertigo are often associated with other otologic symptoms such as hearing loss and tinnitus.
- Central causes of vertigo are often associated with neurologic symptoms such as diplopia, vision loss, unilateral weakness, dysarthria, and ataxia.
- Symptoms of fluctuating hearing loss, vertigo lasting hours, tinnitus, and aural pressure suggest Ménière's disease. This disease is due to an overaccumulation of endolymph in the cochlea.
- Vertigo lasting less than a minute, initiate consistently by changes in head position is most likely BPPV. The pathophysiology involves the presence of a free floating debris, called an **otolith**, in the vestibular apparatus.

PHYSICAL EXAM

- Inspect the tympanic membrane. Assess hearing using the Weber and Rinne tuning fork test. (See Hearing Loss)
- Inspect eyes for nystagmus during an acute attack.
- Perform a neurologic exam, including cranial nerves and peripheral sensation.
- If the vertigo is initiated by changing positions that lasts mere seconds, perform the Dix-Hallpike maneuver to confirm the diagnosis of BPPV.

WORKUP

- Routine laboratory investigations for vertigo are not recommended.
- Blood work can help to rule out other common causes of dizziness, such as anemia and hypothyroidism.
- A battery of specialized electrophysiologic investigations exists for evaluation of vertigo.
  - ENG: This includes caloric testing, where the ear canals are irrigated with cold and hot water. Nystagmus caused by cold water is to the opposite side and hot water is to the same side.

MANAGEMENT

- Most causes of vertigo are benign.
- Unless any red flags exist, reassure the patient and offer symptomatic relief.
- Medications can be used to suppress vertigo during acute attacks lasting more than an hour.
  - Brief episodes will likely end spontaneously before the onset of pharmacologic action.
  - Antihistamines (meclizine, dimenhydrinate) and anticholinergics (scopolamine)

CLINICAL BOX

Dix-Hallpike Maneuver

1. With the patient's head rotated 45° to one side, quickly lie the patient down with the head hanging over the edge of the table. Hold the position for at least 30 s, and note the presence of vertigo and nystagmus.
2. Bring the patient back up to upright position and repeat the maneuver on the opposite side.

CLINICAL BOX

Caloric Testing

COWS—Cold Opposite, Warm Same

SORE THROAT (RHINORRHEA)

RATIONALE

- Coexistence of rhinorrhea and pharyngitis often suggests URTI such as the common cold.
- Pharyngitis may be due to viral and bacterial pathogens. Infections are transmitted through direct contact with infected bodily fluids, such as saliva or nasal secretions.
- Rhinorrhea may be acute, seasonal, and chronic. It is most commonly due to URTIs, sinusitis, and rhinitis.

CAUSAL CONDITIONS

Table **7.9**	Causal Conditions of Pharyngitis and Rhinitis			
	Pharyngitis			**Rhinitis**
Viral	**Bacterial**	**Other**		**Allergic rhinitis**
Adenovirus	GAS	Mycoplasma		Idiopathic rhinitis
Rhinovirus	Group C and G Streptococcus	Candidiasis		Sinusitis
Influenza/parainfluenza	Neisseria gonorrhoeae			CSF leak
Coxsackie	Corynebacterium diphtheria			Foreign body
HSV				
EBV				
CMV				

See also Figure 7.5.

APPLIED SCIENTIFIC CONCEPTS

- The most common agents responsible for a sore throat are adenovirus, EBV, and GAS. Specifically, it is crucial to determine if GAS is the etiologic factor, as it is associated with specific complications, namely glomerulonephritis and rheumatic fever, and requires a course of Abx.
- The **RADTs** is useful as an initial screen for GAS. While the specificity of RADTs exceeds 95%, the sensitivity varies between 65% and 90%.
- If the RADT is positive, the diagnosis is reliable and treatment should be initiated. A negative RADT could have a 10% to 35% false-negative rate. As such, the clinician must wait for the throat culture results to confidently rule out GAS.

APPROACH TO PHARYNGITIS

- The major task is to determine if GAS is the pathogen.
- Appropriate Abx can prevent complications and decrease the duration of symptoms.
- Clinical differentiation of GAS pharyngitis from viral is difficult.
- The presence of rhinorrhea and cough, and absence of fever make the diagnosis of GAS infection less likely. Such patients are most likely to have a viral URTI, and do not require further testing or interventions.
- The Sore Throat Score aids in the diagnosis of GAS pharyngitis. (see Table 7.10)

APPROACH TO RHINORRHEA

- The most common causes: allergic rhinitis, idiopathic rhinitis, and sinusitis.
- Allergic rhinitis (hay fever) affects up to 20% of individuals. There is often a personal and family history of atopy, such as asthma or eczema. It is usually seasonal, and patients also complain of nasal or ocular itching.

C₂LEO Box

Abx Overtreatment

- Acute pharyngitis is one of the most common presenting complaints to the physician's office.
- While the most clinically important pathogen is GAS, this is the causal agent in <10% of cases. However, up to 75% of adults with acute pharyngitis are prescribed Abx.
- The overtreatment of pharyngitis with Abx against the established practice guidelines is a major cause of Abx abuse, leading to bacterial resistance and unnecessary health spending.

ASC Box

Tests for Complications of GAS Pharyngitis

Poststreptococcal glomerulonephritis

- Elevated antistreptolysin O-quantitative titer
- RBC casts on urinalysis

Acute Rheumatic Fever

- Clinical diagnosis on evidence of antecedent pharyngeal GAS infection and two major or one major and two minor Jones criteria
- Major criteria: carditis, polyarthritis, chorea, erythema marginatum, subcutaneous nodules
- Minor criteria: arthralgia, fever, elevated RBC sedimentation, elevated C-reactive protein, prolonged PR interval

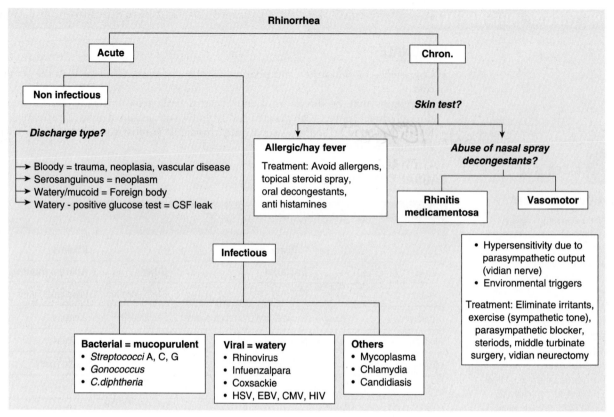

Figure 7.5 Rhinorrhea.

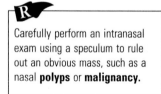

Carefully perform an intranasal exam using a speculum to rule out an obvious mass, such as a nasal **polyps** or **malignancy.**

- Idiopathic rhinitis, or vasomotor rhinitis, is characterized by watery nasal discharge and intermittent congestion that is induced by nonspecific irritants, such as temperature changes or spicy foods.
- Sinusitis leads to nasal obstruction, facial pain, and purulent nasal discharge. Examine the nasal cavity for mucopurulent fluid.

MANAGEMENT

- GAS pharyngitis is treated with a 10-day Abx course. The recommended Abx is **penicillin V** in adults and **amoxicillin** in children.

Table **7.10**	Sore Throat Score in Diagnosis of GAS Pharyngitis
Symptom	**Points**
Cough absent?	1
History of fever >38°C?	1
Tonsillar exudates?	1
Swollen, tender anterior nodes?	1
Age 3 to 14?	1
Age 15 to 44?	0
Age >45?	−1
Score	**Recommended Action**
0−1	No culture or Abx
2−3	Culture all, Abx only if culture is positive
4	Culture all, treat with Abx, discontinue to cultures negative

(Centor RM, Witherspoon JM, Dalton HP, et al. The diagnosis of strept throat in the emergency room. *Med Decis Making.* 1981;1:239–246.)

- Abx prevent the development of acute rheumatic fever, but do not decrease the incidence of glomerulonephritis.
- Incidence of GAS transmission in untreated patients to close contacts is 35%. However, within 24 hours of penicillin administration, the patient becomes minimally contagious. If a close contact experiences pharyngitis, there is a higher likelihood of the causative agent being GAS and should be managed accordingly

SMELL AND TASTE DYSFUNCTION

RATIONALE

- Disorders of taste and smell are common occurrences. Approximately 80% of taste problems are actually secondary to disorders of smell.
  - Total loss of taste rarely occurs due to neural cross innervation.

CAUSAL CONDITIONS

Table **7.11** Causal Conditions of Smell and Taste Dysfunction	
Conductive	**Sensorineural**
The odor cannot reach the olfactory epithelium secondary to nasal obstruction. Inflammatory <ul><li>Allergic rhinitis</li><li>Vasomotor rhinitis</li><li>Nasal polyps</li></ul>	Central neural structures cannot interpret the neural transmission. Degenerative <ul><li>Stroke</li><li>Alzheimer disease</li><li>Parkinson disease</li><li>Multiple sclerosis</li></ul>
Nasal cavity neoplasms	Endocrine/metabolic <ul><li>Diabetes mellitus</li><li>Adrenal hypo/hyperfunction</li><li>Pseudohypoparathyroid</li><li>Hypothyroid</li><li>Renal failure</li><li>Hepatic failure</li></ul>
Congenital <ul><li>Septal deformity</li><li>Choanal atresia</li></ul>	Intracranial neoplasms
Other <ul><li>Foreign body</li></ul>	Other <ul><li>Chemicals</li><li>Drugs</li><li>Head trauma</li></ul>

APPROACH

- Note the time course of the dysfunction.
  - Sudden onset of smell or taste dysfunction could represent viral infection.
  - Gradual loss of smell/taste function suggests allergic rhinitis, nasal polyposis, or neoplasms.
  - Intermittent disruption of function favors the diagnosis of allergic rhinitis.
- Examine oral and nasal cavity.
- Rule out common causes of nasal obstruction, such as nasal polyps and edematous mucosa due to rhinitis.
- Question the patient on the presence of any neurologic symptoms indicative of central disease.
- Perform a neurologic exam, including a thorough evaluation of the cranial nerves.

Any neurologic signs or symptoms warrant an MRI to rule out intracranial pathology, such as a tumor or stroke.

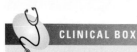

CLINICAL BOX

Samter Triad

Nasal polyposis, ASA sensitivity, asthma

WORKUP

- If the patient complains of chronic nasal obstruction and purulent discharge, obtain a CT scan of the paranasal sinuses to evaluate for sinusitis, polyps or intranasal masses.
- Routine blood work is not indicated, but the clinician may elect to order blood tests to examine for diabetes mellitus, thyroid, and renal function.

MANAGEMENT

- The treatment of smell or taste dysfunction is directed at the causative factor.
- If nasal congestion or nasal polyposis is present, consider intranasal corticosteroid sprays and antihistamines.
- Treatment of acute sinusitis consists of Abx and saline irrigation.
- Polyps and sinus disease that are refractory to medical treatment warrant otolaryngology consultation for surgical intervention.
- Overall, the patient needs reassurance that the disease state is rarely serious or life threatening.

MOUTH PROBLEMS

CLINICAL BOX

Signs of Oral Malignancy

- leukoplakia non-healing oral ulcers

RATIONALE

- Two of the most common diseases affecting the mouth are **odontogenic infections** and **neoplasia**.
- Periodontal diseases affect 15% of the population and have potentially serious complications.
- Oral neoplasms are difficult tumors to treat and signs of oral malignancy must be recognized early.

APPLIED SCIENTIFIC CONCEPTS

- Two main odontogenic infections, dental caries and periodontal disease, both of which arise from bacteria that colonize the teeth surface.
  - Dental caries are caused by bacteria within the plaques, which produce acid. The acid generated on the surface of the tooth by these bacteria demineralizes the enamel coating, and help the bacteria invade the pulp.
  - Bacterial plaques located below the gingival margin may lead to periodontal disease, which are defined as infections of the gum, ligaments, and bones that support the teeth.
- Dental infections that invade through the mandible or maxilla may spread through various fascial planes to cause life-threatening complications, such as sepsis or airway compromise.
- Predisposing factors for odontogenic infections include poor dental hygiene and advanced age, with associated gingival recession. Other predisposing factors include hormonal changes, such as that during puberty or pregnancy, and systemic illnesses that impair the immune system.

ASC Box

Bacteremic Seeding in Patients with Prosthetic Appliances

According to the 2007 AHA guideline for IE prophylaxis, patients with prosthetic heart valves or a prior history of IE undergoing dental procedures should receive prophylactic Abx. The preferred Abx regimen is amoxicillin, or a macrolide or clindamycin if penicillin allergic.

CAUSAL CONDITIONS

Table **7.12**	**Causal Conditions of Mouth Problems**	
Children	**Adults**	**Elderly**

• Teeth abnormalities
  • Caries
  • Eruption
• Gingival overgrowth
  • Idiopathic, genetic, drugs
• Trauma
  • Abuse
  • Accidents
	• Periodontal infections
	  • Dental caries/endodontic infection/periapical abscess
	  • Gingivitis/periodontitis/pericoronitis/periodontal abscess
	  • Fascial space infections/osteomyelitis
	• Oral carcinoma
	  • Premalignant
	    • Leukoplakia/erythroplakia
	  • Malignant
	    • Squamous cell carcinoma
	• Salivary glands
	  • Infections (mumps, bacterial)
	  • Sialolithiasis
	  • Tumor
	• Other
	  • Cellulitis
	  • Trauma
	  • Candida
		• Receding gingival/gums
		• Edentulism

APPROACH

Any suspicious lesions, such as leukoplakia, nonhealing ulcer, or exophytic lesion, should be referred a head and neck oncology surgeon for prompt diagnosis and treatment.

- Inspect and palpate the oral cavity and oropharynx for leukoplakia, ulcers, and asymmetric masses.
- Prolonged use of tobacco (smoke or chewing) and/or alcohol synergistically increase the risk of head and neck cancer.
- Patients with dental disease may present with localized pain, and hypersensitivity to temperature and air. Exam may reveal grossly decayed teeth with erythematous gingiva. Such cases require referral to a dentist for management.

MANAGEMENT

If a patient presents with evidence of complications from a tooth infection, such as neck swelling, trismus, hoarseness, or stridor, an urgent consult to an otolaryngologist is warranted for definitive management.

- The main bacterial pathogens are various serotypes of *Streptococcus mutans. Lactobacilli* are progressive agents due to their acid-producing ability. In acute odontogenic infections, especially periodontal disease, systemic antimicrobials are of benefit.
  - Abx: penicillin, ampicillin-sulbactam, and clindamycin.
- Strategies to prevent odontogenic infections include regular teeth brushing with fluoride toothpaste, flossing, topical antiseptics (i.e., chlorhexidine) and dietary changes to decrease sugar consumption.
- The most significant public health change in decreasing dental caries has been the fluoridation of water supplies.

CHAPTER 8

Family and Community Medicine

Dr. Janna Kasumovic and Dr. Fraser R. Brenneis

PERIODIC HEALTH EXAM

DEFINITION

Patients present when they are asymptomatic in hope of discovering disease in the early stages or in order to prevent disease all together. It is an excellent opportunity for the physician to emphasize preventative medicine.

CHILD AGE 0 TO 3 YR

AT RISK FOR

SIDS (<1 yr), FTT, developmental delay

SCREENING QUESTIONS/MEASUREMENTS

Height, weight, head circumference, diet Hx, birth Hx/pregnancy Hx, developmental milestones, family Hx

LAB WORK/TESTING

TSH, PKU at birth
   As needed
    Some provinces include screening for other metabolic D/O

STRONG EVIDENCE TO RECOMMEND/DISCUSS

Immunization, back to sleep, home safety, smoke-free environment, dental health

CHILD AGE 3 TO 12 YR

AT RISK FOR

Developmental delay, accidents/trauma, visual/hearing loss, obesity

SCREENING QUESTIONS/MEASUREMENTS

BP, nutrition Hx, physical activity Hx, developmental milestones

LAB WORK/TESTING

As needed

STRONG EVIDENCE TO RECOMMEND/DISCUSS

Home safety, nutrition, dental health, immunization

ADOLESCENT 13 TO 24 YR

AT RISK FOR

MVA, substance abuse, STI, obesity, eating D/O

CLINICAL BOX

HEEADSS: Periodic Health Exam

Home—with who, safe

Education—grade, academic success, behavior/punishment

Employment—what, do they need the wage/supporting self

Activities—risky behavior, sports, peer group

Drugs—types, amount, time period

Suicide—mood, self esteem

Sex—with who, activities, safety

SCREENING/MEASUREMENTS

BP, nutrition Hx, physical activity Hx, HEEADSS

LAB WORK

Pap test within 1 yr of becoming sexually active, discussion of HPV vaccination (for age 9–13), and STI as necessary

STRONG EVIDENCE TO RECOMMEND/DISCUSS

Condoms, contraception, avoid risky behavior, seat belts, body image, dental health, immunization

ADULT 24 TO 44 YR

AT RISK FOR

Cancer, IHD, substance abuse, eating D/O, HTN, incontinence

SCREENING/MEASUREMENTS

BP, Psych Hx, social Hx, past medical Hx, current symptoms, depression screen

LAB WORK/IMAGING

Mammography (50 to 69 q 1 to 2 yr), Pap (start of sexual intercourse to age 69 yearly), fasting lipids (men >40 and women postmenopausal or >50 or any age with risk factors q 1 to 3 yr), fasting glucose (>40 q 3 yr or more frequent if risk factors)

STRONG EVIDENCE TO RECOMMEND/DISCUSS:

Breast exam by physician, folic acid if planning pregnancy, smoking cessation, dental health, immunization

ADULT AGE 45 TO 64 YR

AT RISK FOR

Cancer, IHD, substance abuse, obesity, osteoporosis, HTN, incontinence

SCREENING/MEASUREMENTS

BP, Psych Hx, social Hx, past medical Hx, current symptoms

LAB WORK/IMAGING

FOB (start age 50 q 1 to 2 yr), mammogram (yearly 50 to 69 yr), Pap test, DRE and PSA, bone density (if risk factors for osteoporosis, previous fracture or over age 65 q 3 to 5 yr)

STRONG EVIDENCE TO RECOMMEND/DISCUSS

Breast exam by physician, smoking cessation, dental health, Ca^{2+} and Vit D (postmenopausal women), physical activity, heart-healthy diet, immunization.

OVER 65 YR

AT RISK FOR

Falls, polypharmacy, IHD, cancer, visual/hearing loss, incontinence

SCREENING/MEASUREMENTS

MMSE if suspect cognitive decline

LAB WORK/IMAGING

FOB (start age 50 q 1 to 2 yr), mammogram (yearly 50 to 69 yr), Pap test, DRE and PSA, bone density (if risk factors for osteoporosis, previous fracture or over age 65 q 3 to 5 yr)

STRONG EVIDENCE TO RECOMMEND/DISCUSS

Breast exam by physician, smoking cessation, dental health, Ca^{2+} and Vit D (postmenopausal women), physical activity, heart-healthy diet, immunization

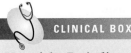

CLINICAL BOX

Use of the Periodic Health Exam

Periodic health exams are no longer encouraged to be overly exhaustive. The physician should focus on and order investigations based on the likelihood of finding an abnormality. This is also the case for the physical exam.

FATIGUE

DEFINITION

The patient complaint of fatigue is common and unfortunately often frustrating for the family physician. It is important for a physician to be able to take an appropriate Hx and conduct a thorough physical exam in order to detect those patients who require further evaluation.

CAUSAL CONDITIONS

Table **8.1**	Fatigue: Causal Conditions by Age-Group	
Child	**Adult**	**Elderly**
Onset (<1 mo is recent, >6 mo is chronic) When noticed most (with activity, time of day, all day) Improvement with rest Physical symptoms worrisome to patient Constitutional symptoms Sleep Hx Diet Hx Past medical Hx Medications		
URTI symptoms	Chest pain	Orthopnea
Diarrhea/vomiting	Myalgias/weakness	PND
Appetite	Bowel function	SOB
Abdominal pain	Sexual function	Chest pain
Voiding concerns	Somnolence	Myalgias/weakness
	Depression screen	Geriatric depression scale

Full Hx and Physical Exam in Fatigue

It is important to perform a full Hx and physical exam of each patient although up to 75% of patients will have a psychological cause.

Management of Psychological or Idiopathic Fatigue

Recommend regular exercise

Sleep hygiene

Keep socially active

APPROACH

PHYSICAL EXAM

- Jaundice
- Conjunctival pallor
- Thyroid exam
- Full cardio exam (CHF signs, murmurs)
- Full pulmonary exam
- Abdominal exam (body habitus, ascites, bruits, spleen size, liver size, tenderness, masses)
- Extremities (joint swelling or dermatological changes)
- Dermatological/MSK exam (rashes, joint tenderness, Musc strength)

Investigation of Fatigue

In the absence of symptoms other than fatigue and a normal physical exam, labwork will be of value in <5% of patients.

Table **8.2**	**Systemic Causal Conditions of Fatigue**
Psychological	Depression Anxiety Mania
Pharmacologic	Hypnotics Antihypertensives Antidepressants Drug abuse Drug withdrawal
Endocrine Metabolic	Diabetes Adrenal insufficiency Hypothyroidism Hyperthyroidism Chronic renal failure Chronic liver failure Hypercalcemia
Cardiac	CHF Endocarditis
Pulmonary	TB/pneumonia COPD
Connective tissue	RA PMR
Neoplastic	Malignancy
Hematologic	Anemia
Infectious	HIV Hepatitis Mononucleosis
Sleep	PLMD/restless leg Apnea Bruxism
Idiopathic	Chronic fatigue syndrome

Table **8.3**	**Approach to Fatigue by Age-Group**		
Age-group	**Child**	**Adult**	**Elderly**
Common conditions	Commonly: Infection Diabetes Anemia	Commonly: Stress/poor sleep Anemia Thyroid disease Depression	Commonly: Infection Chronic disease Myositis Depression Polypharmacy Malignancy
Approach and investigation	Focus on Hx and physical. Labwork can be limited and based on assessment. Possible CBC, glucose.	Focus on Hx and physical. Consider CBC, glucose, TSH. Screen for depression.	Hx and physical to guide labwork. Consider CBC, glucose, TSH, ESR. Screen for depression. Advanced testing as needed. Review medications.

WEIGHT LOSS AND EATING D/O

DEFINITION

Both severe voluntary or involuntary weight loss can indicate a serious psychiatric or medical condition that needs attention. Involuntary weight loss of >5% of baseline is worrisome.

CAUSAL CONDITIONS

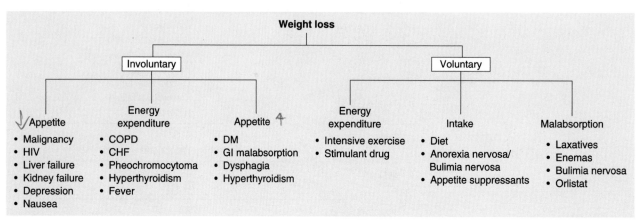

Figure 8.1 Weight loss: causal conditions.

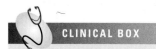

Lab Investigations of Weight Loss

Chosen based on suspected diagnosis

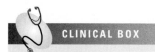

Lab findings of malnutrition

Low prealbumin, low albumin, anemia

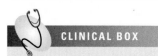

Chronic Disease

Perform a full physical exam looking for signs of chronic disease.

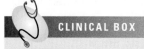

Russell sign

Calluses on the knuckles from self-induced vomiting

APPROACH

Hx

- Voluntary or Involuntary
- Amount of weight lost and over what period of time
- Appetite increased or decreased
- Diet
- Energy level
- Difficulty swallowing
- Vomiting/nausea or diarrhea
- Exercise/activities
- Menstrual Hx
- Chronic medical conditions
- Psych Hx
- Medications/recreational drugs
- Fevers or night sweats
- Is patient concerned about weight loss

PHYSICAL EXAM

Physical signs of eating D/O

Anorexia	Bulimia
Low BP, HR	Russell sign
Dry skin and hair	Enlarged parotid glands
Hair loss	Tooth decay
Peripheral edema	Peripheral edema
Musc wasting	Musc wasting

LAB INVESTIGATION

Anorexia	Bulimia
Low RBC, WBC	Low serum lytes (Na, K)
Low sex hormones	Vomiting: high amylase
High cholesterol	Laxatives: high pH
Low albumin	Low albumin
Low lytes (Na, K, Ca^{2+}, Mg, PO_4)	

HOSPITALIZATION CRITERIA
- <65% Expected weight
- IV fluids required
- Abnormal lytes/pH
- Actively suicidal
- Severe complications
- Patients are best managed with a multidisciplinary approach
- Admission criteria may vary by site

COMPLICATIONS OF EATING D/O
- Arrhythmias
- Sudden cardiac death
- CHF
- Osteoporosis
- Renal failure
- Musc wasting
- Amenorrhea
- GERD
- Seizures
- Pancreatitis

ADVISING HEALTHY WEIGHT LOSS
- Encourage a well-rounded approach of which diet is only a portion.
- Diet involves creating a deficit of 500 to 1,000 kcal/d.
- Aim to achieve weight loss of 1 to 2 lbs/wk.
- Initially, aim to reduce body weight by ~10% from baseline.
- Encourage moderate levels of activity for 30 to 40 min/d, 3 to 5 d/wk.
- Lifestyle therapy should be considered before drug therapy.

APPLIED SCIENTIFIC CONCEPTS

UNDERSTANDING EATING D/O
Anorexia Nervosa—DSMIV Criteria
1. Body weight <85% than expected for age and weight
2. Intense fear of weight gain
3. Denies the serious nature of severe weight loss
4. Absence of three consecutive menstrual cycles

Types of Anorexia Nervosa
- Restrictive—decreased food intake
- Binge eating/purging—binge eating and/or purging behavior

Binging: consuming an abnormally large amount of food in a 2-h period than your average person would

Purging: wanting to remove intake; can be self-induced vomiting, laxatives, diuretics or enemas.

Bulimia Nervosa—DSMIV Criteria
1. Recurrent binge episodes
2. Recurrent episodes of behavior that attempts to compensate the binging

CLINICAL BOX

Anorexia versus Bulimia

Bulimia can appear in patients with a normal weight or in obese patients. Anorexia is always found in patients with extremely low body weight.

CLINICAL BOX

Multifactorial Eating D/O

Eating D/O are often multifactorial and there is often causes from each category in a given patient.

CLINICAL BOX

Management of an Eating D/O

Management of an eating D/O is best done with a multidisciplinary approach. Referral to a specialist is often necessary.

3. Both the above occur at least ×2/wk for 3 mo
4. Self opinion is largely centered around physical appearance.

Types of Bulimia Nervosa

- Purging
- Nonpurging—compensatory behavior is fasting or excessive exercise

RISK FACTORS FOR AN EATING D/O

Table **8.4**	Risk Factors of an Eating D/O	
Environmental	**Biological**	**Psychosocial**
• Career choice (athlete, model) • Industrial society	• Female • Obese • Teens to 20s in age	• Perfectionist • OCD • Personality D/O • Hx sexual abuse • Hx substance abuse

PREOPERATIVE MEDICAL EVALUATION

DEFINITION

A thorough medical examination is required before surgery to detect or know the current status of chronic medical conditions. The management of these conditions can then be maximized before surgery and surgical risk can be minimized.

APPROACH

Hx

Recent Illnesses or Symptoms (Last 3 mo)
- Chest pain (anginal)
- SOB
- Cough
- Peripheral edema
- Palpitations
- Fevers
- Exercise tolerance

When judging a patient's exercise tolerance ask about specific tasks (flights of stairs, blocks walked). Decide if an individual of similar age would be able to do more or less.

Chronic Medical Conditions
- Worsening of symptoms/status
- Last evaluation by specialist
- Last relevant imaging/lab work
- Knowledge of end-organ damage, *Diabetes ?*
- Previous thromboembolism

Medications
- Antihypertensives
- Insulin/hypoglycemics
- β-Blockers
- Anticoagulants
- Home O_2

Allergies
- Medications
- Past RXNs/family RXNs to anaesthetics

Last Menstrual Period
- Chance of pregnancy

Smoking/ETOH
- Frequency/duration
- Amount

PHYSICAL EXAM

Physical exam should focus on the cardiac, pulmonary and vascular exam. The exam should also look for signs of end-organ damage from chronic medical conditions.

INVESTIGATIONS

Male	Female
Hgb	Hgb
Creatinine/CrCl	Creatinine/CrCl
(age >50)	(age >50)
EKG (age >45)	EKG (age >55)
CXR (age >60)	CXR (age >60)
INR	INR
PTT	PTT
Cross match	Cross match
	β-HCG (childbearing age)

Further testing may be necessary if a chronic medical condition has recently changed in status or if abnormalities on physical exam warrant investigation. However, random testing is not cost effective or necessary in a previously healthy patient. A random abnormal test may have no clinical significance and may create unnecessary delay of surgery.

CARDIAC EVALUATION

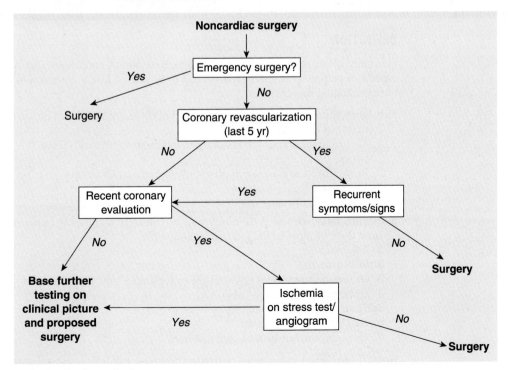

Figure 8.2 Cardiac evaluation.

PULMONARY EVALUATION

Test	When to Order
ABG	CABG, upper abdominal surgery
CXR	Age >60
PFT	Thoracic or upper abdominal surgery, known lung pathology, lung pathology and indeterminate clinical status
Smoking cessation	All patients (8 wk prior)

CLINICAL BOX

General Operative Risk for Surgery

Low—endoscopic, superficial, cataract

Intermediate—carotid endarterectomy, HEENT, intraperitoneal, intrathoracic, orthopaedic

High—emergency, aortic and major vascular, peripheral vascular, prolonged

CLINICAL BOX

Risk of Surgical Procedure

Try to evaluate patients as being increased or average risk for a certain surgical procedure rather than fit or unfit for surgery.

SUBSTANCE ABUSE, ADDICTION, AND WITHDRAWAL

DEFINITION

Substance abuse and addiction are extremely common conditions that affect numerous aspects of patient's lives. Physicians need to be skilled in the detection of addictions and the treatment options.

Substance abuse/addiction: A 12-mo period of clinically significant impairment or distress from one or more of:
1. Recurrent substance use resulting in failure to fulfill major roles (work, school, home)
2. Recurrent substance use in physically hazardous situations
3. Use related legal problems
4. Continued substance use despite social problems from the use

Substance dependence: A 12-mo period of clinically significant impairment or distress from three or more of the following at any time:
1. Tolerance
2. Withdrawal
3. Increasing amount taken over time or for longer time than intended
4. Unsuccessful efforts to cut down
5. Time consumed in attaining substance
6. Past interests diminished
7. Use continued in spite of consequences

Note: These DSMIV criteria can be used as diagnosis guidelines as well as to contrast abuse and dependence

CAUSAL CONDITIONS

Table **8.5**	Common Drugs of Abuse, Addiction, and Dependence
Drug Class	**Examples**
Stimulants	Nicotine
Hallucinogens	Cannabis LSD, Psilocybin (mushrooms), mescaline (peyote), amphetamines, cocaine, PCP
Sedative hypnotics	ETOH, benzodiazepines, barbiturates, rohypnol (date rape drug)
Opioids	Codeine, morphine, heroin
Inhalants	Glue, amyl nitrate, NO
Anesthetics	Ketamine

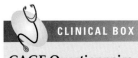

CLINICAL BOX

CAGE Questionnaire

Cut down?

Annoyed by others criticizing your use?

Guilty of your use?

Eye opener?

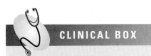

CLINICAL BOX

Addiction versus Dependence

Many patients think addiction and dependence are the same. It is important to explain the difference.

APPROACH

Hx

- CAGE questionnaire
- TWEAK EtOH screening tool in women (more sensitive, particularly in higher use patients)
- Type of drug and route
- Past and recent quantity of use
- Past and recent frequency of use
- Signs of withdrawal/dependence
- Signs of abuse
- Family Hx
- Treatment Hx
- Support network
- Readiness to change

FALLS

DEFINITION

Falls are a very common cause of trauma and can have serious morbidity and mortality for an elderly patient. Falls are very preventable and should not be thought of as an inevitable sign of aging.

CAUSAL CONDITIONS

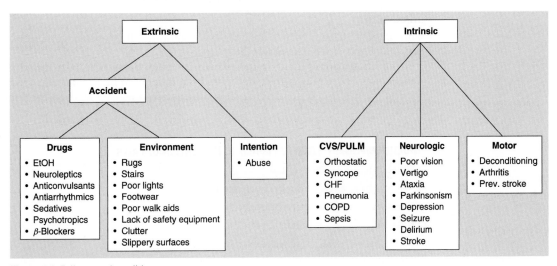

Figure 8.3 Falls: causal conditions.

APPROACH

Hx

- When
- Where
- Symptoms during/before
- Activity before fall
- LOC
- Memory of incident
- Incontinence
- Witness
- How landed
- Able to get up on own
- How long before found
- Previous falls and suspected causes
- General health recently
- Past medication and medical Hx

Physical Exam

- Vitals including postural BP
- Pulse rhythm
- Visual acuity/HEENT exam
- Full CVS and Resp exam
- Abdominal exam
- Musc/joint/bone tenderness
- Joint ROM
- Musc strength
- Skin survey looking for injuries
- CN exam and reflexes
- Screen for ataxia
- Balance and gait (if possible)
- Cognition

Investigations

Always do:

- CBC-D
- Lytes
- BUN
- Creatinine
- Glucose
- Vit B_{12} (in elderly)
- TSH

Further investigations based on Hx and physical findings

Management

Educate patient about what to do in the event of future falls. Consider getting an emergency response button for a patient who lives alone.

The assessment of falls is a time where the entire patient can be assessed for level of functioning. Hx of falls in the elderly has been thought to be a factor that predicts motor vehicle crashes. Safety for driving should be assessed as well as cognitive function and ability to live independently. Some provinces have mandatory reporting laws for unsafe drivers.

Multidisciplinary Team Approach to Prevention of Falls

OT—home safety assessment

PT—rehab/strengthening and balance retraining

Pharmacy—medication recommendations

Physician—optimize medical conditions

CLINICAL BOX

Etiology of falls

Only 20% of falls are due to a single cause—the majority are multifactorial.

PAIN

See also Chapter 12 and Chapter 17

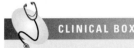

CLINICAL BOX

Exam Pearls

- In chronic pain, perform a complete physical exam.
- When examining an area of pain watch for signs of inflammation, infection, or trauma to skin.
- Determine if there is tenderness to palpation.
- If the area of pain is a joint, elicit ROM and pain with movement.

CLINICAL BOX

Determining the Etiology of Pain

Use of provocative maneuvers can be key for determining cause.

DEFINITION

Pain is a very common complaint seen in a physician's office. It is important for the family doctor to understand the physiology as well as the emotional and subjective experiences of pain in an individual patient. Adequate pain control is important in order to prevent progression of acute pain into a chronic state as well as to prevent unnecessary suffering.

Pain: the unique subjective experience, both somatic and emotional, of nociception or nerve damage

Nociception: neural activity transmitted along pain fibers informing the CNS of tissue damage

APPROACH

Hx

- Onset (gradual or acute, associated with injury)
- Generalized or localized (how specifically can the pain be localized)
- Provoking or alleviating factors
- Quality (stabbing, burning, sharp, dull, cramping)
- Radiation
- Severity (out of 10)
- Timing (association with certain activities, time of day, pattern of the pain)
- Associated symptoms (nausea and vomiting)
- Hx of trauma
- How is the pain affecting function
- Current medications, allergies, and past medical and a Psych Hx

INVESTIGATIONS

Lab and imaging performed on the basis of suspected cause of pain

MANAGEMENT

Note: Many analgesic drugs have similar side effects and therefore combining drugs must be done with care.

Table **8.6**	**Pharmacologic Management of Pain**			
Drug Class	**Action**	**Side Effects**	**Cautions**	**Examples**
Anti-inflammatories	Inhibit Cox 1 and 2—blocks prostaglandin cascade	Gastritis, GI bleeds, renal failure, platelet dysfunction	Patients with known GI bleeds, renal impairment, coagulopathy	ASA, ibuprofen, ketorolac, diclofenac, indomethacin, naproxen, celecoxib
Narcotics	Bind to opioid receptors and mimic endogenous opioids	Dose dependant—constipation, sedation, Resp depression	Potential for addiction and abuse of drug	Codeine, morphine, Demerol, fentanyl, oxycodone, methadone
Acetaminophen	Not anti-inflammatory—possibly involved in NO cycle	Can interact with warfarin	Liver toxicity >4 g/d—lower dose with liver impairment	Tylenol
Antidepressants	Inhibit 5-HT and NE uptake in CNS—for neuropathic pain	Headaches, Drowsiness, dry mouth	Should not be stopped abruptly	Amitriptyline, trazodone, venlafaxine, paroxetine
Anti-convulsants	Blocks Na channels—blocks abnormal depolarization pain nerves	Sedation, Headaches, Nausea	Should not be stopped abruptly	Gabapentin, pregabalin, clonazepam, phenytoin carbamazepine

Principles of Pain Management
- Always try to remove the cause.
- Proper pain management can prolong life.
- If a physician is acting in efforts to relieve pain it is not unethical to prescribe higher-dose opioids.
- Fear of creating opioid dependence should not prevent a physician from properly controlling pain.
- Those with chronic pain are more likely to request euthanasia and physician-assisted suicide. Aggressive pain control can lessen the chance.
- Always consider what psychiatric factors may be playing a role in the patient's experience/management of pain.
- Difficult cases may warrant referral to a pain clinic.
- Remember the patient's family—think of caregiver burnout and depression.

MULTIDISCIPLINARY APPROACH

Pharmacist—medication recommendations

Physical therapist—restore movement/strengthening

Psychiatry/spiritual services—counseling

Physician—surgery/nerve blocks

APPLIED SCIENTIFIC CONCEPTS

Acute: minutes to weeks

Subacute: weeks to months

Chronic: >3 mo

Pain that was once acute can progress down the spectrum to become chronic if adequate control is not achieved initially.

Table **8.7** Nociceptive vs. Neuropathic Pain

Type of Pain	Nociceptive Pain (Protective)			Neuropathic Pain (Pathologic)
Tissue damage	Somatic tissue damage		Visceral tissue damage	Nerve damage (laceration, compression, etc.)
Afferent fibers involved	Myelinated fiber	Unmyelinated fiber	Visceral afferents	Motor or autonomic, CNS or peripheral Abnormal activity from an injured nerve
Pain type	Sharp initial pain	Dull delayed pain	Pain in somatic tissues innervated at same spinal level as transmitting afferents (referred pain)	
Pain localization	Localized pain		Less localized type of referred pain	Tissue damage not always present Not always protective

Table **8.8** Types of Pain

Types of Neuropathic Pain	Mechanism	Examples
Sympathetic	Damage/pressure to PNS	Complex regional pain syndrome, Reflex sympathetic dystrophy
Central	Abnormal CNS activity	Phantom limb pain, Post Stroke or spinal cord injury
Nonsympathetic	Damage/pressure to PNS	Trigeminal neuralgia, Herpes zoster

SLEEP PROBLEMS

DEFINITION

Sleep problems are a common patient complaint. Thorough Hx taking is the key to diagnosis and a good knowledge of management options is important. Poor sleep greatly affects quality of life.

Circadian Rhythm: a cycle of ~24 h that governs numerous physiologic processes including sleep and wakefulness

Circadian Rhythm D/O: D/O related to the timing of sleep in a 24-h d

APPROACH

Hx and Physical Exam

- Onset of problem
- Difficulty falling and/or staying asleep
- Full assessment of sleep environment (where, with television, restless partners, pets)
- Activity before sleep (exercise, drugs, ETOH)
- Chronic medical conditions and their management
- Psych Hx and recent stressors
- Collateral Hx from bed partner (movements during sleep, snoring)
- Physical exam focuses on signs of chronic disease.
- Sleep log may be helpful.

Polysomnography measures sleep stages, airflow, Resp effort, O_2 saturation, limb movements, and brain activity while the patient sleeps. This level of study is not necessary for all patients with sleep problems.

Diagnosis

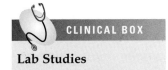

Lab Studies

Not routinely required and should only be ordered if underlying chronic illnesses are suspected

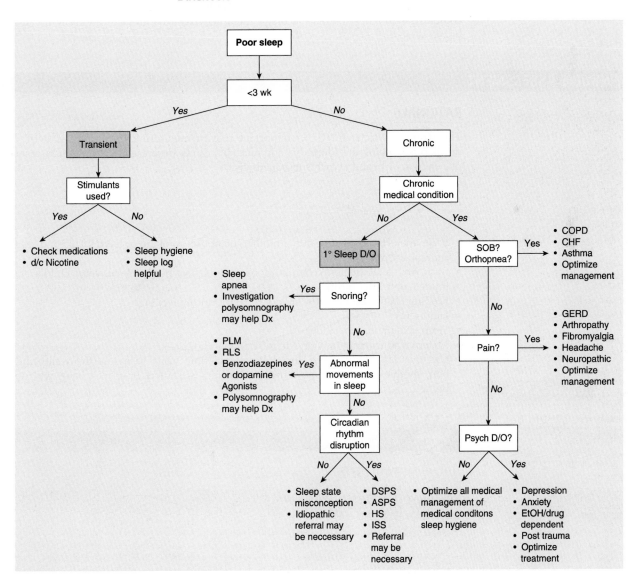

Figure 8.4 Diagnosis and management of sleep D/O.

MANAGEMENT

Sleep Hygiene for All Patients

- Bedtime routine
- Bed only for sleep and intimacy
- Regular wake time schedule
- No naps in late afternoon
- Avoid stimulants before sleep
- Exercise before afternoon
- Try to sleep only when tired
- Avoid heavy meals before bed
- Improve sleep environment (no noise, pets, cool temperature)

CLINICAL BOX

Important Causes of Transient Poor Sleep

Altitude changes, jet lag, changes in sleeping environment, change in work shift, temperature, noise, new onset stressful life event

Pharmacologic therapy is not the first-line treatment of choice. It should always be combined with other nonpharmacologic therapies. The need for medication should always be reassessed.

NEWBORN ASSESSMENT

RATIONALE

The family physician plays an important role in monitoring the health, growth, and development of infants. Morbidity and mortality can be decreased by thorough assessment of a child at birth and at each subsequent visit.

APPROACH

Hx

- Pregnancy Hx (general health of mother, drug use, smoking or ETOH, U/S and results, trauma, hospital/ER visits)
- Birth Hx (fetal distress/complications, long labor, mode of delivery, child's status immediately after birth)
- Feeding Hx (breast or bottle, child's behavior during feeding)
- Family Hx
- Sleep Hx (amount, position)
- Maternal adjustment (anxiety, depression, bonding)
- Use the day of discharge and subsequent clinic visits to assess the well-being of both mother and baby—how mom is feeling will affect how well baby will do at home.

CLINICAL BOX

Newborns should be examined

24 h after birth and/or before discharge

1 wk post discharge

1 mo of age

CLINICAL BOX

Infant Growth Facts

Should return to birth weight within 10 d of birth

Need 120 kcal/kg/d and a term infant should gain 20 to 30 g/d

Population of Children	Screens/Lab Testing
All newborns	TSH, PKU by all provinces (provinces vary greatly in other testing) Full physical exam
Child with family Hx of Sickle cell anemia	Hgb electrophoresis
HIV positive mother	HIV testing
Hepatitis positive mother	HBsAg and/or Hepatitis C PCR
Congenital anomaly	Possible karyotype Possible imaging (ECHO, U/S) (depends on presentation)
Ambiguous genitalia	Karyotype Abdominal U/S

PHYSICAL EXAM

- Caput—birth trauma
- Feel fontanelle
- Sclera —jaundice
- Red reflex
- Patent nostrils anteriorly
- Hearing—startle to sound
- CVS exam—heart sounds, murmurs, cardiomegaly, femoral pulses
- Pulmonary exam
- Umbilical stump for signs of infection
- Musc tone/neurologic (placing response, rooting response, palmar grasp reflex, vertical suspension, Moro reflex, moves all limbs equally?)
- Genital—phenotypic sex, sexual ambiguity, patent anus, descended testis
- Dermatologic (café au lait, ash leaf macules, port wine stains, birth trauma, dermatitis, jaundice)
- Hips—ortolani, Barlow maneuvers
- Abdominal masses
- Neck—thyroid masses

Infant feeding facts
- Breast is best
- Mother's diet should be well rounded—EtOH and recreational drugs will enter breast milk—other drugs vary
- Contraindications to breast-feeding are HIV, chemotherapy/nuclear medicine, illicit drug use, active and untreated TB
- Neonate should not be sleeping through the night—should eat ~q 3 h (more frequent if premature)
- Should be heavily soiling ~five to six diapers a d
- Need to give Vit D supplement with breast-feeding
- Do not need free water—milk or formula is adequate
- No solid foods until 6 mo
- Never prop a bottle
- Mother Risk (www.motherrisk.org) can be useful resource

CLINICAL BOX

Palpation of the Neonate

It is normal to be able to palpate the liver, spleen, and kidneys in a neonate.

CHILDHOOD IMMUNIZATIONS

RATIONALE

Immunization is an important part of preventative medicine for children. Physicians should be knowledgeable about the benefits and risks associated with immunization in order to counsel families.

APPLIED SCIENTIFIC CONCEPTS

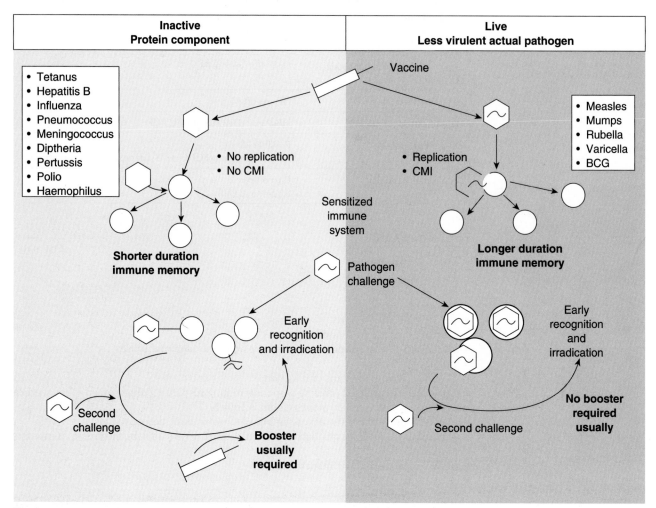

| Inactive Protein component | Live Less virulent actual pathogen |

- Tetanus
- Hepatitis B
- Influenza
- Pneumococcus
- Meningococcus
- Diptheria
- Pertussis
- Polio
- Haemophilus

- No replication
- No CMI

Shorter duration immune memory

- Measles
- Mumps
- Rubella
- Varicella
- BCG

- Replication
- CMI

Longer duration immune memory

Sensitized immune system

Vaccine

Pathogen challenge

Early recognition and irradiation

Second challenge

Booster usually required

Early recognition and irradiation

Second challenge

No booster required usually

Figure 8.5 Vaccines.

MYTHS OF CHILDHOOD IMMUNIZATION

True
- Vaccines cause milder natural infection or none at all.
- Some diseases have been eradicated.
- Herd immunity prevents outbreaks.
- Only true contraindications are:
  - Pregnant or immunocompromised and a live vaccine
  - Anaphylaxis to given vaccine or vaccine constituent

False
- Vaccines cause autism, MS, SIDS, or other chronic illnesses.
- Everyone responds to a vaccine.
- A missed dose means you must restart a vaccine series.

APPROACH

Vaccination schedules vary from province to province. There are also provincial variations in administration (physician vs. public health).

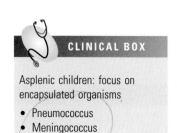

CLINICAL BOX

Asplenic children: focus on encapsulated organisms

- Pneumococcus
- Meningococcus
- Haemophilus

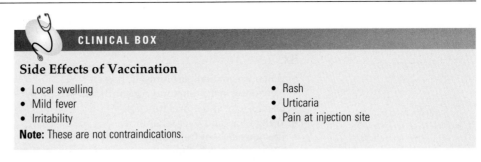

Side Effects of Vaccination

- Local swelling
- Mild fever
- Irritability

Note: These are not contraindications.

- Rash
- Urticaria
- Pain at injection site

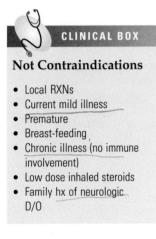

Not Contraindications

- Local RXNs
- Current mild illness
- Premature
- Breast-feeding
- Chronic illness (no immune involvement)
- Low dose inhaled steroids
- Family hx of neurologic D/O

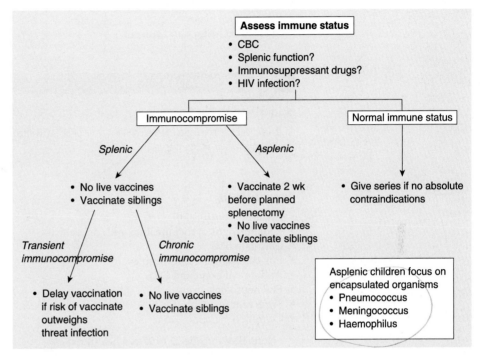

Figure 8.6 Approach to childhood immunization.

FAILURE TO THRIVE: ELDERLY

DEFINITION

FTT in an elderly patient is a decline in function that is often associated with weight loss, energy loss, and depression.

CAUSAL CONDITIONS

Table **8.9**	FTT in the Elderly: Causal Conditions	
Extrinsic Environmental	**Intrinsic**	
	Decreased Energy (Poor Intake)	**Increased Energy Demands**
Isolation	Poor dentition	COPD
Poverty	Malabsorption	Malignancy
Elder abuse	Dysphagia	Hyperthyroidism
Loneliness	Poor access	CHF
	Depression	Fever/inflammatory D/O/chronic infection
	Dementia	
	Anorexia due to chronic illness or medication	

APPROACH

Hx

- When was patient last himself/herself
- New onset symptoms and constitutional symptoms
- Diet history and bowel function
- Weight loss and over what time
- Previous level of functioning (ADLs and IADLs)
- Changes to level of functioning
- Social history (living arrangement, family supports, community supports, finances)
- Past medical history
- Medication history and current

CLINICAL BOX

Elderly with No Support

If the patient has no support in the community he or she will often need to be admitted to allow for further workup and rehab and/or placement.

PHYSICAL EXAM

- Vitals and postural BP
- Look for signs of malnutrition and/or cachexia
- Calculate BMI
- Full cardiac/vascular/Resp exam
- Abdominal exam and DRE
- Full neurologic exam
- Signs of trauma/abuse
- Cognition

    Note: BMI outside 22 to 27 is a health risk.

INVESTIGATION

- CBC-D
- lytes
- BUN
- Creatinine
- Ca^{2+}, Mg, Vit B_{12}
- Liver function tests, liver enzymes
- FOB
- Other investigations as assessment suggests

MANAGEMENT

The geriatric patient can be complex and therefore a multidisciplinary approach to medical optimization is best.

- Pharmacy—medication review
- PT—mobilization
- OT—assess safety for home and assess needs for performing ADLs
- Social work—help with finances and suggestions for placement in the community if cannot return home
- Dietician—assess caloric needs and make recommendations for weight gain
- Speech language pathology—swallowing assessment if dysphagia suspected

    Always try and discover the cause of the function decline and weight loss. Treatment may result in the return of patient to previous level of functioning and restore his or her independence.

    There are numerous community supports to consider that can allow patients to return home with improved safety and quality of life—home care nursing, home personal care, companion care, meals on wheels

Considerations of FTT in the Elderly

Cause of malnutrition/weight loss—chronic illness–related cachexia versus malnutrition due to caloric intake

Other medical conditions—diabetes, renal failure

Nutrient content—proteins, fats, minerals required

Nutrition

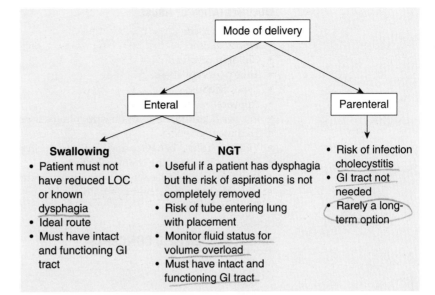

Figure 8.7 Nutrition delivery in the elderly.

FAMILY VIOLENCE

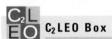

C₂LEO Box

Reporting of Abuse

A physician should be knowledgeable about the laws of reporting in their particular province. All provinces require the reporting of child abuse (direct abuse, abandonment, witnessing abuse in the home, neglect). Some provinces require the reporting of abuse directed against disabled persons and those >60 yr of age. Reporting is to the police or social services.

See also Chapter 19

DEFINITION

Family violence can greatly affect the health of a family. Patients will often hide the fact that they are being abused and therefore it is the physician's duty to create a safe and welcoming environment to allow for such discussions.

Domestic violence: intentionally controlling or violent behavior

CAUSAL CONDITIONS

- Dependant relationship (e.g., parent to child)
- Kinship relationship (e.g., son/daughter to elderly)
- Intimate relationship (e.g., spouse to spouse)

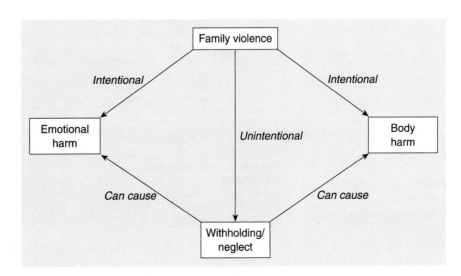

Figure 8.8 Causal conditions: family violence.

APPROACH

DOCUMENTATION OF ABUSE

- Who is abused
- Who is abuser
- Children involved
- Time period of abuse
- Types of abuse
- Appearance of victim
- Injuries (location, description, size, photos if possible)
- Treatment given
- Victim/parent's behavior and attitudes during questioning
- Where is victim going (home, shelter)
- Is patient willing to leave abusive environment
- Did physician report and to whom
- **Be very detailed**

APPLIED SCIENTIFIC CONCEPTS

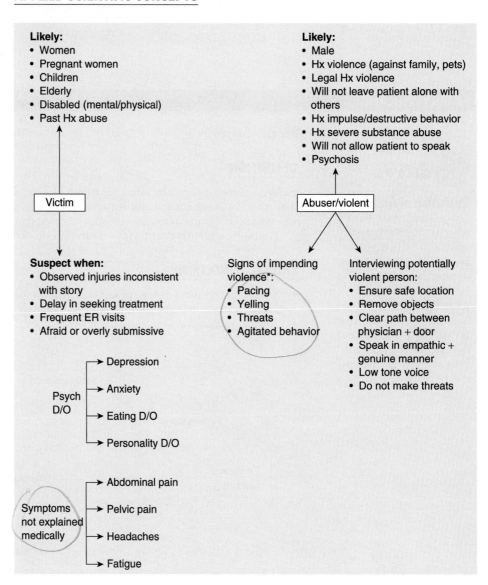

Figure 8.9 Applied scientific concepts: violence.

*Leave immediately and contact security.

ADULT ABUSE/SPOUSAL ABUSE

See also Chapter 19

DEFINITION

Unfortunately, abuse in intimate relationships is not an uncommon occurrence. The family physician can play an important role in helping victims of abuse get the help they need.

CAUSAL CONDITIONS

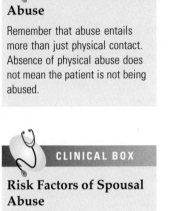

CLINICAL BOX

Abuse

Remember that abuse entails more than just physical contact. Absence of physical abuse does not mean the patient is not being abused.

CLINICAL BOX

Risk Factors of Spousal Abuse

- Younger age
- Common law status
- Partner with substance abuse problem
- Marital separation
- Social isolation
- Hx of previous abuse/assault

Figure 8.10 Adult abuse: causal conditions.

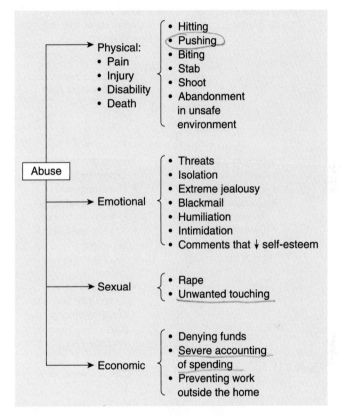

APPROACH

Hx

When you suspect abuse . . .

- Initially approach the subject with open-ended questions:

  "Are you in a relationship at the moment . . . How is the relationship going?"

- As the examination proceeds and rapport is established:

  " When someone talks to me about these symptoms (or "When I see someone with this type of injury") I feel as though I should ask them if anyone in their life is hurting them"

- If the patient admits to being abused or seems open to discussing the topic more specific questioning can be done.

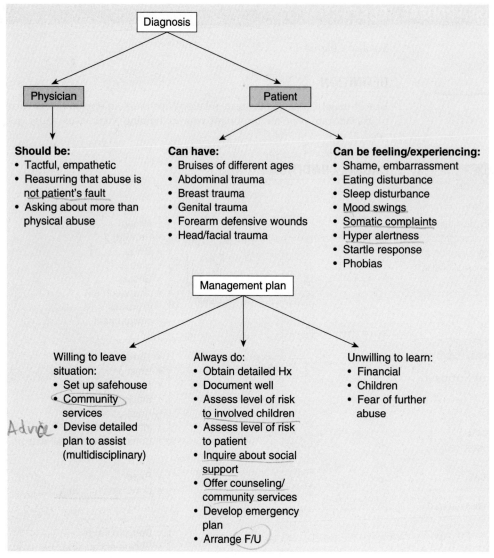

Figure 8.11 Adult abuse: diagnosis and management.

MANAGEMENT

Assessing Safety Risk for Patients Returning Home
- What types of abuse are present
- Severity of injuries and frequency
- Nature of threats (threat of death)
- Presence of supports for victim and proximity to patient's home
- Emergency plan in place
- Children involved

Multidisciplinary Team
- Women's shelters
- Police service
- Counseling
- Child social services

C₂LEO

Reporting adult abuse may be seen as breech of confidentiality if the patient did not give permission.

CHILD ABUSE

CLINICAL BOX

Parental Behavioral Signs

- Refusal to have child interviewed alone
- Inconsistent or implausible Hx
- Vague Hx or none offered
- Changing Hx
- Injuries attributed to siblings
- Bringing child to medical attention late

See also Chapter 19

DEFINITION

Child abuse can take many forms. It is important for any physician who works with children to be astute to possible signs of child abuse in order to reduce morbidity and mortality.

CAUSAL CONDITIONS

CLASSIFICATION OF CHILD ABUSE

Physical: pushing, hitting, biting, locking out of home, Münchhausen by proxy

Sexual: rape, touching

Emotional: isolating, overpressuring, verbal assault, rejecting

Neglect

Denying physical and emotional needs

Denying education and medical attention

APPROACH

HX AND PHYSICAL EXAM

The abuser is often someone the child knows: parent, relative, caretaker, teacher.

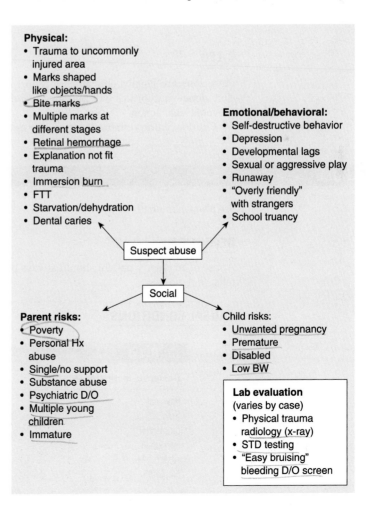

Figure 8.12 Hx and physical exam of child abuse.

MANAGEMENT

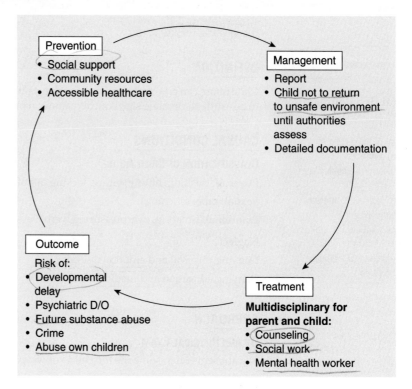

Figure 8.13 Management of child abuse.

C₂LEO

Physicians are legally obligated to report child abuse. Reports can be based on suspicion alone—authorities will investigate and provide further advice. Good faith reporting prevents legal action.

Caution: cultural therapy can appear as abuse—coining, spooning, cupping.

ELDER ABUSE

See also Chapter 19

DEFINITION

Abuse of an elderly patient should always be included in the differential diagnosis of FTT, falls, or depression.

CAUSAL CONDITIONS

Table **8.10** Elder Abuse: Causal Conditions	
Domestic, Institutional	**Self-Neglect**
Physical	Nutrition
Sexual	Personal hygiene
Emotional	Poorly maintained living environment
Economic	Isolation
Abandonment	
Neglect	

Table **8.11**	Signs of Elder Abuse			
Physical Abuse		**Emotional Abuse**	**Neglect**	**Financial Abuse**
Burns		Withdrawn	Dehydration	Lack of essentials
Lacerations		Depression	Malnutrition	Pressure to change
Bruises		Mood changes	Poor hygiene	wills/power of attorney
Not accessing medical services		Caregiver burnout	Weight loss	Loss of property
for injuries or doing so after an			Lack of essentials	Creation of debt in
extended period			(clothing, ADL aids)	patient's name
Caregiver burnout			Caregiver burnout	

CLINICAL BOX

Prevention of Abuse

- Encourage creation of legal documents before functional/cognitive decline.
- Encourage respite for caregivers.
- Community resources
- Encourage social networks/supports

C₂LEO Box

Reporting of Elder Abuse
The abuse of an elderly person is not a specific crime in Canadian law. However, the individual acts inflicted on the person may be criminal. Not all provinces have mandatory reporting of suspected/known elder abuse.

APPROACH

Hx and Physical Exam
It may be difficult to obtain an accurate Hx from a patient with dementia. However demented patients are at significant risk for abuse. Therefore, physicians must rely on other signs and sources to make the diagnosis.

Management
See Adult Abuse/Spousal Abuse for management plan

Resources for Assisting Elders
Local police

Abuse help lines

Social/victims services

Admission to hospital

C₂LEO

Consent to report becomes more difficult in the elderly patient if the patient is deemed incompetent to make decisions. Know the patient's ADs (if available) and decide if a substitute decision maker can be involved. Ensure the decision maker will act in the patient's best interests. Sometimes a court-appointed guardian may be necessary to have a patient removed from an unsafe/unhealthy environment.

DYING AND BEREAVEMENT

C₂LEO Box

Withholding Information
Withholding information from a patient for any reason that would interfere with the patient's ability to make informed life decisions is considered unethical and could result in litigation. Be careful when patients refuse to be informed.

DEFINITION
Regardless of the area of specialization, effective skills for breaking bad news are extremely important. It is also important to realize that end-of-life care needs to be delivered in a manner unique to the individual patients and their families in order to be most effective.

APPROACH

Breaking Bad News
Setting up—private place, seated discussion, minimal interruptions, time available
Patient perceptions—What does the patient already know or understand?
Invitation—Does the patient want basic information or full details of results/condition?
Knowledge—given at patient's level of understanding, accurate, appropriate
Emotions—Acknowledge emotions and allow their expression.
Strategy and summary—Ensure patient understanding and follow-up.

SPIKES

Aspects of SPIKES can be used at any stage of assessing a patient with end-of-life issues. Effective communication and insight into a patient's illness can help guide the creation of an AD or guide future management.

C₂LEO Box

Legal Documents

Fully discuss the advantages and limitations of ADs with patients—the wording of such documents and the situations mentioned in the document are extremely important. There can be some difficulty in honoring ADs if they are too vague or too specific and an unexpected situation occurs.

C₂LEO

ADS

AD is a legal document that states a patient's wishes about his or her medical care. It is created when a patient is deemed competent. The document can be used to guide care once the patient becomes no longer competent. Areas to be addressed include:

- Medical procedures—treatment or diagnostic (intubation, chest tubes, paracentesis)
- CPR/life-sustaining/life-saving measures (ICU, particular drugs)

PROXY DECISION MAKERS

By fully understanding a patient's medical condition and personal values, medical dilemmas can be somewhat anticipated and an AD can be made more effective.

Roles of the physician in end-of-life issues include:

- Delivering accurate medical information in an appropriate manner
- Eliciting the patient's goals in end-of-life care
- Determining a patient's decision-making capacity
- Determining whether an AD is in place and guidance for creation of such a document
- To optimize the patient medically so that he or she can have meaningful and comfortable final days
- Ensuring a multidisciplinary approach to care is given including spiritual and psychological help to patient and family

C₂LEO Box

Capacity and Substitute Decision Makers

Elderly: Determine current mental status. AD?

Adult: Determine current mental status. AD?

Child: Determine legal caregivers. Is child a mature minor and capable of directing his or her own care? AD?

AD naming proxy decision makers

MANAGING PAIN IN THE DYING PATIENT

- Proper management of pain can prolong a patient's life such that he or she may complete important end-of-life tasks. Difficulty in managing pain may warrant referral to a palliative or chronic pain specialist.
- Remember that Resp depression may be a sign of natural death rather than opioid overdose.
- A physician is protected legally if death is hastened secondary to medications for pain management as long as the physician had no intention of causing death. Treating pain is critical in a palliative patient and the hastening of an inevitable death is not considered euthanasia.

HEALTH OF SPECIAL POPULATIONS

DEFINITION

There are many factors that determine the health of a population. Certain populations are more susceptible to particular conditions that are worth remembering and focusing on at a **periodic health exam.**

CAUSAL CONDITIONS

Table **8.12** **Consideration of Select Special Populations**

Population	Causal Factors			Common Diagnoses
	Social Environment	**Genetics**	**Physical Environment**	
People with disabilities	Finances Education/mental capacity Access to health care Community/social supports Caregiver abuse	Down syndrome	Modified environment to accommodate special needs Work conditions Geographic location (rural, urban)	Pressure sores Depression Musc atrophy Obesity Falls Substance abuse Malnourishment Abuse
Children in poverty	Poverty Education Parental support Access to health care Community support Family violence		Geography (safety of neighborhood, homeless) Smoke Clean drinking water and nutritious food	Trauma Poisoning SIDS Low birth weight Infection Substance abuse Child abuse Asthma FTT Psychiatric D/O Poor dentition
Aboriginal populations	Poverty Education Cultural practices (tobacco use) Access to health care Family violence		Housing (reservation, homeless) Northern/isolated community Lack of clean drinking water and nutritious food	Trauma Poisoning SIDS Malignancy COPD Otitis media TB Hepatitis/cirrhosis HIV Suicide/depression Substance abuse Diabetes
Elderly population	Finances Community/social Support Access to health care Caregiver abuse		Housing (independent, assisted) Modified for individual's needs Geographic location (rural, urban)	Falls Arthritis Heart disease Resp disease (COPD, ISLD) Dementia Abuse Incontinence FTT Malignancy PVD Visual/hearing loss Depression Malnourishment Diabetes

HEALTH STATUS ASSESSMENT AND MEASUREMENT

DEFINITION

The interventions and programs designed to create and promote health in a particular community can be evaluated to ensure that the needs of the community are being met. The health status of a community can also be measured in order to decide which interventions are needed.

CONCEPTS

MORTALITY RATES

$$\text{Infant} : \frac{\text{\# Deaths in children} < 1\text{yr in a certain time period and population}}{\text{\# Live Births in that same time period and population}}$$

- **Neonatal:** Change numerator to # Deaths in children <28 d old
- **Perinatal:** Change numerator to # Deaths in fetuses >28 wks GA + infants <7 d old

$$\text{Maternal} : \frac{\text{\# Deaths related to a puerperal cause in a certain time period and population}}{\text{\# Pregnancies in the same time period and population}}$$

$$\text{Proportionate mortality ratio} : \frac{\text{\# Deaths due to a particular cause}}{\text{Total \# deaths in the same time period and population}}$$

$$\text{Crude death rate} : \frac{\text{\# Deaths in population from any cause}}{\text{Total population in that same time period}}$$

$$\text{Age specific death rate} : \frac{\text{\# Deaths in an age} - \text{group in a certain time period and population}}{\text{Average or mid} - \text{year population of that age} - \text{group in the same time period and population}}$$

$$\text{Case fatality rate} : \frac{\text{\# Deaths from illness in certain time period}}{\text{\# People diagnosed with that illness in that time period}}$$

YEARS OF LIFE LOST

$$\text{PYLL} : \text{Life expectancy for population} - \text{age at death of individual}$$

$$\text{For population PYLL} : \frac{\text{Add all PYLL for all members who died}}{\text{Total \# members of population under the age of life expectancy}}$$

SCREENING TESTS

Disease Should Be
- Relatively common
- Serious morbidity and/or mortality
- Treatment available/prognosis improved with early detection

Test Should Be
- Safe
- Cost effective
- Specific > sensitive
- Reliable and valid

A screening test is not a diagnostic test.

CLINICAL BOX

Plain English Definitions

Valid—Does it measure what it claims to?

Reliable—Can it be repeated and the same result obtained?

Predictive value—the probability that a positive test is a true positive case or that a negative test is a true negative case; determined by the sensitivity and specificity and prevalence of the tested condition

Efficacy—the ability to produce a specific result

Efficient—Is the output useful and worth the input?

Compliance—Did someone do as instructed?

Incidence—the # new cases that will occur in a certain time period

Prevalence—the # cases present at a particular time

SENSITIVITY AND SPECIFICITY

Table **8.13**	**Sensitivity and Specificity**	
	Disease Present	**Disease not Present**
Positive test	A	B
Negative test	C	D

Sensitivity – if the condition is there the test will pick it up $= A/(A + C)$

Specificity – if the condition is not there the test will not pick it up $= D/(B + D)$

Positive predictive value : $A/(A + B)$

Negative predictive value : $D/(C + D)$

GENERAL RULES FOR EVALUATING EVIDENCE

- Systematic reviews are better than an individual trial of the same kind.
- Randomized control trials are the best evidence when true randomization and allocation concealment are present.
- Ignore conclusions drawn from a trial that was designed to test something different (ignore secondary findings if study was not originally looking for them)
- Few studies will directly quote useful values. If possible, calculate them yourself to see if you feel the numbers match the conclusions given.
- Try to use EBM whenever possible but there is not always research available to support our decisions.
- When advising patients about a screening test consider incidence and prevalence of disease, specificity and sensitivity, safety, natural Hx of the disease and resources available for diagnosis and treatment.
- When advising patients about a treatment consider the efficacy, efficiency, and likelihood for compliance.

POPULATION HEALTH AND ITS DETERMINANTS

DEFINITION

The social and physical environments are just as important in defining the health of a population as genetics. It is important for the physician to know the social and physical environments of the patient population they serve in order to provide more comprehensive care.

DETERMINANTS OF HEALTH

OVERALL DETERMINANTS OF HEALTH

- Biology
  - Genetics
- Behaviors
  - Coping skills
  - Diet
  - Exercise
  - Substance use
  - Use of medical services
- Physical environment
  - Geographic location
  - Peace
  - Housing
  - Work conditions
- Social environment
  - Employment income
  - Social status
  - Education
  - Culture
  - Religion
  - Health services
  - Support network
  - Family violence

DISEASE PREVENTION

In order to decide which preventative strategies/recommendations to make in a particular population, determine age of members, incidence of a disease, prevalence of a disease, attack rate or create surveys to poll the population as to which behaviors/conditions are an issue.

Table **8.14** Preventative Medicine	
Ask All Patients About	**What You May Learn that Allows for More Effective Preventative Medicine**
Ethnic background and culture	Genetic predispositions Perceptions of disease/illness Willingness to seek medical services
Education	Level of medical knowledge How to effectively communicate
Occupation	Disease predispositions Economic means for health
Religion	Perceptions of disease/illness Which treatments/procedures a patient finds acceptable
Housing/living arrangements	Whether they are living in a safe environment Disease predispositions

Table **8.15**	Disease Prevention		
Type of Prevention	**Level of Action**	**Key Strategies for Prevention**	**Conditions Prevented**
Primary	Before any disease is present	Education Social marketing Public health policy Community organizations	Family violence Outbreaks Many chronic medical conditions Accidental death
Secondary	Very early stages of disease—allows for effective intervention	Education Social marketing Public health policy	Those for which an effective screening test is available
Tertiary	Disease established—treatment and minimize suffering	Education Social marketing Community organizations (support groups)	Hopefully morbidity and mortality reduced

WORK-RELATED HEALTH

DEFINITION

A patient's occupation plays a large role in his or her life. It is important for a physician to know a patient's occupational Hx in order to provide preventative and comprehensive care.

APPROACH

Hx

- What type of work do you do? In the past?
- What type of work activities?
- How long at each job?
- Wore protective gear?
- Current symptoms?
- How long have symptoms been present?
- Are symptoms different at work and home?
- Do you think it is related to your work?
- Anyone else at work with similar symptoms?

CLINICAL BOX

For work places involving chemicals ask about:

- Products manufactured
- Heating sources
- Clean-up practices
- Protocol for handling hazardous substances
- Ventilation
- Protective garments

INVESTIGATION

Table **8.16** Common Occupational Exposures					
Type of Exposure	**Example**	**Protection**	**Occupations at Risk**	**Conditions to Think About**	**Tests**
Inhalants	Volatile chemicals, CO, grain, mold/plant matter, asbestos, smoke, wood, metals	Resp mask Fume hood	Chemist Farmer Fireman Construction Welder Medical Lab Scientist	Asbestosis Mesothelioma Interstitial fibrosis Asthma Lung cancer	CXR
Skin contact	Chemicals Latex Radiation	Gloves Lead barriers Close-toed shoes	Manufacturing X-ray Technician Chemists	Contact dermatitis	Often clinical diagnosis
Blood borne	Virus Bacteria	Gloves Universal precautions	Health care Prostitution Veterinarian	Hepatitis A, B, C HIV Animal bites	Serology
Sound	Machinery Music	Ear plugs	Construction DJ Bartender	Tinnitus Hearing loss	Audiology
MSK	Heavy lifting Repetitive movements Prolonged sitting	Proper technique Rest	Hairdresser Dentist Assembly line	Low back pain Carpal tunnel Cervical strain	Often clinical diagnosis

MANAGEMENT

- Thoroughly document work-related injuries/conditions.
- Treatment should focus on removing the worker(s) from immediate danger, relieving immediate suffering as well as returning function long term.
- Determine fitness to return to work.
- Recommend preventative measures.
- Remember you must obtain consent to release information to WCB or a patient's employer.
- MSDS can be obtained from OHS for particular exposures.
- May warrant referral to an occupational health specialist

CLINICAL BOX

Occupational Exposures

Always think how occupational exposures can be causing a condition in a particular patient with no typical risk factors. For example, the diagnosis of lung cancer in a nonsmoker.

CLINICAL BOX

Prescribing Medication

Always think about a patient's occupation when prescribing medication. For example a medication that causes drowsiness can lead to a fatal mistake at work

OUTBREAK MANAGEMENT

DEFINITION

Physicians play a very large role in the control of an outbreak. They must be able to diagnose the condition, help limit the spread, and report to health authorities.

Outbreak: a greater than expected # epidemiologically linked cases of a particular illness

Case definition: the specific criteria (symptoms, onset) required to label an individual suspicious for or actually infected with the illness in question; can initially be broad but becomes more defined over time

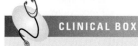

Outbreaks

An outbreak is not limited to only infectious agents. For example, environmental exposures can create an increased # cancers in a particular population.

CLINICAL BOX

Immunizations

Immunization is a major player in outbreak prevention of infectious agents. Important ones to know are measles, mumps, diphtheria, meningitis, and influenza.

APPROACH

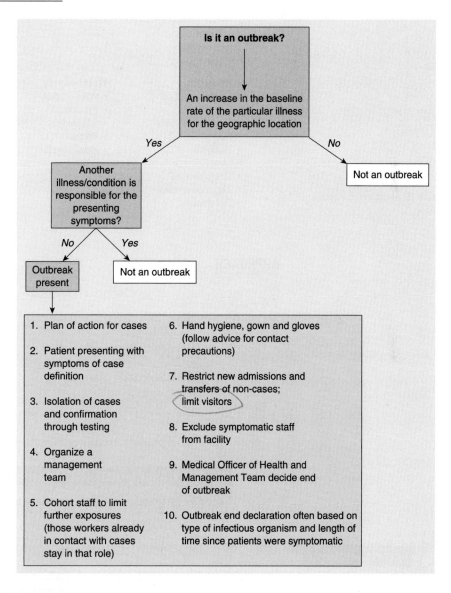

Figure 8.14 Approach to an outbreak.

MANAGEMENT

The Role of Public Health Can Include
- Education
- Immunization/prophylaxis strategies
- Advice for health centers
- Investigate cause of outbreak (travel, food borne)

- Investigate environments involved (restaurants)
- Communication with the public/media

ENVIRONMENT

DEFINITION

The physical environment plays a large role in the development of illness in a population. By understanding the physical environment of a patient population, a physician can better provide preventative and comprehensive care.

CAUSAL CONDITIONS

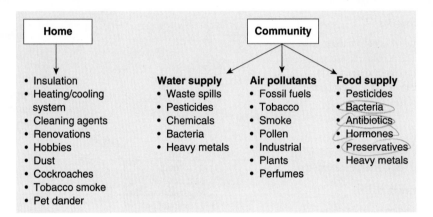

Figure 8.15 Environmental causal conditions.

APPROACH

Hx

- Type of symptoms
- Onset of symptoms
- Relation to work, home, hobbies
- Occurrence after known exposure
- Time to develop after exposure
- Time to resolve after exposure removal
- Progression/frequency of symptoms over time
- Occupational Hx
- Rural or urban home

    Note: Think about possible exposures from the flow chart above.

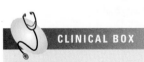

CLINICAL BOX

References

When symptoms are suspected to be due to an environmental cause, further information can be obtained from MSDS, toxicologists, government agencies, or poison control centers.

Table **8.17**	**Symptoms of Environmental Exposure**
Common Symptoms	**Exposures to Think About**
Headaches	Sick building syndrome CO, SO_2 Perfumes Paint/varnishes
Dermatitis	Chemicals (laundry detergents, cleaning agents) Radiation (UV, x-ray) Metals (nickel)
SOB/cough	Tobacco smoke, fertilizers, asbestos, pollen,
Vomiting/diarrhea	Bacterial or chemicals in food Heavy Metals

INVESTIGATION

Table 8.18	Investigation of Select Environmental Exposures		
Exposure	**Symptoms**	**Tests and Treatment**	**Complications**
Lead	Nausea, GI upset, headache, seizures, irritability, Burton line	Chelation therapy Lead blood level	Coma Learning disability
CO	Fatigue, headaches, palpitations, SOB, confusion	CO-Hgb level EKG O_2 Creatinine	Arrhythmias MI ARF Cardiac/Resp arrest Cognitive difficulties Musc necrosis

Authorities may have to be contacted to have an environment inspected and to eliminate other exposures.

CHAPTER 9

Gastroenterology

Michael Tso, Evelyn Wu, Myriam Farah, Eric M. Yoshida,
Michael F. Byrne, and Grace Li

DYSPHAGIA/DIFFICULTY SWALLOWING

DEFINITION

Difficulty swallowing causing sensation of food sticking. Food remains in mouth, pharynx, or esophagus

APPLIED SCIENTIFIC CONCEPTS

2. Pharyngeal phase (1 s)
- Bolus stimulates tactile receptors in pharynx
- Soft palate elevated—complete closure of nasopharynx (prevents regurgitation)
- Elevation of larynx—inhibition of respiration (prevents aspiration)
- Peristaltic action by pharyngeal constrictors propels bolus from pharynx to cricopharyngeal sphincter
- Cricopharyngeal sphincter relaxes —food enters esophagus
- Soft palate and larynx releases
- Reflexive control involving CN V, X, XI, XII and central inhibition of respiration

1. Oral preparatory phase
- Convert food to semisolid state **(bolus)**
- Bolus propelled toward the pharynx
- Affected by poor dentition, salivary gland disorders, neurologic disorders, tounge weakness
- Voluntary control involving CN V, VII, and XII

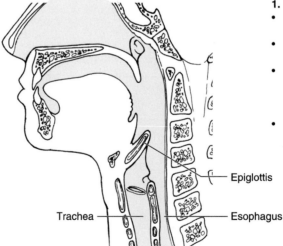

3. Esophageal phase (8–20 s)
- Transit time from cricoesphageal to gastroesophageal junction

Figure 9.1 Phases of swallowing.

CAUSAL CONDITIONS

Table **9.1**	Oropharyngeal vs. Esophageal Dysphagia

Oropharyngeal dysphagia

Neuromuscular

CNS	Cranial nerves	Myopathic	Functional
• Cerebral palsy • CNS tumor • Head trauma • Parkinson • Dementia • CVA	• Laryngeal nerve palsy • Polio • MS • ALS • Diabetes	• Polymyositis • Myasthenia • Dermatomyositis	• Xerostomia

Esophageal dysphagia

Mechanical			Motility	
Intrinsic				
Intermittent	Progressive	Extrinsic	Intermittent	Progressive
• Lower esophageal ring or web	• Peptic stricture • Carcinoma	• Mediastinal mass (goiter, tumor)	• Diffuse esophageal spasm	• Scleroderma • Achalasia

APPROACH

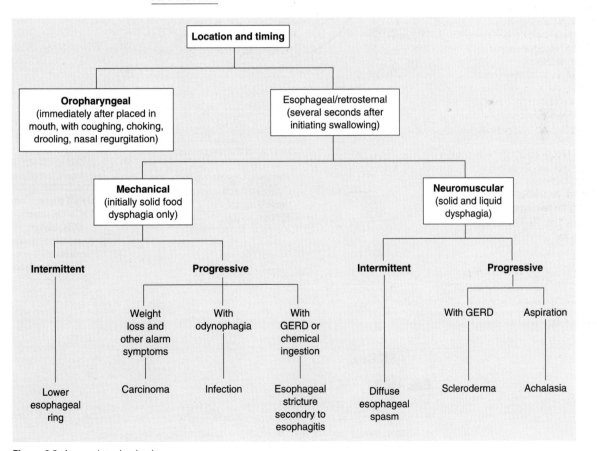

Figure 9.2 Approach to dysphagia.

VOMITING/NAUSEA

RATIONALE

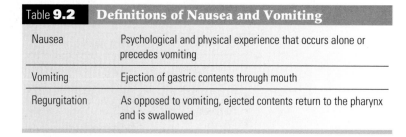

Table **9.2**	**Definitions of Nausea and Vomiting**
Nausea	Psychological and physical experience that occurs alone or precedes vomiting
Vomiting	Ejection of gastric contents through mouth
Regurgitation	As opposed to vomiting, ejected contents return to the pharynx and is swallowed

> **R**
>
> Severe vomiting can cause fluid and electrolyte imbalances.

APPLIED SCIENTIFIC CONCEPTS

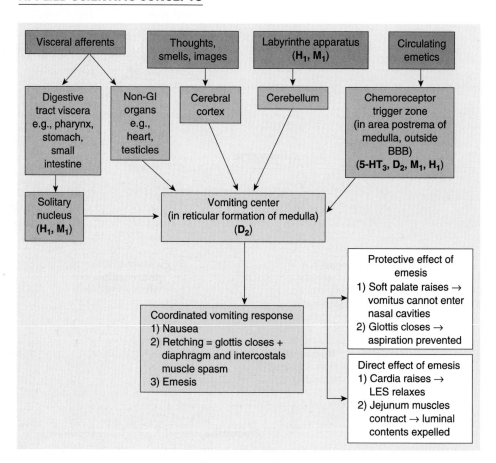

Figure 9.3 Physiology of vomiting. Adapted with permission from Brunton LL, Lazo JS, Parker KS, eds. *Goodman and Gilman's Pharmacological Basis of Therapeutics*. New York: McGraw-Hill; 2006.

ASC Box

Bile Acids

- Bile acids promote formation of micelles.
- Micelles consist of a core triglycerides and cholesterol esters surrounded by phospholipids.
- Micelles have ↑ surface area for hydrolysis by pancreatic lipase.
- **Enterohepatic circulation**: Bile acids are actively reabsorbed in the terminal ileum, enter the portal circulation, and are then secreted into bile again.

CAUSAL CONDITIONS

Table **9.3**	System-Based Differential Dx of Nausea and Vomiting	
System		**Differential Dx**
CNS		• Elevated ICP (infection, tumors) • Vestibular nerve lesion • Brain stem lesion • Psychiatric issue
GI	UGI	• Acute gastroenteritis • Gastroparesis/postoperative/nonulcer dyspepsia • Neoplasm • PUD • Gastric outlet obstruction • GERD
	Lower GI	• Acute infectious enteritis • IBD • Obstruction • Neoplasm
	Other GI	• Hepatobiliary disease • Acute hepatitis/cholecystitis • Acute pancreatitis • Peritoneal irritation
Endocrine/metabolic		• Diabetes • Hypercalcemia • Uremia • Pregnancy
CA		• Paraneoplastic syndrome • Hypernephroma • Ovarian CA • Gastric CA
Systemic		• Sepsis (pyelonephritis, pneumonia) • Acute inferior myocardial infarct • Chemotherapy • Food poisoning

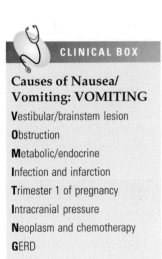

CLINICAL BOX

Causes of Nausea/ Vomiting: VOMITING

Vestibular/brainstem lesion

Obstruction

Metabolic/endocrine

Infection and infarction

Trimester 1 of pregnancy

Intracranial pressure

Neoplasm and chemotherapy

GERD

APPROACH

INVESTIGATIONS

- General lab tests: CBC, electrolytes, tests of renal function, glucose, thyroid function tests, liver biochemical tests, serum amylase and lipase levels
- Specific lab tests: Tailor lab test to clinical suspicions to determine etiology for specific Rx.

TX

Manage the combined fluid and electrolyte depletion that may occur following vomiting by:

- Volume assessment by evaluation of jugular venous pressure, vitals, skin turgor, mucus membranes
- Restore volume depletion by administration of isotonic normal saline.
- Evaluation of Na, Cl, HCO_3, K and correction through appropriate replacement

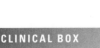

CLINICAL BOX

$$\Delta Na = (140 - P_{Na}) \times TBW$$

ΔNa = Sodium deficit (in mEq/L)
P_{Na} = Plasma sodium concentration
TBW = Total body water (in L, ↓ if dehydrated)

Table **9.4**	Approach to Nausea and Vomiting			
Etiology	**Hx**	**Physical**	**Labs/Imaging**	**Tx**
Chemotherapy	CA	—	—	Ondansetron, glucocorticoids
Pregnancy	Occurs in morning	—	β-Human chorionic gonadotropin	Antihistamine (may be teratogenic)
Drug/toxin (e.g., lithium, digoxin, mushrooms)	Full med and social Hx	—	Drug screen	Discontinue use if possible, or use central antiemetic
DKA	Diabetes mellitus, polyuria, polydipsia	Fruity breath, abdominal pain, volume depletion	Glucose, serum and urinary ketones, electrolytes	DKA Tx (IVFs and insulin)
↑ ICP	Headache, visual field change, Hx of space-occupying lesion/hydrocephalus/trauma	Neurologic impairment	Head CT or MRI	Correct underlying condition
Labyrinthe disorder	Vertigo, tinnitus	Neurologic impairment	—	Correct underlying condition
Delayed GI emptying	Occurs after meals, partially digested food particles, Hx of diabetes or scleroderma, early satiety, weight loss	—	UGI series/barium, motility studies, endoscopy to rule out structural causes	Meds (domperidone, erythromycin, maxeran) Feeding tube/TPN
Obstruction	Abdominal distention, pain, inability to pass gas or bowel movements	Absent bowel sounds, acute abdomen, and hemodynamic instability if perforated	Abdominal 3 views/CT scan	Supportive (NPO, IV fluids, NG decompression) Surgical (OR)
Infection/Inflammation	Pain in affected organ	Fever, abdominal guarding	CBC, liver biochemical tests, serum amylase and lipase	Correct underlying condition
Myocardial ischemia	Chest pain	Cardiovascular exam	ECG	Correct underlying condition

CHRONIC ABDOMINAL PAIN

RATIONALE

- Recurrent or continuous pain >3 to 6 mo, a common complaint (in 20% to 40% of adults)
- Distinguish organic from functional pain by Hx and physical exams.

CAUSAL CONDITIONS

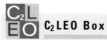 **C₂LEO Box**

Truth Telling

- After diagnosing carcinomatosis, although the patient requires family support for optimal care, they may ask the doctor to not inform their family.
- Respect the patient's wishes over that of the family.
- Understand the patient's personal and cultural context in his or her decision.
- Always seek patient consent for disclosure.

APPROACH

INVESTIGATIONS

If inconclusive and age <50 yr, do a plain abdominal film to investigate for bowel obstruction. If not present, then try an antispasmodic to relieve pain/diarrhea Sx.

Table **9.5**	Differential Dx of Chronic Abdominal Pain by Quadrant			
Upper Quadrants		**System**	**Pathology**	
			Organic	Nonmalignant
	Dyspepsia/Epigastric	Bowel disease	• PUD • GERD • Gastric CA	• Nonulcer dyspepsia
		Pancreatic disease	• Chronic pancreatitis • Pancreatic CA	
	RUQ	Biliary disease	• Biliary colic/ choledocholithiasis • Chronic cholecystitis	• Sphincter of Oddi dysfunction
		Hepatic disease	• Hepatomegaly (fat infiltration/ granuloma/congestion) • Malignancy (primary or sec- ondary)	
Lower Quadrants		Bowel disease	• Crohn disease (right) • UC • Diverticulitis (left)	• IBS
		Genitourinary disease	• Endometriosis • Ovarian cyst/torsion	• Urinary tract infection/stones
		Hernia	• Inguinal • Femoral	
Diffuse/Local Pain			• Lymphomas/neoplasms (e.g., spinal cord) • Diabetes mellitus • Chronic uremia • Degenerative disc disease	• Lactose intolerance • Abdominal wall injury • Somatization

Tx

1. Nutritional: ↑ Fiber and try lactose-free diet. Limit aggravating food (e.g., fatty food, chocolate, mint)
2. Psychological: Stress Tx (e.g., relaxation techniques, biofeedback)
3. Patient education: If pain is nonorganic, reassure that disease is benign and will not alter life expectancy.
4. Med and Surgical: Tailor to specific etiology.
5. Narcotics
   • Initial: Consider short-term hospitalization NPO, short-acting opiates, NSAIDs, amitriptyline
   • Maintenance: Long-acting opiates if pain is persistently severe
   • Complications: Constipation (use fiber supplement, laxative)

Table **9.6**	GERD vs. PUD	
	GERD	**PUD**
Pathophysiology	1. Hypotensive LES 2. Transient LES relaxation 3. Hiatus hernia	1. *H. pylori* infection 2. Iatrogenic (NSAIDs, anti-Plt drugs) 3. Other (a growing population are developing ulcers that are not related to *H. pylori* or NSAIDs)
Tx	1. Lifestyle: Elevate head of bed, ↑ salivation to neutralize acid (chew gum, stop smoking/drinking) 2. Med: ↓ acid production (PPI or H_2RA receptor antagonist), ↑ LES tone (cisapride) 3. Surgical: reduce hiatus hernia, ↑ LES tone by fundoplication	1. Eradicate *H. pylori* (antibiotics) 2. Discontinue NSAIDs if possible 3. ↓ Acid production (H_2RA, PPI)

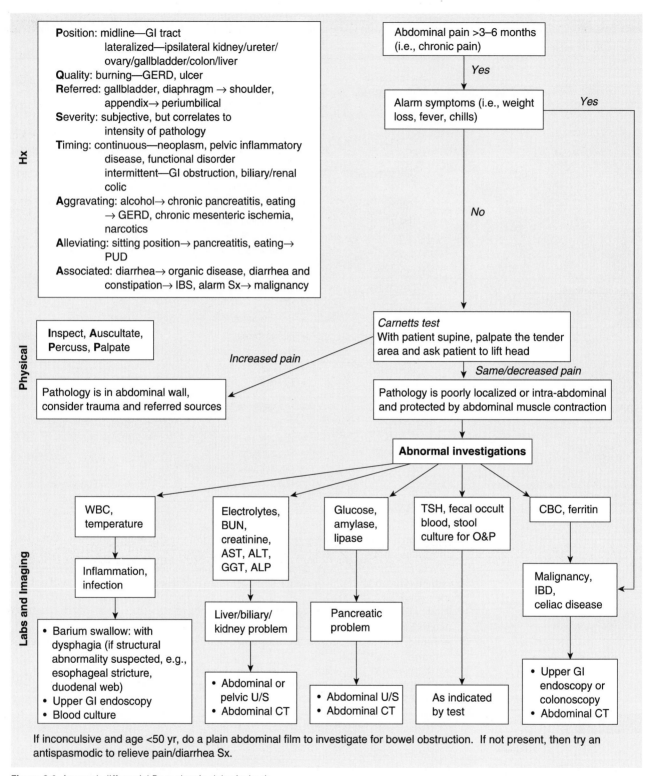

Hx

Position: midline—GI tract
            lateralized—ipsilateral kidney/ureter/
            ovary/gallbladder/colon/liver
Quality: burning—GERD, ulcer
Referred: gallbladder, diaphragm → shoulder,
            appendix→ periumbilical
Severity: subjective, but correlates to
            intensity of pathology
Timing: continuous—neoplasm, pelvic inflammatory
            disease, functional disorder
            intermittent—GI obstruction, biliary/renal
            colic
Aggravating: alcohol→ chronic pancreatitis, eating
            → GERD, chronic mesenteric ischemia,
            narcotics
Alleviating: sitting position→ pancreatitis, eating→
            PUD
Associated: diarrhea→ organic disease, diarrhea and
            constipation→ IBS, alarm Sx→ malignancy

Abdominal pain >3–6 months
(i.e., chronic pain)

Yes

Alarm symptoms (i.e., weight
loss, fever, chills) → *Yes*

No

Physical

Inspect, Auscultate,
Percuss, Palpate

Increased pain

Pathology is in abdominal wall,
consider trauma and referred sources

Carnetts test
With patient supine, palpate the tender
area and ask patient to lift head

Same/decreased pain

Pathology is poorly localized or intra-abdominal
and protected by abdominal muscle contraction

Abnormal investigations

Labs and Imaging

WBC,
temperature

↓

Inflammation,
infection

↓

• Barium swallow: with
dysphagia (if structural
abnormality suspected, e.g.,
esophageal stricture,
duodenal web)
• Upper GI endoscopy
• Blood culture

Electrolytes,
BUN,
creatinine,
AST, ALT,
GGT, ALP

↓

Liver/biliary/
kidney problem

↓

• Abdominal or
pelvic U/S
• Abdominal CT

Glucose,
amylase,
lipase

↓

Pancreatic
problem

↓

• Abdominal U/S
• Abdominal CT

TSH, fecal occult
blood, stool
culture for O&P

↓

As indicated
by test

CBC, ferritin

↓

Malignancy,
IBD,
celiac disease

↓

• Upper GI
endoscopy or
colonoscopy
• Abdominal CT

If inconclusive and age <50 yr, do a plain abdominal film to investigate for bowel obstruction. If not present, then try an
antispasmodic to relieve pain/diarrhea Sx.

Figure 9.4 Approach differential Dx to chronic abdominal pain.

BLOOD FROM GI TRACT

RATIONALE

- UGI bleed usually manifests as **hematemesis** (vomiting blood or coffee-ground material) and/or **melena** (black, tarry stools)
- Lower GI bleed usually manifests as **hematochezia** (bright red blood or dark red blood or clots PR)
- **Occult GI bleed** (i.e., normal stool color) may be suggested by positive commercial fecal occult blood tests (i.e., **Guaiac smear test**) for occult blood or presence of iron-deficiency anemia.

CLINICAL BOX

Bleeding Variances
- Melena seen in 5% to 10% of patients with slow colorectal/small bowel bleed
- Hematochezia can be seen in massive UGI bleed

CAUSAL CONDITIONS

Table **9.7**	Upper vs. Lower GI Bleed
Hematemesis	• **See upper GI bleed**
Melena	• UGI bleed • consider possibility of slow transit lower GI bleed
Hematochezia/bright red	• **See lower GI bleed** • Left colon (75% colon, 20% UGI/small intestine) • Consider possibility of massive and vigorous UGI bleed
Dark red, mixed with stool	• Right colon

HEMATEMESIS

RATIONALE

- UGI bleed defined as blood originating proximal to ligament of Treitz (duodenal-jejunal junction)
- May result in hematemesis, melena (requires >50 mL of blood), and/or hematochezia (vigorous UGI bleed)
- Requires urgent workup and Rx; can be self-limited
- Urgency and type of resuscitation dependent on total blood loss, cause of bleeding, and presence of any comorbidities

APPLIED SCIENTIFIC CONCEPTS

PATHOPHYSIOLOGY OF HELICOBACTER PYLORI INFECTION

- Specific adherence to gastric epithelium through bacterial **adhesins** (does not invade systemically); disrupt mucous layer
- Liberate enzymes/toxins such as urease, phospholipases, catalase, LPS
- Virulent strain: **VacA**+ (passive urea transporter which ↑ gastric permeability and create favorable basic environment for *H. pylori*) and **CagA**+ (necessary for VacA expression)
- Pathogenesis: host immune response → chronic inflammation and acid peptic damage (inflammatory cytokines such as IL-1, IL-6, **IL-8**, TNF-α) and antibody response (IgA and IgG to CagA that activate complement and neutrophils) → chronic gastritis
- Progression: 1) ASx; 2) PUD; 3) atrophic gastritis; 4) intestinal metaplasia/gastric CA; 5) gastric lymphoma

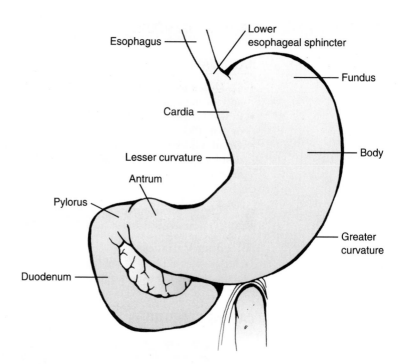

Figure 9.5 Normal gastric anatomy.

Table **9.8**	Normal Gastric Histology and Function	
	Anatomic Location	**Secretions**
Mucous surface cells (goblet cells)	Surface simple columnar layer	Secrete mucus
Mucous neck cells	Line upper walls of gastric glands	Secrete mucus
Parietal (oxyntic) cells	Scattered along neck and lower walls of gastric glands mainly in fundus/body	Secrete HCl and intrinsic factor
Chief (peptic or zymogen) cells	Line lower walls of gastric glands mainly in fundus/body	Secrete pepsinogen
Enteroendocrine cells (i.e., G cells)	Located mainly in antrum/pylorus	Secrete hormones such as **gastrin**

Table **9.9**	Effects of NSAIDs on Gastric Physiology
Cox-I Dependent	**Cox-I Independent (Direct Topical Effect)**
<ul><li>PGE_2 ($\downarrow$ GI mucosal protection)<ul><li>$\downarrow$ Gastric mucosal blood flow</li><li>$\downarrow$ mucus secretion</li><li>$\downarrow$ Stabilization of cell membranes and tight junctions</li><li>$\downarrow$ Duodenal HCO_3^- secretion</li><li>$\uparrow$ Gastric acid secretion</li></ul></li><li>TXA_2 ($\downarrow$ Plt adhesiveness/hemostasis)</li></ul>	<ul><li>NSAIDs are weak organic acids that become trapped in gastric mucosal epithelial cells and build up to cause local toxic effects.</li><li>$\uparrow$ Glutathione to scavenge superoxide radicals (anticarcinogenic)</li></ul>

CAUSAL CONDITIONS

CLINICAL BOX

Differential Dx of UGI Bleed: GUM BLEEDING

Gastritis

Ulcer

Mallory-Weiss

Biliary (hemobilia)

Large varices

Esophageal ulcer/**e**sophagitis

Enteroaortic fistula (aortic graft)

Duodenitis

Inflammatory bowel disease

Neovascularization (AVM)

Gastric CA

Table **9.10**	Differential Dx of UGI Bleed
Mechanism	**Causes (Incidence)**

Ulcerative/erosive	• PUD (esophageal vs. gastric vs. duodenal) (55%)
	• Infectious (*H. pylori*)
	• Drugs (NSAIDs)
	• Stress ulcer
	  • Cushing ulcer: associated with ↑ ICP
	  • Curling ulcer: associated with severe burns or other severe physiologic stress
	• Zollinger-Ellison syndrome (hypersecretion of gastrin from gastrinoma)
	• Nonulcerative esophagitis/gastritis
	  • Peptic
	  • Infectious
	  • Drugs

Portal HTN	• Varices (15%)
	  • Esophageal
	  • Gastric
	  • Duodenal

Trauma/postsurgery	• Mallory-Weiss tear (5%)
Tumor (5%)	• Benign • Malignant
Vascular malformation	• Angioma • Dieulafoy lesions (small ectatic arterial malformations)
Hepatobiliary	• Hemobilia • Neoplasia • Biliary inflammation • Hepatic artery aneurysm • Iatrogenic (i.e., complication of core liver biopsy)

APPROACH

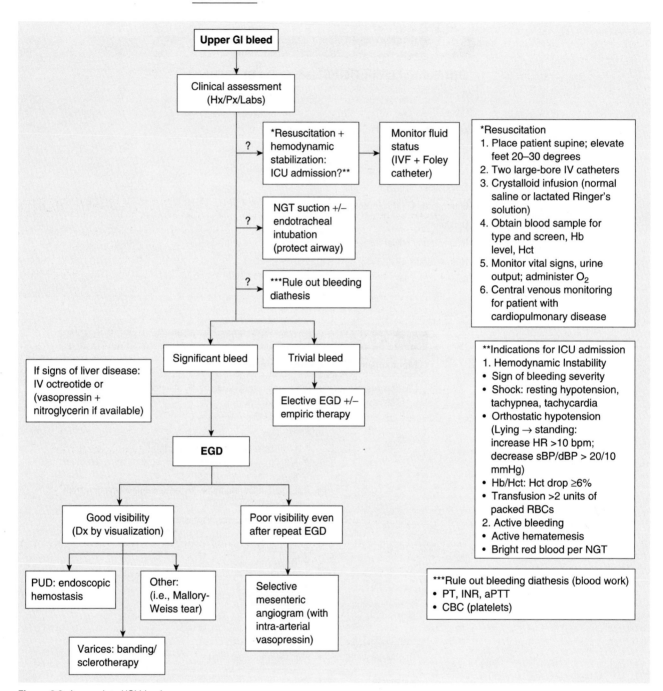

Figure 9.6 Approach to UGI bleed.

Risk Factors

EtOH, cigarettes, aspirin/NSAIDs, anticoagulants (i.e., warfarin), steroids, trauma, vomiting, Hx of UGI bleed, Hx of PUD, liver disease, esophageal varices, portal HTN, splenic vein thrombosis, AAA repair (aortoenteric fistula), burns

Lab Tests

CBC, Hct, type and cross, Chem-7 (Na^+, K^+, Cl^-, HCO_3^-, creatinine, BUN, glucose), LFTs, bilirubin, amylase, PT/INR/aPTT

UGI Bleed Outcomes

- 80% to 85% of patients spontaneously stop bleeding.
- Overall 10% mortality rate from acute UGI bleed

H. pylori Rx (7 d)

1. Bismuth triple Rx
   - Bismuth, 2 tab q.i.d.
   - Metronidazole, 250 mg t.i.d.
   - Tetracycline, 500 mg q.i.d.
2. PPI triple Rx
   - PPI (i.e., omeprazole 20 mg) b.i.d.
   - Amoxicillin, 1,000 mg b.i.d.
   - Clarithromycin, 500 mg b.i.d. **or** metronidazole, 500 mg b.i.d.
3. Quadruple Rx
   - PPI (i.e., omeprazole 20 mg) b.i.d.
   - Bismuth, 2 tab q.i.d.
   - Metronidazole, 250 mg t.i.d.
   - Tetracycline, 500 mg q.i.d.

HIGH RISK CRITERIA FOR REBLEED

1. Old age
2. Comorbid conditions
3. Clinical evidence of aggressive bleed
4. Size (>2 cm)
5. Onset of bleeding in hospital
6. Diagnostic appearance:
   - Ulcer base with recent, adherent clot
   - Ulcer base with visible vessel
   - Ulcer base with blood oozing or spurting

TX

Table **9.11**	**Mechanism of Selected Drugs in GI Bleed**
Octreotide	↓ Portal pressure by inhibiting vasoactive peptides such as substance P and glucagon and ↓ splanchnic blood flow in treating variceal hemorrhage
Vasopressin	↓ Portal pressure by mesenteric vasoconstriction receptors in treating variceal hemorrhage
PPI (i.e., omeprazole)	Inhibits gastric H^+/K^+ pump, resulting in ↓ gastric acid secretion
H₂RA (i.e., ranitidine)	H₂RA on parietal cells to ↓ gastric acid secretion; first-line Rx for GERD

PUD

- Pharmacologic Rx: *H. pylori* eradication, continued PPI or H₂RA
- Stop NSAID, anticoagulant, EtOH ingestion
- Endoscopic Rx:
  - Injection: saline and epinephrine
  - Coagulative diathermy: bipolar or multipolar electrocoagulation; heater probe
  - Hemoclips
  - Radiologic arterial embolization
  - Surgery for refractory bleeding: oversewing of bleeding site; resection of ulcer

ESOPHAGEAL VARICES

- Pharmacologic Rx (in acute setting only): (vasopressin/terlipressin + nitroglycerin) or somatostatin/octreotide for 3 to 5 d
- **Sengstaken-Blakemore balloon**: compression
- Endoscopic Rx:
  - Sclerotherapy
  - Rubber band ligation
  - TIPS
  - Surgical decompressive portal-systemic shunt
  - Liver transplant

MALLORY-WEISS TEAR

- Endoscopic injection of saline and epinephrine
- Endoscopic thermal electrocautery
- Radiologic arterial embolization
- Surgery: refractory bleed

STRESS ULCER PROPHYLAXIS

- PPI (PO recommendation)
- H₂RA (IV recommendation)
- Antacids
- Sucralfate
- PG analog
- Enteral nutrition or TPN

HEMATOCHEZIA

Critical to have early identification of colorectal CA (second most common cause of CA-related mortality after lung CA)

RATIONALE

Lower GI bleed defined as blood originating distal to ligament of Treitz (duodenal-jejunal junction)

- May result in melena and/or hematochezia
- Lower GI bleed < UGI bleed (20% vs. 80%)
- Affects mainly elderly patients (10% to 20% morbidity/mortality)

CAUSAL CONDITIONS

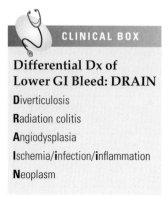

CLINICAL BOX

Differential Dx of Lower GI Bleed: DRAIN

Diverticulosis
Radiation colitis
Angiodysplasia
Ischemia/infection/inflammation
Neoplasm

Table **9.12** Differential Dx of Lower GI Bleed	
Mechanism	**Causes (Incidence)**
Diverticulosis (40%)	• Mostly right colon; most common cause of massive lower GI bleed (painless)
Angiodysplasia (25%)	• May be anywhere in small or large intestine

Other	• Anorectal disease (<50 y.o.)
	  • Hemorrhoids
	  • Fissures
	• Colorectal CA/polyps (if >50 y.o. 10%–20%)
	• Enterocolitis
	  • Ischemia
	  • Infectious
	  • IBD
	• Other
	  • Small bowel neoplasms/ulcers
	  • Meckel diverticulum
	  • Traumatic rectal injuries

Tumor (5%)	• Benign • Malignant
Vascular malformation	• Angioma • Dieulafoy lesions (small ectatic arterial malformations)
Hepatobiliary	• Hemobilia • Neoplasia • Biliary inflammation • Hepatic artery aneurysm • Iatrogenic (i.e., complication of core liver biopsy)

CLINICAL BOX

Limitations of Fecal Occult Blood Testing as a Screen for Colorectal CA

- Relatively low sensitivity (35% to 80%)
- Relatively low specificity (i.e., does not indicate etiology at all)
- High false-positive and false-negative rate
- Poor participation and compliance after positive test
- Lack of follow-up by physicians

APPROACH

SCREENING FOR COLORECTAL CA

1. ASx without first-degree family Hx
   - Annual DRE at 40 y.o.
   - Annual fecal occult blood test at 40 y.o.
   - Consider colonoscopy at 50y
2. ASx with first-degree family Hx
   - Colonoscopy at 40 y.o. (if relative <55 yr)

Table **9.13**	Risk Factors for Colorectal CA and Diverticulosis	

Colorectal CA	Diverticulosis
• Polyps • FAP • HNPCC • IBD: UC > Crohn • Previous colorectal CA, breast CA	• Chronic constipation • CT disorders i.e., Marfan Sx • Meds: corticosteroids, NSAIDs
• Diet: low-fiber, high-fat • Old age • Family Hx	

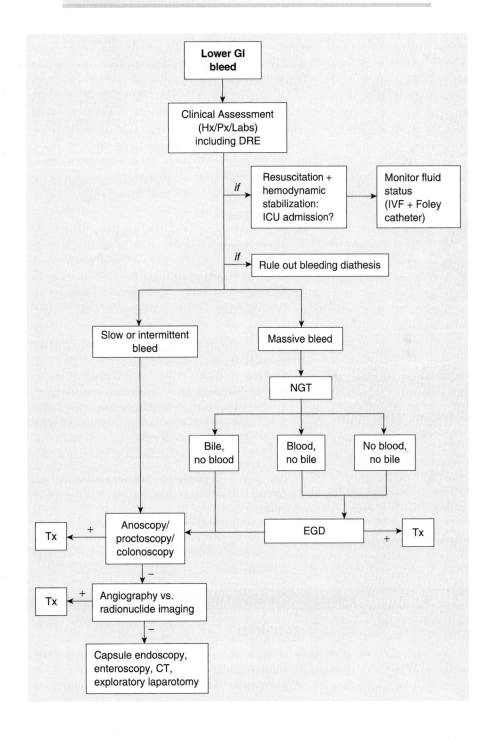

Figure 9.7 Approach to lower GI bleed.

Table **9.14**	Radiologic Imaging vs. Angiography	
	Radiologic Imaging	**Angiography**
Detection limit	• Bleeding rate of 0.1–0.5 mL/min	• Bleeding at the rate of 1.0–1.5 mL/min
Sensitivity and Specificity	• More sensitive than angiography • Less specific than angiography, colonoscopy	• 100% specific; poor sensitivity
Advantages	• Noninvasive • Sensitivity	• No bowel prep • Accurate localization • Therapeutic intervention (intra-arterial vasopressin)
Disadvantages	• Poor localization • Only localize to abdominal area	• Complications: • Arterial thrombosis embolization • Renal failure
Types	• 99mTc sulphur colloid • 99mTc pertechnate-labeled autologous RBCs	
Recommended for	• After colonoscopy • Before angiography to confirm presence of bleeding and/or location	After colonoscopy

INVESTIGATIONS

- CBC, Hct, type and cross, Chem-7 (Na$^+$, K$^+$, Cl$^-$, HCO$_3^-$, creatinine, BUN, glucose), PT/INR/aPTT
- Acute bleed: assess vital signs, check CBC, type and cross in anticipation of immediate or future blood transfusion.
- Chronic bleed: confirm that patient is hemodynamically stable, assess hemoglobin, MCV and iron studies; consider specialty referral for definitive Dx and Rx

Tx

- Immediate Rx: two large bore IVs for resuscitation with normal saline or transfusion of packed red cells as needed
- Med Rx:
  - Mild/moderate IBD: mesalamine suppository/enema; sulfasalazine; corticosteroids
  - Severe IBD: corticosteroids, cyclosporine, infliximab
  - Ischemic colitis: conservative Tx; consider surgery as last resort
  - Infectious colitis: antibiotics
- Colonoscopic Rx: laser, electrocoagulation, local epinephrine injection (rare situations, usually diagnostic only)
- Consider angiography Rx: intra-arterial vasopressin (vasoconstriction), **selective arterial embolization** (e.g., coils, gelfoam) for acute lower GI bleed
- Surgery
  - Bleeding site known: segmental resection of bowel
  - Bleeding site unknown: exploratory laparotomy +/− total abdominal colectomy (ileorectostomy)

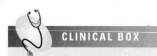

CLINICAL BOX

Outcomes of GI Bleeding
- 80% to 90% of lower GI bleeding stop spontaneously with resuscitation.
- 10% of patients require surgery (consider risks of emergent and nonemergent surgery)

ACUTE DIARRHEA

RATIONALE

- Diarrhea is very common worldwide; morbidity and mortality are significant, even in North America.
- Physicians will have to decide which patients presenting with acute diarrhea will have the need for further investigations/Rx and which patients will have self-limiting conditions.

Table **9.15**	**Definitions of Diarrhea**
Acute	>2 d, ≤2 wk >3 stools/d or >200 g stools/d, likely infectious etiology
Persistent	>2 wk
Chronic	>4 wk; likely noninfectious etiology
Pseudodiarrhea	↑ Frequency, normal consistency, normal stool weight (i.e., thyrotoxicosis, acute IBS-like episodes, proctitis, neurologic impairment, impaction)

CAUSAL CONDITIONS

The etiology of true acute diarrhea can be described by two main categories: infectious versus noninfectious (including osmotic).

APPROACH

Hx

- Onset, duration, frequency
- Stool characteristics
- Fever
- Med Hx (including prescription and OTC meds)
- Dietary Hx, that is, unpasteurized/pasteurized dairy products and chicken/meat/fish and shellfish (e.g., cooked, uncooked, meals prepared in a restaurant, social gathering etc.)
- Exposure, that is, occupation, travel, pets, hobbies, sexual partners (e.g., fecal-oral route of infectious transmission, HIV risk factors etc.), other known individuals afflicted (i.e., may point to common-source infectious outbreak)

PHYSICAL EXAM

- Signs of volume depletion
- Abdominal exam: peritoneal signs

CLINICAL BOX

Timing of Onset

1. <6 h: preformed toxin, that is, *S. aureus*, *B. cereus*
2. 8 to 16 h: *C. perfringens*
3. >16 h: bacterial or viral

CLINICAL BOX

Public Health Notification

- Patient's occupation involves food handling, day cares, direct patient contact.
- When a public food service facility is identified as the potential cause
- Patient is suspected to be part of a community outbreak.

CLINICAL BOX

Signs of Volume Depletion

- ↓ Skin turgor
- Orthostatic hypotension
- Tachycardia
- Diaphoresis
- Vasoconstriction (↓pulse pressure with ↑diastolic pressure)
- Altered mental status

Table **9.16**	**Differential Dx of Acute Diarrhea**		
	Major Causes		
Infectious	Diarrhea predominant		Small bowel Bacteria (i.e., *C. perfringens*, *V. cholera*, *E. coli*, *Salmonella*, *Yersinia*)[a] Viruses (i.e., **Norovirus**/Norwalk, rotavirus)[b] Parasites (i.e., *Giardia*) Drugs, toxins Large bowel Bacteria (i.e., *Shigella*, *Campylobacter*, *E. coli* 0157:H7, *Salmonella*, *C. difficile*)[a]
	Nausea/vomit predominant		• Bacteria (i.e. *B. cereus*, *S. aureus*)
Drugs	• Antibiotics (*C. difficile* negative), digoxin, laxatives		
Food/additives	• Lactose intolerance (e.g., dairy products) • Sorbitol (osmotic)		

[a]Majority of severe acute diarrhea
[b]Majority of self-limited acute diarrhea

INVESTIGATIONS

Bacterial versus Viral

Bacterial → ↑WBC, left shift, neutropenia in salmonellosis

Viral → normal WBC differential or lymphocytosis

Indications for O&P Testing
- Persistent diarrhea
- Travel, especially mountainous regions
- Exposure to infant day care
- AIDS
- Waterborne outbreak
- Bloody diarrhea with few leukocytes → amebiasis

Criteria for Further Diagnostic Evaluation

One or more of the following:
- Watery diarrhea with signs of dehydration or volume depletion
- Stools containing blood and/or mucus
- Fever with temperature >38.5°C
- >6 Unformed stools/d for >2 d
- Severe abdominal pain with age >50 yr
- Recent antibiotic use or hospitalized patient
- Age >70 yr or immunocompromised

Table **9.17** Investigations for Acute Diarrhea	
Test	**Rationale**
CBC with differential, electrolytes, renal function	—
Abdominal x-ray	—
Fecal leukocytes or **lactoferrin assay**	• Test for inflammatory process
Fecal occult blood test	• Test for inflammatory process
ELISA for *C. difficile* toxins A and B	• Previous antibiotic use, nosocomial infection
Stool culture for bacteria	• Routine: *Shigella, Campylobacter, Salmonella* • Special: *Aeromonas, Yersinia* (traveller's diarrhea), *Listeria, E. coli* 0157:H7, *Vibrio*
O&P—three specimens at least 24 h apart	• Generally not cost-effective without clinical suspicion • Routine: *Giardia, Cryptosporidium, E. histolytica, Cyclospora*
Proctoscopy or flexible Sigmoidoscopy +/− mucosal biopsy	• Uncommonly used in acute setting • Visually distinguish infectious diarrhea from IBD

Tx
- If meds/food additives (i.e., dairy products in lactose intolerance, sorbitol etc.) are suspected cause—discontinue and observe
- General Diet recommendations
  - Anorexic: short period of liquids consumption only
  - Starches, grains, bananas, soup, boiled vegetables, salt

Volume Repletion As Appropriate
- Oral rehydration:
  - Contain NaCl, KCl, glucose or sucrose, trisodium citrate or NaHCO$_3$
  - Reduce hospitalization, easy to administer, but difficult to monitor absorption
- IV rehydration
  - Easy to monitor absorption, but requires hospitalization
- Vitamin and mineral repletion
- Sx Rx
  - Patient with no fever, nonbloody diarrhea: antimotility agent loperamide (Imodium)
  - Bismuth subsalicylate (Pepto-Bismol)
  - Diphenoxylate (Lomotil)
- Probiotics
- Referral to gastroenterology if diarrhea persists and lab tests are negative

Antibiotic Rx (for Infectious Etiology)
- Generally not required
- Diarrhea usually self-limited and should be avoided in *E. coli* 0157:H7
- Indication: traveler's diarrhea, invasive bacterial (fever, blood), hospitalization, elderly, immunocompromised
- Empiric Rx:
  - First-line: fluoroquinolone (i.e., ciprofloxacin 500 mg b.i.d) 3 to 5 d
  - -Second line: azithromycin 500 mg PO q.d. for 3 d **or** erythromycin 500 mg PO b.i.d. for 5 d

CHRONIC DIARRHEA

RATIONALE

- ↓ Fecal consistency for >4 wk; likely noninfectious etiology
- Affects ~5% of the population

APPLIED SCIENTIFIC CONCEPTS

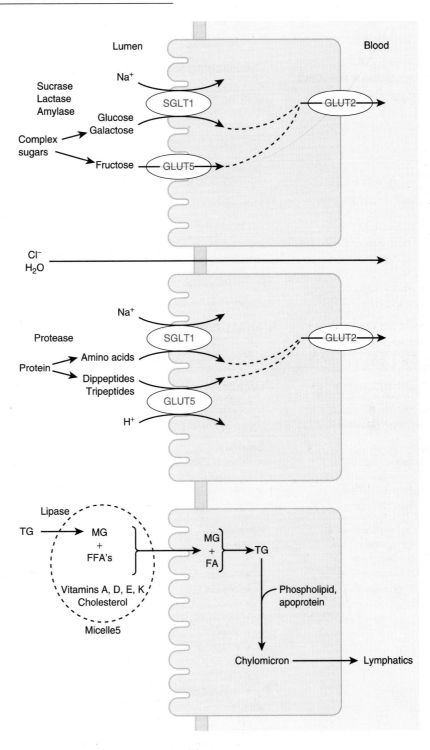

Figure 9.8 Major nutrient transport systems of the small intestine.

- **Maldigestion**: impaired digestion of nutrients within the intestinal lumen or at the brush border
- **Malabsorption**: impaired absorption of nutrients
  - **Global** malabsorption: Impaired absorption of almost all nutrients due to diffuse mucosal disease or reduced surface area, that is, Celiac disease
  - **Partial/isolated** malabsorption: impaired absorption of specific nutrients, that is, pernicious anemia
- Small intestinal epithelium have specialized transport processes to absorb nutrients
- Absorptive surface area is ↑ by intestinal villi and microvilli

ASC Box
Components of Fat Digestion and Absorption

- Mastication and gastric mixing
- Lingual lipase and gastric lipase
- Pancreatic lipase (with colipase)
- Pancreatic HCO_3^- secretion for optimal fat digestion
- Large intestine mainly involved in water reabsorption
- Bile acids promote formation of micelles

ASC Box
Pharmacological Rx of Nausea and Vomiting

Pharmacologic Rx	
Drug class	Drug example
5-HT_3 antagonist	Ondansetron
D_2 antagonist	Metoclopramide (crosses BBB, acts at vomiting center) Domperidone (does not cross BBB, acts at chemoreceptor trigger zone)
H_1 antagonist	Diphenhydramine
M_1 antagonist	Scopolamine
CB_1 agonist	Dronabinol

(Adapted with permission from Brunton LL, Lazo JS, Parker KS, eds. *Goodman and Gilman's Pharmacological Basis of Therapeutics.* New York: McGraw-Hill; 2006.)

CAUSAL CONDITIONS

Table 9.18 Differential Dx and Common Sx of Chronic Diarrhea

Steatorrhea/Secretory	Large Bowel	Small Bowel
Oily, foul, difficult to flush; indicates malabsorption	Small volume, bloody (if inflammatory), painful cramps, tenesmus, urgency	Large volume, watery, weight loss, malnourished

Luminal phase
 • *Substrate hydrolysis*
   • Pancreatic insufficiency
 • *Fat solubilization*
   • Liver cholestasis
	Secretory
	 • Secretory villous adenoma
	 • Collagenous colitis
	 • Bile salt malabsorption
		Osmotic
		 • Mg, phosphate, sulphate
		 • Carbohydrate malabsorption

Mucosal malabsorption
 • Celiac disease
 • Ileal disease/resection
 • Bacterial overgrowth
 • Radiation enteritis
 • Amyloid/CT diseases
	Inflammatory
	 • *IBD*
	   • UC
	   • Crohn colitis
	 • *Infectious*
	   • Pseudomembranous colitis
	   • TB
	   • Viral
	   • Amebiasis
	 • *Other*
	   • Radiation
	   • Ischemic colitis
	
	 Motility
	 • IBS
	 • Hyperthyroidism
		Secretory
		 • *Neuroendocrine Tumors*
		   • Gastrinoma
		   • VIPoma
		   • Carcinoid
		   • Mastocytosis
		 • *Mucosal*
		   • Crohn
		   • Celiac sprue
		   • Whipple disease
		   • Lymphoma
		
		 Disordered motility
		 • Diabetic autonomic neuropathy
		 • Hyperthyroidism
		 Infectious
		 • Giardia
		 • HIV-associated infections

APPROACH

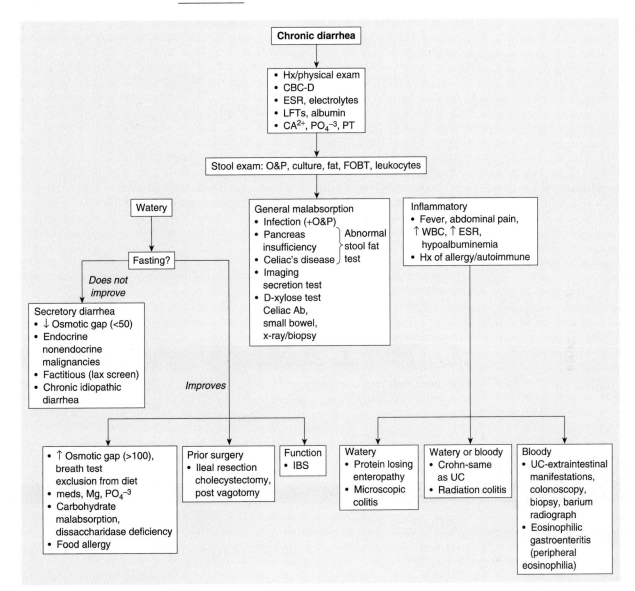

Figure 9.9 Approach to Dx of chronic diarrhea.

CLINICAL BOX

Extraintestinal Manifestations of IBD: "A SICK APE"

Aphthous ulcers (Crohn disease)

Sclerosing cholangitis (UC or Crohn colitis)

Iritis

Clubbing of fingers

Kidney (oxalate renal stones— Crohn disease)

Arthritis, ankylosing spondylitis

Pyoderma gangrenosum

Erythema nodosum

CLINICAL BOX

$$\text{Osmotic gap} = OG = [290 \text{ mOsm/kg} - 2(Na^+ + K^+)]$$

- OG <50 → secretory diarrhea
- OG >100 → osmotic diarrhea

IBS

Rome criteria for IBS: recurrent abdominal pain or discomfort at least 3 d/mo in the last 3 mo associated with two or more of the following:

- Improvement with defecation
- Onset associated with alteration in stool frequency
- Onset associated with alteration in stool form (appearance)

Table **9.19**	IBD Endoscopy	
Crohn		**UC**
Transmural inflammation of small bowel, colon, or both with skip areas of normal bowel		Mucosal/submucosal inflammation of rectum spreading proximally in a continuous manner without skip areas; may have backwash ileitis

TX

INITIAL

- Volume repletion and diet recommendations (see Acute Diarrhea—Tx)
- Treat specific cause if known (e.g., immunosuppressive Rx for IBD)
- Empiric Rx recommended when:
  1. Awaiting diagnostic testing
  2. Unclear Dx, or
  3. No specific/effective Rx available
- For unexplained steatorrhea, therapeutic trials of pancreatic enzyme replacement and conjugated bile acid supplementation
- Probiotics

CLINICAL BOX

Referral to Gastroenterology
- If diarrhea is bloody or associated with constitutional Sx (e.g., weight loss, fever)
- Etiology unknown despite extensive testing and therapeutic trials

PEDIATRIC DIARRHEA

Complications include **hypovolemia** (↓ effective intravascular volume) and **dehydration** (loss of water in excess of solute); children are more susceptible than adults. There is potential for developing electrolyte abnormalities and significant morbidity and mortality.

RATIONALE

- Diarrhea can be described as frequent, watery stools and is a frequent med concern in pediatrics.
- Most cases are mild and self-limited.

APPLIED SCIENTIFIC CONCEPTS

Table **9.20**	Differences in Fluid Loss and Their Effects	
	Secretory diarrhea (i.e., *V. cholera* infection)	Majority of bacterial and viral enteritis (i.e., Rota virus)
Fluid loss	$[Na^+] + [K^+]$ in diarrhea isotonic to plasma	$[Na^+] + [K^+]$ in diarrhea is hypotonic to plasma
Effects	Initially, more hypovolemia than dehydration	Initially, more dehydration than hypovolemia
Na	Hyponatremia	Hypernatremia especially in pediatric population
pH	Acidosis as a result of HCO_3^- loss	Acidosis
K	Normal serum $[K^+]$ to eliminate acidosis, despite total body K^+ depletion; hypokalemia after acidosis is corrected	Hypokalemia

CAUSAL CONDITIONS

Table **9.21** Differential Dx of Pediatric Diarrhea	
Age	**Causes**

Neonatal	• Diet-related
	   • Milk protein intolerance
	   • Overfeeding
	• Necrotizing enterocolitis

Older child (see Acute Diarrhea)	• Infectious
	   • Bacterial gastroenteritis
	   • Viral gastroenteritis
	   • Food poisoning
	• Malabsorption
	   • Lactase deficiency
	   • Cystic fibrosis
	   • Celiac disease
	   • Primary immunodeficiencies (HIV)
	• Other
	   • Drugs
	   • Laxative abuse
	   • IBD

APPROACH

Hx

- Estimated onset if suspected source known:
  - <1 h—chemical
  - <6 to 7 h—toxin
  - >15 h—bacteria, viruses
- Other known cases (food-borne outbreak)
- Duration
- Diet Hx, travel Hx
- Stool characteristics and bowel habits
- Fever, abdominal cramps, vomiting
- Weight loss, ↓ urine output, ↑ thirst, lethargy

PHYSICAL EXAM

- Vital signs (tachycardia, hypotension), height, weight
- External: drug mucous membranes, ↓ skin turgor, cold extremities, fontanelle (infants only), clubbing, capillary refill
- Signs of dehydration, that is, sunken eyes, sunken anterior fontanelle
- Wheezing

Table **9.22** Investigation for Pediatric Diarrhea		
Stool	**Blood**	**Advanced**
Leukocytes/lactoferrin, pH	CBC	3-d stool fat collection or **stool elastase**
Fat globules	ESR	Stool electrolytes, osmolality
O&P	Electrolytes (Na, K, Cl, HCO_3^-)	H_2 breath test
Cultures	BUN	Sigmoidoscopy, colonoscopy +/− biopsy
C. difficile toxin (antibiotic-mediated, nosocomial)	Creatinine	Barium studies Hormonal studies: VIP, gastrin, secretin, 5-HIAA assays

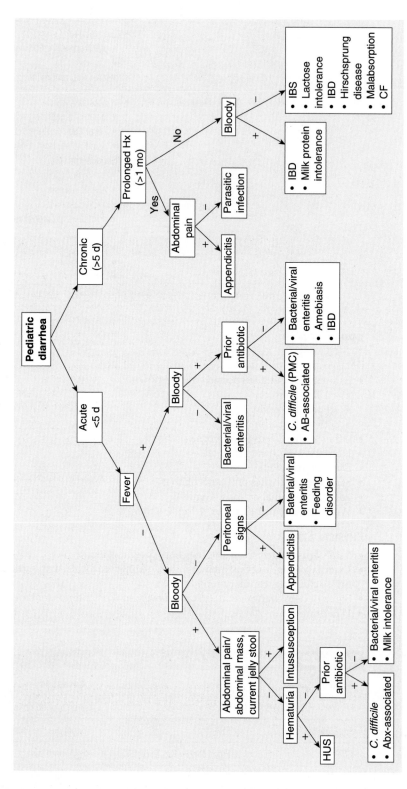

Figure 9.10 Approach to Dx of pediatric diarrhea.

TX

Table **9.23** Canadian Pediatric Society Rehydration Guidelines	
No dehydration	• Replenish ongoing losses with ORS i.e., Pedialyte, Gastrolyte
Mild dehydration <5%	• Rehydrate with 50 mL/kg ORS over 4 h • Replenish ongoing losses with ORS
Moderate dehydration 5%–10%	• Rehydrate with 100 mL/kg ORS over 4 h • Replenish ongoing losses with ORS
Severe dehydration >10%	• Resuscitate with IV normal saline **or** Ringer lactate (20–40 mL/kg) for 1 h • Reassess and repeat administration if necessary • Rehydrate and replenish ongoing losses with ORS

Age-appropriate diet following rehydration

Table **9.24** Specific Guidelines	
Recommendation	**Notes**
Limit carbonated drinks and fruit juices	Excessive sugar, low electrolyte content
Limit plain water in acute gastroenteritis	May cause hyponatremia and hypoglycemia
Ensure adequate fat intake	Nutritional
Carbohydrate intolerance	Limit lactose/sucrose
Predigested formula i.e., Pregestimil, Alimentum	Malabsorption (weight loss, fatty stools)
Antibiotics i.e., metronidazole + (ampicillin or TMP-SMX)	Intestinal bacterial overgrowth
Consider congenital defect in transport proteins, need nutritional support	Secretory diarrhea during first month of life

CLINICAL BOX

Referral to Pediatric Gastroenterologist

Patient with persistent diarrhea (>2 wk) and normal initial screening tests

ADULT CONSTIPATION

RATIONALE

Definition is patient and physician-dependent and includes:

- Infrequent bowel movements (<3 times/wk) for at least 12 wk
- Straining, hard stools, incomplete evacuation, anorectal obstruction, and/or manual maneuvers for 25% of defecations
- Patient does not meet criteria for IBS
- In patients >65 yr, almost 1/3 complain of constipation.

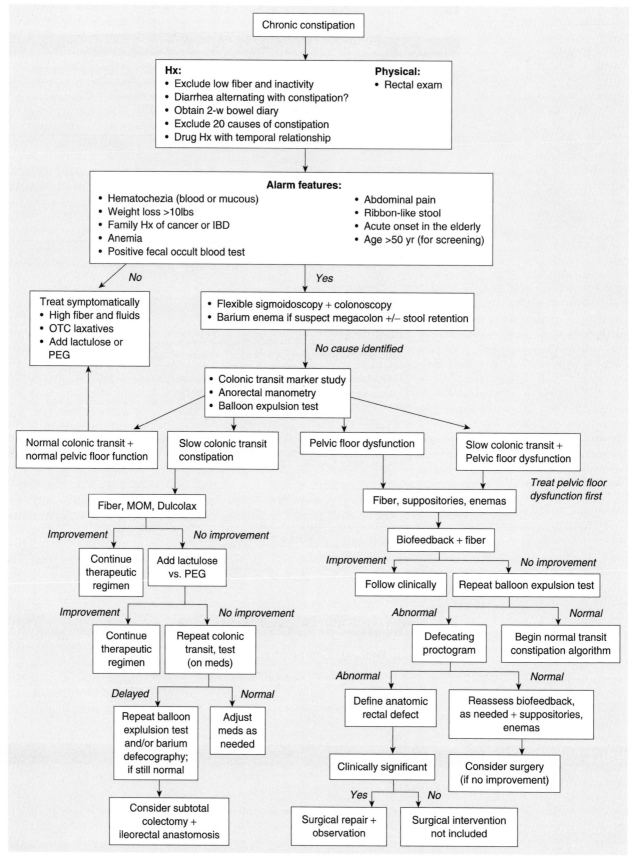

Figure 9.11 Approach to adult constipation. (Adapted from American Gastroenterological Association. Medical Position Statement: guidelines on constipation. *Gastroenterology*. 2000;119:1761.)

CAUSAL CONDITIONS

Table **9.25** Differential Dx of Constipation	
Disordered Lower Intestinal Motility	**2° Constipation**
Diet (↓ calorie, ↓ fiber, or ↓ fluid intake)	Neurogenic —central
Inactivity	• MS
Drugs	• Parkinson
• Analgesics	• Spinal cord injury
• Anticholinergics (e.g., antihistamines, antispasmodics, antidepressants, antipsychotics)	Neurogenic —peripheral
	• Autonomic neuropathy
	• Diabetes mellitus
• Cation-containing (e.g., iron supplements, aluminum)	• Hirschsprung disease
	• Intestinal pseudo-obstruction
• Neurally active (e.g., opiates, antihypertensives)	Metabolic
	• Hypercalcemia
Idiopathic	• Hypokalemia
• 70%—IBS	• Hypothyroidism
• 15%—Pelvic floor dysfunction (dyssynergic defecation)	Pregnancy
	Obstructing lesions
• 10%—Normal/slow colonic transit	• Anorectal (e.g., fissures, hemorrhoids, strictures)
	• Colorectal (e.g., neoplasm, inflammatory disease, diverticular disease)
	• Bowel obstruction

PEDIATRIC CONSTIPATION

RATIONALE

- Altered frequency and consistency of stool, or difficulty in the passage of stools that leads to incomplete evacuation of the lower bowels, resulting in <3 stools/wk for at least 2 wk
- Constipation accounts for 3% to 5% of physician visits by children.
- Major cause of chronic abdominal pain in children
- Painful defecation has been proposed as the primary precipitant of constipation and encopresis.

CLINICAL BOX

Stool Retention Clues: RAP SOS

Refusal to go

Access (limited) to toilets

Postures (that scream for **SOS**):

Standing with legs crossed

r**O**cking

Squeezing gluteal muscles

CAUSAL CONDITIONS

Table **9.26**	**Differential Dx of Pediatric Constipation**		
	Older Child		**Neonate/Infant**
Dietary/ Functional	Dietary: • Malnutrition • Insufficient fiber • Insufficient fluid	Other: • Psychological • Developmental delay • Inactivity • Fear of anal fissures	• Malnutrition (↓ stool volume) • Insufficient fiber (↓ stool bulk) • Excessive/early introduction of cow's milk • Milk intolerance or allergy
Anatomic	• Hirschsprung disease • Bowel obstruction/pseudo-obstruction		• Anus (atresia, stenosis, imperforation) • Intestinal (atresia, stenosis, Hirschsprung disease) • Abdominal muscles (absent/abnormal/enteric myopathy)
Neurologic	• Spinal cord disorders (e.g., meningomyelocele) • Amyotonia congenita (**Oppenheim syndrome**) • Guillain-Barré syndrome		
Metabolic	• Hypothyroid • Diabetes insipidus/mellitus • Hypercalcemia • Hypokalemia • Meds		

CLINICAL BOX

Functional Constipation

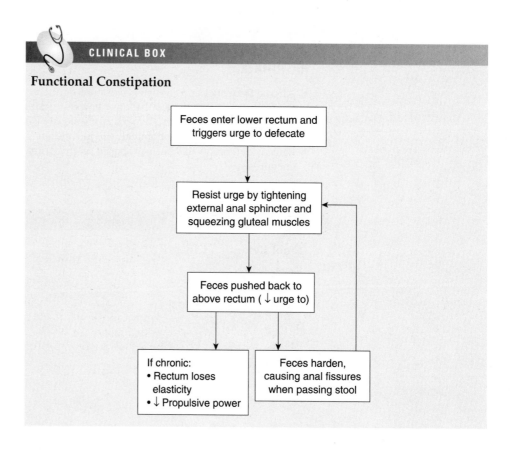

APPROACH

Differentiate functional (95%) from organic (5%) causes for appropriate investigations and Rx:

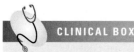

Special Considerations

HX of Abuse and Other Mental Disorders

Consider psychological Rx

Mental Disability

Constipation common if feeding with enteral formula

Prevention regime

Older Children

Regular follow-up

Address psychosocial concerns

Positive reinforcement beneficial

Table **9.27** Differentiating Function and Organic Constipation	
Suggests Functional Constipation	**Suggests Organic Constipation**
• Pass stools within 48 h of birth • Large, hard stools • Encopresis (fecal soiling) • Fluctuating pain with stool passage • Blood on tools (anal fissure) • Diet: low fiber, low fluids and/or high dairy • Avoiding toilets or withholding • Toilet training practices • Fecal impaction	• No stools within 48 h of birth, fever, failure to thrive, bloody diarrhea, bilious vomiting, "pencil-thin" stools → **Hirschsprung disease** • Fatigue, cold intolerance, bradycardia → **hypothyroidism** • Polyuria, polydipsia → **diabetes insipidus** • Abdominal distension → **pseudo-obstruction** • Congenital anatomic malformations • ↓ Reflexes/tone, no anal wink → **spinal cord anomaly**
Treat symptomatically (see Rx of Functional Constipation)	Consult with specialist

TX

RX OF FUNCTIONAL CONSTIPATION

North American Society for Pediatric Gastroenterology and Nutrition

Fecal Disimpaction
- **If large:** mineral oil and isotonic saline, then hypertonic phosphate enema after 1 to 3 h
- **If small:** isotonic saline or phosphate enema
- **If difficult to clear:** milk of Mg
- Combination Rx (can be repeated as necessary)
  - D 1—mineral oil + isotonic saline = hypertonic phosphate enema
  - D 2—bisacodyl suppository
  - D 3—bisacodyl tablet every 12 to 24 h

Follow-up/Maintenance (Up to 2 yr): Behavioral Modification
- Routine toilet patterns (best immediately after meals)
- Regular exercise (to stimulate bowel motility)
- Positive reinforcement: Encourage days with no fecal soiling.
- Educate parents and child on the importance of maintenance and adherence.
- Evaluate social and psychological effects of chronic constipation.
- Diet (↑ soluble fiber and fluids; ↓ sugar, fat, starch, insoluble fibers)
- Diary of stool movement frequency, consistency and amount (for med adjustment)

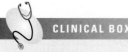

Efficacy of Rx

1 yr—30% to 50%

5 yr—48% to 75%

Table **9.28**	**Rx Agents for Constipation**	
	Disimpaction	**Maintenance**
Mineral oil (first-line Rx for fecal impaction)		
Oral	5–10 mL daily ↑ Dose by 5 mL/d until stool soft + no encopresis	[a]1–3 mL/kg/d —
Rectal enema	30–60 mL, then isotonic saline + hypertonic phosphate in 1–3 h	—
[a]Osmotic laxatives (first-line Rx for maintenance)		
PEG—PO or NG	25–40 mL/kg/h	[a]1 g/kg/d Maximum 17 g/d
Sorbitol—PO (70% solution)	—	[a]1–3 mL/kg/d
Lactulose—PO (10 g/15 mL)	—	2.5–10 mL/dose in 3 to 4 equally divided doses
Sodium phosphate—PR	Used in conjunction with isotonic saline 1–3 h after mineral oil enema OTC: 66 mL in one enema	—
Mg salts		
Magnesium citrate—PO (290 mg/5 mL)	<6 yr: 2–4 mL/kg/dose >6 yr: 100–150 mL/dose	—
Magnesium hydroxide—PO (400 mg/5 mL)	—	<2 yr: 0.5 mL/kg/dose OD [b]2–5 yr: 5–15 mL/d [b]6–12 yr: 15–30 mL/d [b]>12 yr: 30–60 mL/d
Stimulant laxatives (OTC)		
Bisacodyl	PO: 5 g every 12–24 h (combo Rx d 3) PR: 10 mg every 12–24 h (combo Rx d 2)	[a]PO: 5–15 mg/d [a]PR: 5–10 mg/d
Senna	—	[b]2–6 yr: 2.5–7.5 mL/d [b]6–12 yr: 5–15 mL/d

[a]Risk of electrolyte and/or fluid imbalances. Use with caution in patients with diabetes or renal impairment
[b]Doses can be given once daily or divided BID

FECAL/STOOL INCONTINENCE

RATIONALE

- Definition: continuous passage of fecal material (>10 mL) for >1 mo
- Minor incontinence: inadvertent soiling with liquid stool
- Major incontinence: involuntary excretion of feces
- Affects self-confidence and may lead to social isolation
- Second leading cause of nursing home placement
  - In the elderly, comorbidities include urinary incontinence, inactivity, diarrhea, and enteral tube feeding.

APPLIED SCIENTIFIC CONCEPTS

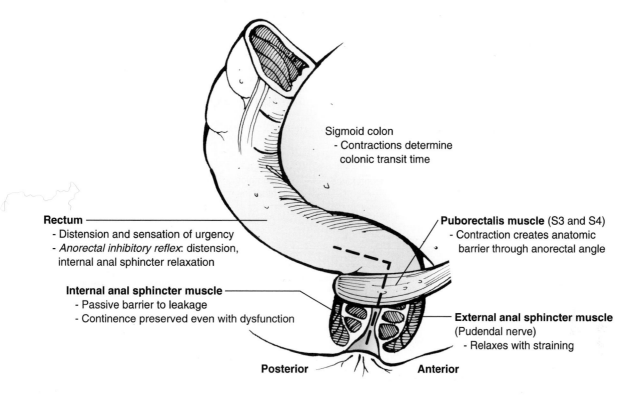

Sigmoid colon
- Contractions determine colonic transit time

Rectum
- Distension and sensation of urgency
- *Anorectal inhibitory reflex*: distension, internal anal sphincter relaxation

Internal anal sphincter muscle
- Passive barrier to leakage
- Continence preserved even with dysfunction

Puborectalis muscle (S3 and S4)
- Contraction creates anatomic barrier through anorectal angle

External anal sphincter muscle (Pudendal nerve)
- Relaxes with straining

Posterior   Anterior

Figure 9.12 Anatomy of the distal colon, rectum, and anal canal.

ASC Box

Other Factors in Maintaining Continence

- Mental function
- Stool volume and consistency

ASC Box

Anorectal Angle

Angle between longitudinal axis of rectum and anal canal

- At rest: 80° to 110°
- To avoid defecation: <80°
- With straining: >110°

CAUSAL CONDITIONS

Table **9.29** **Differential Dx of Fecal Incontinence**	
Pelvic Floor Intact	**Pelvic Floor Affected**
Neurologic	**Trauma**
• Age-related (e.g., dementia, strokes)	• Pelvic fracture
• Neuropathy (e.g., diabetes mellitus, congenital megacolon, Hirschsprung disease)	• Anorectal surgery (for fistulas, hemorrhoids)
• Congenital anomalies (e.g., myelomeningocele)	• Vaginal delivery
• MS	**Nerve/sphincter damage**
• Tumors of CNS (brain, spinal cord, cauda equina)	• Vaginal delivery
• Trauma to CNS	• Descending-perineum syndrome
Overflow	• Rectal prolapse
• Fecal impaction or encopresis	• Chronic straining (↓ sensitivity)
• Tumors of rectum	
Diarrhea	**Malformation**
• Infection	• Congenital anorectal malformation
• IBD	
• Overuse of laxatives	

APPROACH

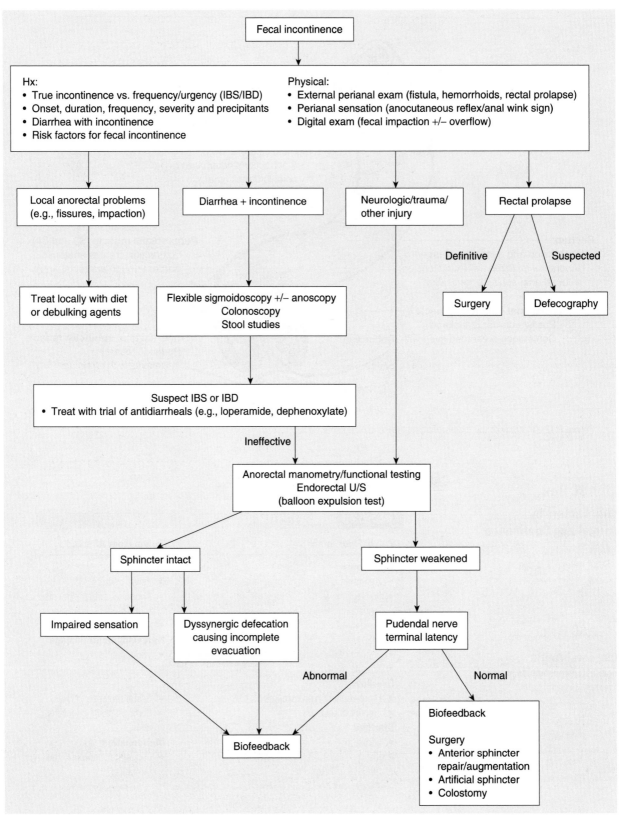

Figure 9.13 Approach to fecal incontinence.

ADULT HEPATOMEGALY

RATIONALE

- Hepatomegaly is a sign in which the liver can be palpated below the costal margin.
- The liver edge may be palpated without actual hepatic enlargement; liver span needs to be estimated.
- The cause of hepatomegaly and the extent of the disease are required to establish a prognosis.

CAUSAL CONDITIONS

Table **9.30**	**Differential Dx of Hepatomegaly**
	Major Causes
Congestive	• Right heart failure • Budd-Chiari syndrome

Infiltrative	• Malignant
	  • Metastatic CA
	  • Lymphoproliferative
	  • Leukemia
	  • Leukemia
	  • Polycythemia
	• Nonmalignant
	  • Fat (**most commonest cause**)—alcoholic and nonalcoholic
	  • Cysts
	  • Hemochromatosis
	  • Wilson disease
	  • Myeloid metaplasia
	  • Amyloid
	  • Metabolic myopathies

Proliferative	• Infectious
	  • Acute viral
	  • TB
	  • Pyogenic abscess
	  • Echinococcus
	• Inflammatory
	  • Alcoholic/chronic hepatitis
	  • Sarcoidosis
	  • Histiocytosis X
	• Neoplastic (primary hepatocellular CA)
	• Benign tumors
	  • Hepatic adenoma
	  • Cavernous hemangioma
	  • Focal nodular hyperplasia

APPROACH

Hx

- Sx of CHF—fatigue, SOB, chest pain, orthopnea, palpitations, dizziness, fainting, cough
- Abdominal pain, onset of jaundice
- Fever, malaise, weight gain/loss
- Travel Hx, occupation, infectious disease exposure
- Coexisting med problems: diabetes mellitus, obesity, dyslipidemia
- Family Hx, that is, hemochromatosis, Wilson disease
- Meds and allergies
- Intake of EtOH; IV drug use; HIV status
- Vaccinations

Table **9.31**	**Physical Exam for Hepatomegaly**
Vital signs	
Fever, tachycardia	Hepatitis, liver abscess, sepsis
Tachypnea and/or Cheyne-strokes respiration	Heart failure, sepsis
HTN	Heart failure
Examine skin and mucosa	
Cold clammy skin and cyanosis	CHF
Warm and clammy skin, petechiae, rash, splinter hemorrhages	Sepsis
Jaundice	Hepatic involvement, malignancy
Spider nevi, palmer erythema	Stigmata of chronic liver disease
Dupuytren contractures	Alcoholic liver disease
↑ JVP, peripheral edema, orthopnea, lower lobe rales, gallop rhythm, S_3	CHF
Weight (estimate BMI)	Fatty infiltration
Lymphadenopathy	Infections
Abdominal exam	
Abdominal distension, positive fluid wave test, dull percussion	**Ascites**

CLINICAL BOX

Liver Texture

Firm	Infiltrative diseases
Hard	Neoplasia
Nodular	Cirrhosis; however cirrhosis usually results in a small "shrunken" liver

CLINICAL BOX

Hepatomegaly associated with splenomegaly

- Hematologic and myeloproliferative disorders
- Lymphoma
- Leukemia

R

Consider liver biopsy (only in consultation with gastroenterologist/hepatologist or hepatobiliary surgeon—risk of bleeding, seeding of malignancy along needle track etc.)

INVESTIGATIONS

- CBC, PT/aPTT/INR
- Albumin
- Electrolytes, renal function (creatinine, BUN), fasting glucose
- -LFTs: ALT, AST, GGT, ALP
- Iron studies: ferritin, transferrin, TIBC
- ECG, CXR, echocardiogram (if cause is thought to be primary cardiac hepatic congestion)
- Abdominal U/S and Doppler studies of hepatic vasculature
- Abdominal CT, MRI
- Blood cultures for aerobic, anaerobic, and fungal microorganisms

Tx

- Tx depends on underlying cause.
- Consult gastroenterologist or hepatologist in patients with liver disease.
- Consult hepatobiliary surgeon if hepatobiliary neoplasm
- Consult cardiologist in patients with CHF and infectious disease specialist in patients with sepsis.

Table **9.32**	**Liver Examination**
Liver Span Percussion, Palpation, Auscultation	**Liver Displacement vs. Enlargement**
Liver tenderness	Inflammatory processes including hepatitis, abscess or congestion from Budd-Chiari syndrome (i.e., hepatic vein thrombosis)
Pulsatile liver	Right-sided heart failure and hepatic congestion
Hepatic bruits and rubs	Hepatic neoplasia, abscesses, inflammation
Liver texture	See Clinical Box Liver Texture

ABNORMAL LIVER FUNCTION TESTS

RATIONALE

- Abnormal LFTs are commonly found on routine screening in ASx patients.
- Intensive workup is not necessary until LFTs are more than twofold the upper limit of normal for over 6 mo

APPLIED SCIENTIFIC CONCEPTS

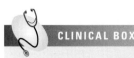

CLINICAL BOX

Abbreviations for LFTs

ALT = Alanine aminotransferase

AST = Aspartate aminotransferase

ALP = Alkaline phosphatase

GGT = Gamma glutamyl transpeptidase

IVIg = Intravenous immunoglobulin

INR = International normalized ratio

LFT = Liver function test

Table **9.33**	Differentiating LFT	
System Affected	**LFT**	
Hepatocyte injury	• ↑↑AST (also in skeletal and heart muscle) • ↑↑ALT (liver specific)	• ↑GGT + ↑ALP (because ALP also in bone, gut, placenta)
Cholangiocyte injury	• ↑↑GGT + ↑↑ALP	• ↑Cholesterol (chronic)
Liver biosynthesis	• ↑INR (advanced disease)	• Albumin (chronic disease)
Liver metabolic capacity	• ↑Bilirubin	• Bile acids (not a routine LFT)

↑, increase and ↑↑, higher increase.

Table **9.34**	Differentiating Viral Hepatitis			
	Transmission	**Prophylaxis Indications**	**Prevention**	**Natural Hx**
Hepatitis A	• Fecal-oral • Parenteral (uncommon)	• Vaccine: travel to developing countries, chronic liver disease, HIV+, homosexual • IVIg: postexposure (if <2 wk)	• Wash hands before handling food • Vaccine	• Incubation: 2–4 wk • Sx: ASx, GI illness, jaundice • Chronic carrier: n/a • Mortality: 0.1%, usually from fulminant hepatitis
Hepatitis B	• Sexual • Vertical • Parenteral	• Vaccine: health care workers, chronic liver disease, IV drug user • IVIg: newborns (if mother is HBsAg+), postexposure	• Condoms • Vaccine before travel to endemic areas (SE Asia, Africa) • Public health: vaccinate all children	• Incubation: weeks to 6 mo • Acute Sx: fever, arthralgia, rash (maculopapular or urticaria) • Chronic: usually ASx • Mortality: <1% have fulminant hepatitis, ↑HCC risk
Hepatitis C	• Parenteral • Intranasal cocaine • Sexual (uncommon) • Prevalence: 1%	• Vaccine: n/a • IVIg: n/a	• Abstinence from IV drugs, cocaine, dirty tattoo needles	• Incubation: 5–10 wk • Sx: few, 80% become chronic • Chronic: slowly progressive • Morbidity: cirrhosis

C₂LEO Box

HCV: Informing Contacts

Risk of transmission of HCV infection between monogamous stable sexual partners is low (~1% annually). The decision to inform contacts regarding this potential for infection rests with the physician and patient.

APPROACH

Hx

- Sx:
  - Jaundice, pruritus, rash
  - Arthralgias, myalgias
  - Fever, weight loss, abdominal pain, chills
  - Changes in bowel/urinary patterns (acholic stool, dark urine)
- Social Hx: EtOH, illicit drug use (cocaine)
- Parenteral exposures: transfusion, IV drug use, tattoos, sexual activity
- Other exposures: recent travel Hx, sick contacts, food, toxins

PHYSICAL EXAM

CLINICAL BOX

Stigmata of Chronic Liver Disease

Clubbing, Dupuytren contractures, palmar erythema, asterixis, parotid gland enlargement, spider angiomas, gynecomastia, caput medusa, testicular atrophy

Table **9.35**	Physical Findings with Abnormal LFT
Malignancy	Left supraclavicular (Virchow) node
	Periumbilical (Sister Mary Joseph) nodule
Abdomen	Hepatomegaly or tenderness
	Ascites
	Splenomegaly
	Prominent abdominal collateral vessels (including caput medusae)
Sx of hepatic congestion	JVD
	Pleural effusion (advanced cirrhosis)

INVESTIGATIONS

Table **9.36**	Abnormal Lab Investigations
Liver test	**Found in**
AST	Liver, heart, skeletal muscle, kidney and brain
ALT	Liver (predominantly)
ALP	Hepatic canalicular membrane, bone, intestines, kidney and placenta
GGT	Hepatocytes, biliary epithelial cells
Other tests	
Albumin	↓ In chronic liver failure
PT	↑ If ↓ production of coagulation factors
Bilirubin	Both conjugated and unconjugated forms

Indications of Abdominal Ultrasound
- Abdominal, flank or back pain (with clinical indications)
- Palpable abnormalities
- Abnormal lab values suggesting abdominal pathology
- Detect ascites in abdominally obese.
- Locate appropriate site for paracentesis.
- Detect hepatic malignancy (primary or metastatic)

Indications for Ascitic Fluid Tap (Both Diagnostic and Therapeutic)
- New-onset ascites (inpatient or outpatient)
- Worsening ascites
- Anyone with ascites showing signs/Sx of infection (fever, hypotension, peripheral leukocytosis, encephalopathy, acidosis)

CLINICAL BOX

Contraindications for Ascitic Fluid Tap

Absolute: clinically evident fibrinolysis or DIC

Relative: coagulopathy

Indications for Liver Biopsy
- Unexplained abnormal liver enzymes
- Unexplained hepatosplenomegaly
- Unexplained intrahepatic cholestasis
- Suspected malignancy
- Dx and/or staging alcoholic liver disease, NASH, or chronic hepatitis

CAUSAL CONDITIONS/PATTERNS OF LIVER INJURY

Table **9.37**	Hepatocellular (Predominantly ↑ AST, ALT)
Drugs and toxins	• EtOH, acetaminophen, NSAIDS, antibiotics, statins, antiepileptics • Suspect EtOH if AST:ALT is >2:1
Nonalcoholic steatohepatitis	• Suspect if obese, diabetic and has hyperlipidemia
Viral (hepatitis A, B and C)	• Rare: hepatitis D and E, CMV, EBV, HSV, VZV
Less common	• Muscle disorders (polymyositis, seizures, strenuous exercise) • Measure creatine kinase, lactate dehydrogenase • Hyperthyroidism • Celiac disease • Adrenal insufficiency • Genetic conditions (hemochromatosis, Wilson disease, α_1-antitrypsin deficiency) • Autoimmune hepatitis

Table **9.38**	Cholestatic (Predominantly ↑ ALP, GGT)
Biliary dilatation (extrahepatic cholestasis)	• May require other imaging (ERCP, MRI, or CT scanning) to identify site of obstruction • Choledocholithiasis (most common cause) • PSC • Malignancy (pancreatic, gallbladder, ampullary and cholangiocarcinoma)
No biliary dilatation (intrahepatic cholestasis)	• Drug-induced cholestasis (steroids, chlorpromazine, imipramine, antibiotics) • PBC • PSC • Hepatitis • Others: TPN, nonhepatobiliary sepsis, postoperative, paraneoplastic syndrome

Table **9.39**	Isolated Hyperbilirubinemia (↑ Bilirubin; Other Liver Tests Relatively Normal)	
↑ Unconjugated bilirubin	Overproduction	Hemolysis, ineffective erythropoiesis, hematoma resorption, pulmonary embolism
	Problems with conjugation	• ↓ Bilirubin UDP-GT activity • Gilbert syndrome, Crigler-Nijjar syndrome, drug-induced
↑ Conjugated bilirubin (problems with excretion)		Dubin-Johnson syndrome, Rotor syndrome

Table **9.40**	Infiltrative (↑ ALP; Other Liver Tests Relatively Normal)
Granulomatous disease	Tuberculosis, histoplasmosis, sarcoidosis
Malignancy	HCC, lymphoma, metastatic
Others	Abscess formation, meds, idiopathic

Table **9.41**	Complications of Liver Disease
Sequelae	**Pathophysiology**
Jaundice and pruritus	Deposition of bilirubin
Peripheral edema and ascites	↓ Oncotic pressure from ↓ albumin
Coagulopathy	↓ Coagulation factors
Hepatic encephalopathy	↓ Liver detoxification → accumulation of toxins in blood and brain
Sensitivity to meds	↓ Clearance
Varices	Portal HTN
Insulin resistance and diabetes mellitus	Loss of liver function in glucose deregulation by multiple pathways
HCC	End-stage neoplasia by multiple pathways
Others	↓ Immune system, impotence, kidney dysfunction, osteoporosis

Jaundice can represent med emergency: massive hemolysis, ascending cholangitis, acute hepatic failure.

ADULT JAUNDICE

 C₂LEO Box

Doctor–Patient Relationship

Maintain a nonjudgmental attitude toward all patients and care for their med conditions, even if such conditions are considered self-inflicted or the result of life style (i.e., EtOH or drugs in cirrhosis).

RATIONALE

- Jaundice (or icterus) is the yellowish appearance in the skin, sclera, and mucous membrane that results from bile pigment deposition.
- Underlying cause varies from hemolysis to hepatobiliary disease
- Evaluation usually not urgent

APPLIED SCIENTIFIC CONCEPT

See Figure 9.14.

CAUSAL CONDITIONS

See Table 9.42.

APPROACH

See Table 9.43.

 CLINICAL BOX

LFTs

1. **Direct** (measured) = conjugated bilirubin (normal values 0 to 4 μmol/L) **Total** (measured) = conjugated + unconjugated bilirubin (normal values 2 to 14 μmol/L) **Indirect** (calculated) = unconjugated bilirubin = total − conjugated bilirubin
2. A**L**T is more **L**iver specific than AST
3. ↓ Serum albumin—chronic only (>90% hepatic function impairment) ↑ INR—acute/chronic (>90% hepatic function impairment)

C₂LEO Box

Competency and Capacity to Give Consent

Patients with liver disease may lack the capacity to give consent and the physician should be able to conduct an assessment of the patient's competency and capacity to give consent:

- Conscious
- Cognitive ability
- Psychiatric condition
- Emotional status/maturity
- Patient subject to coercion or threat

See Figure 9.15.
See Table 9.44.

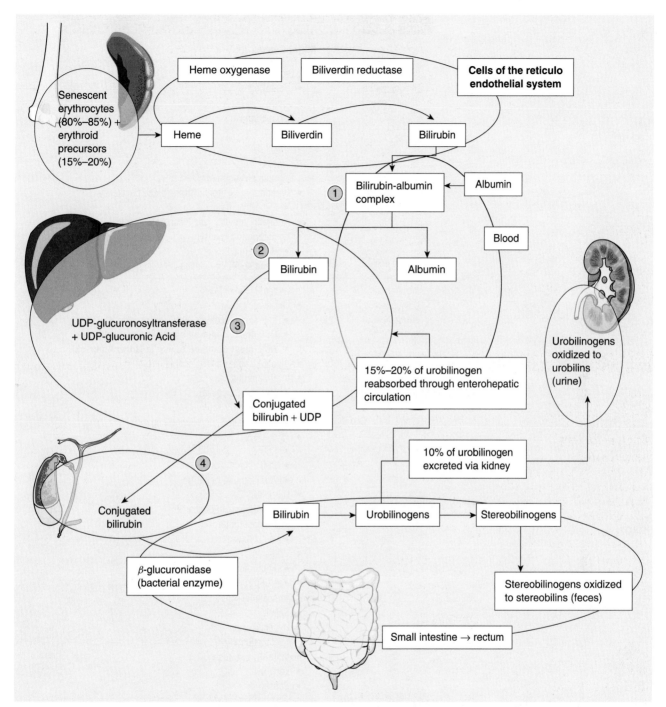

Figure 9.14 The production, metabolism, and excretion of bilirubin. There are four stages of bilirubin metabolism by the liver—(**1**) uptake from the circulation, (**2**) intracellular storage, (**3**) conjugation with glucuronic acid, and (**4**) biliary excretion.

Table **9.42**	**Differential Dx of Jaundice**
	Major Causes

Prehepatic Unconjugated bilirubinemia	• ↑ Production
	  • Hemolysis
	  • Ineffective erythropoiesis
	• ↓ Hepatic uptake
	  • CHF
	  • Drugs
	  • Sepsis
	• ↓ Bilirubin conjugation
	  • Hereditary glucuronosyltransferase deficiency
	    • Gilbert syndrome
	  • Neonatal jaundice (see Neonatal Jaundice)
	  • Acquired glucuronosyltransferase deficiency
	    • Breast milk
	    • Hepatocellular disease

Intrahepatic Conjugated bilirubinemia	• Intrahepatic cholestasis
	  • End-stage cirrhosis (any etiology)
	    • End-stage alcoholic cirrhosis
	    • HBV (**most common cause in the world**)
	    • HCV (**most common cause in North America**)
	  • Alcoholic hepatitis (reversible or fatal)
	  • Viral hepatitis
	    • HAV (acute cause)
	    • Chronic HBV, HCV
	    • Non-A, non-B, non-C viral hepatitis
	  • AI
	    • PBC
	    • PSC
	    • Autoimmune hepatitis
	  • Hereditary
	    • α_1 Antitrypsin deficiency
	    • Hemochromatosis
	    • Wilson disease
	  • Drugs
	    • Erythromycin
	    • OCPs
	• Hepatocellular injury
	  • Sepsis
	  • Hypoperfusion
	• Miscellaneous
	  • Infiltrative states
	  • Fatty liver
	  • Sepsis

Posthepatic Extrahepatic cholestasis	• Intraductal obstruction
	  • Gallstones
	  • Sclerosing cholangitis
	  • Pancreatitis
	  • Biliary malformation
	    • Stricture
	  • Malignancy
	    • Cholangiocarcinoma
	• Compression of biliary ducts
	  • Malignancy

Table **9.43**	**Focused Liver Hx and Characteristic Findings on Physical Exam**
Hx	**Findings on Physical Exam (Complications of Liver Disease)**
<ul><li>Onset of jaundice</li><li>Meds</li><li>IV drugs</li><li>EtOH</li><li>Blood transfusions</li><li>Sexual activity</li><li>Immunization status</li><li>HIV status</li><li>Past med Hx</li><li>Family Hx</li><li>Travel</li><li>Toxic exposure</li><li>Associated Sx<ul><li>Abdominal pain</li><li>Anorexia</li><li>Weight loss</li><li>Fevers/chills</li><li>Change in urine</li><li>Change in stool</li><li>Dyspepsia</li><li>Pruritus</li></ul></li></ul>	<ul><li>Abdominal distension (ascites)</li><li>Asterixis ("liver flap")</li><li>Bruising</li><li>Fever</li><li>Gynecomastia</li><li>Hepatomegaly vs. small liver</li><li>Jaundice</li><li>JVD</li><li>Kayser-Fleischer rings</li><li>Lymphadenopathy</li><li>Orthostasis</li><li>Palmar erythema</li><li>Peripheral edema</li><li>Skin rashes, spider angiomas, caput medusae</li><li>Splenomegaly</li><li>Testicular atrophy</li><li>Charcot triad for choledolithiasis (RUQ pain, fever, jaundice)</li></ul>

Table **9.44**	**Tx of Common Hepatobiliary Conditions**
Etiology	**Rx**
Biliary obstruction	<ul><li>**ERCP** + therapeutic intervention: biliary stone removal, sphincterotomy, biliary stent placement; risk of pancreatitis or perforation</li><li>**Surgical Tx**: resection of obstructing tumor such as CA at head of pancreas, ampullary tumor, cholangiocarcinoma if respectable; cholecystectomy after ERCP</li></ul>
Chronic cholestatic liver disease	<ul><li>PSC: ursodeoxycholic acid</li><li>PBC: ursodeoxycholic acid</li></ul>
End-stage liver disease	<ul><li>Autoimmune hepatitis: corticosteroids</li><li>Chronic HBV: antiviral Rx (**Lamivudine, Adefovir**)</li><li>Chronic HCV: not treated in end-stage, but otherwise antiviral Rx (**pegylated interferon-α with ribavirin**)</li><li>Alcoholic hepatitis: prednisone or pentoxifylline</li><li>All: transplant assessment; Rx of end-stage cirrhosis manifestations (lactulose for encephalopathy, diuretics for ascites, etc.); acute viral hepatitis may be observed (but not treated)</li></ul>
Acute hepatic failure	<ul><li>Investigation of underlying causes (i.e., viral hepatitis [No Rx for acute HAV, HBV], drug hepatotoxicity [*N*-acetyl cysteine for acetaminophen OD], acute autoimmune disease, acute Wilson disease)</li><li>Observation for decompensation</li><li>If decompensation occurs, then transplant assessment; critical care referral if in coma</li></ul>

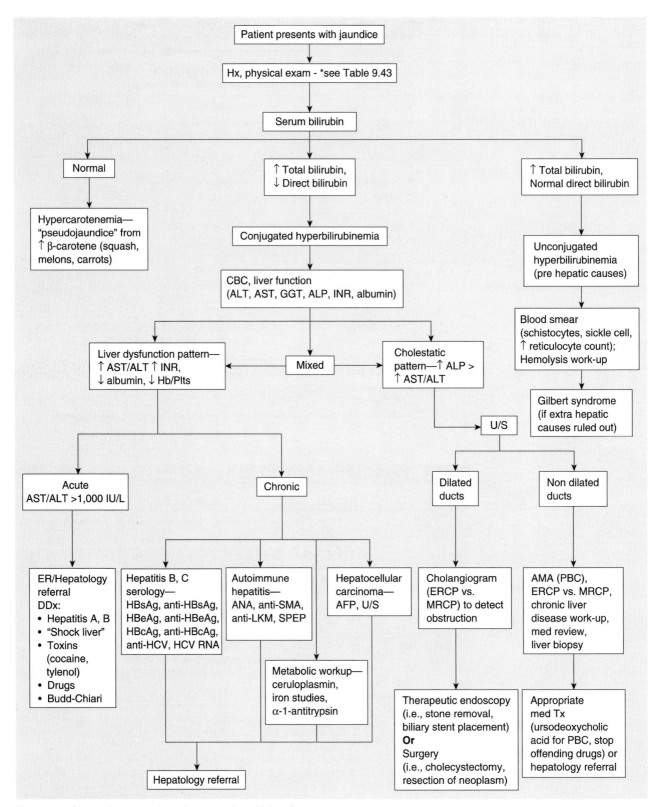

Figure 9.15 Diagnostic workup of a patient presenting with jaundice.

NEONATAL JAUNDICE

See also Chapter 18.

RATIONALE

Table **9.45**	Types of Jaundice
Physiologic jaundice	• Unconjugated bilirubinemia resulting from ↑ **breakdown of fetal RBCs** and **immature hepatic functioning** (i.e., ↓ ligandin causing ↓ bilirubin uptake by hepatocytes, ↓ activity of glucuronyl transferase) • Transient (72–96 h of age) and usually medically inconsequential • Present in up to 65% of term neonates
Hyperbilirubinemia	In infants ≥35 wk gestation: TSB >95th percentile based on Bhutani nomogram (see Investigations)
Severe hyperbilirubinemia	**TSB >340 μmol/L** at any time during first 28 d of life
Conjugated hyperbilirubinemia	Never physiologic

Unconjugated bilirubinemia may deposit in the relatively immature CNS resulting in bilirubin-induced neurologic dysfunction; acutely it is called **acute bilirubin encephalopathy** and may progress to the chronic and permanent **kernicterus.**

CAUSAL CONDITIONS

Table **9.46**	Differential Dx of Neonatal Jaundice	
		Causes

Unconjugated hyperbilirubinemia	↑ **Bilirubin production**	**Hemolytic causes: Coombs positive**
		• Isoimmune
		  • Rh, ABO, other blood antigens
		  • Autoimmune (i.e., SLE)
		• Acquired RBC defect (i.e., drugs)

		Hemolytic causes: Coombs negative
		• RBC membrane defect
		  • Elliptocytosis
		  • Pyknocytosis
		• RBC enzyme deficiency
		  • Pyruvate kinase deficiency
		  • G6PD deficiency
		• Hemoglobinopathy
		  • Thalassemia
		• Microangiopathy
		• HUS

	↓ **Bilirubin conjugation**	• Metabolic/genetic
		  • Gilbert syndrome
		  • Criggler-Najjar syndrome
		  • Hypothyroidism
		• Physiologic jaundice **or** breast milk jaundice

	GI causes	• Pyloric stenosis • Meconium ileus • Sequestered blood

Conjugated hyperbilirubinemia	↓ Bilirubin uptake	• Infections
		  • Sepsis
		  • Neonatal hepatitis
		  • Toxic (TPN)
		• Metabolic/genetic
		  • Galactosemia
		  • Gaucher disease
		  • Niemann-Pick disease
		  • ↓ Y protein

CLINICAL BOX

Causes of Nonphysiologic Jaundice: JAUNDICE

Jaundice visible within 24 h

A sibling with neonatal jaundice

Unrecognized hemolysis; **U**DP-GT deficiency

Nonoptimal feeding; **n**ear-term

Deficiency in G6PD

Infection or **i**nfant of diabetic mother

Cephalhematoma/bruising/polycythemia

East Asian, Mediterranean or Native American

APPROACH

Hx

- Onset
  - Jaundice in the **first 24 h** is more likely to be nonphysiologic.
- Neonate's weight curve, adequacy of breast-feeding
- Stool color
- Obstetric Hx
- Family Hx of hematologic disorders; previously affected children
- Maternal blood type and antibody status
- Meds

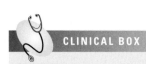

Rapid onset of jaundice is more life threatening.

Physical Exam

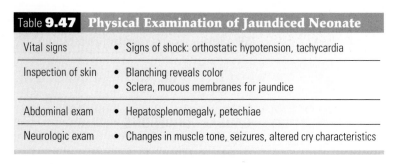

Table **9.47**	**Physical Examination of Jaundiced Neonate**
Vital signs	• Signs of shock: orthostatic hypotension, tachycardia
Inspection of skin	• Blanching reveals color • Sclera, mucous membranes for jaundice
Abdominal exam	• Hepatosplenomegaly, petechiae
Neurologic exam	• Changes in muscle tone, seizures, altered cry characteristics

Signs of acute bilirubin encephalopathy: severe jaundice, lethargy, poor sucking, hypotonia progressing to hypertonia, high-pitched cry, fever, eventually seizures and coma

Investigations

- TcB and TSB in all neonates within 72 h of delivery; immediate testing if clinical jaundice detected
- Measure serum conjugated bilirubin in neonates with severe/prolonged hyperbilirubinemia
- **Bhutani nomogram**: displays normal TSB percentiles for hours-of-age
- Blood type and Rh status in mother and neonate
- CBC, Hct
- Serum albumin (bilirubin/albumin ratio)
- Direct Coombs test
- LFTs: AST, ALT, GGT, ALP
- Galactosemia screen: reducing substance in urine
- **G6PD** screen
- Thyroid function
- **ETCO** breath test
  - Measures breakdown of heme into bilirubin and carbon monoxide
  - Not universally available
- U/S of liver and biliary apparatus

CLINICAL BOX

G6PD Screen

Especially in Middle Eastern, Mediterranean, African, SE Asian origins and in any neonate with severe hyperbilirubinemia

Tx

- Improve frequency and effectiveness of breast-feeding and/or infant formula supplementation (water or dextrose water)
- Adequate follow-up and consultation with pediatric gastroenterologist to determine etiology

Phototherapy — Prevention and First-Line Intervention

- Exposure to light of a specific wavelength reduces TSB mainly through **structural isomerization to lumirubin**, which is more soluble and is excreted into bile and urine
- Generally very safe and inexpensive
- Potential for retinal damage prevented with eye protection
- **Bronze baby syndrome** may develop: grayish-brown discoloration of skin, serum, and urine secondary to impaired biliary excretion of bile pigment photoproducts

EXCHANGE BLOOD TRANSFUSION

Last resort intervention; Rx of isoimmune hemolysis and neurologic signs secondary to hyperbilirubinemia

- Removes bilirubin from the circulation
- Most effective method for rapid bilirubin removal
- Rarely performed; risk assessment unclear

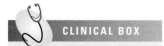

Complications of exchange blood transfusion: infection, coagulopathy, graft-versus-host disease, necrotizing enterocolitis

PHARMACOLOGIC

- **IVIg** (1 g/kg)
  - Given to neonates with positive direct Coomb test; reduces need for exchange transfusion
  - Ursodeoxycholic acid: ↑ bile flow; Rx of cholestatic jaundice

GI-ASSOCIATED HYPOMAGNESEMIA

See also Hypomagnesium in Chapter 13.

CLINICAL BOX

Hypomagnesemia Is Often Overlooked

Serum Mg levels are not routinely measured. Be alert in cases of alcoholism and GI/renal problems.

RATIONALE

- Hypomagnesemia is defined as low levels of Mg in the blood ($[Mg^{2+}]$ serum ≤ 0.6 mmol/L); normal plasma Mg concentration is 0.7 to 0.9 mmol/L
- Serum levels of Mg are not a reliable indicator of total body levels of Mg.
- Can occur without Mg deficiency and vice versa.
- ~10% of hospitalized patients have hypomagnesemia, with an incidence of >60% in severely ill patients.
- There is a frequent association with hypokalemia and hypocalcemia.

APPLIED SCIENTIFIC CONCEPTS

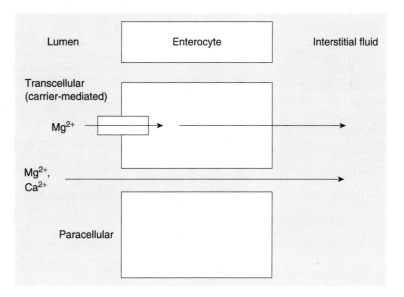

Figure 9.16 Transport of Mg in the ileum/jejunum.
There are two modes of Mg absorption:
1. Paracellular, diffusible pathway that is competitive with Ca^{2+} ions
2. Transcellular, carrier-mediated process that is saturable and not competitive with Ca^{2+}.

Mg handling in the intestinal tract:

- Average dietary intake of Mg is ~300 to 500 mg/d from a variety of sources including vegetables.
- Only ~ one third of the ingested Mg is absorbed in the GI tract—occurs mainly in the ileum, but may also occur in the jejunum.

CAUSAL CONDITIONS

Table **9.48** Differential Dx of Hypomagnesemia
GI causes
1. Marked ↓ in dietary intake (alcoholism, malnutrition, nausea/vomiting/NG suction)
2. Diarrhea (acute/chronic); malabsorption and steatorrhea, short gut
3. Acute pancreatitis
See Chapter 13 for renal causes.

APPROACH

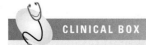

Hypomagnesemia Signs

Chvostek sign: abnormal momentary contraction of ipsilateral facial muscles in response to a tap on the facial nerve at the angle of the jaw

Trousseau sign: carpal spasms in response to 3 min of suprasystolic pressure on the brachial artery. Movements are manifested as wrist/MCP flexion, PIP/DIP extension, and adduction of thumb and fingers.

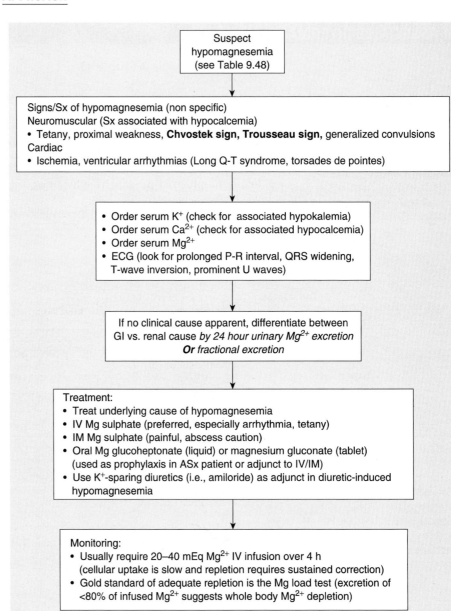

Figure 9.17 Approach to hypomagnesemia. (Adapted from Rao SS. Diagnosis and management of fecal incontinence. *Am J Gastroenterol*. 2004;99:1585.)

ALLERGIC REACTIONS/FOOD ALLERGIES, INTOLERANCE, ATOPY

See also Allergy in Dermatology, Respirology, and Anaphylaxis in Chapter 5.

RATIONALE

- Patients with a single allergic reaction often present with other atopic conditions (e.g., asthma, allergic rhinitis).
- Family Hx or respiratory atopy is positive in 50% of patients with atopic dermatitis.

APPLIED SCIENTIFIC CONCEPTS

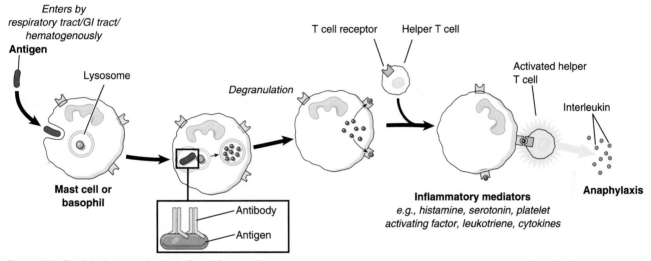

Figure 9.18 Physiologic mechanism and effects of mast cells.

Table **9.49**	**Physiologic Sx of Anaphylaxis**
System	**Sx**
Psychologic	Anxiety, chest tightness, dyspnea, ↓ level of consciousness
Respiratory	Fullness in throat, hoarse voice, respiratory distress
Vascular	Circulatory arrest, hypotension, syncope, tachycardia
Skin	Pruritus, cutaneous flushing, urticaria, angioedema
GI	Nausea, vomiting, diarrhea

CAUSAL CONDITIONS

Table **9.50**	**Allergy vs. Intolerance**	
	Allergy	**Intolerance**
Immune-mediated?	Yes	No
Sx	Skin, GI, respiratory	Mainly GI
Reaction to small amount of food?	Yes	No
Example	Peanut allergy	Lactose intolerance

Table **9.51**	Presentations by System
System	**Condition**
Skin	• Dermatitis/atopy/pruritus • Urticaria • Angioedema
Respiratory	• Rhinorrhea • Angioedema • Wheezing
GI tract	• Food intolerance • Celiac disease

APPROACH

Table **9.52**	Common Allergens: Their Possible Effects on Susceptible Children	
Common Allergen	**Specific Reaction**	**Long-term Tx**
Food	GI (vomiting, diarrhea), skin (rashes), and airways	Avoidance
Environment	Rhinorrhea, bronchoconstriction	Avoidance, oral antihistamine, β-adrenergic agonist, anticholinergic
Insect sting	Localized pain and swelling, angioedema	Ice, oral antihistamine, antivenom Rx
Drugs (e.g., penicillin)	Varies depending on drug, e.g., malaise, fever, skin eruption, Stevens-Johnson syndrome	Avoidance
Latex	Skin eruption	Avoid latex and cross reacting foods (banana, kiwi, avocado, chestnut)

CLINICAL BOX

Acute Tx of anaphylaxis: AEIOUS

Antihistamine-H$_1$ blocker:
• Diphenhydramine 25 to 50 mg IV),
• H$_2$ blocker (ranitidine 50 mg IV)

Albuterol—2.5 to 5 mg in saline nebulizer

Epinephrine—0.3 to 0.5 mg IM thigh

Intubate—if airway involved or swelling

Oxygen—100%

Upright (if severe bronchospasm) or recumbent position

Saline—normal saline, 1 to 2 L rapid bolus

Steroid—consider methylprednisone 125 mg IV

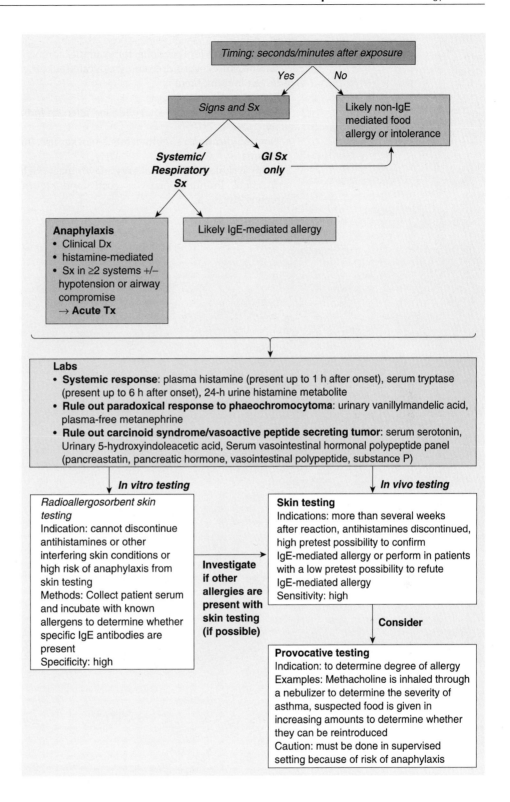

Figure 9.19 Approach to anaphylaxis.

TX

1. Patients with Hx of anaphylaxis should be referred to an allergist.
2. Education
   - Counsel the patient, parents, and school about allergy recognition and acute Tx.
   - Suggest risk reduction strategies (e.g., how to read food ingredient labels, inform of drug classes at risk for cross-reaction allergies, ↓ exposure to trigger).
3. Epinephrine: Provide an annual prescription for epinephrine, to be carried at all times.

4. Med
   - Sx-based long-term options, for example, adrenergic agonist, anticholinergic, antihistamine, glucocorticoid, cromolyn glycate, leukotriene receptor modifiers, theophylline.
5. Allergen immunotherapy
   - Consider allergen extracts.
   - Indications: environmental allergies, allergen-induced asthma, insect venom sensitivity.
   - Contraindications: simultaneous ß-blocker use, initiation during pregnancy, unstable asthma
6. Social/psychologic: Severe allergy may impact quality of life by limiting diet, exercise, and school. Immunotherapy is costly and requires time commitment, causing the caregiver stress.

CHAPTER 10

General Surgery

Ahmed Kayssi, Jaskaran Kang, Dr. Yen Dang, and Dr. Ralph George

ABDOMINAL DISTENSION

DEFINITION

Abdominal distension presents in a large number of diverse pathologies, including:

- Ascites
- Bowel obstruction
- Pelvic masses
- Organomegaly

CAUSAL CONDITIONS

ASCITES

In an average adult ascites must be >1.5 L for clinical diagnosis.

BOWEL DILATION

- Mechanical obstruction
  - Adhesion
  - Volvulus
  - Malignancy
  - Intussusception
  - Constipation
  - Intestinal pseudo-obstruction
    - Acute
- Toxic megacolon
  - Ogilvie syndrome (trauma/surgery, medical illness/drugs, retroperitoneal hemorrhage)
  - Chronic intestinal pseudo-obstruction
    - Myopathic (scleroderma, familial)
    - Enteric neuropathic (diabetes, amyloid, paraneoplastic, narcotics)
    - Extrinsic neuropathic (MS, spinal injury, stroke)
    - Other paralytic ileus
      - *C. difficile*
      - Peritonitis
      - Postoperative
      - Hypothyroid
      - Hypokalemia

OTHER

- Pelvic mass
  - Pregnancy
  - Ovarian mass
  - Bladder

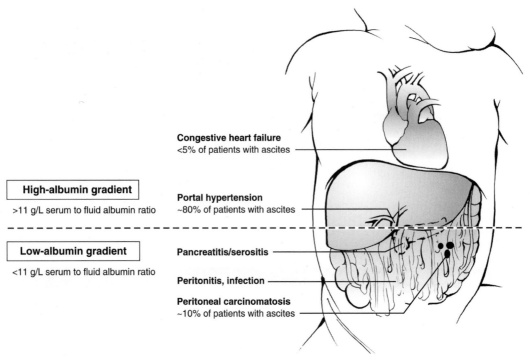

Figure 10.1 Causes of ascites.

CLINICAL BOX

Useful Diagnostic Tests

- AXR
- Abdominal CT
- Abdominal U/S
- Paracentesis
- Cytology and cell block examination of ascitic fluid

- Fibroids
- Malignancy
- Bowel
  - Feces
  - IBD
  - Flatus
  - Malabsorption
  - Constipation
  - Mass/Organomegaly
    - See Abdominal Mass

APPROACH

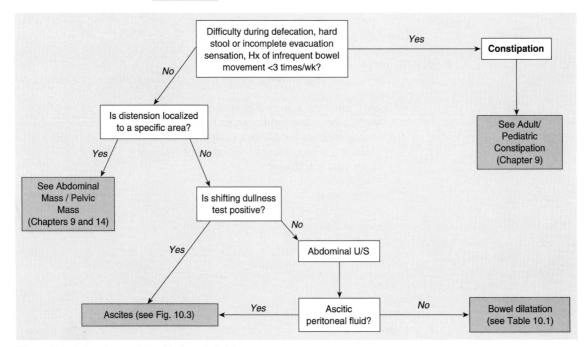

Figure 10.2 Approach to patient with distended abdomen.

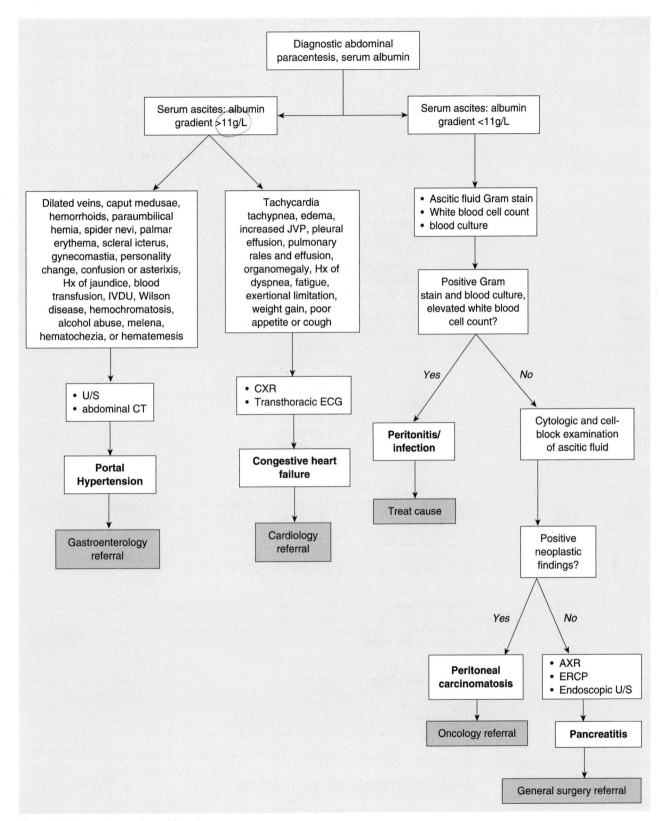

Figure 10.3 Approach to patient with ascites.

Table **10.1** Approach to Patient with Bowel Dilatation				
Condition	**Colicky Pain?**	**Signs/Symptoms**	**Workup**	**Management**
Myopathic or neuropathic chronic intestinal pseudo-obstruction	+	Constipation, obstipation, N/V, anorexia, weight and muscle loss, distended bladder, mydriasis, ptosis, and external ophthalmoplegia, Hx of diabetes, amyloid disease, cancer, narcotic use, MS, spinal injury or stroke	Antroduodenal manometry	Gastroenterology referral
Ogilvie syndrome		Hx of trauma, fractures, surgery, narcotics and anticholinergic medication use, spinal cord injury, cardiovascular disorder or severe medical illness with long bedrest	AXR	
Adhesions		Hx of bowel surgery		General surgery referral
Large bowel obstruction		Diffuse tenderness, Hx of constant pain with intermittent to little vomiting		Urgent general surgery referral
Intussusception		Pediatric patient, Dance sign, Hx of URTI, rectal bleeding, and/or lethargy		Urgent pediatrics referral
Paralytic ileus	−	No bowel sounds on auscultation, no passage of flatus		Bowel rest
Toxic megacolon		Fever, hypotension, tachycardia, Hx of IBD, recent travel, exposure to *C. difficile* or antibiotic use, chemotherapy, immunosuppression, leukocytosis, anemia, dehydration, altered mental status, electrolyte abnormality		Treat cause; general surgery referral if condition worsens

+ = present; − = absent.

Table **10.2** Cirrhotic versus Malignant Ascites		
	Ascites Cirrhotic	**Malignant**
Treatment aim	Curative	Palliative
Paracentesis	Yes	Yes
Pharmacotherapy	Steroids, antivirals, β-blockers, diuretics, broad-spectrum antibiotics	Chemotherapy, diuretics
Lifestyle modifications	Alcohol and smoking cessation, reduced sodium diet, and fluid intake	Subject to cancer management approach
Surgical intervention	None	Peritoneovenous shunting for refractive ascites
Liver transplant	May be beneficial	Not indicated

MANAGEMENT OF BOWEL OBSTRUCTION

- Gastrointestinal drainage
- Fluid and electrolyte replacement
- Indwelling catheter
- Serial electrolyte measurements
- Hematocrit and white blood cell counts

- Central venous or pulmonary artery catheter
- Prophylactic broad-spectrum antibiotics
- Surgical relief

CLINICAL BOX

Shifting Dullness Test

- Percuss supine abdomen to determine areas of dullness
- Roll patient onto the left decubitus position
- Percuss previously outlined areas of dullness
- Shifting of dullness to areas of previous tympany suggests ascites

ERCP

- Endoscopic injection of dye at the site of pancreatic duct and biliary tree opening
- Used in diagnosing and treating biliary and pancreatic duct problems

ANTRODUODENAL MANOMETRY

- Intraluminal pressure recordings of the stomach and the small bowel
- Used in evaluating the muscular activity of the gut

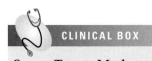

CLINICAL BOX

Serum Tumor Markers

- Colonic
  - CEA
- Pancreatic
  - CEA, CA 19-9
- Hepatoma
  - AFP
- Ovarian
  - CA-125

CLINICAL BOX

Bowel Obstruction Symptoms

- Constipation/obstipation
- Distension
- Pain
- Vomiting

APPLIED SCIENTIFIC CONCEPTS

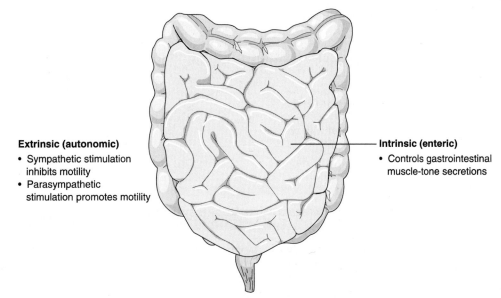

Extrinsic (autonomic)
- Sympathetic stimulation inhibits motility
- Parasympathetic stimulation promotes motility

Intrinsic (enteric)
- Controls gastrointestinal muscle-tone secretions

Figure 10.4 Innervation of the gut.

INTERSTITIAL CELLS OF CAJAL

- Intestinal pacemaker cells
- Connect enteric nerves and intestinal smooth muscles
- Coordinate function of both intrinsic and extrinsic neurons

ABDOMINAL MASS

DEFINITION

Abdominal mass is important as it can be caused by:

1. Organomegaly
2. Neoplastic processes
3. Growth of pelvic structures
4. Infective or other pathological process in the abdominal cavity

CAUSAL CONDITIONS

ORGANOMEGALY

- Hepatomegaly
- Splenomegaly
- Enlarged kidneys
  - Cysts
  - Hydronephrosis
  - Tumors

NEOPLASMS

- Lymphoma/sarcoma
- Gastrointestinal tumors
  - Gastric
  - Pancreas
  - Colon
  - Hepatoma
- Gynecologic tumors
  - Ovarian
  - Uterine
- Neuroblastoma

OTHER

- Pelvic organs in abdomen
  - Pregnancy
  - Bladder
- Pancreatic pseudocyst
- Abdominal aortic aneurysm
- Abdominal wall masses

APPROACH

CLINICAL BOX

Mass Size and Malignancy

>4 cm on radiologic studies is 93% sensitive and 76% specific in detecting an adrenocrotical carcinoma.

CLINICAL BOX

Signs of Symptomatic Abdominal Aortic Aneurysm

1. General diffuse abdominal, low-back or flank pain
2. Pulsatile paraumbilical mass
3. Systolic bruit over the abdominal aorta
4. Tenderness over affected area on palpation
5. Abdominal fullness sensation
6. Leg swelling

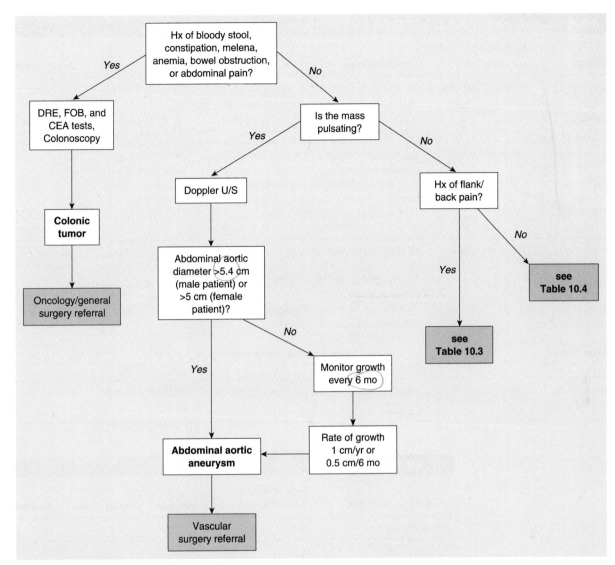

Figure 10.5 Approach to patient with abdominal mass.

Table **10.3**	Approach to Patient with Flank or Back Pain			
Condition	**Signs/Symptoms**		**Workup**	**Management**
Renal tumor	Hx of hematuria, hypertension		Kidney U/S, abdominal CT	Urology referral
Gastric tumor	Hx of bloating, premature satiety, dysphagia, anorexia, melena, hematemesis, and epigastric pain		FOB test, double contrast radiographic examination ± endoscopy	General surgery referral
Renal cyst	Hx of nephrolithiasis, hematuria, renal infection, polyuria, end-stage renal disease, renal failure, hypertension, dialysis		Kidney U/S and CT	Nephrology referral
Hydronephrosis	Hx of N/V, worsening pain with consumption of fluids, radiates to ipselateral testes/labia, hematuria			
Sarcoma	Lower extremity edema, Hx of dysphagia, constipation, melena, nonspecific abdominal pain, early satiety, or sensation of fullness		AXR and CT	Oncology referral

Table **10.4**	Approach to Abdominal Mass by Location			
Condition	**Anatomical Location**	**Signs/Symptoms**	**Workup**	**Management**
Hepatomegaly	Right subcostal area	Palpable lower border of liver, liver span ≥ 12 cm	Hepatic U/S and CT	See Chapter 9—Hepatomegaly
Hepatoma		Jaundice, scleral icterus, deep palpation-induced pain, Hx of right shoulder pain	AFP serology, Hepatic U/S and CT	General surgery referral
Pancreatic tumor	Left subcostal area	Recent onset of diabetes mellitus, darkening urine, changing color stools	CA 19-9 serology, abdominal U/S and CT	General surgery referral
Pancreatic pseudocyst		Hx of acute or chronic pancreatitis, abdominal trauma	Abdominal U/S and CT	
Splenomegaly		Positive Castell sign, palpable spleen		See Chapter 11—Splenomegaly
Uterine tumor	Suprapubic area	Hx of abnormal vaginal bleeding ± discharge	Endometrial biopsy	Gynecology referral
Ovarian tumor		Hx of abdominal pain, bloating, irregular menses or change in bowels	CA-125 serology	
Pregnancy		Hx of fatigue, breast tenderness or enlargement, N/V, increased urination, amenorrhea	hCG test, suprapubic U/S	See Chapter 14—Antepartum Care
Enlarged bladder		Hx of urinary frequency, dysuria, change in urine appearance	Bladder U/S	Treat cause
Neuroblastoma	Crosses the midline	Irregular abdominal mass, exclusively in pediatric patients	CBC, ESR, AXR, and CT	Oncology referral

Table **10.5**	Biopsies			
Pathologic Condition	**Type of Biopsy Percutaneous**	**Endoscopic**	**Laparoscopic**	**Endometrial**
Hepatomegaly	X			
Enlarged kidneys	X			
Lymphomas[a]	X	X	X	
Sarcomas[a]	X	X	X	
Gastrointestinal cancers		X		
Ovarian cancer			X	
Uterine cancer				X
Neuroblastoma	X			
Abdominal wall mass	X			

X is a checkmark to indicate biopsy performed.
Biopsies are not indicated for pelvic organ enlargement or in abdominal aortic aneurysms.
[a]Type of biopsy used depends on mass location.

ABDOMINAL MASS–ADRENAL MASS

DEFINITION

Located in the adrenal medulla or cortex, most are nonfunctioning and are found incidentally during radiologic investigation of the abdomen. Functioning masses must be surgically removed.

CAUSAL CONDITIONS

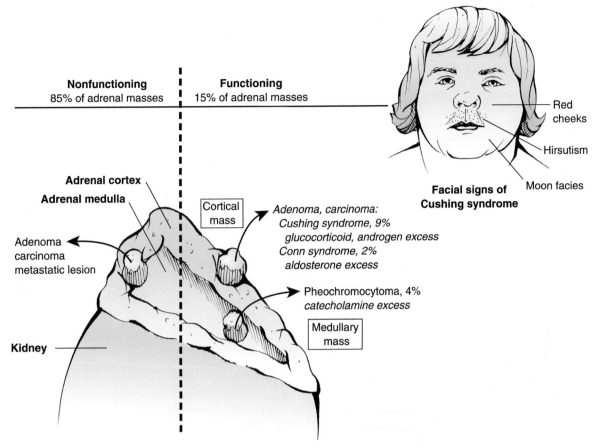

Figure 10.6 Adrenal masses.

(From Bickley, LS and Szilagyi, P. *Bates' guide to physical examination and history taking*, 8th ed. Philadelphia: Lippincott Williams & Wilkins; 2003.)

  CLINICAL BOX

Fine Needle Biopsy

- Differentiates between primary and metastatic adrenal tumors.
- Cannot differentiate between a benign adrenal mass and rare adrenal carcinomas.
- Use has fallen with advances in imaging modalities.
- Indicated if there is suspicion of cancer outside the adrenal gland and in staging of a known cancer.
- Pheochromocytoma should be first ruled out before fine needle biopsy to prevent progression to a hypertensive crisis.

  CLINICAL BOX

Classic Triad of Pheochromocytoma

1. Episodic headaches
2. Sweating
3. Tachycardia

APPROACH

RADIOLOGIC FEATURES OF ADRENAL MASSES

Benign Adenomas
- Round and homogeneous density
- Smooth contour and sharp margination
- Unilateral
- <4 cm
- Low unenhanced CT attenuation values <10 HU

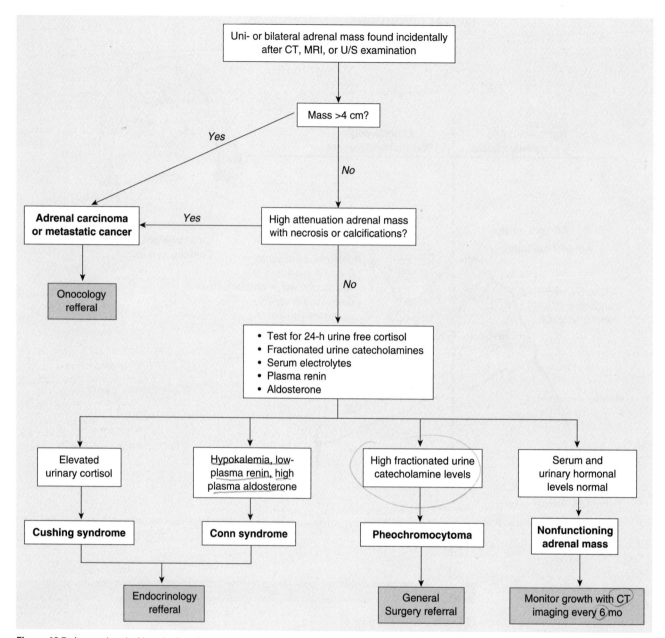

Figure 10.7 Approach to incidental adrenal mass discovery in asymptomatic patient.

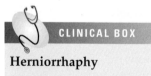

CLINICAL BOX

Herniorrhaphy

Herniorrhaphy is the most common general surgical procedure.

Pheochromocytoma
- Enhanced with intravenous contrast on CT
- Cystic and hemorrhagic changes
- May be bilateral and variable in size

Adrenocortical Carcinoma
- Irregularly shaped and inhomogeneous density
- Central areas of low attenuation due to necrosis
- Calcification observed in 30% of patients
- Unilateral
- >4 cm
- High unenhanced CT attenuation values >10 HU

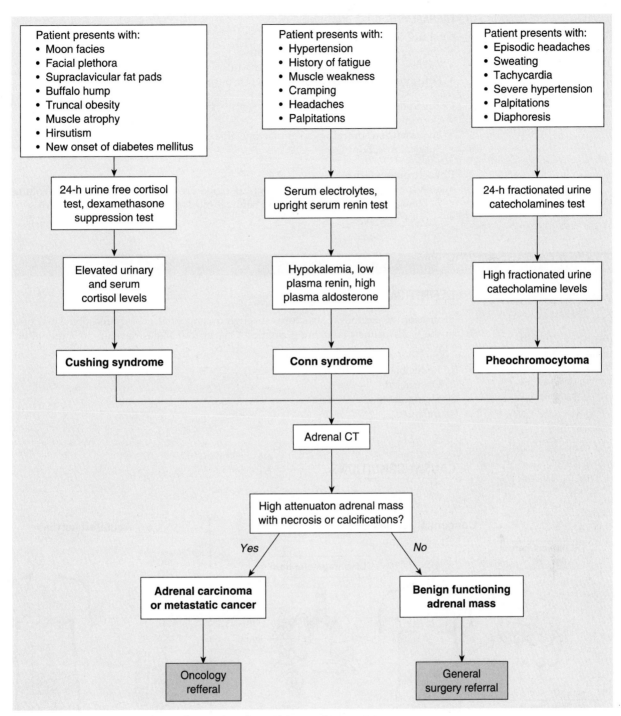

Figure 10.8 Approach to adrenal mass discovery in patient with hormonal excess state.

Adrenal Metastases
- Irregularly shaped and inhomogeneous density
- Larger masses are invasive, irregular, and may present with central necrosis or hemorrhage
- Bilateral
- High unenhanced CT attenuation values >10 HU

MANAGEMENT OF A FUNCTIONING MASS

Cushing Syndrome
- Unilateral adrenalectomy often curative
- Medical treatment if surgery unsuccessful
- Ketoconazole used to control hypercortisolism

Conn Syndrome
- Correction of hypokalemia
- Hypertension control with spirolactone, thiazides, or ACE inhibitors
- Surgical resection

Pheochromocytoma
- α- Adrenergic receptor blocker to control blood pressure and restore plasma volume
- β- Blockers should never be started before α-blockers to avert hypertensive crisis
- Surgical resection

ABDOMINAL MASS – HERNIA

CLINICAL BOX

Common Types of Hernia

Indirect inguinal: Sac lies within the spermatic cord.

Direct inguinal: Sac parallels the spermatic cord.

Femoral hernia: Sac descends through the femoral canal beneath the inguinal ligament.

DEFINITION

Protrusion of peritoneal structures through a congenital or acquired abnormal opening in the walls of their containing cavities. One in four males develop an inguinal hernia. May be:

1. Reducible or irreducible (incarcerated)
2. Obstructed
3. Strangulated
4. Inflamed

CAUSAL CONDITIONS

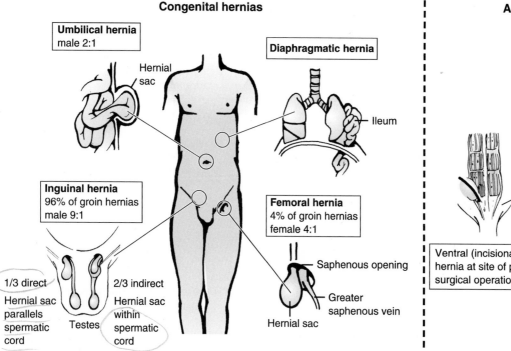

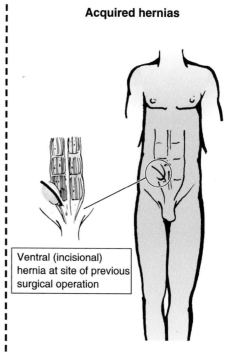

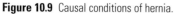

Figure 10.9 Causal conditions of hernia.

Peritoneal Signs

- Guarding
- Rebound tenderness

Hernias in Males

- Indirect inguinal hernias more frequent in males for embryological reasons
- Related to failure of *processus vaginalis* closure in the male embryogenesis

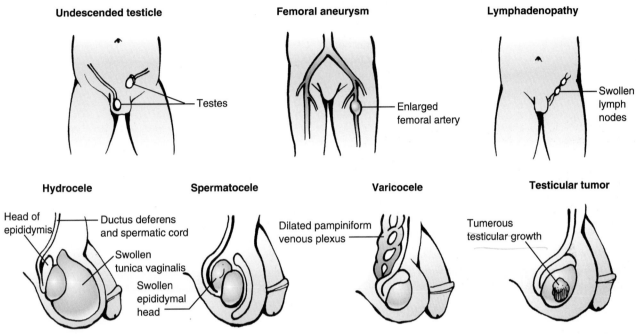

Figure 10.10 Differential diagnosis of a mass in the groin.

APPROACH

MANAGEMENT

1. Asymptomatic reducible hernias treated through open or laparoscopic surgery
2. Irreducible hernias at a high risk for strangulation and must be treated urgently

UNTREATED HERNIAS COMPLICATIONS

1. Incarceration, obstruction, and strangulation
2. Herniation of the female genitalia, pregnancy in a hernial sac
3. Involvement of the hernial sac in disease processes (e.g., carcinoma, peritonitis, acute appendicitis, endometriosis)
4. Rupture of the hernia, spontaneous or traumatic
5. Urinary tract complications, hernia of the bladder, the ureter, and of a urinary ileal conduit
6. Testicular strangulation (infants, adults with large giant inguinoscrotal hernias)

FACTORS AFFECTING POSTOPERATIVE RECURRENCE

Aberrant Collagen States or Metabolic Disorders

1. Ehler–Danlos syndrome
2. Osteogenesis imperfect

Compromised Tissue Healing

1. Malnutrition
2. Compromised or suppressed immunity

Increased Intra-Abdominal Pressure

1. Obesity
2. Ascites

3. Peritoneal dialysis
4. Chronic cough
5. Intraperitoneal mass
6. Organomegaly
7. Pregnancy
8. Constipation
9. Straining on urination
10. Prostatism
11. Lifting heavy weights

Iatrogenic Factors
1. Postoperative infection
2. Failure to repair internal inguinal ring
3. Damage to floor of inguinal canal
4. Use of absorbable sutures
5. Inadequate sac reduction

INVESTIGATIONS

Cough impulse: Patient should stand erect. Coughing results in mass swelling and increase in tension.

Transillumination: Serous-containing enlargements (e.g., hydrocele or spermatocele) will light up brightly.

Herniography: Uncommon, used in investigating hidden hernias.

Ultrasonography. See Figure 10.11.

ACUTE ABDOMINAL PAIN

CLINICAL BOX

Causes of Abdominal Pain in Special Patients

Elderly
• Biliary tract disease
• Malignancy
• Bowel obstruction
• Complications of peptic ulcer disease
• Hernia-related pain

Immunocompromised patients
• Graft-versus-host disease
• Cytomegalovirus infection
• Neutropenic enterocolitis

DEFINITION

Defined as pain <6 h; may be due to:

1. Intra-abdominal inflammation
2. Referred pain
3. Abdominal wall pain

DESCRIBING ABDOMINAL PAIN

• **Colicky:** stretch of hollow muscular organ
• **Constant:** chemical irritation or stretch of a solid organ
• **Referred:** due to neuronal pathways shared by somatic and visceral afferent nerves

CAUSAL CONDITIONS

EXTRA-ABDOMINAL CAUSES
Abdominal Wall
• Rectus muscle hematoma

Genitourinary
• Testicular torsion

Infectious
• Herpes zoster

Metabolic
• Alcoholic ketoacidosis
• Diabetic ketoacidosis
• Porphyria
• Sickle cell disease

Thoracic
• Myocardial infarction
• Pneumonia

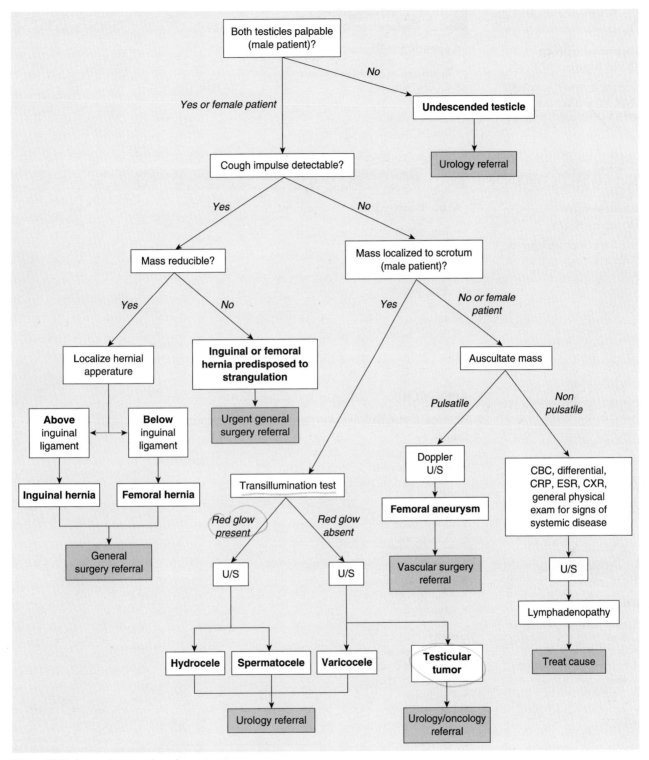

Figure 10.11 Approach to mass in groin.

- Pulmonary embolism (PE)
- Radiculitis

Toxic
- Black widow spider bite
- Heavy metal poisoning
- Methanol poisoning
- Scorpion sting

Ruptured Spleen (Kehr Sign)

Onset of acute pain at the edge of the left shoulder in supine patient with elevated legs.

Appendicitis Signs

- Tenderness along McBurney point
- Rovsing sign
- Psoas sign
- Obturator sign

Cholecystitis (Murphy Sign)

Inspiratory arrest secondary to RUQ costal margin palpation in supine patient.

Acute Pancreatitis Management

- **P**ain control
- **A**rrest shock
- **N**asogastric tube for vomiting
- **C**alcium monitoring
- **R**enal evaluation
- **E**nsure pulmonary function
- **A**ntibiotics
- **S**urgery or special procedures

APPROACH

HYPERCALCEMIA/HYPERPARATHYROIDISM COMPLICATIONS

Stones
- Nephrolithiasis
- Nephrocalcinosis

Bones
- Osteitis fibrosa cystic
- Pseudogout
- Osteoporosis

Moans
- Peptic ulcer disease
- Acute pancreatitis
- Constipation

Groans
- Altered consciousness
- Decreased concentration
- Personality change
- Psychosis
- Depression

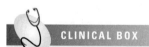

DRE

- Used to assess sphincter tone.
- Can reveal masses in the anorectum or adjacent structures.

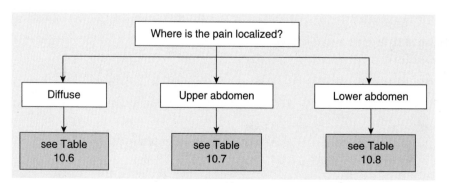

Figure 10.12 Approach to patient with acute abdominal pain.

APPLIED SCIENTIFIC CONCEPTS

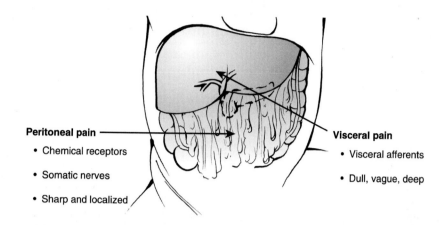

Peritoneal pain
- Chemical receptors
- Somatic nerves
- Sharp and localized

Visceral pain
- Visceral afferents
- Dull, vague, deep

13 Neurologic basis of
pain.

CTAL PAIN

DEFINITION

- Caused by infectious, dermatologic, or anorectal disease
- May require urgent surgical referral

CAUSAL CONDITIONS

ANORECTAL DISEASE

- Abscess (related to IBD)
- Fistula (related to IBD)
- Fissures
- Hemorrhoids
  - Internal hemorrhoid
  - External hemorrhoid
- Chemotherapy
- Neuropathic
- Psychological
- Coccygeal pain
- Other pelvic floor muscle syndromes

DERMATOLOGIC DISEASE

- Psoriasis
- Contact/atopic dermatitis
- Malignancy
- Ulcer

INFECTIONS

- Sexually transmitted diseases (STD)
- Bacterial infections
- Fungal infections
- Parasitic infections

APPROACH

CLINICAL BOX

Anoscopy and Sigmoidoscopy

- Anoscopy: viewing hemorrhoids or potential erosions in the mucosal wall
- Sigmoidoscopy: detecting friability or ulceration within the rectal mucosa

Table **10.6** **Approach to Patient with Diffuse Abdominal Pain**

Condition	Peritoneal Signs?	Clinical Onset	Other Signs	Workup	Management
Abdominal aortic aneurysm	+	Sudden	Tearing abdominal and lumbar pain, pulsating periumbilical mass, hypotension	None	Urgent vascular surgery referral
Perforated viscus		Sudden or gradual Colicky abdominal pain disproportionate to physical findings, Hx of occult blood stool	Syncope or vomiting, shallow thoracic respirations	Abdominal CT	Urgent general surgery referral
Small bowel obstruction		Intermittent, colicky, postprandial	Recurring cramps every 3–10 min, vomiting, crescendo–decrescendo rushes of high-pitched peristalsis sounds coincident with pain onset. Hx of surgery	See Abdominal Distension	
Bacterial peritonitis		Sharp, constant	Pain worsened by movement, presence of ascites, Hx of cirrhosis, fever, altered mental status	Paracentesis of ascetic fluid	Treat cause
Gastroenteritis	−	Diarrhea with cramping pain	Vomiting. Hx of contaminated food or water consumption or travel, poor skin turgor, hyperactive bowel sounds, orthostatic or generalized hypotension	Blood and stool bacterial cultures	
Irritable bowel syndrome		Episodic crampy pain in at least 12 wk, which need not be consecutive in the preceding 12 mo	2/3 of the following: Relieved by defecation, onset associated with changes in stool frequency, onset associated with changes in stool form	None	Education, reassurance, dietary/lifestyle changes. Gastroenterology if condition worsens
Constipation		Sudden or gradual	Hx of infrequent bowel movement <3/wk, difficulty during defecation	See Chapter 9—Adult/Pediatric Constipation	
Ketoacidosis		Gradual Hypertension, ostealgia, easy fatigability, generalized weakness, mild cognitive impairment	Hx of diabetes or alcoholism, tachypnea, tachycardia, orthostatic hypotension, fruity breath	Urinalysis, blood work	Treat cause

+ = present; − = absent.

Table **10.7**   Approach to Patient with Upper Abdominal Pain

Condition	Peritoneal Signs?	Clinical Onset	Other Signs	Workup	Management
Pancreatitis	+	Constant mid-epigastric pain, radiates to left shoulder region and back	N/V, tachycardia, hypotension, hypoxemia, Hx of alcohol abuse, gallstones, medication use	Abdominal U/S, serum enzyme tests	Treat cause
Cholangitis		RUQ pain	Jaundice, chills and fever (Charcot triad), signs of CNS depression		Gastroenterology referral
Cholecystitis		RUQ pain rising over 2–3 min to an intense plateau that is maintained for >20 min, radiates to shoulder or back	Recurrent attacks 1–6 h after meals lasting >12 h, positive Murphy sign		General surgery referral
Appendicitis[a]		Dull ache and tenderness along McBurney point	Anorexia, N/V, guarding, positive Rovsing, psoas, and obturator signs	Abdominal CT	
Peptic ulcer disease/gastritis	−	Burning epigastric pain after eating, relieved by food and antacids	Hx of belching, bloating, abdominal distension, food intolerance, chronic NSAID/aspirin use	CBC, gastroscopy, serology	Treat cause
Acute hepatitis		RUQ pain	Hepatomegaly, jaundice, Hx of anorexia, N/V, fatigue, malaise, arthralgias, myalgias, headache, photophobia, pharyngitis, cough, and/or coryza	Serum aminotransferase levels	
Biliary colic		Progressive aching, cramping epigastric or RUQ pain a few hours after a meal and lasting 0.5–6 h	No signs of systemic disease	Abdominal U/S	Supportive treatment. General surgery referral if condition worsens
Splenic infarct		LUQ pain	N/V, fever, chills, chest pain, positive Kehr sign	Abdominal CT	
Gastroesophageal reflux disease		Epigastric pain	Hx of heartburn, regurgitation of digested food, angina-like chest pain	24-h esophageal pH test	Education, reassurance, dietary/lifestyle changes; general surgery referral if condition worsens
Hepatic abscess		RUQ pain	Fever, chills, nausea, anorexia, and weight loss	Abdominal CT, CBC, serum enzyme tests	General surgery referral
	LUQ pain and tenderness	Fever, splenomegaly. Hx of infection, embolic disease, trauma, malignant hematologic conditions, or immune-suppression			

+ = present; − = absent.
[a]Appendicitis typically presents as diffuse central abdominal pain that later localizes to the RLQ.

Table **10.8**   Approach to Patient with Lower Abdominal Pain

Condition	Peritoneal Signs?	Clinical Onset	Other Signs	Workup
Diverticulitis	+	Persistent LLQ pain	Abdominal distension, N/V, constipation, anorexia, fever	Abdomina
Appendicitis[a]		Dull ache and tenderness along McBurney point	Anorexia, N/V, guarding, positive Rovsing, psoas, and obturator signs	
Incarcerated hernia		Lower abdominal pain	Painful enlargement of previous hernia, abdominal distension, N/V, constipation, anorexia	None
Ectopic pregnancy		Sudden cramping genital pain in pregnant female patient	Vaginal bleeding	Pelvic
Pelvic inflammatory disease/salpingitis		Lower abdominal, bilateral adnexal, and cervical motion tenderness	Temperature >38° C, cervical/vaginal discharge	Pelvi sme
Ovarian torsion		Sudden, severe unilateral lower abdominal pain that worsens intermittently Breast tenderness, N/V, fatigue, abdominal distension	N/V, fever, Hx of recent strenuous physical activity	Pel Do
Mesenteric lymphadenitis	−	Mild RLQ pain	N/V before pain onset, fever, diarrhea, anorexia, current or Hx of URTI	
		Fever, limitation of hip movement, Hx of Crohn disease, or appendicitis		
Inflammatory bowel disease		Crampy RLQ pain	Diarrhea, rectal bleeding, tenesmus, occult blood loss, anemia, weight loss, fever	
Urinary tract infection		Lower abdominal aching pain	Dysuria, urgency, urge incontinence, fever	
Renal colic		Intermittent sudden onset of severe flank pain originating at the costovertebral angle and radiating anteriorly in waves to the groin	N/V	

[a]Appendicitis typically presents as diffuse central abdominal pain that later localizes to the RLQ.

Figure 10 abdominal

ANOR

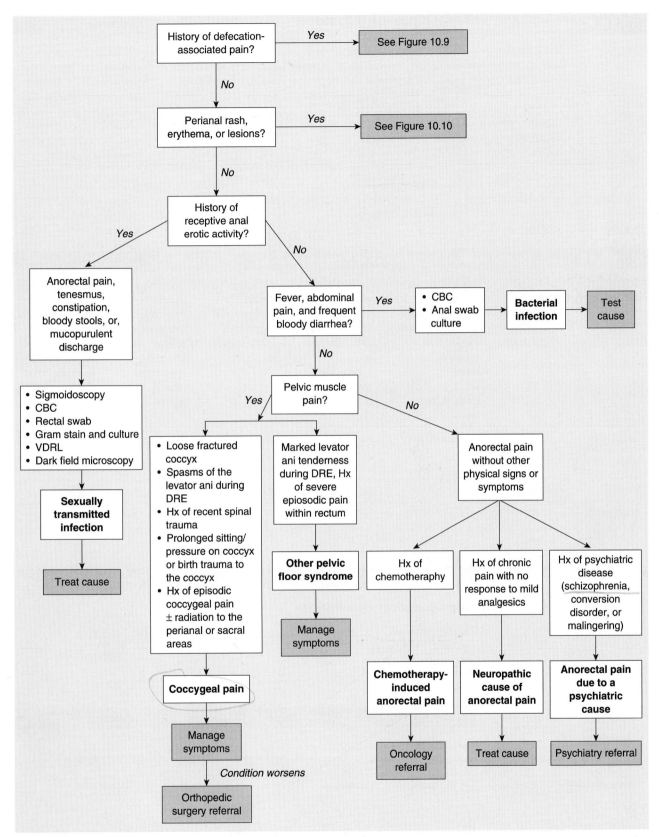

Figure 10.14 Approach to patient with anorectal pain.

Table **10.9**	Approach to Patient with Defecation-Associated Pain			
Description	One or more para-anal openings, palpable cord-like para-anal tract, Hx of previous abscesses, intermittent or constant purulent or serous anginous discharge from para-anal opening	Tender anorectal mass, fever, DRE reveals a tender fluctuant mass on rectal wall, Hx of continuous deep seated pain and rectal discomfort that worsens with ambulation or straining	Anal canal tear along posterior or anterior midline, bleeding, hypertrophic papillae, skin tags, Hx of hard, large, painful stools, "knife-like" pain lasting up to several hours post defecation	Painful, bluish perianal swellings, skin tags, sensation of incomplete defecation, pruritus, bloody stools, or prolapsed mass. Hx of pregnancy, constipation, or portal hypertension; anoscopy shows anal swellings
Diagnosis	Anorectal fistula	Anorectal abscess	Anal fissures	External hemorrhoids
Management	General surgery referral	Urgent general surgery referral	Manage symptoms	Manage symptoms

Table **10.10**	Approach to Patient with Perianal Rash, Erythema, or Lesions					
Clinical presentation	Sharply demarcated inflamed, bright red pruritic perianal lesions	Papulovesicles with surrounding erythema, weeping and crusted lesions, Hx suggestive of chronic contact with potentially allergic agents (eg., latex condoms, sanitary wipes)	Generalized xerosis, erythematous, lichenified, pruritic patches and papules; Hx of asthma, allergic rhinoconjunctivitis	Single of multiple papillary eruptions, Hx of receptive anal activity, immuno-suppression	Ulcerating anal or perianal lesion, Hx of bleeding, HPV infection, receptive anal intercourse, or cancer (especially cervical, vulvar, or vaginal)	Symmetric sharply demarcated erythematous rash, Hx of recurrent anal pruritis and rash, contact sport participation
Investigation		Closed patch test	Antibody serology	Acetowhitening test, anoscopy	Malignancy	Potassium hydroxide wet mount of scales
Diagnosis	Psoriasis	Contact dermatitis	Atopic dermatitis	HPV	Malignancy	Fungal Infection
Management		See Chapter 4—Skin Rash: Papules			Oncology referral	Treat cause

Infectious Agents

Sexually transmitted
- *N. gonorrhoeae*
- *C. trachomatis*
- HSV
- Syphilis

Bacteria
- *Salmonella*
- *C. difficile*
- *Shigella*
- *Campylobacter*

Fungi
- *Tinea* (ringworm)

Parasites
- *E. vermicularis* (pinworm)

Management of Hemorrhoids
- Oral fiber intake, stool softeners, or supplements
- Toilet retraining
- Treatment of underlying disease

Sitz Bath
- Patient sits in bath and the buttocks and hips are covered with warm water
- For management of hemorrhoid pain

CHAPTER 11

Hematology

Surabhi Rawal, Dr. Sapna Rawal, and Dr. Ahmed Galal

SPLENOMEGALY

CLINICAL BOX

Major Causes of Splenomegaly

ICE MASS:

Infectious

Congestive splenomegaly/
Chronic liver disease

Extramedullar hematopoiesis

Malignancy

Amyloidosis

Sarcoidosis, **S**torage disease

RATIONALE

Splenomegaly is usually suggestive of an underlying disorder, rather than a 1° splenic pathology. Therefore, Rx is aimed at the underlying etiology.

CAUSAL CONDITIONS

Table **11.1**	Causal Conditions of Splenomegaly	
Demand for ↑ splenic function	Clearance of abnormal RBCs	• Abnormalities of RBC shape (hereditary spherocytosis/elliptocytosis) • Hemoglobinopathies (thalassemias) • Nutritional anemias
	Infection	• Acute (infectious mononucleosis, hepatitis, SBE) • Chronic (TB, AIDS, malaria, brucellosis, syphilis) • Bacterial septicemia • Splenic abscess
	Autoimmune	• RA (Felty syndrome) • SLE • Collagen vascular diseases • Drug reactions
	Extramedullary hematopoiesis	• Myelofibrosis • Marrow toxicity (chemotherapeutic agents, radiotherapy) • Marrow infiltration (solid tumors, leukemia, storage diseases)
Altered splenic circulation		• Cirrhosis • Portal vein obstruction • Splenic vein obstruction • CHF
Splenic infiltration		• Storage diseases (Niemann-Pick, Gaucher, nonlipoid) • Amyloidosis • Malignancy (leukemias, lymphomas, metastases) • Splenic cysts • Myeloproliferative disorders

APPROACH

See Figure 11.1.

CLINICAL BOX

Hypersplenism

- Cytopenia 2° to splenomegaly of most etiologies
- Key features are splenomegaly, hyperplastic bone marrow, modest pancytopenia
- Occasional RBC spherocytosis, typically reticulocytosis
- Treat underlying disease

- Avoid splenectomy when possible to avoid risk of OPSI
- If necessary administer vaccines versus *Strep pneumo*, *HiB*, *N. meningitidis*, and annual influenza vaccine and prophylactic Abx Tx

CLINICAL BOX

Dx of Splenomegaly on Exam

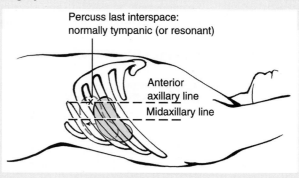

Percuss last interspace: normally tympanic (or resonant)

Anterior axillary line
Midaxillary line

Castell method: If the spleen is normal, percussion in the lowest intercostal space (eighth to ninth) in the left anterior axillary line of the supine patient elicits a resonant note throughout the respiratory cycle. If percussion on full inspiration produces a dull note (Castell sign), this is suggestive of splenic enlargement.

BLEEDING TENDENCY/BRUISING

RATIONALE

Bleeding that is spontaneous or excessive/delayed in relation to the inciting trauma must be examined for underlying pathology.

APPLIED SCIENTIFIC CAUSES

See Figure 11.2.

CAUSAL CONDITIONS

The clinical history should consider likely etiologies:

1. Personal history of bleeding diathesis
2. Family history of bleeding diathesis
3. Medication use

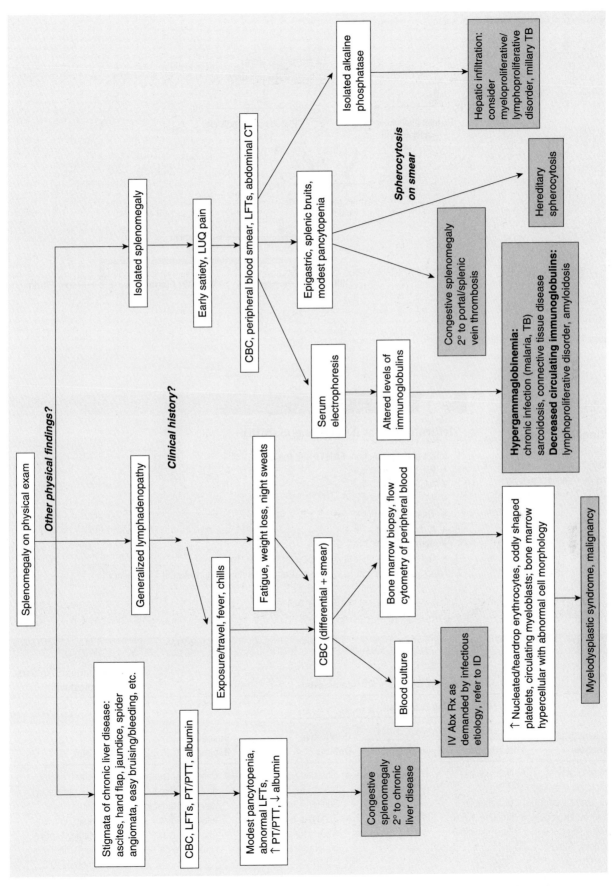

Figure 11.1 Approach to splenomegaly.

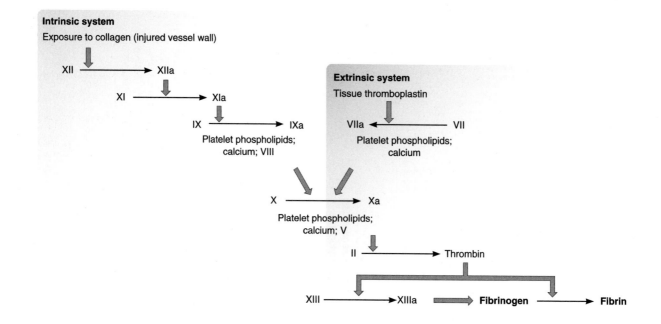

Figure 11.2 Coagulation cascade.

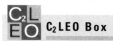 **C₂LEO Box**

Reporting Child Abuse
Children with extensive bruises may represent child abuse and there may be a requirement for reporting.

CLINICAL BOX

Medications that Affect Coagulability

1. Affect platelet function: **FANTAS**tic **Q**ueen
   - **F**olate antagonists
   - **A**SA
   - **N**SAIDs
   - **T**hiazide diuretics
   - **A**lcohol abuse
   - **S**ulfa/β-lactam Abx
   - **Q**uinidine
2. Affect coagulation pathway: Abx that affect gut flora and induce Vit K deficiency

Table 11.2 Causal Conditions of Bruising and Bleeding

	Purpuric Disorders (1° Hemostasis)					Coagulation Disorders (2° Hemostasis)
	Platelet Plug Formation					
	Quantitative Defects			Qualitative Defects	Vascular Response	Fibrin Clot
↓ Production	↑ Destruction	Splenomegaly				
• ↓ Megakaryopoesis (aplastic anemia, toxic, displacement) • Ineffective megakaryopoesis (B₁₂/folate deficiency, folate antagonist)	• Nonimmune (TTP/HUS, DIC, infection) • Immune (ITP, SLE, quinidine)	• ↑ Sequestration	• Inherited (von Willebrand, Bernard Soulier, Glanzmann • Acquired (uremia, ASA, NSAIDs, antiplatelet agents)	• Congenital (collagen disease, hereditary hemorrhagic telangiectasia) • Acquired (vasculitis, steroids)	• Inherited (factor VIII, IX deficiency) • Acquired (liver disease, Vit K deficiency, anticoagulants, inhibitors) • Fibrinolysis (DIC, inhibitors)

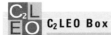
C₂LEO Box

Prenatal Dx and Counseling

- Counseling on prenatal Dx of sickle cell disease and thalassemia should be nondirective and not restricted to those willing to have an abortion.
- Reproductive decisions must not be forced by the results of tests.
- Because the only pragmatic options for mothers are abortion or no children, it is vital that women not be pressured into prenatal Dx.

APPROACH

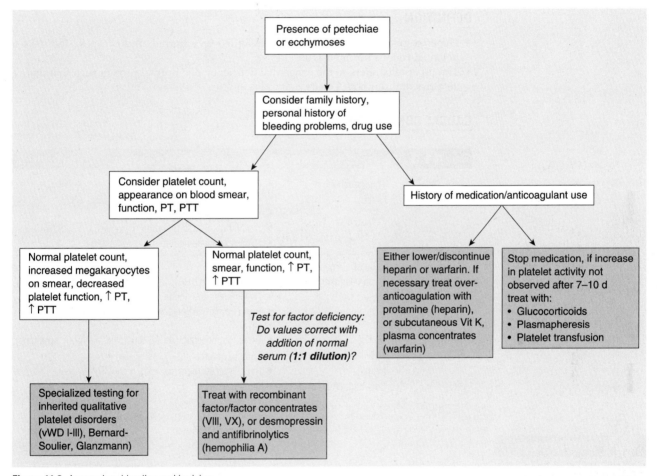

Figure 11.3 Approach to bleeding and bruising.

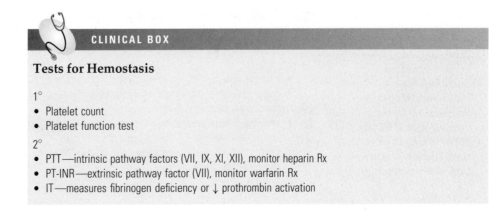

CLINICAL BOX

Tests for Hemostasis

1°
- Platelet count
- Platelet function test

2°
- PTT—intrinsic pathway factors (VII, IX, XI, XII), monitor heparin Rx
- PT-INR—extrinsic pathway factor (VII), monitor warfarin Rx
- IT—measures fibrinogen deficiency or ↓ prothrombin activation

PTT 1:1 Dilution

If PTT corrects with 1:1 dilution = absolute deficiency in factor level

If PTT remains high = factor inhibitor present

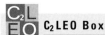

C₂LEO Box

Blood Transfusion Refusal

In patients who are bleeding but refuse blood transfusion, it must be determined whether the decision can be justified within the context of a relatively stable set of values. If a coherent and consistent justification does not exist, identify a substitute decision maker.

HYPERCOAGULABLE STATE

DEFINITION

- Hypercoagulable conditions may be inherited or acquired, and can pose the risks of potential venous thrombosis and PE.
- Thrombophilia refers to the congenital deficiency of a normal protein such that there is an ↑ risk of thrombotic events.

CAUSAL CONDITIONS

Table **11.3**	Causal Condition for Hypercoagulable State	
Inherited	Thrombophilia (<50-yr old)	• Antithrombin deficiency • Protein C, S deficiency • Factor V Leiden (APC resistance) • Prothrombin 20210 mutation • Hyperhomocysteinemia
Acquired disorders /risk factors	Cellular elements (hypercoagulability)	• Malignancy • Pregnancy, OTC, HRT, tamoxifen • Hyperhomocysteinemia • Hyperviscosity (Waldenström, multiple myeloma, PCV) • HIT • Other (antiphospholipid Ab syndrome, nephrotic syndrome)
	Vascular endothelium (injury)	• Surgery, trauma • Hyperhomocysteinemia
	Circulatory (hemostasis)	• Surgery, trauma • Pregnancy • Immobilization • CHF, atrial fibrillation

CLINICAL BOX

HIT with Subsequent Thrombosis

- Patient has Ab against the PF4–heparin complex.
- Leads to ↓ in platelet count (<150,000/mm³ or <50% of baseline) and a 30-fold ↑ in risk of thrombosis.
- Discontinue heparin—cannot replace with LMWH (cross-reactivity), warfarin (skin necrosis), ASA, or IVC filter.
- Instead, switch to either direct thrombin inhibitors or heparinoid anticoagulation.

APPROACH

CLINICAL BOX

Clinical Screening Tests for Thrombosis

1. Initial tests
   - Inherited defects: APC resistance (factor V Leiden), prothrombin 20210 mutation, factor VIII level
   - Acquired defects/risk factors: antiphospholipid Ab (lupus anticoagulant, anticardiolipin Ab)
2. Postrecovery testing
   - Inherited defects: antithrombin activity, protein C activity, protein S activity, free and total levels (varies with levels of C4 binding protein)
   - Cannot be performed during acute event because levels fluctuate with active thrombosis and are suppressed by warfarin Rx.

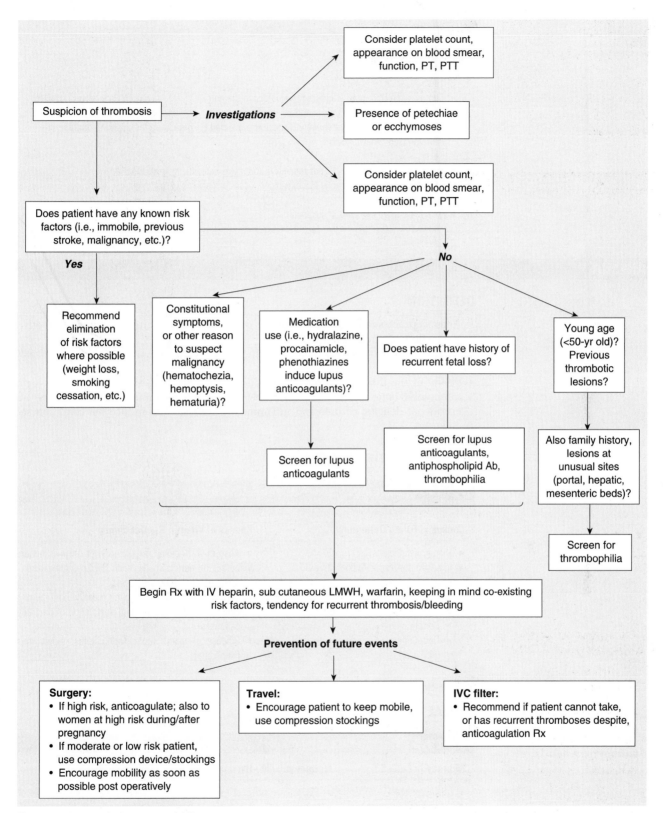

Figure 11.4 Approach to hypercoagulability states.

CLINICAL BOX

Diagnostic Testing

1. 1° Tests
- Compression U/S: gold standard in veins above the calf
- Pulmonary angiography: gold standard for PR
- Spiral CT: becoming more commonly used in suspected CT but cannot be used in patients with compromised renal function

2. 2° Tests
- Contrast venography: if U/S not feasible/informative but difficult for patient
- MRI: accurate as venography but expensive, used for patients with pregnancy, poor renal function, or contrast agent allergy
- V/Q scan: routinely used in suspected PE

ANEMIA

DEFINITION

- Anemic processes reduce the number of circulating erythrocytes, either through ↓ production or ↑ destruction.
- Anemias are usually classified according to MCV, which is an assessment of RBC size.
- In any of the three categories (microcytic, macrocytic, and normocytic), 1° etiologies can involve bone marrow and erythrocyte abnormalities, immunologic disorders, and nutritional deficits; chronic and inflammatory diseases can induce the condition secondarily.

APPLIED SCIENTIFIC CONCEPTS

Table **11.4** Megaloblastic Anemia—Caused by Vitamin B_{12} or Folate Deficiency	
Causes of Folate Deficiency	**Causes of Vitamin B_{12} Deficiency**

• Dietary insufficiency
• Impaired absorption (inflammation/resection)
• Systemic causes:
  • ↑ Consumption due to pregnancy
  • Certain medications
  • Certain medical conditions (i.e., psoriasis)
	• Absorption depends on secretion of intrinsic factor by gastric parietal cells; if Vit B_{12} compound taken up in terminal ileum
	• Impaired parietal cell function (gastrectomy, pernicious anemia—autoimmune destruction of parietal cell mass
	• Disease of distal ileum (Crohn ileitis, tapeworm, lymphoma)

CLINICAL BOX

Principal Causes of Microcytic Anemia: TAILS

- **T**halassemia
- **A**nemia of chronic disease/inflammation
- **I**ron-deficiency anemia
- **L**ead toxicity-associated anemia
- **S**ideroblastic anemia

CAUSAL CONDITIONS

Table **11.5** Causal Conditions of Anemia		
Microcytic (<80 fL)	**Normocytic (80–100 fL)**	**Macrocytic (>100 fL)**
• Thalassemias • Anemia of chronic disease/inflammation • Iron deficiency • Lead toxicity-associated anemia • Sideroblastic anemia	• EPO deficiency (renal insufficiency, anti-EPO Ab) • Bone marrow aplasia/hypoplasia (1°, 2° from drugs, toxins, infections, radiation) • Myelofibrosis • Myelophthisis	• Megaloblastic (Vit B_{12}, folate deficiency) • Nonmegaloblastic (drugs—chemotherapeutic, immunosuppressive)

APPROACH

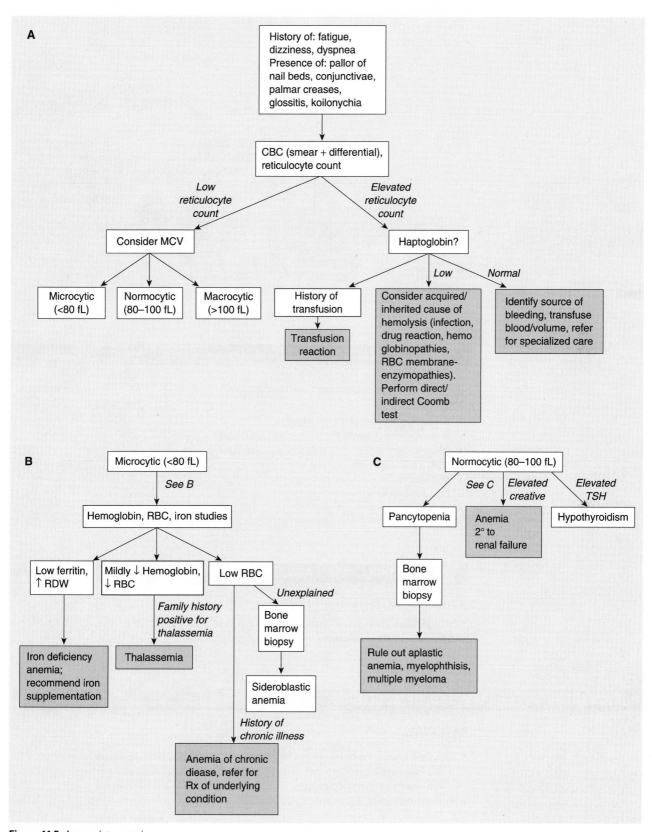

Figure 11.5 Approach to anemia.

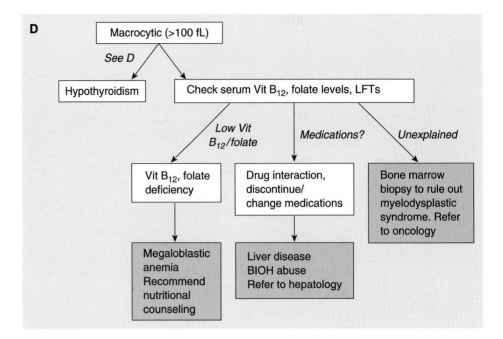

Figure 11.5 (*Continued*).

CLINICAL BOX

Drugs that can induce megaloblastic anemia (depress/affect metabolism of Vit B_{12} or folate): **PAM ASA MOM**

- **P**yrimidine analogs (5-FU, zidovudine)
- **A**nticonvulsants (phenytoin, phenobarbital, primidone)
- 6-**M**ercaptopurine and other purine analogs (acyclovir)
- **ASA**
- **M**ethotrexate
- **O**ral contraceptives
- **M**etformin

CLINICAL BOX

Confirm Baseline Levels of B_{12}

Do not administer folic acid without confirming Vit B_{12} levels; normalized folate will resolve the anemia and mask Vit B_{12} deficiency, allowing hemopathy to progress.

POLYCYTHEMIA VERA/ELEVATED HEMOGLOBIN

RATIONALE

- Elevated hemoglobin levels (>185 g/L [men], >165 g/L [women]) can be attributed to:
  - PCV, a myeloproliferative disorder with clonal expansion of erythroid, myelocytic, and megakaryocytic lineages
  - Erythrocytosis, 2° to underlying systemic processes

APPLIED SCIENTIFIC CONCEPTS

- Hemoglobin and hematocrit **measure the ratio of RBC mass to plasma volume**; therefore, they are sensitive to changes in either one.
- Determination of polycythemia **must be based on direct assessment of RBC mass and plasma volume**. "True" polycythemia involves an absolute ↑ of RBC mass, whereas "relative" polycythemia (Gaisböck) is a ↓ in volume.
- Erythropoiesis begins with a pluripotent hematopoietic stem cell and follows a hierarchic process of lineage commitment and differentiation.

CAUSAL CONDITIONS

Table **11.6** Causal Conditions of PCV		
True Polycythemia		
Appropriate ↑ EPO (2° Erythrocytosis)	**Inappropriate ↑ EPO**	**Relative Polycythemia**
• Hypoxemia (living at high altitude, COPD, congenital cardiac anomalies) • Hemoglobinopathies (with an ↑ affinity for O_2)	• PCV • Renal pathology (renal artery stenosis) • Malignancy (renal cell, hepatocellular, ovarian, uterine tumors) • Cerebral hemangioma • ↑ Carboxyhemoglobin (chronic smoking, exposure to carbon monoxide)	• ↓ Plasma volume (burns, diarrhea) • Stress (Gaisböck)

CLINICAL BOX

Characteristics of PCV

60 Jewish men HATE BIG Spleens

- **60** (median age of Dx)
- **Jewish men** (slight predominance)
- **H**eadache (2° to ↓ cerebral circulation)
- **A**bdominal discomfort
- **T**ired (↑ risk of TIA)

- ↓ **E**xercise tolerance and ↑ **E**pistaxis
- **B**lurred vision and ↑ **B**lood viscosity
- **I**tchy (pruritus 2° to histamine release)
- **G**outy arthritis and **G**I bleeding
- **BIG Spleens** (splenomegaly)

CLINICAL BOX

Criteria for PCV

Requires three major criteria or first two major and any two minor criteria.

Major
1. ↑ RBC mass (≥36 mL/kg [♂], ≥32 mL/kg [♀])
2. Normal SaO_2 (≥92%)
3. Splenomegaly

Minor
1. ↑ Platelets (>400,000/μL)
2. ↑ WBC (>12,000/μL)
3. ↑ Leukocyte alkaline phosphatase
4. ↑ Vit B_{12}

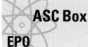

ASC Box

EPO

Stimulation: ↓ in oxygenation of blood

Production: peritubular kidney cells

Action: bone marrow, ↑ RBC production

APPROACH

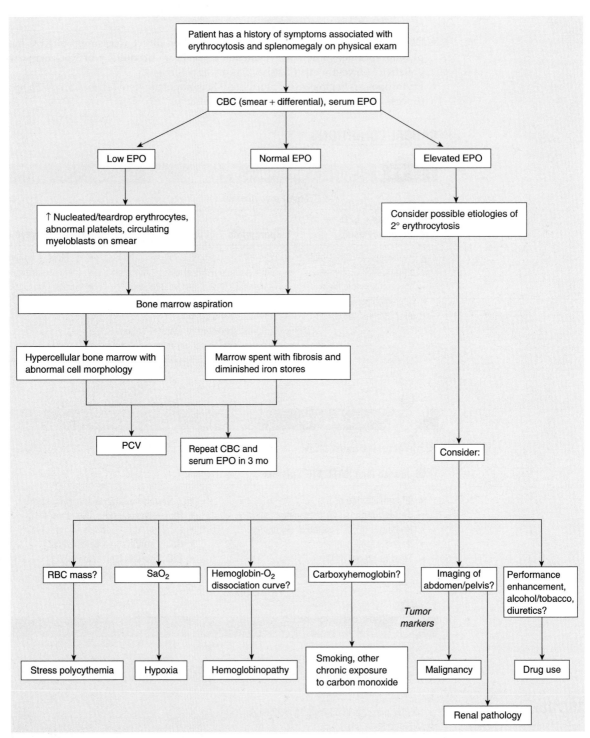

Figure 11.6 Approach to PCV.

LYMPHADENOPATHY

DEFINITION

- The normal immune response promotes lymph node enlargement, through the proliferation of its cellular elements.
- Except for the inguinal nodes, diameters >1 cm are considered abnormal.

• The location of the enlarged node is helpful in localizing the site of foreign antigen invasion; generalized lymphadenopathy suggests systemic involvement.

ADVANCED SCIENTIFIC CONCEPTS

• Lymphatic system consists of lymph nodes and vessels as well as the thymus, spleen, and Peyer patches in the gut.

For a simplified schematic of immune system, see Figure 15.10.

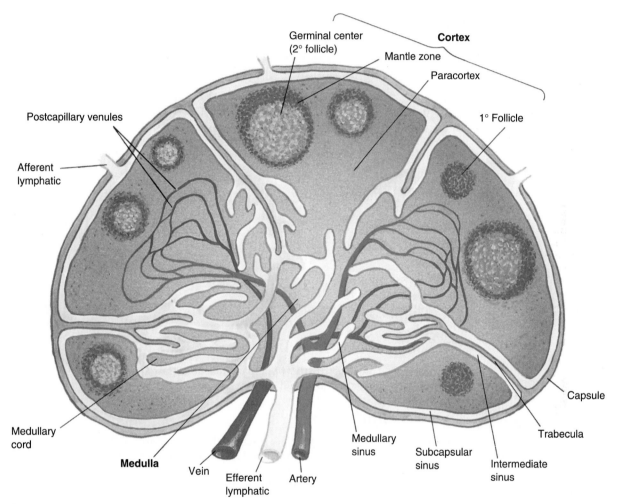

Figure 11.7 Anatomy of a normal lymph node. (Image from Rubin E, Farber JL. *Pathology*, 3rd ed. Philadelphia: Lippincott Williams & Wilkins; 1999.)

CAUSAL CONDITIONS

CLINICAL BOX

Most Common Etiologies of Lymphadenopathy

U MIND?

• **U**nexplained
• **M**etastatic carcinoma/sarcoma
• **I**mmune system malignancies (leukemia, lymphoma) and **I**nflammatory conditions (collage diseases, vasculitides, amyloidosis, sarcoidosis)
• **N**eoplasms (all other tumors)
• **D**rainage of local infection or **D**isseminated infection

Table **11.7**	**Causal Conditions of Lymphadenopathy**
Endo	• Thyroid pathology (inflammation, hyperthyroidism) • Adrenal insufficiency
Infectious	• Viral (EBV, CMV, hepatitis, HIV) • Bacterial (pyogenic bacteria, syphilis, TB) • Fungal (histoplasmosis) • Parasitic (toxoplasmosis)
Immune/inflammation	• Collagen diseases (RA, SLE, Kawasaki, Sjögren) • Serum sickness • Drug reactions (phenytoin, allopurinol) • Sarcoidosis • Amyloidosis
Hematologic malignancy	• Leukemia (AML/CML, ALL/CLL) • Lymphoma (non–Hodgkin) • Hemoglobinopathies (Waldenström, multiple myeloma)
Other malignancy	• Breast/lung carcinoma • Kaposi sarcoma • Head/neck CA
Storage diseases	• Gaucher, Niemann-Pick

APPROACH

See Figure 11.8.

FEVER IN THE IMMUNE COMPROMISED HOST/RECURRENT FEVER

DEFINITION

Compromised immunity ↑ susceptibility to infection. The etiology and severity of immuno-suppression predispose to certain types of causative organism and particular sites.

APPLIED SCIENTIFIC CONCEPTS

- Thermoregulation is centrally regulated in the preoptic area of the hypothalamus, which stimulates various heat-retention and dissipation responses to maintain a thermal set point.
  - Pyrogenic cytokines released by mononuclear phagocytes have the capacity to raise this set point.
- RES includes the spleen, lymph nodes, liver, marrow, and lung in its tissue component and macrophages and monocytes in its cellular component.
- Spleen has two components:
  - White pulp produces lymphocytes.
  - Red pulp filters blood and contains phagocytes that ingest/phagocytose circulating microorganisms and eliminates senescent RBCs.

CAUSAL CONDITIONS

CLINICAL BOX

Typical Infectious Organisms in CMI Defects versus Asplenia/ Hypogammaglobinemia

CMI defects: predispose to infection with intracellular pathogens

- Bacteria (*L. monocytogenes, Salmonella* spp., *Legionella* spp., and mycobacterial spp.)
- Fungal (*C. neoformans, Candida* spp., *P. jirovecii/carinii*)
- Parasitic (*T. gondii*)
- Viral (varicella-zoster, HSV, CMV)

Hypogammaglobinemia and asplenia predispose to infection with encapsulated bacteria: *Strep pneumo, H. influenza, N. meningitidis*

ASC Box

Complement and Immune Dysfunction

Normally involved in inducing inflammation, leukocytosis; protective against viruses, improves bacterial opsonization, produces bacterial cell wall/membrane lysis.

Inherited complement deficiencies: predispose to frequent and recurrent infections with encapsulated bacteria

Acquired complement deficiencies: can develop with rheumatologic disorders (SLE)

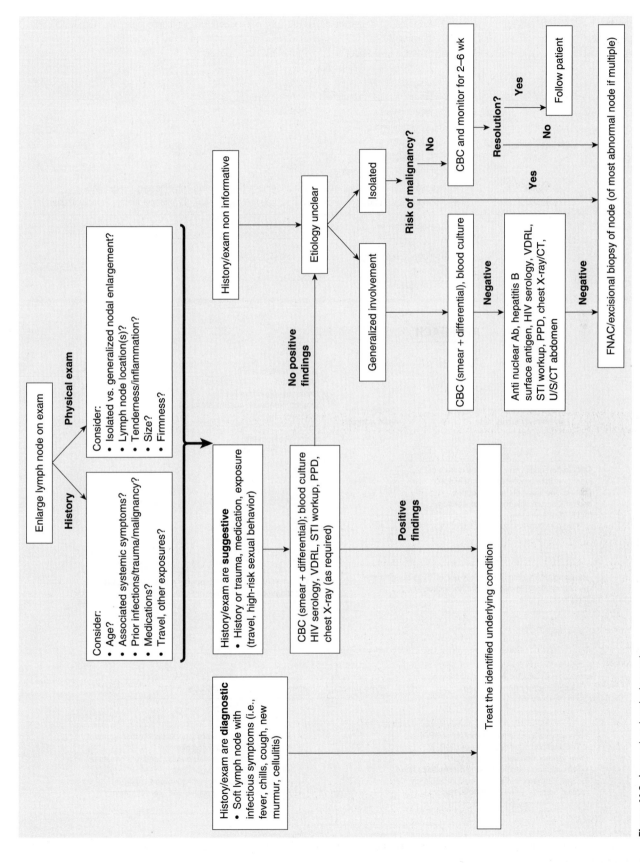

Figure 11.8 Approach to lymphadenopathy.

Table **11.8**   **Causal Conditions of Fever in the Immunocompromised Host**

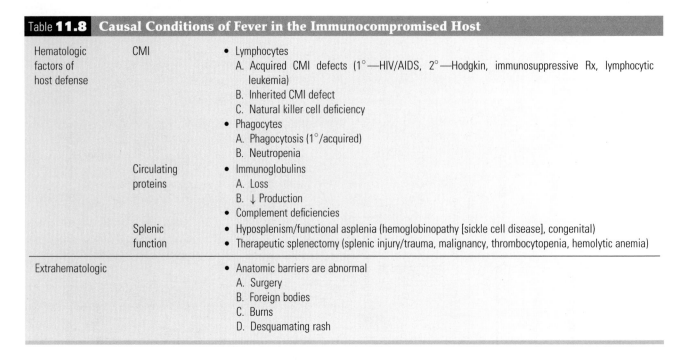

Hematologic factors of host defense	CMI	• Lymphocytes
		  A. Acquired CMI defects (1°—HIV/AIDS, 2°—Hodgkin, immunosuppressive Rx, lymphocytic leukemia)
		  B. Inherited CMI defect
		  C. Natural killer cell deficiency
		• Phagocytes
		  A. Phagocytosis (1°/acquired)
		  B. Neutropenia

	Circulating proteins	• Immunoglobulins
		  A. Loss
		  B. ↓ Production
		• Complement deficiencies

	Splenic function	• Hyposplenism/functional asplenia (hemoglobinopathy [sickle cell disease], congenital) • Therapeutic splenectomy (splenic injury/trauma, malignancy, thrombocytopenia, hemolytic anemia)

Extrahematologic		• Anatomic barriers are abnormal
		  A. Surgery
		  B. Foreign bodies
		  C. Burns
		  D. Desquamating rash

APPROACH

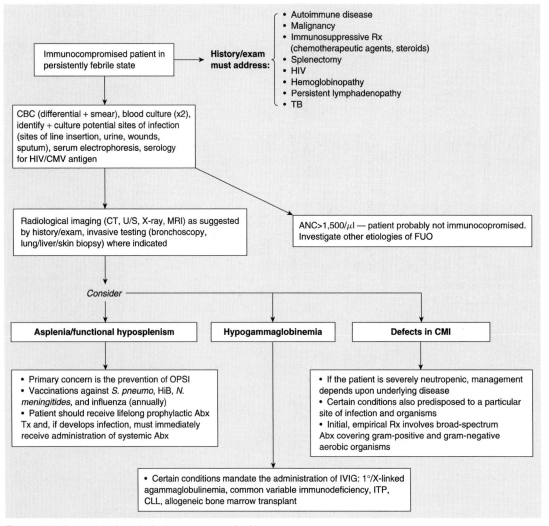

Figure 11.9 Approach to fever in the immunocompromised host.

Table **11.9**	Classical Findings in Neutropenic Patients and Their Associated Pathogens
Physical Exam	
Oral mucositis	Viridans streptococci, HSV, Candida spp.
Black eschar	Aspergillus, mucor
Necrotizing skin lesions	*P. aeruginosa*, aspergillus
Subcutaneous nodules (nontender)	Nocardia, cryptococcus
Skin papules (nontender)	Candida
RLQ abdominal tenderness (+/−) pan, distention, bloody diarrhea)	Typhlitis (neutropenic enterocolitis) 2° to pseudomonas, *E. coli*, Clostridium spp.
Perineal tenderness	Gram-negative bacilli, anaerobes
Inflammation/pain at IV, catheter site	Coagulase negative staph, corynebacterium, Bacillus spp.
Chest radiography	
Localized infiltrate	Bacterial/mycobacterial pathogens
Nodular infiltrate	Nocardia, filamentous fungi
Cavitary lesions	Aspergillus
Diffuse interstitial infiltrate	*P. jirovecii*, viral pathogen
Fever	
Fever persists after 1 wk of antimicrobial Rx	Filamentous fungal infection
Fever persists after resolution of neutropenia	Hepatosplenic candidiasis

ASC Box

T Cells

- 1° Mediators of CMI
- Ab production requires intact T-cell number and function (stimulation of B-cell proliferation by IL-2)

ASC Box

Humoral Immunity

Measurement of specific Ab titers indicates infection with specific pathogens and level of function of the humoral immune system.

FEVER OF UNKNOWN ORIGIN

CLINICAL BOX

Classes of Drugs Associated with Fever

- Antimicrobials
- Anticonvulsants
- Antihistamines
- Cardiovascular drugs
- H2 blockers
- Herbal remedies
- Iodides
- NSAIDs
- Phenothiazines
- Salicylates

See also Chapter 18.

DEFINITION

- Documented 3 or more wk without Dx after 1 wk of investigation
- Fever is a feature of not only most infectious conditions but also a feature of noninfectious processes.

APPLIED SCIENTIFIC CONCEPTS

- Fever: body temperature ($\geq 38.3°$C)
- Hyperpyrexia: excessive fever ($>41.5°$C) caused by ↑ in body's thermal set point Hyperthermia: ↑ in body temperature beyond the body's thermal set point
- Exogenous pyrogens: substances (notably microbial cell wall components, LPS) that induce the formation of endogenous pyrogens from host cells (primarily macrophages)
- Pyrogenic cytokines: cytokines (primarily IL-6) that act on the preoptic hypothalamus to ↑ body temperature by releasing PGE_2
- Antipyretics inhibit synthesis of PGE_2
  - Corticosteroids inhibit phospholipase A_2
  - ASA, NSAIDs inhibit cyclooxygenase

CLINICAL BOX

Avoid Pharmacological Dx

Using response to medication as a means to establish Dx is discouraged:

- Illness may temporarily respond to corticosteroids, but eventually worsens due to induced immunosuppression.
- Abx use is often unspecific and impedes Dx of many infectious processes.

CAUSAL CONDITIONS

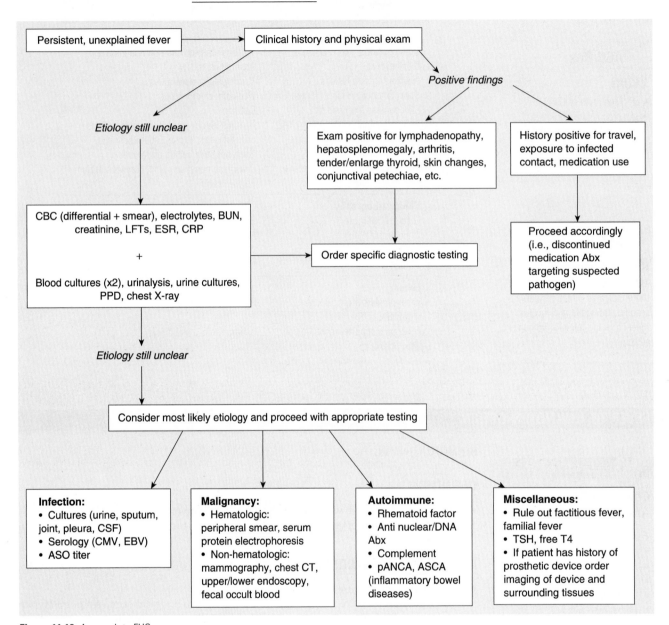

Figure 11.10 Approach to FUO.

Table **11.10**	Causal Conditions by Etiology for FUO
Infection	• Upper/lower respiratory tract infection • Abdominal abscess (hepatic, splenic, intestinal, renal) • SBE, TB, bacteremia, travel/HIV-associated infections • Osteomyelitis • Meningitis, cerebritis
Inflammatory/ autoimmune	• RA • IBD • Collagen vascular disease (SLE, vasculitis), granulomatous disease (sarcoidosis, temporal arteritis) • Thyroiditis • Glomerulonephritis
Malignancy	• Leukemia, lymphoma • 1° Tumors in colon, pancreas; hepatoma, renal cell CA • Metastases
Miscellaneous	• DVT, PE • Drug induced • Complications of hepatic disease (cirrhosis, hepatitis) • Hyperthyroid • Familial mediterranean fever • Factitious

WHITE BLOOD CELL ABNORMALITIES

DEFINITION

- **Neutropenia** (ANC <1,500/μL): Defects in neutrophils (PMNLs) may be due to 1° or underlying pathology, or 2° to medication use, and lead to compromised immunity.
- **Neutrophilia** (ANC >7,700/μL]: Common etiologies include infection (leading to ↑ production, release), and benign reactive neutrophilia, 2° to epinephrine release, common with vigorous exercise and stress (↑ demargination).

CLINICAL BOX

Extramedullary Hematopoiesis

Characteristic signs on blood smear: **My Pro TSN-rbc**
- **My**elocytes
- **Pro**myelocytes
- **T**ear-drop **S**haped and **N**ucleated **r**ed **b**lood **c**ells

Extensive extramedullary hematopoiesis can cause **A-SHOPS**
- **A**scites
- **S**pinal cord compression
- **H**ypertension (intracranial, pulmonary, portal)
- **O**bstruction (intestinal, ureteric)
- **P**ericardial tamponade
- **S**kin nodules

APPLIED SCIENTIFIC CONCEPTS

- Neutrophils are derived from a common progenitor that also gives rise to erythrocytes, megakaryocytes, eosinophils, basophils, and monocytes.
  - Proliferation of the common progenitor is stimulated by IL-3 and GM-CSF.
  - Later differentiation is regulated by granulocyte colony-stimulating factor.

- Production of granulocytes involves movement from marrow to blood to tissue.
  - The peripheral neutrophil count reflects equilibrium between several compartments.
  - WBC count and differential measures only neutrophils in the circulating pool during their brief 3- to 6-h period of transit from the bone marrow to tissue.
- PMN granules contain toxic substances.
- Neutrophils migrate to sites of infection or inflammation via paracellular and transcellular routes through endothelial cell layers.

CAUSAL CONDITIONS

ASC Box

Leukemoid Reaction

- Persistent neutrophilia with WBC counts from 30,000 to 50,000/μL, circulating neutrophils tend to be mature and not clonally derived (contrast with leukemia)
- Most frequently associated with septicemia and severe bacterial infections, including shigellosis, salmonellosis, meningococcemia
- If 12% of all cells are immature, then it is known as **left shift** and indicates a rapid release of cells from bone marrow
- May see ↑ in band forms and in metamyelocytes/myelocytes, which usually do not circulate.
- Higher degree of left shift is associated with more immature neutrophil precursors and suggests serious bacterial infection, trauma, burns, surgery, acute hemolysis, or hemorrhage.

Table **11.11**	Causal Conditions for WBC Abnormalities
Neutropenia (ANC <1,500/μL, isolated— no other cell lines)	
↑ Destruction	• Autoimmune disorders (SLE, Felty, Wegener granulomatosis) • Splenic/lung trapping • Drugs (sulfa-containing Abx, α-methyldopa)
↓ Production	• Marrow invasion (aplastic anemia, tumor, myelofibrosis) • Infection (TB, infectious mononucleosis, viral hepatitis, AIDS) • Drugs (alkylating agents, antimetabolites, anti-inflammatory agents, antipsychotics) • Nutritional deficiency (Vit B$_{12}$, folate—especially in alcoholics) • Idiopathic, cyclic neutropenia
Transient neutropenia (peripheral pooling)	• Overwhelming bacterial infection • Hemodialysis • Cardiopulmonary bypass
Neutrophilia (ANC >7,700/μ L)	
↑ Production	• Hypersensitivity states • Myeloproliferative diseases (myelocytic leukemia, PCV) • Bacterial, fungal, occasionally viral infections • Collagen vascular diseases • Glucocorticoids • Thermal injury • Tissue necrosis
↑ Marrow release	• Acute infection (endotoxin) • Glucocorticoids • Thermal injury
↓ Margination	• Drugs (epinephrine, glucocorticoids, NSAIDs) • Stress, vigorous exercise
Miscellaneous	• Metastatic CA • Metabolic disorders (ketoacidosis, eclampsia, acute poisoning/renal failure) • Acute hemorrhage/hemolysis • Lithium

APPROACH

See Figure 11.11.

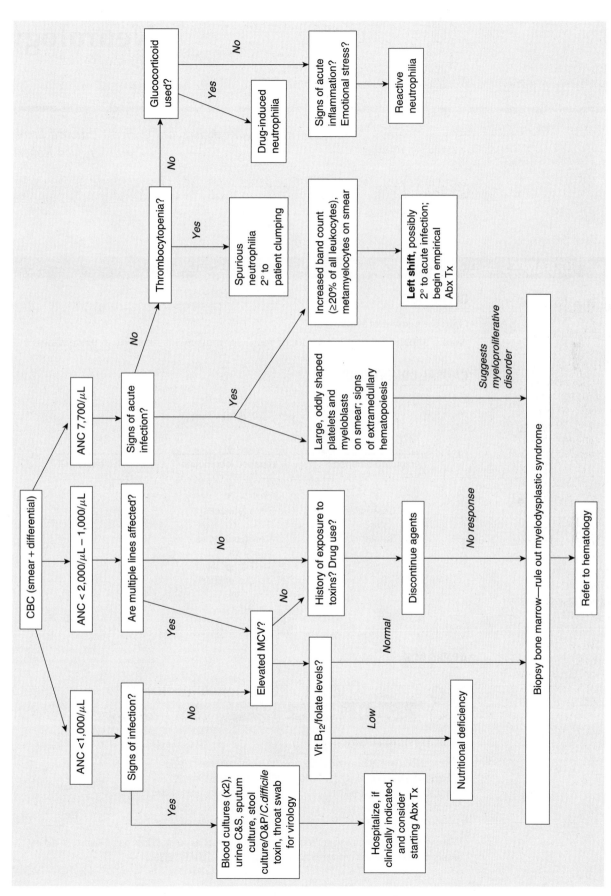

Figure 11.11 Approach to WBC abnormalities.

CHAPTER 12

Neurology

Dr. Hernish Jayant Acharya, Dr. Scott Edward Jarvis,
and Dr. Ted Roberts

GAIT DISTURBANCES AND ATAXIA

DEFINITION

Gait: the manner of walking

Ataxia: impaired ability to coordinate muscular movements resulting in unsteadiness

CAUSAL CONDITIONS

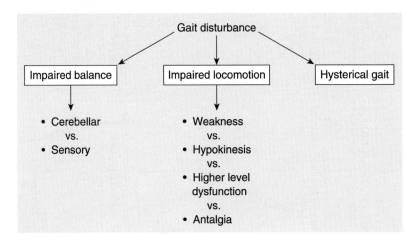

Figure 12.1 Classification of gait disturbance.

APPROACH

CLINICAL BOX

Fx of Hysterical Gait

Incongruous with known gait D/Os	Abrupt onset
Bizarre presentation	Extreme slowness
Variable, inconsistent pattern	Unusual or uneconomic posture
Nonphysiologic pattern	Exaggerated effort
Rare falls or injuries	Sudden buckling of the knees

(Adapted from Snijders A, van de Warrenburg B, Giladi N, et al. Neurological gait disorders in elderly people: Clinical approach and classification. *Lancet Neurol.* 2007;6(1):63–74.)

Table **12.1**	Approach to Gait Disturbance		
	Clinical fx	**Investigations**	**Management**
Impaired balance			
1. Cerebellar			
A. Midline lesion (tumor, hemorrhage, MS, drugs, tox)	Ataxia, nystagmus, disequilibrium, wide based, reeling, ↑ stride to stride variability, abnormal postural sway	MRI, tox screen, EtOH level	If mass lesion, consult neurosurgery. If drug/tox related, refer to emergency
B. Hereditary	Wide based, unsteady gait, uncoordinated limbs and speech, FHx	Genetic testing available for some, vitamin B_{12}, TSH	Refer to neurology, genetic counseling
i. Catalytic/inborn errors			Refer to neurology
• Intermittent	Examples: Hartup disease, Tay-Sachs, Niemann-Pick, Lesch Nyhan, Wilson		Genetic counseling
• Progressive			
ii. Progressive degenerative	Examples: Friedrich ataxia, ataxia telangectasia, spinocerebellar ataxia, prion disease		Refer to neurology
• Recessive			
• Dominant			
• X-linked/ mitochondrial			
2. Sensory			
A. Vestibular	Vertigo, N/V, no Δ in dark	MRI, TSH, B_{12}, Cr, LFTs	Refer to neurology
B. Proprioceptive	Patient may compensate by watching feet, positive Romberg, impairment worse in dark	MRI, TSH, B_{12}, Cr, LFTs	Refer to neurology, PT/OT
C. Visual	Poor visual acuity, poor peripheral vision	Snellen chart	Corrective visual aid. Refer to ophthalmology
Impaired locomotion			
1. Weakness	See Hemiplegia/Hemisensory loss topic		
2. Hypokinetic	See Movement D/Os topic		
3. Higher level dysfunction (frontal lobes, basal ganglia, thalamus, midbrain, tumor, dementia, hydrocephalus)	Abnormal cognitive testing, abnormal corrective response to perturbation, bizarre gait, worse in unfamiliar environment	MRI, cognitive testing	Refer to neurology, OT
4. Antalgia (MSK D/O, arthropathies, deformities)	Hx of MSK disease, improves with analgesia, normal neurologic exam	As per clinical situation	As per clinical situation

HEADACHE

DEFINITION

Headache (h/a) can be $2°$ to severe disease requiring emergent management.

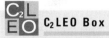 **C₂LEO Box**

Physician Legal Responsibility
Physicians are legally bound to perform complete clinical assessment on all patients presenting with h/a.

APPLIED SCIENTIFIC CONCEPTS

Brain parenchyma is not pain sensitive.

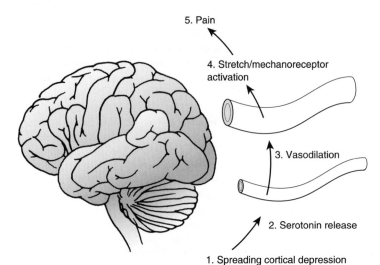

Figure 12.2 Neurovascular/serotonin theory of migraine pathophysiology.

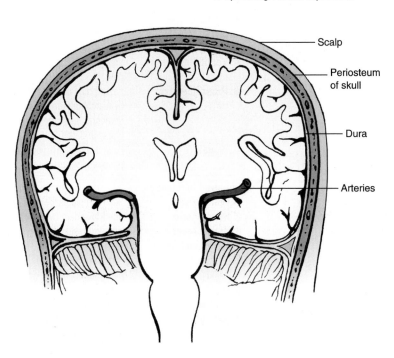

Figure 12.3 Cranial pain sensitive structures.

CAUSAL CONDITIONS

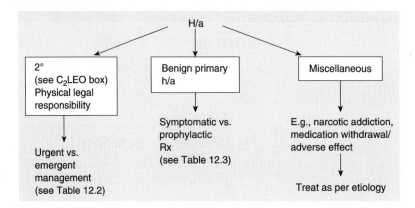

Figure 12.4 Approach to h/a.

- First
- Worst
- Different
- Persistent
- >50 yr
- Worse in recumbency
- Worst in A.M.
- Hx trauma, cancer
- Abnormality on neurologic exam
- Fever
- Meningismus
- Hypercoagulable state
- Sudden onset
- Pregnant

APPROACH

CLINICAL BOX

Clinical Signs Suggestive of ↑ ICP

"Put on your thinking cap, **COG CAP**"

Cushing triad (bradycardia, HTN, widened pulse pressure)

Ocular palsies

GI: N/V

Consciousness, altered LOC

A.M. h/a, worse in recumbency

Papilledema

CLINICAL BOX

Hypercoagulable W/U

CBC, INR, PTT

Fibrinogen

Protein C, protein S

Activated protein C resistance (factor V Leiden)

Antiphospholipid antibodies

Anticardiolipin antibodies

Lupus anticoagulant

Hyperhomocysteinemia

Prothrombin G20210A mutation

Antithrombin III deficiency

Pregnancy test

Malignancy w/u

Table **12.2** Red Flag H/A Should be Evaluated in a Hospital Setting			
	Clinical Fx	**Lab/Radiologic Fx**	**Management**
Vascular			
SAH	Sudden onset, preceded by Valsalva, meningismus	CT: acute blood in subarachnoid space / LP: xanthochromia	Refer to neurosurgery
Temporal arteritis	>50 yr, monocular blurred vision, tenderness over TA, proximal muscle tenderness	↑ ESR	TA biopsy, high-dose corticosteroids
Venous thrombosis	Diffuse h/a, Hx clot, hypercoagulable state, low flow state	Abnormal hypercoagulable w/u (see clinical box Hypercoagulabe w/u), MRV: thrombosis	Anticoagulation
Intracranial hematoma	Hx trauma, bleeding diathesis / Acute: rapidly progressive neurologic deficit / Chron.: h/a may be only sign/symptom	CT: epidural/subdural blood	Refer to neurosurgery
Severe arterial HTN (malignant HTN)	HTN, encephalopathic, papilledema, Hx cocaine, amphetamine, MAOI	Positive drug screen, urine metanephrines	Management based on etiology
Nonvascular			
↑ CSF pressure	See clinical box Hypercoagulable w/u	CT: slit-like ventricles, obliteration of fourth ventricle	Refer to neurosurgery
Intracranial infection			
• Meningitis	Febrile, sepsis, meningismus, rash, ↓ LOC	Bacterial: ↑↑ protein, ↓ gluc., ↑↑ WBCs / Viral: ↑ protein, gluc. normal, ↑ WBCs	Immediate broad-spectrum IV antibiotics, do not wait for LP/CT
• Mass lesion, e.g., abscess, tumor	Gradually progressive h/a, focal neurologic findings, sepsis	CT: ring-enhancing lesion	Refer to neurosurgery and ID

Table **12.3** Fx of Benign Primary H/A		<8 d/mo (Symptomatic)	>12 d/mo (Prophylactic)
Migraine	N/V, photo/phonophobia, aura (e.g., scintillating scotoma), worse with activity	Triptans, DHE	Propranolol, TCAs, AEDs
Tension type	Later in the day, no associated symptoms/signs Dull, aching, band-like h/a associated with stress	NSAIDs, acetaminophen	TCAs, AEDs
Cluster	♂ > ♀, severe stabbing, periorbital pain with ipsilateral autonomic signs (tearing, miosis, hydrosis, conjunctival injection), seasonal recurrence of multiple episodes with intermittent remission	O₂, triptans, DHE	Steroids (short term), verapamil, methysergide, lithium
Medication overuse	Early morning h/a Only resolved by next dose of narcotic, ergotamine, triptan, OTC analgesic, etc.	Drug holiday, d/c offending agent if possible	

HEMIPLEGIA/HEMISENSORY LOSS

DEFINITION

Hemiplegia: loss of power on the left or right side of the body

Hemisensory loss: loss of sensation on the left or right side of the body

APPLIED SCIENTIFIC CONCEPTS

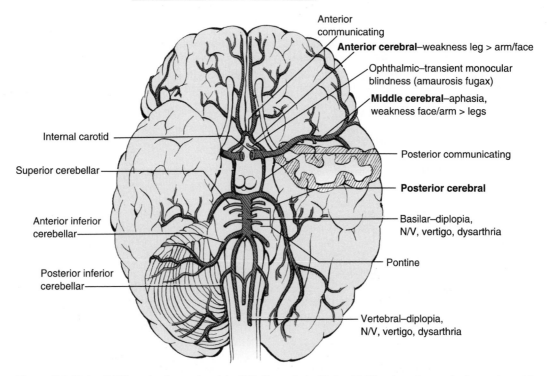

Figure 12.5 Circle of Willis and major arteries of the CNS. Shown is the Circle of Willis, where the anterior (internal carotid) circulation meets the posterior (vertebrobasilar) circulation. Important clues for localizing lesions in the CNS vasculature include weakness (leg > arm = face)—contralateral ACA; weakness (face = arm > leg) ± aphasia—contralateral MCA (aphasia if the lesion is on the dominant side); transient monocular blindness (amaurosis fugax)—ipsilateral ICA (with emboli to the ophthalmic artery); and dysarthria, diplopia, vertigo, N/V—vertebrobasilar circulation.

Figure 12.6 Effect of CO_2 in CNS vasculature. CO_2 is a potent vasodilator. Therefore, decreasing CO_2, by hyperventilation or ↑ tidal volume, will cause vasoconstriction, leading to ↓ blood flow and a ↓ ICP. Therefore, in the management of acute ICH, for example, it is important to keep pCO_2 from 30 to 35. Remember: ↓ CO_2 → ↓ blood flow → ↓ ICP. Note: When monitoring ICP, one may also measure the MAP and then calculate the CPP using the formula CPP = MAP − ICP.

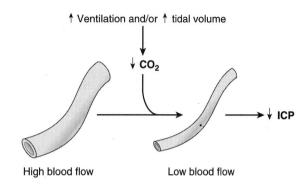

Figure 12.7 Cardiac sources of thromboembolism. DCM; PFO allows right-sided thrombus through congenital heart defect. Note: Implication of PFO in stroke etiology requires two additional fx to be present: (a) DVT and (b) RA pressure > LA pressure (e.g., RV hypertrophy) to allow right to left flow of clot through the PFO. PFO is present in 20% to 25% of the general population.

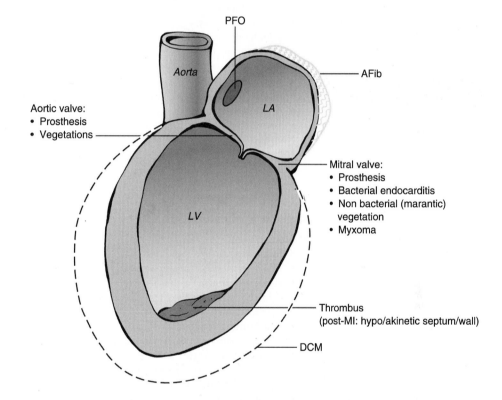

CAUSAL CONDITIONS

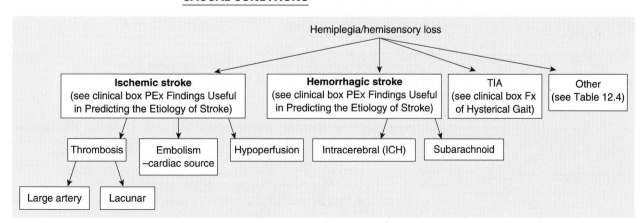

Figure 12.8 Approach to hemiplegia/hemisensory loss.

APPROACH

Dx

Onset of clinical symptoms in ischemic and hemorrhagic strokes:

- Ischemic stroke: develops over minutes to hours
- Thrombotic stroke: maximal at onset
- Lacunar stroke: stuttering progression ± periods of improvement/deterioration common
- ICH: develops over minutes to hours
- SAH: abrupt, severe "thunderclap" h/a, other symptoms within hours
- TIA: onset and resolution of symptoms within 1 h (was previously defined as a neurologic deficit <24-h duration)

RFs for hemorrhagic stroke

- **Modifiable**
  - **HTN**
  - **Smoking**
  - Atherosclerosis
  - Bleeding diathesis
  - ↑ EtOH consumption
  - **Cocaine**, amphetamines
  - Trauma
  - Vasculitis
  - Aneurysm (surgery)
  - AVM (surgery)
  - Tumors (surgery)
- **Nonmodifiable**
  - **↑ Age**
  - **FHx**
  - Inherited blood dyscrasias
  - Amyloid angiopathy

RFs for ischemic stroke

- **Modifiable**
  - **Smoking**
  - **DM2**
  - **Hyperlipidemia**
  - Obesity
  - Physical inactivity
  - Oral contraceptives
  - Cardiac sources of thromboembolism: see Figure 12.8
  - Atherosclerosis* (intracerebral [ICA] and extracerebral [ECA])
  - Obstructive sleep apnea (independent RF; mechanisms unclear†)
  - Elevated homocysteine‡
  - Elevated CRP‡
- **Nonmodifiable**
  - **↑ Age**
  - **Previous stroke/TIA**
  - **FHx**
  - ♂ sex§
  - Ethnicity
  - Hypercoagulable states: see clinical box Hypercoagulable w/u
  - Hypoperfusion: cardiac arrest, acute MI, tamponade, PE
  - Sickle cell disease

---

* Mechanisms = (a) perfusion failure (e.g., carotid stenosis [ECA]), (b) plaque rupture (local thrombosis [ICA] +/− distal arterioarterial thromboembolism [ICA and ECA]), and (c) occlusion of small artery origins (ICA)

† Proposed mechanisms include hypercoagulability, acute hemodynamic Δs during apnea, ↓ cerebral blood flow, paradoxical embolization, and atherosclerosis development.

‡ Elevated homocysteine and CRP are **associated** with ↑ risk of stroke, and can be lowered medically, but there are currently no RCTs to support lowering them for stroke risk reduction.

§ Postmenopausal women have the same stroke risk as men.

| Table **12.4** | Common Causes of Hemiplegia/Hemisensory Loss and Differentiating Factors |

	Symptom Onset	Duration of Deficit	LOC	H/A	Vision Δ	Aphasia
Stroke (hemorrhagic)	Immediate See clinical box Clinical Signs Suggestive of ↑ ICP	Hours to permanent.	Confused/ disoriented with ICH Possible ↓ LOC with SAH	Sudden, severe h/a. "Worst ever" with SAH	Diplopia, field cuts common, depending on lesion location	Uncommon
Stroke (ischemic)	Immediate	<1 h for TIA	Typically alert	Possible, not frequent		Common with dominant side lesion
Postictal (Todd paresis)	Postseizure (typically clonic, GTC)	Minutes to hours. Can be up to 48 h.	Confusion/ drowsiness —lasting up to hours	Common	Possible, likely with occipital lobe seizure	Possible, uncommon
Hemiplegic migraine	During aura	Plegia/paresis may outlast h/a	Can be ↓	Yes	Nystagmus can occur, photophobia	Common
Hypoglycemia	Within hours of ↓ gluc.	<24 h (once gluc. corrected)	Confusion common, coma possible	Common	Diplopia can occur	Uncommon, transient
Inflammatory (MS)	Can be abrupt, but typically over days	Deficit may be permanent or resolve completely	↓ LOC, h/a, vision Δ (common) and aphasia can all occur in MS, but will not be due to the same lesion causing hemiplegia/hemisensory loss			
Viral encephalitis	Over days	Depends on latency to Rx, can be permanent	Confusion → delirium → lethargy → coma	Common	Photophobia, nystagmus, diplopia (2° ocular palsy)	2° ↓ LOC
Trauma, acute SDH	Abrupt, or following lucid interval (SDH)	Can be permanent	Initially alert, then rapid ↓ LOC with acute SDH	Severe	Common—diplopia	Common
Mass lesion (tumor, abscess, Chron. SDH)	Gradual onset (days to weeks)	Until lesion removed, some permanent	Gradual ↓ LOC with Chron. SDH	Common, may become severe	Depends on lesion location	Common

Conversion D/O is a common cause of hemiplegia/hemisensory loss, but is considered a Dx of exclusion. Suggestive of conversion D/O:
- Pattern of weakness cannot be explained by a single lesion
- Give-way weakness and discontinuous power during strength testing
- Sensory Δs do not correspond to dermatomes

Syncope does not cause hemiplegia or hemisensory loss, and can generally be differentiated from seizures by considering the criteria in Table 12.16

INVESTIGATIONS

Standard w/u for stroke/TIA patients

- CBC, Lytes, Cr, BUN, gluc., INR, PTT
- LFTs, CK (before starting statin Rx)
- Fasting lipid profile, fasting gluc.
- Tox screen if suspected in SAH
- ESR, CRP if inflammatory process suspected
- EKG
- Noncontrast CT head

If clinically suspicious of hemorrhage, and CT head is negative for acute bleed, do LP for xanthochromia (xanthochromia present in all SAH ≥2 wk postbleed)

Imaging studies in stroke/TIA patients:

- **Noncontrast CT**—always done. Differentiates hemorrhagic stroke from ischemic stroke (blood is white on CT). Faster as an initial screen in patients with acute symptoms, less susceptible to motion artifact, and cheaper than MRI. Used to determine whether tPA is given.
- **CT angiography**—gold standard for imaging atherosclerosis and dissection in carotid, vertebral, and basilar arteries. Highly effective for identifying site of intracranial vascular lesions. Requires injection of dye (potentially nephrotoxic).

PEx Findings Useful in Predicting the Etiology of Stroke

Retinal hemorrhages—HTN and diabetic retinopathy

Purpura, ecchymoses—platelet D/O, coagulation D/O, vascular disease

Carotid bruit*—extracranial carotid stenosis

Retro-orbital bruit—intracranial atherosclerosis

Osler nodes, Janeway lesions, Roth spots, splinter hemorrhages, petechiae—endocarditis

DVT findings (in combination with PFO)—thromboembolism

- **MRI**—superior to CT for detecting aneurysms, AVMs, other structural lesions. Much more sensitive than CT for acute ischemic Δs (within the first few hours of stroke) and superior for imaging the posterior fossa. MRI–DWI can detect early ischemic Δs within 10 min of an event. PWI is employed to demonstrate penumbral tissue at risk. GRE–MRI has the highest sensitivity for detecting early hemorrhagic Δs.
- **MR angiography**—useful in identifying extracranial arterial dissections. Less information on intracranial vascular lesions than CT angiography, but **does not require injection of dye**.
- **Conventional angiography**—gold standard for identifying AVMs, aneurysms, requires dye injection.
- **TTE**—noninvasive examination of the heart for cardiac sources of emboli and wall motion abnormalities.
- **TEE**—typically performed after TTE is invasive but has a much higher yield in detecting atrial thrombi, atheromatous aortic disease, valvular disease, and PFO.
- **Carotid Doppler ultrasound**—rapid, noninvasive, dye-free initial assessment of carotid artery stenosis. High sensitivity and specificity for carotid stenosis ≥50%. Does not accurately assess stenosis <50% nor is it useful for assessing vertebral circulation. Useful for screening stroke/TIA patient for carotid stenosis—guides and accelerates clinical decision to use angiography.

STROKE PREVENTION

- Surgical management (carotid endarterectomy) if:
  - Symptomatic (i.e., patient has had stroke/TIA)
  - ≥70% carotid stenosis (determined by angiography or noninvasive imaging)
  - Performed within 2 wk of stroke/TIA
  - Acceptable surgical risk
- Medical management
  - **Primary prevention**
    - Lifestyle modifications (smoking cessation, regular exercise, weight loss, diet modifications, EtOH consumption one to two drinks per day)
    - BP: maintain BP ≤140/90, ≤130/80 for diabetics (first line = ACEI/ARB, diuretics)
    - Lipids: LDL ≤4 mmol/L, TC/HDL ≤5 if no RFs; LDL ≤2 mmol/L, TC/HDL ≤4 if multiple RFs. Initiate statin at low dose (e.g., simvastatin 20 mg qHS) and titrate up as needed. If needed, add on additional agent—ezetimibe, fibrate, niacin
    - DM: maintain tight glycemic control; targets = fasting BG <7, HbA$_{1C}$ ≤7.0%
    - Afib: target INR 2.5, range 2.0 to 3.0
  - **2° Prevention (i.e., following a TIA)**
    - All of the above
    - **ASA 81 mg daily**
    - **Clopidogrel (Plavix) 75 mg daily as monotherapy is not superior to ASA, but is recommended over ASA for patients with PVD**
    - **ASA 81 mg + clopidogrel 75 mg daily if evidence of large vessel disease (e.g., carotid or vertebral artery stenosis)**
    - **Aggrenox** (dipyridamole 200 mg + ASA 25 mg) b.i.d. may be superior to ASA—can be used instead of ASA, but not in addition to ASA
    - **Lipids: target LDL <2.0, TC/HDL ≤4**

Medical and Surgical Management of Acute ICH

- Ensure airway patency, intubate for GCS <8, adequate oxygenation
- Treat HTN only if severe and persistently elevated. Goals: sBP ≤220 mm Hg and dBP ≤120 mm Hg[†]. Use labetolol 10 mg IV q5-10 min and enalapril 2.5 mg. For refractory HTN, consider nitroprusside, hydralazine, clonidine. Do not drop BP more than 25% from baseline in the first 24 h.
- Correct coagulation abnormality (FFP, vitamin K[‡])

---

[*] Carotid bruit—high predictive value for moderate to severe **extra**cranial atherosclerosis, but poor predictive value for **intra**cranial atherosclerosis.

[†] Elevated BP is necessary to maintain cerebral perfusion following insult and will naturally trend down in most cases without medication.

[‡] Note that vitamin K even given IV (vs. SC) does not act to acutely reduce an elevated INR.

- If GCS <9, consider ICP monitor (with ventricular catheter)
- If ↑ ICP (on monitor, and look for midline shift, herniation, mass effect) Rx include:
  - Intubate and hyperventilate with target Paco$_2$ 30 to 35 mm Hg (see Figure 12.6)
  - Drain CSF through ventricular catheter
  - Furosemide and either mannitol or hypertonic saline
  - Elevate head of bed 30 to 45 degrees (reverse Trendelenberg)
- Craniotomy/evacuation of hematoma to reduce risk of brain herniation (from cerebellar lesion >3 cm, hemorrhage 2° structural lesion, lobar hemorrhage in young patients).

Medical Management of Acute Ischemia/TIA

- Ensure airway patency, all patients on O$_2$
- IV fluids only if hypotense, avoid D5 W
- tPA if no contraindications and time from onset <3 h [Notes: (a) if tPA to be given, risk of ICH makes BP control critical—keep sBP ≤185 and (b) no additional anticoagulants within 24 h of tPA administration]
- Treat HTN only if severe and persistently elevated, as for ICH (above)
- Treat arrhythmias appropriately (or consult)
- Treat Lyte abnormalities
- Avoid hyperthermia (acetaminophen 650 mg PO/PR q4 h, cooling fan)
- ASA 160 mg loading dose, then 81 mg q.d. (hold for 24 h post-tPA)
- Admit to stroke unit

POSTSTROKE REHAB

- Passive movement of paralyzed limbs should begin within 2 d of the event, regardless of pain, to avoid contractures and potential CRPS
- Intense PT results in better recovery
- SLP for dysphagia early in recovery to assess risk of aspiration
- Brain tissue remodeling and reorganization continues for months poststroke—most hemiplegics recover some ability to walk by 6 mo.

HOARSENESS/DYSPHONIA/SPEECH AND LANGUAGE ABNORMALITIES

DEFINITION

Language D/O: impaired comprehension, form, content, or function of language

Speech D/O: correct word choice and syntax, impaired articulation

Hoarseness: Δ in quality of voice

APPROACH

Determine if speech apparatus is intact (i.e., language vs. speech D/O)

CLINICAL BOX

Functions of Larynx/Hypopharynx

Cough production

Protection of airway

Voice generation

CLINICAL BOX

Conservative Management for Speech D/Os

Voice rest, fluids, humidity, antireflux, smoking cessation

If conservative measures fail >2 wk, refer for laryngoscopy to R/O neoplasm (RF: smoker/drinker/Asian descent)

Table **12.5** Language D/Os		
Classification	**Common Etiologies**	**Management**
Language D/Os		
Developmental	Learning disability, ADHD	Refer to pediatrics, SLP
Degenerative	Mucopolysaccharidosis, aphasia	Refer to neurology, SLP
Neglect/abuse/head trauma		SW, refer to pediatrics/ neurology, SLP
Speech D/Os		
A. Articulation D/O		
1. Nasal/badly articulated/slurred		
• Dysarthria ± dysphagia	CVA, tumour, CP	Refer to emergency/neurology
• Hearing impairment	Cerumen impaction	Disimpaction, SLP
	Sensorineural loss	Refer to audiology
• Soft palate paralysis	MG, MS, cleft lip/palate	Refer to neurology/ENT
• Bulbar/psuedobulbar palsy	ALS	Refer to neurology
• Tongue paralysis/ macroglossia	Cranial polyradiculitis, allergic edema, CVA	Refer to emergency/neurology
2. Speech apparatus lesions/hoarseness		
• Inflammation	Infection, allergy, voice abuse, smoking, EtOH, GERD	Treat as per cause, see clinical box Conservative Management for Speech D/Os
		If persists >2 wk, refer to ENT
• Neoplasms	Laryngeal benign/malignant neoplasms	Refer to ENT for laryngoscopy
i. Recurrent nerve palsy	Para/thyroidectomy, tumor	Refer to ENT
ii. Hyperfunction	Muscle tension, spasmodic dysphonia	Refer to neurology/ENT
3. Silent/non-speaking	Catatonia, depression, brainstem	Refer to psychiatry/neurology/ pediatrics

APPLIED SCIENTIFIC CONCEPTS

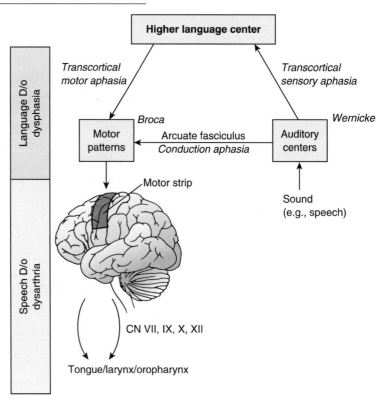

Figure 12.9 Schematic of language and speech dysfunction.

DELIRIUM: ALTERED MENTAL STATUS

DEFINITION

Delirium: Medical emergency characterized by acute, fluctuating disturbance of consciousness with reduced ability to focus, sustain, or shift attention.

Affects 10% to 15% of elderly at presentation to hospital and up to 30% as inpatients. Dementia is a major RF for delirium (acute Δ in behavior in demented patient may represent delirium).

APPROACH

PREVENTION

- Sleep hygiene
- Reduce immobility
- Vision correction
- Hearing aides
- Prevent dehydration
- Provide orienting stimuli (pictures, clock, window [for sunlight])
- Avoid polypharmacy

Dx

- MMSE
- Confusion assessment method
- Collateral Hx

Table **12.6**	Etiology, Investigations, and Management of Delirium	
Etiology	**Investigations**	**Management**
Systemic		
Deficiency		
Hypoxemia		
Global ischemia	Sao_2, ABG	Supplement O_2, consult neurology
Severe anemia	CBC	Varies with cause, transfusion
Endocrine deficiency		
Hypoglycemia	Gluc.	50 mL D50 W IV
Hypothyroid	TSH	Synthroid
Hypopituitary	Consult endocrinology	Thiamine 100 mg IM/IV several days
Thiamine deficiency		
Lytes	Na^+, K^+, Ca^{2+}, Mg^{2+}, PO_4	Determine underlying cause, correct Lytes
Excess		
Drugs/Tox	EtOH level, other drug levels formal drug review	ABCs, stop absorbption, antidote, supportive care, consult ICU, d/c anticholinergic medications
Organ failure		
Uremia	Urea, Cr	Consider dialysis, consult nephrology
Hepatic failure	ALT, AST, ALP, albumin, coagulation studies	Consult gastroenterology
CHF	CXR, ECHO	Consult internal medicine
Hypercarbia	ABG	Supplemental O_2, hyperventilate, correct acid–base abnormality
Sepsis	SWU	ABCs, antibiotics, antifungals, antivirals
Lytes	Lytes, Ca^{2+}, Mg^{2+}, PO_4	Determine underlying cause, correct Lytes
Local CNS		
Infectious	SWU, LP	ER, consult neurology
Vascular event	CT head	ER, consult neurology/neurosurgery
Postictal	CT head, EEG	Consult neurology
Neoplasm	CT/MRI	Consult neurosurgery

APPLIED SCIENTIFIC CONCEPTS

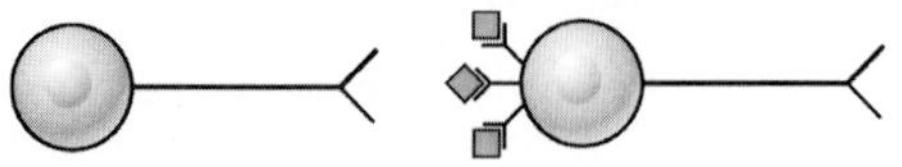

Presynaptic   **Postsynaptic**

↓ Acetylcholine production via:
- Hypoxia
- Hypoglycemia
- Thiamine deficiency

- Anticholinergic drugs worsen delerium

Figure 12.10 Acetylcholine in the pathophysiology of delirium.

Observational evidence implicates Ach dysfunction in the pathophysiology of delerium

DEMENTIA: ALTERED MENTAL STATUS

DEFINITION

Dementia: reversible or irreversible impairment of higher intellectual functions in the absence of impairment in arousal

APPROACH

Establish cognitive decline (patient and collateral Hx)
- Cognitive Hx (serial MMSE, memory, perception, language, visuospatial function, judgement)
- Functional Hx (basic and instrumental ADLs, family involvement)

R/O reversible causes (10% to 15%)

CLASSIFICATION OF DEMENTIA

Primary
- Alzheimer

2°
- Vascular
  - Multiinfarct
  - Vasculitis
- CNS condition
  - Parkinson disease
  - Dementia with Lewy bodies
  - Huntington chorea
  - Brain trauma
  - Frontal lobe dementia
- Potentially reversible—toxic/medication
  - EtOH/drugs (tox screen)
  - Heavy metals
- Mass lesions/neoplasms (CT/MRI)
  - CNS neoplasms
  - Chron. subdural hematoma
  - Normal pressure hydrocephalus
- Chron. infections
  - HIV (CD4 count, viral load)
  - Syphilis (VDRL)
  - CJD (MRI)
  - Chron. meningitis (LP)
- Endocrine/metabolic/vitamin deficiency
  - Hypothyroidism (TSH)
  - Hypo-/hyperparathyroidism (Ca^{2+}, PTH)

- B_{12}/thiamine deficiency (B_{12} level)
  - Lyte disturbance (Lytes)
- Depression

MANAGEMENT

- Patient education/counseling appropriate to cognitive function/level of disability
- Elicit patient/family wishes, community support, functional status of patient
- Consider interdisciplinary approach (OT, psychology, etc.)
- Consider consulting neurology for medical management

COMA: ALTERED MENTAL STATUS

DEFINITION

Coma: state of pathological, unarousable unconsciousness

CAUSAL CONDITIONS

Table **12.7** Localizing Brain Involvement in Altered Mental State				
Focal			**Diffuse**	
Imaging: CT/MRI PEx: response to painful stimuli and tone, brainstem reflexes			Investigations: Sao$_2$, ABG, CBCD, Lytes, Ca^{2+}, Mg^{2+}, vitamin B$_{12}$, urea, ALT, AST, albumin, SWU, urinalysis (+ketones, C&S), TSH, CT head	
Symmetric, normal	**Asymmetric, abnormal**	**Deficiencies**		**Excesses**
Bilateral hemispheric hemorrhage, infarction, mass, neoplasm, abscess, trauma	**Brainstem** Hemorrhage, infarction, mass (herniation), trauma	Hypoxemia, hypocarbia, Lyte deficiency, hypoglycemia, hypothermia, vitamin B$_{12}$/thiamine myxedema		Uremic/hepatic encephalitis, metabolic acidosis, DKA/HONK, ↑ Lytes, hyperthermia, thyroid storm, drug/tox

APPROACH

INITIAL MANAGEMENT

- ABCs, consider intubation if GCS ≤ 8
- Manage ↑ ICP
- Manage seizures
- Manage infections
- Restore Lyte/acid–base balance
- Control body T
- Administer thiamine
- Consider narcotic antagonist
- Consider selective benzodiazepine antagonist
- Consider 50% dextrose

MOVEMENT DISORDERS

DEFINITION

Movement D/Os describe a variety of abnormal movements of the body that have a neurologic basis.

APPLIED SCIENTIFIC CONCEPTS

Extrapyramidal clinical symptomatology results from basal ganglia dysfunction.

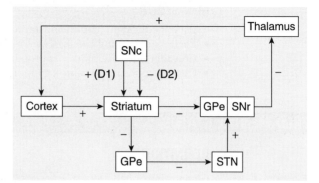

Figure 12.11 Basal ganglia circuitry. Parkinson disease: ↓ dopamine from the SNc through D1 and D2 to the striatum switches the balance of activity in the direct and indirect pathways, leaving the indirect pathway ↑ and the direct ↓.

CAUSAL CONDITIONS

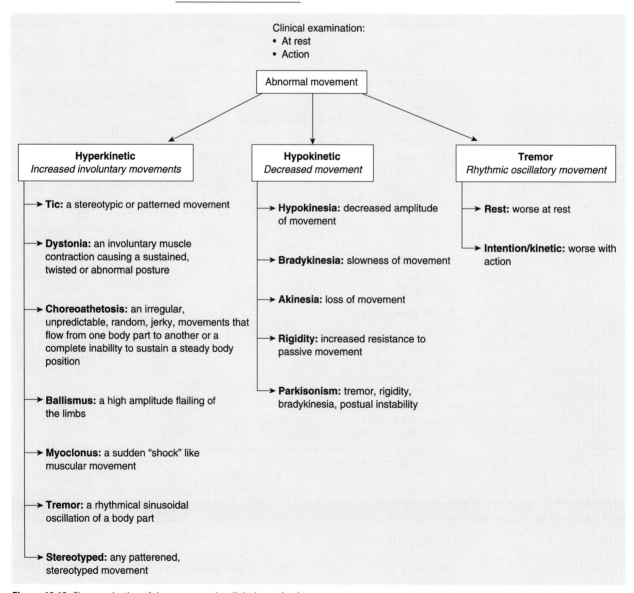

Figure 12.12 Characterization of the movement by clinical examination.

APPROACH

CLINICAL BOX

Possible Tests in Abnormal Movements

CBC, Lytes, Cr, BUN, LFTs

Peripheral smear—neuroacanthocytosis

TSH—hypo- or hyperthyroidism

Gluc.

EEG

Wilson tests—serum ceruloplasmin (↓), serum, urine copper (↑), slit lamp for Kayser-Fleischer rings. If positive, test family.

Table 12.8 Differential Dx of Hyperkinetic Movement D/Os

Phenomenology	Clinical/Labor Findings	Management
Hyperkinetic		
Tic		
A. Primary		
1. Tourette syndrome	Childhood onset, multifocal tics, >1yr	Refer to pediatric neurology
2. Huntington disease	Onset in third decade, insidious onset of chorea/cognitive decline, FHx	Refer to neurology, genetic counselling
B. 2°		
1. Infection		
Encephalitis	Acute onset febrile illness, white count	Referral for LP/imaging, acyclovir
C. Other		
Creutzfeldt-Jacob	Rapidly progressive psychiatric/behavioral symptoms	Referral to neurology for LP, imaging, EEG
Sydenham chorea	1–6 wk post GAS pharyngitis	Referral to pediatrics for w/u of rheumatic fever
Drugs	Methylphenidate, pemoline, amphetamines, cocaine	Remove offending drug
Dystonia		
A. Primary	Only dystonia −/+ tremor, develop over months to years	
1. Sporadic	no FHx	
2. Inherited	FHx	
B. 2°	Dopamine antagonist, evidence of brain insult	
C. Dystonia plus syndromes	Additional neurologic symptoms, e.g., Parkinsonism, myoclonus	
Stereotypies	With autism or mental retardation, failure to achieve/regression of developmental milestones	Refer to pediatrics/pediatric neurology
Chorea/athetosis/ballismus	May be part of Huntington disease, but has many neurologic causes	Neuroleptics for symptomatic control, refer to neurology for assessment
Essential tremor	FHx, inability to take soup with a spoon, better with EtOH	If severe, trial of propranolol, R/O Wilson disease
Myoclonus	Can occur alone or in combination with other neurologic disease	Refer to neurology for assessment (many etiologies, symptomatic control can require polypharmacy)

Table 12.9 Differential Dx of Hypokinetic Movement D/Os

Phenomenology	Clinical/Lab Findings	Management
Hypokinetic		
Parkinson disease	Tremor, rigidity, bradykinesia Postural instability	Trial of L-Dopa or dopamine agonist Refer if Dx unclear
Wilson disease	See clinical box Possible Tests in Abnormal Movements	
Huntington disease	Onset in third decade, insidious onset of chorea/cognitive decline, FHx	Refer to neurology, genetic counseling

Table **12.10**	Differential Dx of Tremors		
Phenomenology	**Clinical/Lab Findings**		**Management**
Tremor			
Resting (Parkinson disease, Wilson disease)	Rest tremor, rigidity, bradykinesia, postural instability		Trial of L-Dopa or dopamine agonist Refer if Dx unclear
Essential tremor	See clinical box Possible Tests in Abnormal Movements FHx, inability to take soup with a spoon, better with EtOH		If severe, trial of propranolol, R/O Wilson disease
Intention/kinetic (cerebellar disease)	Ataxia, nystagmus, dysdiadochokinesis		Refer to neurology for imaging and Rx
MS	Multiple neurologic deficits disseminated in time and space		Refer to neurology for imaging and Rx
Midbrain stroke	Acute onset, vascular RFs		Refer to neurology for imaging and Rx
Trauma	Hx of trauma, external signs		ATLS, rehab
Enhanced physiologic	Worse with anxiety, fever, fatigue, caffeine, EtOH withdrawal, FHx		TSH, gluc.
Peripheral neuropathy	Sensory/motor findings in typical distribution, EtOH Hx		TSH, DM screening, EtOH counseling

NUMBNESS/TINGLING/ALTERED SENSATION

DEFINITION

Sensory complaint

- Positive: **parasthesia/dysasthesia**
  - Detectable on exam (tingling, pins and needles, burning, knifelike)
- Negative: **hypoesthesia**
  - Difficult to detect on exam (numbness, diminution/absence of feeling)

CAUSAL CONDITIONS

See Figure 12.13.

APPROACH

Table **12.11**	Localize the Lesion			
	Distribution of Symptoms	**Associated Fx**	**Common Etiologies**	**Investigations**
Cerebral cortex	Unilateral arm/face ± leg (follows homunculus)	Hemiplegia, apraxia, aphasia, neglect, impaired, two- point discrimination, agraphesthesia	Stroke, demyelination, tumor	CT/MRI
Brainstem	Arm/body/leg and contralateral face	Diplopia, vertigo, dysphagia, dysarthria	Stroke, demyelination, tumor	MRI
Spinal cord/ radiculopathy	Dermatomal distribution, sensory level	Back pain, bowel/bladder dysfunction	Cord infarction, tumor, MS, syringomyelia, B_{12} deficiency	MRI, EMG/NCS, B_{12} level
Peripheral nerve (Mononeuropathy)	One peripheral nerve distribution	Sensory ± motor	Carpal tunnel, ulnar neuropathy	EMG/NCS
Peripheral nerve (Polyneuropathy)	Stocking/glove	Sensory ± motor	DM, uremia, vasculitis, B_{12} deficiency, HIV, Lyme disease, EtOH, paraneoplastic, amyloid	HbA_{1c}, B_{12} level, HIV viral load, CD4 count, TSH

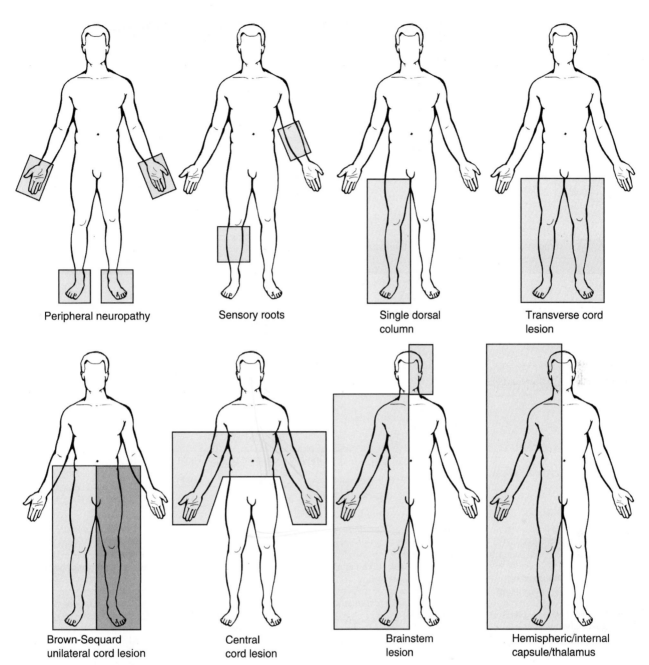

Peripheral neuropathy

Sensory roots

Single dorsal column

Transverse cord lesion

Brown-Sequard unilateral cord lesion

Central cord lesion

Brainstem lesion

Hemispheric/internal capsule/thalamus

Figure 12.13 Patterns of sensory loss.

CLINICAL BOX

Management of Mononeuropathy (e.g., Carpal Tunnel Syndrome)

Hx and PEx suggestive of mononeuropathy

R/O EtOH, DM, TSH abnormalities, mass effect, vasculitis (ESR, CRP), sarcoidosis (SPEP), uremic neuropathy (Cr, urea), lupus (RF, ANA)

R/O subacute ascending neuropathy with areflexia (GBS)

Determine functional limitations

Conservative Rx: task modification, wrist splints (carpal tunnel syndrome)

If conservative measures fail: EMG/NCS

If severe/axonal loss: surgical release

NEUROPATHIC PAIN AND COMPLEX REGIONAL PAIN SYNDROME

DEFINITION

Neuropathic pain: Pain resulting from dysfunction/disruption of either the central or peripheral nervous system.

CAUSAL CONDITIONS

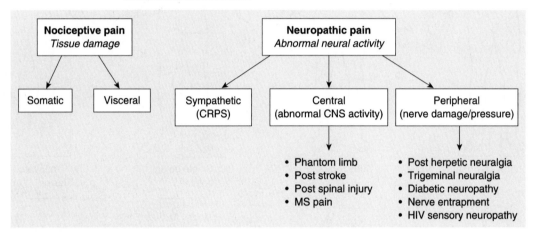

Figure 12.14 Classification of pain.

APPROACH

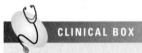

CLINICAL BOX

Symptoms of Neuropathic Pain

Description: burning, sharp, stabbing, shooting, electrical shock

Allodynia: painful response to a stimulus which is not normally painful (e.g., light touch, cool air)

Hyperalgesia: ↑ pain in response to a stimulus which is normally nominally painful (e.g., pin prick)

Figure 12.15 Pharmacological Rx of neuropathic pain.

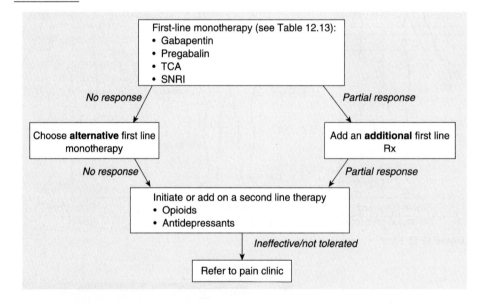

Table **12.12**	Differentiating Diabetic Neuropathic Pain from Diabetic Vascular Pain	
	Neuropathic Pain	**Vascular Pain**
Location	Distal (feet, ankles)	Calves
Timing	Constant	With activity
Perception	Sharp, burning, tingling	Deep pain
At rest	Worse	Better

Table **12.13**	Condition-Specific First-Line Neuropathic Pain Agents	
Condition	**Agent**	
Postherpetic neuralgia, focal neuropathy	Lidocaine (5%) patch, capsaicin	
Trigeminal neuralgia	Carbamazepine, phenytoin, baclofen	
Phantom limb	Preamputation administration of local anesthetic	

MANAGEMENT

Second-line neuropathic pain agents:

Opioids—tramadol, oxycodone, hydrocodone, hydromorphone, morphine, transdermal fentanyl, methadone

Antidepressants—bupropion, citalopram, paroxetine, imipramine

CLINICAL BOX

Peripheral Nerve Injuries—Seddon Categories

Neurapraxia (focal demyelination)
- Temporary conduction block/paralysis occurs
- Complete recovery is typical

Axonotmesis (axonal destruction with preservation of myelin)
- Prolonged conduction block/paralysis
- The recovering axon can follow an intact myelin base to reestablish connectivity
- Complete recovery is possible

Neurotmesis (complete transection)
- Prolonged/permanent conduction block/paralysis
- Loss of myelin base to guide axon
- Neuroma* formation results
- Complete recovery unlikely without surgery

COMPLEX REGIONAL PAIN SYNDROME

DEFINITION

A condition of chron. neuropathic pain, developing over months, which affects an extremity and **cannot be localized to a peripheral nerve or root territory**. May or may not have an obvious etiology. All tissue types in the vicinity are affected. Severe and permanent Δs may occur within 1 yr of disease onset.

- CRPS Type I—no definable lesion/insult, previously known as **reflex sympathetic dystrophy**
- CRPS Type II—a definable lesion/insult, previously known as "causalgia"

APPLIED SCIENTIFIC CONCEPTS

See Table 12.14.

_____

* Neuroma: following injury, multiple axon sprouts emerge from the proximal axon stump. Without guidance (i.e., a myelin sheath to follow) sprouts grow haphazardly and can tangle, resulting in a neuroma. Neuromas exhibit abnormal excitability and discharges, including spontaneous activity, ↑ mechanosensitivity (elicited by Tinel sign), and ↑ pain/heat sensitivity.

Table **12.14** CNS Excitatory and Inhibitory NTs		
NT	**Mechanism and Effect**	**Pharmacology**
Glutamate (major excitatory NT in the CNS)	Released from presynaptic vesicles → binds to postsynaptic receptors → opening of Na^+ and Ca^{2+} channels causing membrane **depolarization** → **excitation of the postsynaptic neuron**	PCP and ketamine antagonize the effect of glutamate in some areas of the CNS. Many pharmaceuticals designed to antagonize glutamate have been developed but none have been clinically useful without neurotoxic effects
GABA (major inhibitory NT in the CNS)	Released from presynaptic vesicles → activates postsynaptic K^+ and Cl^- channels → membrane **hyperpolarization** → postsynaptic Na^+ and Ca^{2+} channels harder to open → **inhibition of the postsynaptic neuron**	Many drugs agonize the GABA receptors or ↑ the available amount of GABA, resulting in antianxiety and anticonvulsant effects. These include ethanol, benzodiazepines, zopiclone, barbiturates, propofol, baclofen, carbamazepine, phenytoin
Glycine	Acts like GABA, but primarily found in the brainstem, spinal cord, retina	Strychnine is a glycine receptor antagonist

CAUSAL CONDITIONS

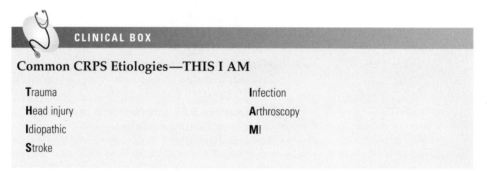

CLINICAL BOX

Common CRPS Etiologies—THIS I AM

Trauma	**I**nfection
Head injury	**A**rthroscopy
Idiopathic	**M**I
Stroke	

APPROACH

Dx

Dx of CRPS is based largely on the clinical exam, but investigations may include:

- Plain radiograph—detects patchy/localized bone demineralization during the chron. stage (>1 yr)
- Bone scintigraphy—mineralization phase shows ↑ uptake during the subacute stage (<1 yr)

Table **12.15** Clinical Findings in CRPS (in Addition to Neuropathic Pain, Allodynia, Hyperalgesia[a])				
Vasomotor/ Sudomotor[b]	**Skin**	**Hail, Nails**	**Muscle and Joint**	**Bone**
Edema	Thickened	↑ Hair growth, then loss	Wasting	Patchy, then severe demineralization
Δ Color: red, then cyanotic	Mottled Contractures	Nails grow fast, then slow	↓ Strength stiffening ↓ ROM	
Δ T: warm, then cool Hyper, then hypohidrosis				

[a]Allodynia, and hyperalgesia occur early in the onset, but tend to fade after a year.
[b]Vasomotor and sudomotor activities, are initially subject to ↑ blood flow, followed by ↓ blood flow, as mediated by abnormal SNS activity.

- Regional sympathetic nerve block—can be diagnostic and therapeutic. Degree of pain relief and improvement in clinical symptoms (↑ ROM, ↑ exercise tolerance) suggests both the degree of SNS involvement and the potential benefit of permanent sympathectomy.

MANAGEMENT

Few Rx exist for CRPS. Early interventions include passive mobilization following injury/stroke, and vitamin C.

SEIZURES (EPILEPSY)

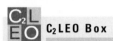 **C₂LEO Box**

Exception to Duty of Confidentiality
Reporting incomplete seizure control to the authorities may be an exception to the duty of confidentiality. This represents a legal requirement in some jurisdictions in the interest of public health, but physicians must recognize reasonable disclosure and reveal only necessary information to third parties.

DEFINITION

Seizure: Transient neurologic dysfunction resulting from excessive/abnormal electrical discharges of cortical neurons.

Epilepsy: Chron. condition of recurrent unprovoked seizures.

CAUSAL CONDITIONS

SEIZURES CLASSIFIED BY ETIOLOGY

Epileptic
- Young
  - Congenital malformation → MRI, EEG → refer to neurology/neurosurgery
  - Inborn errors of metabolism → refer to pediatrics/pediatric neurology
  - Febrile seizures
    - Typical—<15 min, one event in 24 h, generalized, no neurologic Hx, normal pre/post neuro exam
    - Atypical—>15 min, more than one event in 24 h, focal, known neurologic Hx, abnormal pre/post neuro exam
- Adult
  - Tumor, stroke, trauma, abscess → CT/MRI → refer to neurology/neurosurgery
  - Drug intoxication or withdrawal → tox screen, drug levels → refer to emergency, d/c offending agent
- Elderly
  - Cerebral degeneration, vascular, tumor → CT/MRI → refer to neurology/neurosurgery
  - Drug reactions, intoxication, withdrawal → tox screen, drug levels → refer to emergency, d/c offending agent

Nonepileptiform
- Physiologic—must correct underlying pathology
  - Metabolic
    - Thyroid ↓/↑ → TSH, treat
    - Hyponatremia, hypocalcemia → Lytes, treat
    - Hypoglycemia or NKH → gluc., treat
    - Uremia → urea, treat
    - Hyperthermia → vitals, treat as hyperthermia
  - Hypoxemic
    - Find cause of hypoxemia and treat, refer to emergency
  - Nonphysiologic (psychogenic)

SEIZURES CLASSIFIED BY TYPE

Partial—initial signs/symptoms consistent with activation of a localized area within one hemisphere

- Simple—no alteration of LOC
  - Motor—signs/symptoms consistent with activation of motor cortex
  - Somatosensory—signs/symptoms consistent with activation of sensory cortex
  - Autonomic—signs/symptoms consistent with activation of central autonomic network or higher order autonomic control areas (e.g., insula, prefrontal cortices)
- Complex—alteration of LOC

- 2° Generalized—initial signs/symptoms consistent with simple partial seizure (aura), later signs/symptoms consistent with generalized seizure, associated with spread of cortical activation

  Generalized—initial signs/symptoms consistent with activation of both cerebral hemispheres, always associated with a loss of consciousness

- **Convulsive**—episode of excessive abnormal muscle contraction, usually bilateral
  - **Myoclonic**—sudden, brief (<100 ms), involuntary contraction of muscle(s)
  - **Clonic**—myoclonus which is regular and repetitive, involves same muscle groups, 2 to 3 Hz, prolonged
  - **Tonic**—sustained muscle contraction lasting seconds to minutes
  - **Tonic-clonic**—sequence consisting of tonic phase followed by clonic phase (formerly, grand mal)
  - **Atonic**—sudden loss of muscle tone lasting >1 to 2 s
- **Nonconvulsive**—episode without abnormal muscle contraction
  - **Absence**
    - **Typical**—brief (seconds) loss of consciousness without conspicuous convulsions, with accompanying generalized 3 Hz spike and slow wave discharges on EEG
    - **Atypical**—as above with abnormality of tone, 2 Hz spike and slow wave on EEG

APPROACH

Dx

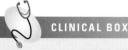

Psychosocial Impact of Seizures

Seizures affect all domains of patient life. Physicians should provide education and support.

Driving—patient must be seizure free for period of time (jurisdiction specific)

Lifestyle

Occupation—professional drivers, airline pilots, and armed forces personnel will need to reconsider profession

Sports/leisure—isolation sports, cycling, swimming must be reconsidered/modified

General—avoid sleep deprivation, limit EtOH intake, shower/bath taken with bathroom door unlocked, women of childbearing age require contraception and specialist review of long-term management

Table 12.16 Is This a Seizure?

	Preictal	Intraictal	Postictal
Syncope	• Lightheadedness • Diaphoresis • Prolonged standing • Chest pain • Palpitations • Bradycardia • Hypotension	• Urinary incontinence • Pallor • Flaccidity	Rapid resolution with recumbency
Seizure	• Déjà vu/jamais vu • Aphasia • Olfactory aura • Epigastric sensation	• Tongue biting • Urinary incontinence • Unilateral head turning • Automatism • Cyanosis	• Post-event delerium • Focal neurologic symptoms (Todd paresis)

Convulsive syncope, which mimics GTC, can occur with cerebral hypoperfusion and subsequent CNS disinhibition of peripheral neurologic activity during syncope.

Table 12.17 Fx Suggesting Pseudoseizures

Historical	Clinical
Associated with psychiatric Dx	Asynchronous limb movements
Hx of sexual/physical abuse	Avoidance behavior
No Hx of injury from seizure	Closed eyes, restricted eye opening
No response or worsening with AED	Dystonic posturing (e.g., opisthotonus)
Personal/family/professional experience with seizures	Emotional/situation trigger
Lab	Pelvic thrusting
Typical seizure without electrical correlate on EEG	Side-to-side head movements
Prolonged seizure (>2–3 min)	Provoked by suggestion
	Seizure only occurring in presence of others
	Gradual onset, gradual cessation
	Ictal crying
	Nonphysiologic progression

Table **12.18**	AEDs			
Seizure Type	**Drug**	**Action**	**Contraindications**	
Absence	Ethosuximide	Ca^{2+} channel modulator	GI upset, sedation, ataxia, rash, h/a, blood dyscrasia	
Myoclonic	Valproate	↑ GABA	GI upset, tremor, sedation, weight gain, hair loss, pancreatitis, hepatic dysfunction	
GTC	Lamotrigine	Na^+ channel antagonist, ↓ glutamate	Dizziness, ataxia, rash, SJS	
	Topiramate	Na^+/Ca^{2+} channel modulation causing ↓ glutamate	Ataxia, confusion, glaucoma renal stones	
Focal ± generalization	Carbamazepine	Na^+ channel antagonist	GI upset, diplopia, ataxia, sedation, rash, blood dyscrasia, hepatic dysfunction	

CLINICAL BOX

Emergency Rx of Tonic-Clonic Seizures

- Remove immediate danger (fire, water, machinery)
- When seizure ceases → lateral decubitus (recovery position)
- Ensure airway clear (do not insert anything into mouth)
- Patient should be accompanied during ictal state
- Consider O_2, AED levels
- If convulsion continues >5 min or recurs without period of normal LOC, summon emergency Rx, consider Rx for status epilepticus

MANAGEMENT

AEDs affect voltage-gated Na^+ channels, GABA metabolism, Ca^{2+} currents, and a variety of other mechanisms *in vitro*. They work by similar complex mechanisms *in vivo*.

MANAGEMENT OF STATUS EPILEPTICUS

Time 0 min:
1. ABCs, vitals, O_2
2. IV N/S at low infusion rate
3. 50 mL of D50 W IV and thiamine 100 mg IV/IM
4. EEG to record as soon as possible
5. Lorazepam 0.1 mg/kg IV at 2 mg/min
6. If seizure persists, fosphenytoin* 18 mg/kg IV at 150 mg/min
7. If seizure persists, fosphenytoin* 7 mg/kg IV at 150 mg/min

Time 20 min:
1. If seizure persists, intubate, Foley, EEG
2. Phenobarbital 20 mg/kg IV at 100 mg/min (loading dose)

Time 40 min:
1. If seizures persists, phenobarbital infusion 5 mg/kg IV, then IV push (≤100 mg/min) until seizure ceases
2. Monitor through EEG, continue phenobarbital at 1 mg/kg/h
3. If seizure stops, ↓ rate q4-6 h

    If phenobarbital ineffective, consider propofol (bolus 1 mg/kg IV over 5 min, then 2 to 15 mg/kg/h IV infusion), midazolam (bolus 200 μg/kg IV, then 1 to 10 μg/kg/min infusion), or pentobarbital (5 mg/kg IV bolus, then 1 to 3 mg/kg/h IV infusion)

WEAKNESS (PARESIS/PARALYSIS), LOSS OF MOTION

DEFINITION

Paresis: partial loss of power

Paralysis (plegia): full loss of power

Loss of motion: reduced ROM

---

* If fosphenytoin is not available, use phenytoin (same dose) 50 mg/min.

APPROACH

Dx

Table **12.19**	Localization of Weakness		
	Distribution of Weakness	**Common Etiology**	**Investigations and Additional Fx**
1. UMN			
• Cortex	Contralateral distal	Stroke, MS, trauma	CT/MRI
• Descending motor pathways	Contralateral	Stroke	CT/MRI
• Brainstem	Long tract and bulbar findings	Stroke, MS	MRI
• Spinal cord	Sensory level bowel/bladder dysfunction	Trauma, MS, transverse myelitis	MRI, LP
2. LMN			
• Anterior horn cell	UMN/LMN mixed	ALS, polio	No sensory findings, EMG/NCS, MRI, FVC
• Nerve root	Back pain with radiation dermatomal sensory	Herniated disc, OA, degenerative disc	X-ray, CT/MRI, myotomal motor
• Plexus	Multiple root distribution	Brachial neuritis, trauma, DM	EMG/NCS, gluc.
• Peripheral nerve	Glove and stocking Peripheral nerve Sensory and motor	DM thyroid EtOH	EMG/NCS TSH, gluc., LFTs FVC GBS
3. NMJ	Proximal > distal fatigability	MG, LES, botulism	See clinical box PEx Findings Useful in Predicting the Etiology of Stroke
4. Muscle	Tender, FHx, bilateral, symmetrical, proximal	Myositis, rhabdomyolysis, myodystrophy	Myositis, ESR, EMG/NCS, muscle biopsy, muscle enzymes

CLINICAL BOX

Grading the Motor Exam

Check for full ROM before motor exam

Strength

0—no contraction

1—flicker

2—no active movement against gravity

3—active movement against gravity (3– or 3+ **are not used**)

4—active movement against resistance (4– and 4+ can be used)

5—normal power

Reflexes

0, absent

1+, present but small, may only be brought out by distraction*

2+, normal range

3+, hyperactive without clonus

4+, hyperactive with clonus

Table **12.20**	UMN versus LMN Lesion	
	UMN	**LMN**
Strength	↓	↓
Tone	↑	↓
Bulk	Normal, then ↓	↓
Reflexes	↑	↓
Fasciculations	Absent	Present

MANAGEMENT

Initial Management of GBS (after ABCs)

• Admit
• Swallowing assessment
• AAT
• Neurovitals q2 h
• FVC q6 h, call MD if <20 mL/kg
• Heparin 5000 IU SC b.i.d.
• Consider IVIg or plasmapheresis
• Consult neurology

---

* Distraction preoccupies the patient, thereby minimizing conscious inhibition of the reflex.

Initial Management of MG (after ABCs)

- Admit
- Swallowing assessment
- AAT
- Neurovitals q2 h
- FVC q6 h, call MD if <20 mL/kg
- Heparin 5000 IU SC b.i.d.
- CXR
- CT chest (R/O thymoma)
- EMG/NCS
- AChR antibodies
- Consider pyridostigmine, corticosteroids, IVIg
- Consult neurology

CLINICAL BOX

Hemiplegia/Paraplegia Rehab

Acute goals: maintain ROM, prevent contracture, prevent pressure ulcers, and prevent disuse atrophy

Long-term goals (hemiplegia): improve sensorimotor control, treat spasticity, speech/language rehab, patient education, home and environmental modifications; consider consultation with physiatrist

Long-term goals (paraplegia): physical skills training, wheelchair skills, patient education, home and environmental modifications, driver training, vocational training; consider consultation with physiatrist.

CHAPTER 13

Nephrology

Ning Zi Sun, Michelle-Lee Jones, Dr. Oliver Haw For Chin,
and Dr. Tomoko Takano

ABNORMAL SERUM HYDROGEN ION CONCENTRATION

RATIONALE

- Severe acidemia/alkalemia can exist without specific symptoms.
- Must ascertain the etiology as metabolic versus respiratory versus both
- Treatment of underlying causes is key

APPLIED SCIENTIFIC CONCEPTS

ASC Box

AG (8 to 12 mmol/L)

- Accounts for unmeasured plasma anions
- $= [Na^+] - ([Cl^-] + [HCO_3^-])$
- ↑ AG → 2° to ↑ in unmeasured anions or ↓ in unmeasured cations
- ↓/narrow AG can be seen with MM and lithium intoxication (presence of unmeasured cations), and hypoalbuminemia (loss of anionic protein) → for every ↓ in serum albumin by 1 g/dL, the AG falls by 2.5 mEq/L
- ↑ AG usually with metabolic acidosis but can be seen with many acid–base disorders.

ASC Box

Urinary [Na⁺] versus [Cl⁻] as a Surrogate for Volume Status

- Usually, Δ in volume status → similar Δ in both renal Na and Cl excretion
- With metabolic alkalosis, Na is excreted in excess alongside HCO_3 → Cl is a better surrogate for volume status.
- With metabolic acidosis, Cl is excreted in excess alongside of NH_4^+ → Na is a better surrogate for volume status.

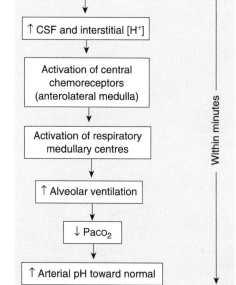

Figure 13.1 Respiratory response to acidosis—effects within minutes. The opposite applies in the event of ↓ $PaCO_2$ and ↓ [H⁺]
Δ Minute ventilation is proportional to Δ $PaCO_2$
If ↑↑↑ $PaCO_2$ → respiratory center depression → ↓ alveolar ventilation → **CO₂ narcosis** (confusion, headache, coma).

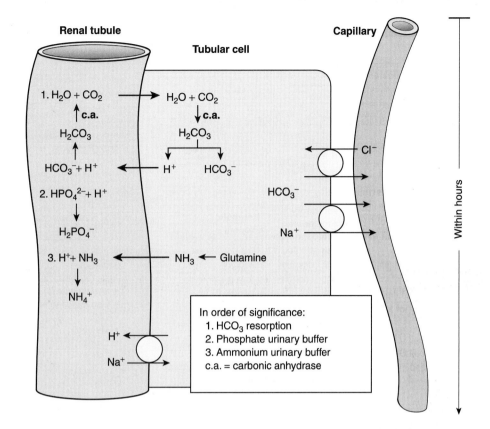

Metabolic Alkalosis

- Initiating factors → pathological generation of HCO_3^- within the body (e.g., vomiting, NG suction, exogenous alkali, diuretics)
- Maintenance factors → disorders that promote renal conservation of HCO_3^- (e.g., volume depletion leading to ↑ HCO_3^- resorption and ↑ H^+ excretion through activation of renin-angiotensin-aldosterone system)

Figure 13.2 Renal response to acidosis—effects within hours.

In the figure:

Renal tubule — Tubular cell — Capillary — Within hours

1. $H_2O + CO_2$ (↑ c.a.) → H_2CO_3 → $HCO_3^- + H^+$

2. $HPO_4^{2-} + H^+$ → $H_2PO_4^-$

3. $H^+ + NH_3$ → NH_4^+

Tubular cell: $H_2O + CO_2$ (↓ c.a.) → H_2CO_3 → H^+ and HCO_3^-

NH_3 ← Glutamine

H^+ ← / Na^+ →

Cl^-, HCO_3^-, Na^+

In order of significance:
1. HCO_3 resorption
2. Phosphate urinary buffer
3. Ammonium urinary buffer
c.a. = carbonic anhydrase

CAUSAL CONDITIONS

Table 13.1   Causal Conditions of Blood pH Abnormalities

Metabolic acidosis	↑ AG	Excess acid	External—ethylene glycol, salicylate, methanol, early toluene, Fe, isoniazid
			Internal—lactic acidosis (2° to infection or ischemia), ketoacidosis
	Normal AG	↓ Renal acid excretion	Renal failure/uremia
		Renal HCO_3 loss	Interstitial nephritis, renal tubular acidosis, posthypocapnea
		GI HCO_3 loss	Diarrhea, pancreatic fistulas
Metabolic alkalosis	↑ ECV, Cl^--resistant	Hypertensive	Conn syndrome, Cushing syndrome, Liddle syndrome
		Normotensive	Bartter syndrome, Gitelman syndrome
	↓ ECV, Cl^--responsive	Renal loss of acid (diuretics)	
		GI loss of acid (vomiting, gastric fistulas/drainage)	
		Exogenous ingestion (HCO_3, other bases)	
Respiratory acidosis	Neuromuscular	Encephalitis, phrenic nerve injury, bulbar palsy, myasthenia, GBS, curare-like drugs, botulism	
	Pulmonary	COPD, asthma, interstitial disease, type II respiratory failure, upper airway obstruction, fibrosis, OSA	
	Chest wall	Obesity, kyphoscoliosis, flail chest	
	Respiratory center depression	Narcotics, anesthetics, CNS trauma/disease	
	Excess CO_2 production	Thyroid storm, protracted seizures, malignant hyperthermia	
Respiratory alkalosis	Hypoxemia	Type I respiratory failure, high altitude	
	Metabolic	Metabolic acidosis, hepatic failure	
	Cardiopulmonary	Pneumonia, asthma, CHF/pulmonary edema, fibrosis, PE	
	CNS disorders	Subarachnoid hemorrhage, infection, hyperventilation syndrome, tumor, CVA	
	Drugs	Salicylates, xanthine, β-agonists, progesterone	
	Miscellaneous	Pregnancy, fever, pain, excess mechanical ventilation	
Mixed acid–base disturbances			

APPROACH

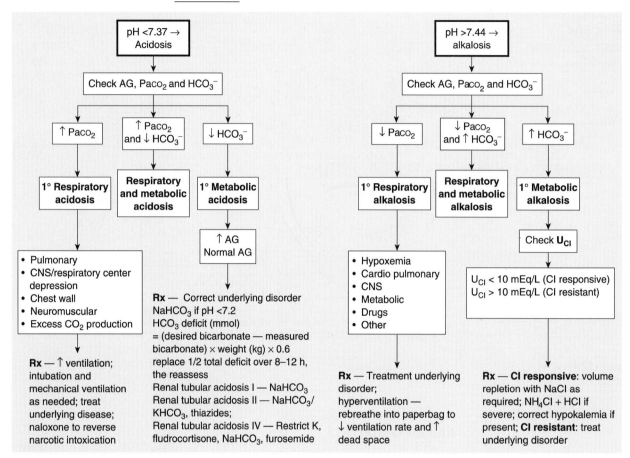

Figure 13.3 Approach to abnormal blood pH.

Table **13.2**	**Expected Compensation for Acid–Base Disturbances**		
Metabolic Acidosis		**Metabolic Alkalosis**	
Expected PaCO$_2$ = (1.5 × [HCO$_3^-$]) + 8 ± 2 ↓ in PaCO$_2$ = Δ [HCO$_3^-$] × 1.2 ± 2		Expected PaCO$_2$ = (0.7 × [HCO$_3^-$]) + 21 ± 2 ↑ in PaCO$_2$ = Δ [HCO$_3^-$] × 0.6	
Respiratory acidosis		Respiratory alkalosis	
Acute	Chronic	Acute	Chronic
↑ [HCO$_3^-$] = Δ PaCO$_2$ / 10	↑ [HCO$_3^-$] = 4 (Δ PaCO$_2$ / 10)	↓ [HCO$_3^-$] = 2 (Δ PaCO$_2$ / 10)	↓ [HCO$_3^-$] = 5 (Δ Paco$_2$ /10)

HYPOMAGNESEMIA

CLINICAL BOX

Hypomagnesemia

- Serum [Mg$^+$] <1.5 mEq/L or 0.75 mmol/L
- Normal = 1.5 to 2.0 mEq/L or 0.75 to 1 mmol/L or 1.7 to 2.4 mg/dL

Also see Chapter 9.

RATIONALE

- ≈10% of hospitalized and >60% of critically ill patients
- Commonly associated with hypokalemia and hypocalcemia (chronic hypomagnesemia → ↓ PTH secretion and ↓ bone response to PTH)

APPLIED SCIENTIFIC CONCEPTS

RENAL HANDLING OF Mg

- ≈70% of plasma Mg is filterable, the rest is bound to albumin (therefore, must multiply PMg by 0.7 when calculating FEMg)

CLINICAL BOX

Common Associations Seen with Hypomagnesemia

- Malnutrition
- Alcoholism
- Electrolyte imbalances
- Diuretics
- Large volumes of IV fluids
- Nephrotoxic agents
- Cisplatin

- ≈95% of filtered Mg is reabsorbed under physiologic conditions (60% to 70% at the TAL, 15% to 25% at the PCT, 5% to 10% at the DCT)
- ECF expansion ↑ renal Mg excretion and ↓ Mg resorption in the loop of Henle
- ↓ GFR → ↓ filtered Mg load → ↓ fractional Mg reabsorption
- Hypercalcemia and hypermagnesemia → ↓ Mg reabsorption
- Phosphate depletion → ↑ urinary Mg excretion
- Chronic metabolic acidosis → ↑ Mg excretion
- Chronic metabolic alkalosis → ↓ Mg excretion
- Intracellular Mg depletion may be present with low normal serum Mg levels
- Hypomagnesemia can exacerbate digitalis toxicity

CAUSAL CONDITIONS

GI losses—see Chapter 9—Mg concentration serum, abnormal/hypomagnesemia

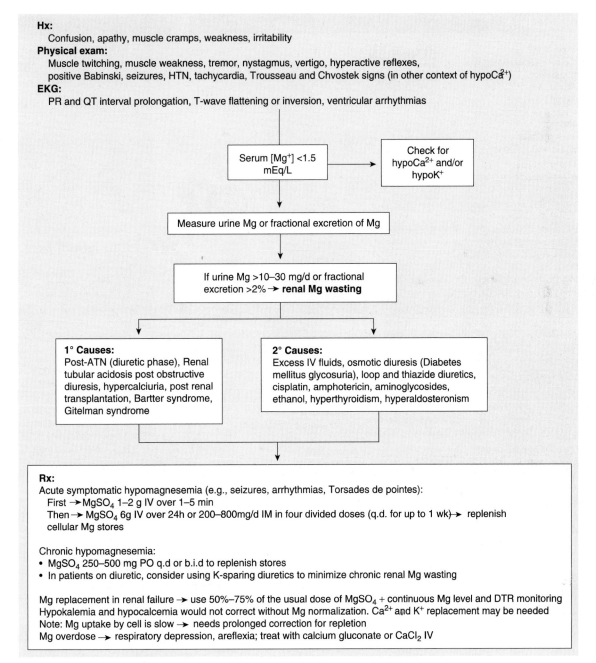

Hx:
Confusion, apathy, muscle cramps, weakness, irritability
Physical exam:
Muscle twitching, muscle weakness, tremor, nystagmus, vertigo, hyperactive reflexes, positive Babinski, seizures, HTN, tachycardia, Trousseau and Chvostek signs (in other context of hypoCa²⁺)
EKG:
PR and QT interval prolongation, T-wave flattening or inversion, ventricular arrhythmias

Serum [Mg⁺] <1.5 mEq/L → Check for hypoCa²⁺ and/or hypoK⁺

Measure urine Mg or fractional excretion of Mg

If urine Mg >10–30 mg/d or fractional excretion >2% → **renal Mg wasting**

1° Causes:
Post-ATN (diuretic phase), Renal tubular acidosis post obstructive diuresis, hypercalciuria, post renal transplantation, Bartter syndrome, Gitelman syndrome

2° Causes:
Excess IV fluids, osmotic diuresis (Diabetes mellitus glycosuria), loop and thiazide diuretics, cisplatin, amphotericin, aminoglycosides, ethanol, hyperthyroidism, hyperaldosteronism

Rx:
Acute symptomatic hypomagnesemia (e.g., seizures, arrhythmias, Torsades de pointes):
First → MgSO₄ 1–2 g IV over 1–5 min
Then → MgSO₄ 6g IV over 24h or 200–800mg/d IM in four divided doses (q.d. for up to 1 wk) → replenish cellular Mg stores

Chronic hypomagnesemia:
• MgSO₄ 250–500 mg PO q.d or b.i.d to replenish stores
• In patients on diuretic, consider using K-sparing diuretics to minimize chronic renal Mg wasting

Mg replacement in renal failure → use 50%–75% of the usual dose of MgSO₄ + continuous Mg level and DTR monitoring
Hypokalemia and hypocalcemia would not correct without Mg normalization. Ca²⁺ and K⁺ replacement may be needed
Note: Mg uptake by cell is slow → needs prolonged correction for repletion
Mg overdose → respiratory depression, areflexia; treat with calcium gluconate or CaCl₂ IV

Figure 13.4 Approach to hypomagnesemia.

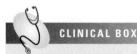

CLINICAL BOX

Check for hypomagnesemia in patients with ventricular arrhythmias (particularly if ischemia + diuretic use).

EKG Δs $2°$ to hypomagnesemia are the same as those $2°$ to hypokalemia.

Table **13.3**	**Renal Losses of Mg**
Diuretics	Thiazides, Loop
Volume expansion	Diabetes mellitus, hyperthyroidism, hypercalcemia, Conn syndrome
Tubular dysfunction	Cyclosporin, ethanol, amphotericin, aminoglycosides, cisplatin, ATN (diuretic phase), tubulointerstitial disease, Bartter syndrome, Gitelman syndrome

APPROACH

See Figure 13.4.

HYPERKALEMIA

DEFINITION

Serum $[K^+] > 5.0$ mEq/L

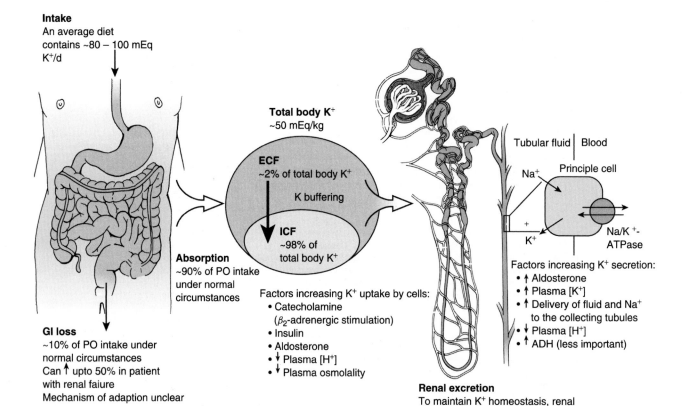

Intake
An average diet contains ~80 – 100 mEq K^+/d

Total body K^+
~50 mEq/kg

ECF
~2% of total body K^+

K buffering

ICF
~98% of total body K^+

Absorption
~90% of PO intake under normal circumstances

Factors increasing K^+ uptake by cells:
• Catecholamine (β_2-adrenergic stimulation)
• Insulin
• Aldosterone
• ↓ Plasma $[H^+]$
• ↓ Plasma osmolality

GI loss
~10% of PO intake under normal circumstances
Can ↑ upto 50% in patient with renal faiure
Mechanism of adaption unclear

Tubular fluid | Blood

Principle cell

Na^+

K^+

Na/K^+-ATPase

Factors increasing K^+ secretion:
• ↑ Aldosterone
• ↑ Plasma $[K^+]$
• ↑ Delivery of fluid and Na^+ to the collecting tubules
• ↓ Plasma $[H^+]$
• ↑ ADH (less important)

Renal excretion
To maintain K^+ homeostasis, renal excretion = GI K^+ absorption (K^+ from alternative routes if applicable) The principle cells of the distal and cortical collecting tubules are the main players in K^+ secretion, which in turn is the most important determinant of renal K^+ excretion.

Figure 13.5 K^+ handling.

APPLIED SCIENTIFIC CONCEPTS

K Adaptation

- Renal response to prolonged (>20 d) ↑ in K^+ load (e.g., from ↑ dietary intake)
- Significant ↑ in the efficiency of renal K^+ excretion
- Mediated by enhanced activity of Na/K-ATPases of renal principal cells
- Manifested by gradual return of $[K^+]$ and aldosterone level to near normal
- Reabsorption of K^+ in the PCT and the loop of Henle remains, however, at a constant rate

CAUSAL CONDITIONS

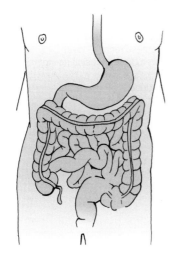
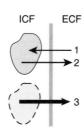
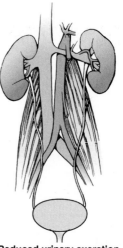

ICF   ECF

Increased intake
(usually associated with impaired excretion)
- Increased dietary intake
- Excessive PO or IV K^+ supplementation

Redistribution
1. Decreased entry into cells
   - Insulin deficiency
   - Digitalis overdose
   - β-Blocker toxicity
2. Increased exit from cells
   - Non anion gap metabolic acidosis
   - Hyperosmolarity (e.g., hyperglycemia)
   - Exercise
3. Cell lysis
   - Rhabdomyolysis
   - Trauma/crush syndrome
   - GI bleeding
   - Intravascular hemolysis
   - Tumor lysis

Reduced urinary excretion
Decreased GFR
- ARF/CRF
Decreased secretion (TTKG <4)
- Hypoaldosteronism
   - Type 4 renal tubular acidosis
   - Aldosterone deficiency
   - Aldosterone resistance
   - Adrenal insufficiency
   - Dysfunction of distal renal tubule
- Drugs
   - NSAIDs
   - ACEI or ARB
   - K^+-sparing diuretics
   - Heparin
Decreased tubular flow rate
- Severe effective volume depletion
- Severe cardiomyopathy

Figure 13.6 Causal conditions of hyperkalemia.

APPROACH

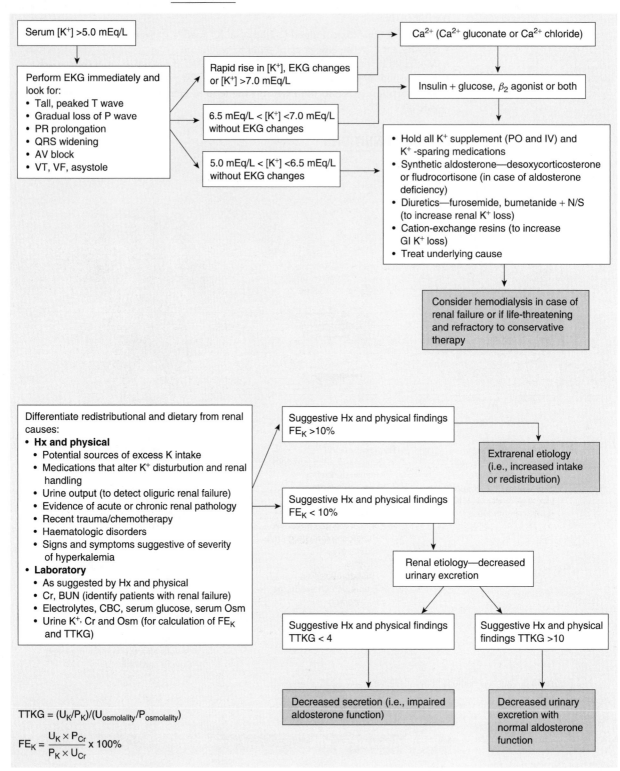

Figure 13.7 Approach to hyperkalemia.

EFFECTS OF HYPOKALEMIA ON EKG

- Hyperkalemia: symmetrically peaked T waves
- Severe hyperkalemia (>8 mEq/L): sine wave

HYPOKALEMIA

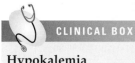

Hypokalemia

Serum [K⁺] <3.5 mEq/L

RATIONALE

- Common incidental finding on routine serum electrolytes and EKG
- Severe deficits likely chronic and symptoms tend to develop late

APPLIED SCIENTIFIC CONCEPTS

See Chapter 13—Hyperkalemia.

CAUSAL CONDITIONS

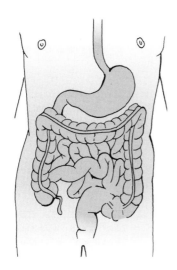

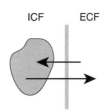

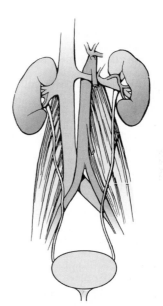

Decreased intake (<1 g/d; rare cause of hypokalemia)
- Starvation
- Anorexia nervosa
- Clay ingestion

Increased GI loss
- Infectious diarrhea
- Villous adenoma
- Laxative abuse
- Tube drainage
- Enteropathy 2° to chemo- or radiotherapy

Redistribution
- Insulin therapy
- Alkalemia
- β-Adrenergic drugs
- Verapamil intoxication
- Chloroquine intoxication
- Delirium tremens (through sympathetic activation → β-adrenergic stimulation)
- Hyperthyroidism (rare; predilection for Asian parents)
- Rapid hematopoiesis (eg., treatment of severe pernicious anemia with vitamin B₁₂)
- Barium poisoning
- Refeeding syndrome

Increased renal loss
High tubular flow rate
- Non-K⁺-sparing diuretics
- Bartter syndrome (hereditary dysfunction of Na transporters in the loop of Henle)
- Gitelman syndrome (hereditary dysfunction of Na transporters in early distal tubule)

High tubular [K⁺] (TTKG >4)
- Hyperaldosteronism (1° or 2°)
- Adrenal hyperplasia
- Pseudohyperaldosteronism
- Cushing syndrome
- Ectopic ACTH
- Juxtaglomerular tumor

Figure 13.8 Causal conditions of hypokalemia.

APPROACH

MANAGEMENT

- Step 1: reduce/stop redistribution or loss of K⁺
  - Correct any abnormalities in acid–base balance
  - Replace Mg⁺⁺ if concomitant deficit
  - Use propranolol for nonspecific β-adrenergic blockade
  - For patients on diuretics, consider adding a K⁺-sparing diuretics (with close monitoring of serum [K⁺] and renal function)

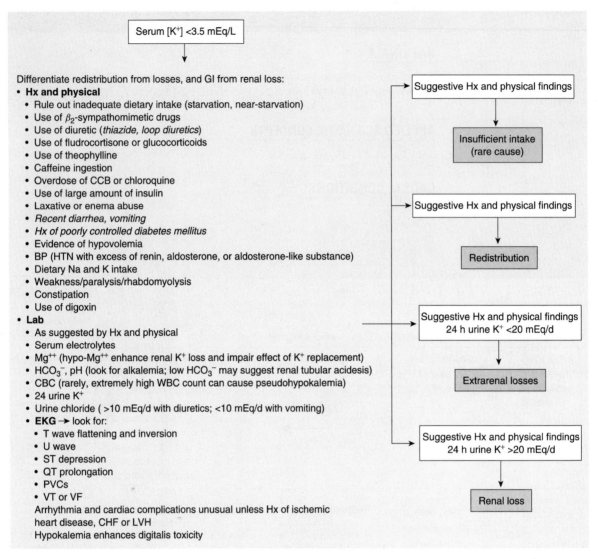

Figure 13.9 Approach to hypokalemia.

- Hold/↓ dose of offending drug(s)
- Treat causative disorder(s) when possible
- Step 2: K⁺ replacement
  - PO (preferred route): potassium chloride (most commonly used), potassium phosphate (if concomitant hypophosphatemia), or potassium bicarbonate (if concomitant metabolic acidosis; rarely used)
  - IV (when there is impaired GI function or evident neuromuscular manifestation of hypokalemia): rate ≤20 mmol/ h
  - Monitor serum [K⁺], EKG, and urine output

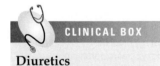

Diuretics

Loop or thiazide diuretics → chloride depletion → hypovolemia and metabolic alkalosis → K⁺ depletion by three mechanisms:

- ↑ Flow and delivery of NaCl to CCD
- Alkalemia → redistributive hypokalemia
- Hypovolemia → activation of renin-angiotensin-aldosterone pathway

HTN

When HTN is a prominent feature, consider:

- Renin excess (e.g., renovascular HTN, renin-secreting tumor)
- Aldosterone excess (1° aldosteronism)
- Excess of aldosterone-like substances (e.g., Cushing syndrome, fludrocortisone ingestion, congenital adrenal hyperplasia)

- Aim to correct the deficit slowly over days to weeks (hyperkalemia is an important side-effect especially common in redistributive hypokalemia)
- Consider instructing patient to ↑ intake of K⁺-rich food

PROTEINURIA

RATIONALE

Proteinuria usually incidental discovery (positive dipstick); if persistent → likely impaired glomerular permselectivity

APPLIED SCIENTIFIC CONCEPTS

See Figure 13.10.

CAUSAL CONDITIONS

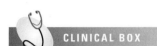

Definitions

Proteinuria → urinary total protein excretion >150 mg/d with ≥30 mg/d albumin

Microalbuminuria → 30 to 300 mg/d albumin

Nephrotic proteinuria → >3.5 g/d total protein

Severity

- >2 g/d → likely glomerular disease
- 0.15 to 2 g/d → likely tubular proteinuria, overflow proteinuria, or mild glomerular disease

Table **13.4**	Causal Conditions of Proteinuria	
Benign		
Transient or intermittent proteinuria (<5%) with fever, dehydration, intense exercise, emotional upset, heat injury, inflammation		
Orthostatic proteinuria (5% of adolescents): >50 mg/8 h while upright		
Persistent		
Glomerular ↑ Glomerular capillary permeability to protein (often related to structural injury)	Active (contain cells, casts, etc.) urine sediment	1°: IgA nephropathy, mesangiocapillary glomerulonephritis, membranoproliferative glomerulonephritis 2°: SLE, anti-GBM disease, postinfectious (streptococcal, hepatitis C, bacterial endocarditis), drugs, Henoch-Schönlein purpura, Wegener granulomatosis, cryoglobulinemia
	Nonactive urine sediment	1°: minimal Δ disease, membranous glomerulonephropathy, focal segmental glomerulosclerosis 2°: diabetic nephropathy, 2° focal segmental glomerulosclerosis, amyloid, hypertensive nephrosclerosis
Tubular ↓ Proximal tubule reabsorption of filtered proteins		Tubulointerstitial disease (causes include NSAID, penicillin derivative and diuretic use; chronic pyelonephritis; Fanconi syndrome; radiation; Sickle cell disease; acute hypersensitivity interstitial nephritis, heavy metals; hypercalcemia; hyperuricemia and obstructive uropathy)
Overflow Overproduction of low molecular weight protein		Plasma cell dyscrasias (MM, MGUS, amyloidosis, etc.) lymphomas, leukemias, hemoglobinuria, myoglobinuria

APPROACH

NEPHRITIC SYNDROMES

- **Berger disease/IgA nephropathy**
- Postinfectious glomerulonephritis
- Goodpastures syndrome
- Alport syndrome
- Wegener granulomatosis
- Membranoproliferative nephropathy

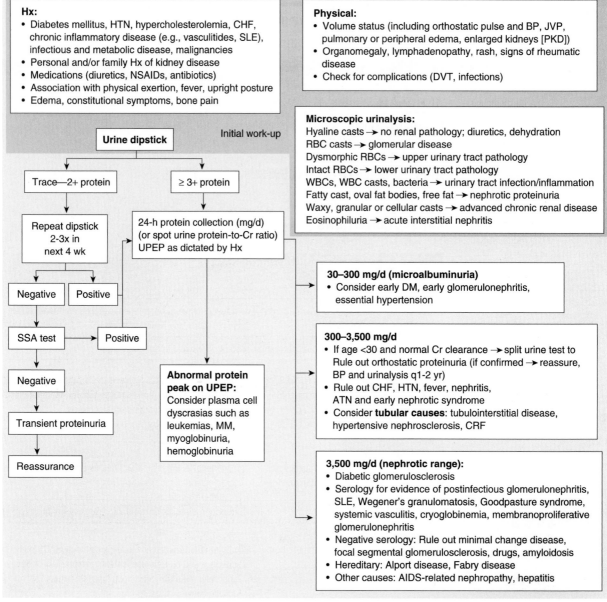

Hx:
- Diabetes mellitus, HTN, hypercholesterolemia, CHF, chronic inflammatory disease (e.g., vasculitides, SLE), infectious and metabolic disease, malignancies
- Personal and/or family Hx of kidney disease
- Medications (diuretics, NSAIDs, antibiotics)
- Association with physical exertion, fever, upright posture
- Edema, constitutional symptoms, bone pain

Physical:
- Volume status (including orthostatic pulse and BP, JVP, pulmonary or peripheral edema, enlarged kidneys [PKD])
- Organomegaly, lymphadenopathy, rash, signs of rheumatic disease
- Check for complications (DVT, infections)

Urine dipstick   Initial work-up

Microscopic urinalysis:
Hyaline casts → no renal pathology; diuretics, dehydration
RBC casts → glomerular disease
Dysmorphic RBCs → upper urinary tract pathology
Intact RBCs → lower urinary tract pathology
WBCs, WBC casts, bacteria → urinary tract infection/inflammation
Fatty cast, oval fat bodies, free fat → nephrotic proteinuria
Waxy, granular or cellular casts → advanced chronic renal disease
Eosinophiluria → acute interstitial nephritis

Trace—2+ protein

≥ 3+ protein

Repeat dipstick 2-3x in next 4 wk

24-h protein collection (mg/d) (or spot urine protein-to-Cr ratio) UPEP as dictated by Hx

Negative   Positive

SSA test → Positive

Negative

Transient proteinuria

Reassurance

Abnormal protein peak on UPEP:
Consider plasma cell dyscrasias such as leukemias, MM, myoglobinuria, hemoglobinuria

30–300 mg/d (microalbuminuria)
- Consider early DM, early glomerulonephritis, essential hypertension

300–3,500 mg/d
- If age <30 and normal Cr clearance → split urine test to Rule out orthostatic proteinuria (if confirmed → reassure, BP and urinalysis q1-2 yr)
- Rule out CHF, HTN, fever, nephritis, ATN and early nephrotic syndrome
- Consider **tubular causes:** tubulointerstitial disease, hypertensive nephrosclerosis, CRF

3,500 mg/d (nephrotic range):
- Diabetic glomerulosclerosis
- Serology for evidence of postinfectious glomerulonephritis, SLE, Wegener's granulomatosis, Goodpasture syndrome, systemic vasculitis, cryoglobinemia, membranoproliferative glomerulonephritis
- Negative serology: Rule out minimal change disease, focal segmental glomerulosclerosis, drugs, amyloidosis
- Hereditary: Alport disease, Fabry disease
- Other causes: AIDS-related nephropathy, hepatitis

Figure 13.10 Approach to proteinuria.

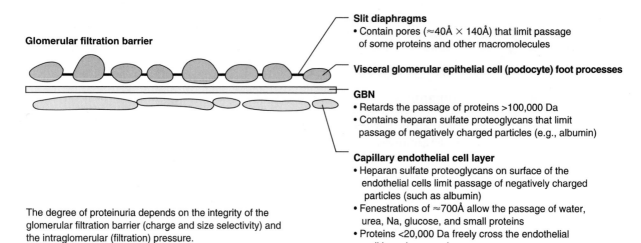

Glomerular filtration barrier

Slit diaphragms
- Contain pores (≈40Å × 140Å) that limit passage of some proteins and other macromolecules

Visceral glomerular epithelial cell (podocyte) foot processes

GBN
- Retards the passage of proteins >100,000 Da
- Contains heparan sulfate proteoglycans that limit passage of negatively charged particles (e.g., albumin)

Capillary endothelial cell layer
- Heparan sulfate proteoglycans on surface of the endothelial cells limit passage of negatively charged particles (such as albumin)
- Fenestrations of ≈700Å allow the passage of water, urea, Na, glucose, and small proteins
- Proteins <20,000 Da freely cross the endothelial cell layer in general

The degree of proteinuria depends on the integrity of the glomerular filtration barrier (charge and size selectivity) and the intraglomerular (filtration) pressure.

Figure 13.11 Glomerular filtration barrier of macromolecules.

Patients with **nephrotic range proteinuria** have significantly **higher risk of progression to renal failure** than those with mild proteinuria.

Normally Excreted Proteins

- 40% Tamm-Horsfall muco-proteins
- 40% Albumin
- 20% Igs

NEPHROTIC SYNDROMES

- **Membranous nephropathy**
- **Diabetic nephropathy**
- Minimal Δ disease
- Lupus nephritis
- Focal segmental glomerular sclerosis
- Renal amylodosis
- Membranoproliferative nephropathy

MANAGEMENT

- If HTN → BP control
  - Target BP <125/75 mm Hg
  - ACEIs and ARBs preferred (have a proteinuria-reducing effect independent of anti-HTN effect)
- If normotensive at low-dose ACEIs or ARBs as tolerated
- If fluid overload/edema at salt and water restrictions ± diuretics (with caution)
- If diabetic → tight glucose control
- If 1° glomerular disease → treat with corticosteroids, diuretics, cytotoxic agents, antihypertensives, and plasmapheresis as appropriate
- Dietary protein restrictions of 0.8 to 1 g/kg/d (controversial)
- Consider treating 2° lipid abnormalities if persistent (particularly if other risk factors for CVD)
- Consider anticoagulant prophylaxis if a second risk factor for venous thrombosis develops

HYPERNATREMIA

Hypernatremia

[Na] $_{serum}$ >145 mEq/L

Hypernatremia is rarely due to Na gain → check for water loss first. For patients at the extremes of age, there may be:

- Difficulty acquiring/asking for water impaired thirst mechanism (elderly)

RATIONALE

Uncommon: mainly in elderly and pediatric populations

CAUSAL CONDITIONS

Table **13.5**	**Causal Conditions of Hypernatremia**
Water depletion (dehydration)	Impaired thirst perception, ↓ water intake ↑ Loss
Na gain	Hypertonic solutions (e.g., tube feeding/IV), excess dietary salt intake, hypertonic dialysis, 1° hyperaldosteronism, Cushing syndrome
Renal loss	Diabetes insipidus, osmotic diuresis (glucose, mannitol, urea), diuretics, ATN (diuretic phase), postobstructive diuresis
GI loss	Diarrhea, vomiting (with more water than NaCl loss; mostly seen in infants)
Other losses	Sweating, burns, dermal and respiratory insensible losses; hypernatremia mainly seen in unconscious or incapacitated patients due to concomitant lack of access to water

$$\text{Water deficit} = [(\text{Plasma [Na]} - 140)/140] \times \text{TBW}$$

$$\text{TBW} = 0.4 - 0.6 \times \text{lean body mass}$$

APPROACH

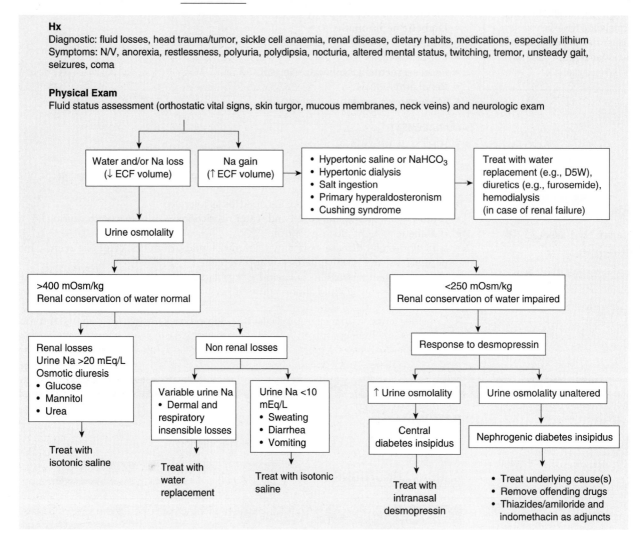

Hx
Diagnostic: fluid losses, head trauma/tumor, sickle cell anaemia, renal disease, dietary habits, medications, especially lithium
Symptoms: N/V, anorexia, restlessness, polyuria, polydipsia, nocturia, altered mental status, twitching, tremor, unsteady gait, seizures, coma

Physical Exam
Fluid status assessment (orthostatic vital signs, skin turgor, mucous membranes, neck veins) and neurologic exam

Water and/or Na loss (↓ ECF volume)

Na gain (↑ ECF volume)

- Hypertonic saline or NaHCO$_3$
- Hypertonic dialysis
- Salt ingestion
- Primary hyperaldosteronism
- Cushing syndrome

Treat with water replacement (e.g., D5W), diuretics (e.g., furosemide), hemodialysis (in case of renal failure)

Urine osmolality

>400 mOsm/kg
Renal conservation of water normal

<250 mOsm/kg
Renal conservation of water impaired

Renal losses
Urine Na >20 mEq/L
Osmotic diuresis
- Glucose
- Mannitol
- Urea

Non renal losses

Response to desmopressin

Variable urine Na
- Dermal and respiratory insensible losses

Urine Na <10 mEq/L
- Sweating
- Diarrhea
- Vomiting

↑ Urine osmolality

Urine osmolality unaltered

Treat with isotonic saline

Treat with water replacement

Treat with isotonic saline

Central diabetes insipidus

Nephrogenic diabetes insipidus

Treat with intranasal desmopressin

- Treat underlying cause(s)
- Remove offending drugs
- Thiazides/amiloride and indomethacin as adjuncts

Figure 13.12 Approach to hypernatremia.

CLINICAL BOX

Overly rapid replacement of water losses → cerebral edema → impaired mental status, headaches, memory loss, seizures, coma

Correct water deficit slowly over at least 48 to 72 h (aim to ↓ [Na$^+$] by 0.5 to 1 mmol/L/h).

Use ¼ or ½ N/S for treatment of hypovolemic hypernatremia.

Use D5 W and concomitant diuretics for treatment of hypervolemic hypernatremia.

CLINICAL BOX

Serum Na$^+$ >150 mEq/L → refer

- Hypervolemic hypernatremia, severe dehydration or altered mental status → admit
- Isolated hypernatremia has no specific effect on EKG

HYPONATREMIA

RATIONALE

- Frequent incidental finding in asymptomatic patients
- Most common electrolyte abnormality in hospitalized patients (2% prevalence)
- Severe (<120 mmol/L) or abrupt hyponatremia → ↑ risk of neurologic complications (due to cerebral edema)
- Pediatric cases often iatrogenic

APPLIED SCIENTIFIC CONCEPTS

Na$^+$ is the predominant ECF cation and key in determining plasma osmolality (see Figure 13.13).

HYPO-OSMOLAR HYPONATREMIA

- Water intake > renal excretory capacity of max 1 L/h (e.g., 1° polydipsia): absolute ADH inhibition → ++ dilute urine (Osm$_{urine}$ <100 mmol/kg, specific gravity <1.003)
- Water retention 2° to impaired renal water excretion (as in CHF): sustained ADH secretion → impaired renal free water excretion

  Either SIADH or ↓ ECV can lead to inability to suppress ADH.

CONDITIONS ASSOCIATED WITH SIADH

- CNS (**meningitis**, encephalitis, brain abscess, brain tumor, **CVA, subarachnoid hemorrhage, subdural hematoma, head trauma, etc.**)
- Pulmonary (**pneumonia, asthma, COPD**, tuberculosis, pulmonary abscess, aspergillosis, acute respiratory failure, atelectasis, pneumothorax, positive pressure ventilation, etc.)
- Tumor (especially small cell lung CA, etc.)
- Endocrine (hypothyroidism, hypopituitarism, Addisons disease)
- Surgery (trans-sphenoidal pituitary surgery, major abdominal or thoracic surgery)
- Drugs (**SSRIs**, MAOIs, TCAs, opioids, carbamazepine, oxcarbazepine, cyclophosphamide, vincristine, vinblastine, **chlorpromamide**, bromocriptine, amiodarone, ecstasy, nicotine, haloperidol, **thiazide diuretics**; exogenous vasopressin, desmopressin, and oxytocin)
- Others (HIV, hereditary SIADH, protracted exercise, emotional stress, **extreme pain, severe nausea**)

CLINICAL BOX

Plasma osmolality (mOsm/kg) = 2[Na$^+$] + [glucose] + [urea] (all units in mmol/L)

CAUSAL CONDITIONS AND APPROACH

- Hx (see Figure 13.14)
  - Recent fluid losses/shifts
  - Use of hypotonic fluids
  - Drugs (especially diuretics)
  - Hx of CHF, cirrhosis, nephrotic syndrome
  - Hx suggestive of possible SIADH
- Physical exam
  - Neurologic status—mental status, muscle weakness
  - Volume status
- Note: Premenopausal women are particularly susceptible to the effects of cerebral oedema.

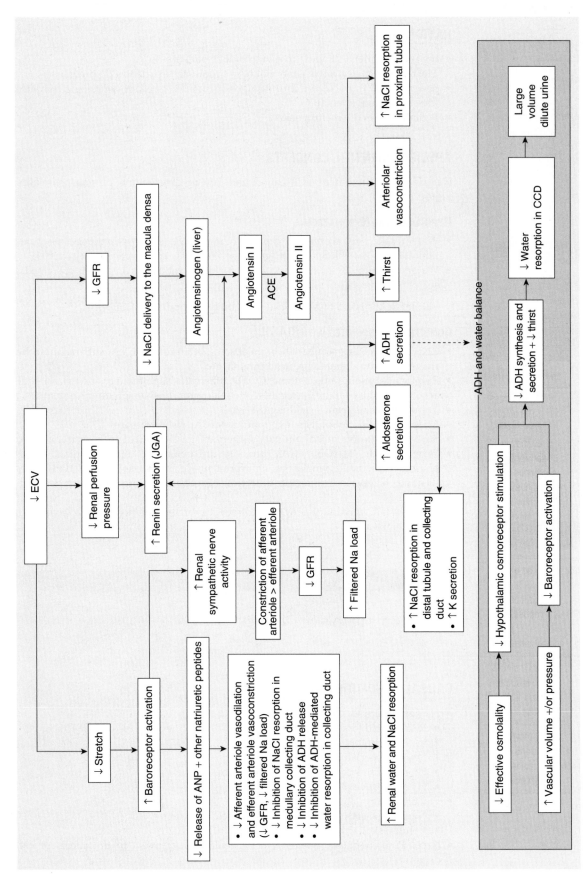

Figure 13.13 Renal Na$^+$ and water control.

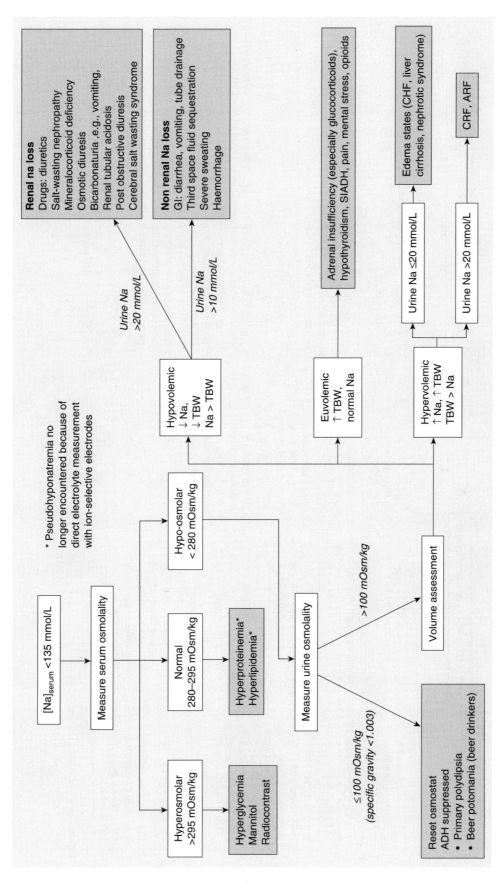

Figure 13.14 Causal conditions and approach to hyponatremia.

351

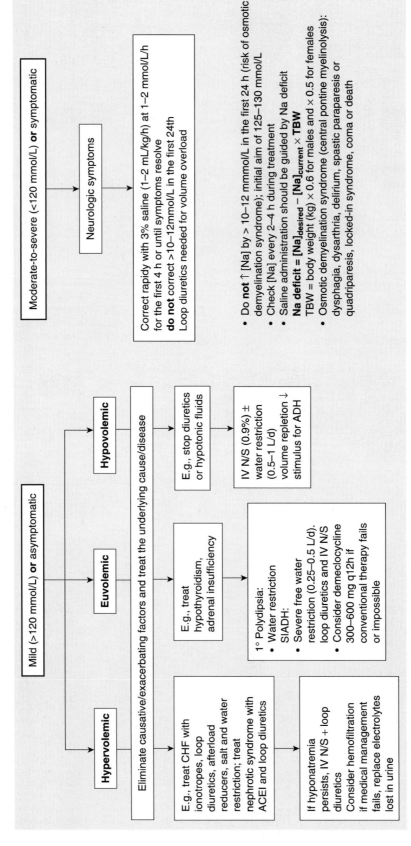

Figure 13.15 Management of hyponatremia.

Mild (>120 mmol/L) **or** asymptomatic

Eliminate causative/exacerbating factors and treat the underlying cause/disease

Hypervolemic

E.g., treat CHF with ionotropes, loop diuretics, afterload reducers, salt and water restriction; treat nephrotic syndrome with ACEI and loop diuretics

If hyponatremia persists, IV N/S + loop diuretics
Consider hemofiltration if medical management fails, replace electrolytes lost in urine

Euvolemic

E.g., treat hypothyroidism, adrenal insufficiency

1° Polydipsia:
• Water restriction
SIADH:
• Severe free water restriction (0.25–0.5 L/d), loop diuretics and IV N/S
• Consider demeclocycline 300–600 mg q12h if conventional therapy fails or impossible

Hypovolemic

E.g., stop diuretics or hypotonic fluids

IV N/S (0.9%) ± water restriction (0.5–1 L/d)
volume repletion ↓ stimulus for ADH

Moderate-to-severe (<120 mmol/L) **or** symptomatic

Neurologic symptoms

Correct rapidly with 3% saline (1–2 mL/kg/h) at 1–2 mmol/L/h for the first 4 h or until symptoms resolve
do not correct >10–12mmol/L in the first 24th
Loop diuretics needed for volume overload

• Do **not** ↑ [Na] by > 10–12 mmmol/L in the first 24 h (risk of osmotic demyelination syndrome); initial aim of 125–130 mmol/L
• Check [Na] every 2–4 h during treatment
• Saline administration should be guided by Na deficit
Na deficit = [Na]$_{desired}$ **− [Na]**$_{current}$ × **TBW**
TBW = body weight (kg) × 0.6 for males and × 0.5 for females
• Osmotic demyelination syndrome (central pontine myelinolysis): dysphagia, dysarthria, delirium, spastic paraparesis or quadriparesis, locked-in syndrome, coma or death

ACUTE VERSUS CHRONIC

- Acute
  - If mild (120 to 130 mmol/L) → asymptomatic or nausea, malaise, anorexia, headache, lethargy, weakness, confusion
  - If abrupt and severe (<120 mmol/L) → delirium, neuromuscular hyperexcitability, seizures, coma, respiratory arrest, death
  - Complications → brainstem herniation; hypothalamic and posterior pituitary infarction
- Chronic
  - Cerebral adaptation → often asymptomatic (even with [Na] as low as 110 mmol/L)
  - If symptomatic, nausea, fatigue, gait instability, amnesia, confusion, lethargy, muscle cramps

MANAGEMENT

See Figure 13.15.

ACUTE RENAL FAILURE

DEFINITION

Sudden and rapid (hours to days) fall in GFR leading to accumulation of nitrogenous waste products.

Common clinical manifestations → azotemia (due to ↓ GFR, associated with ↑ urea and Cr) and often abnormal urine volume (anuria—urine output < 100 mL/24 h or oliguria—urine output between 100 and 400 mL/24 h)

APPLIED SCIENTIFIC CONCEPTS

$GFR = K_f (\Delta P - \Delta \pi)$. Determinants of GFR → properties of the glomerular filtration barrier (surface area and permeability → ultrafiltration coefficient K_f), hydrostatic and oncotic pressure gradients (ΔP and $\Delta \pi$) between glomerular capillary and Bowman space.

Tubuloglomerular feedback: Na^+ delivery to macula densa regulates afferent arteriolar tone. ↑ Delivery → vasoconstriction

Glomerulotubular balance: Proximal tubule tends to reabsorb a constant proportion (rather than amount) of the glomerular filtrate.

Renal portal circulation: afferent arteriole → glomerular capillaries → efferent arteriole → vasa recta

Systemic and local factors (sympathetic discharge, myogenic autoregulation, tubuloglomerular feedback, prostaglandins, angiotensin II) help maintain constant GFR through regulation of afferent and efferent arteriolar tones.

Counter-current flow in the vasa recta → pO_2 is higher in renal cortex and lower in renal medulla.

Being located in outer medulla and having the highest rate of energy-dependant solute transport, the medullary portions of the proximal tubule and of the TAL are the most vulnerable to ischemic injury (ischemic ATN).

CAUSAL CONDITIONS

See Figure 13.16.

APPROACH

STEP 1A: DIFFERENTIATE ACUTE VERSUS CHRONIC VERSUS ACUTE ON CHRONIC

- Determine duration of problem
- Review of lab records
- Search for evidence of CRF (anemia, neuropathy, renal osteodystrophy, small scarred kidneys on ultrasound or renal isotope scan)

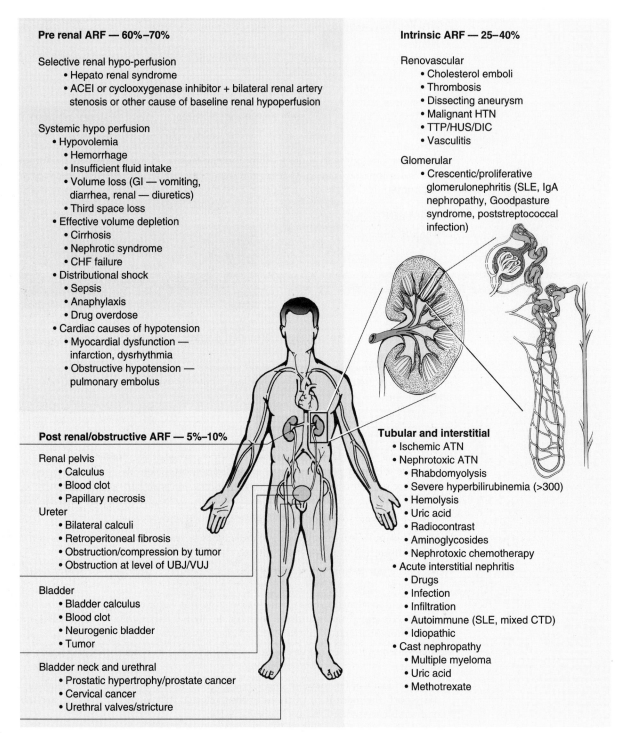

Pre renal ARF — 60%–70%

Selective renal hypo-perfusion
- Hepato renal syndrome
- ACEI or cyclooxygenase inhibitor + bilateral renal artery stenosis or other cause of baseline renal hypoperfusion

Systemic hypo perfusion
- Hypovolemia
  - Hemorrhage
  - Insufficient fluid intake
  - Volume loss (GI — vomiting, diarrhea, renal — diuretics)
  - Third space loss
- Effective volume depletion
  - Cirrhosis
  - Nephrotic syndrome
  - CHF failure
- Distributional shock
  - Sepsis
  - Anaphylaxis
  - Drug overdose
- Cardiac causes of hypotension
  - Myocardial dysfunction — infarction, dysrhythmia
  - Obstructive hypotension — pulmonary embolus

Post renal/obstructive ARF — 5%–10%

Renal pelvis
- Calculus
- Blood clot
- Papillary necrosis

Ureter
- Bilateral calculi
- Retroperitoneal fibrosis
- Obstruction/compression by tumor
- Obstruction at level of UBJ/VUJ

Bladder
- Bladder calculus
- Blood clot
- Neurogenic bladder
- Tumor

Bladder neck and urethral
- Prostatic hypertrophy/prostate cancer
- Cervical cancer
- Urethral valves/stricture

Intrinsic ARF — 25–40%

Renovascular
- Cholesterol emboli
- Thrombosis
- Dissecting aneurysm
- Malignant HTN
- TTP/HUS/DIC
- Vasculitis

Glomerular
- Crescentic/proliferative glomerulonephritis (SLE, IgA nephropathy, Goodpasture syndrome, poststreptococcal infection)

Tubular and interstitial
- Ischemic ATN
- Nephrotoxic ATN
  - Rhabdomyolysis
  - Severe hyperbilirubinemia (>300)
  - Hemolysis
  - Uric acid
  - Radiocontrast
  - Aminoglycosides
  - Nephrotoxic chemotherapy
- Acute interstitial nephritis
  - Drugs
  - Infection
  - Infiltration
  - Autoimmune (SLE, mixed CTD)
  - Idiopathic
- Cast nephropathy
  - Multiple myeloma
  - Uric acid
  - Methotrexate

Figure 13.16 Causal conditions of ARF.

STEP 1B: DIFFERENTIATE PRERENAL VERSUS INTRINSIC VERSUS POSTRENAL ARF AND IDENTIFY CAUSE

Step 1a: Differentiate acute vs. chronic vs. acute chronic
- Determine duration of problem
- Review of lab records
- Search for evidence of CRF (anemia, neuropathy, renal osteodystrophy, small scarred kidneys on ultrasound or renal isotope scan)

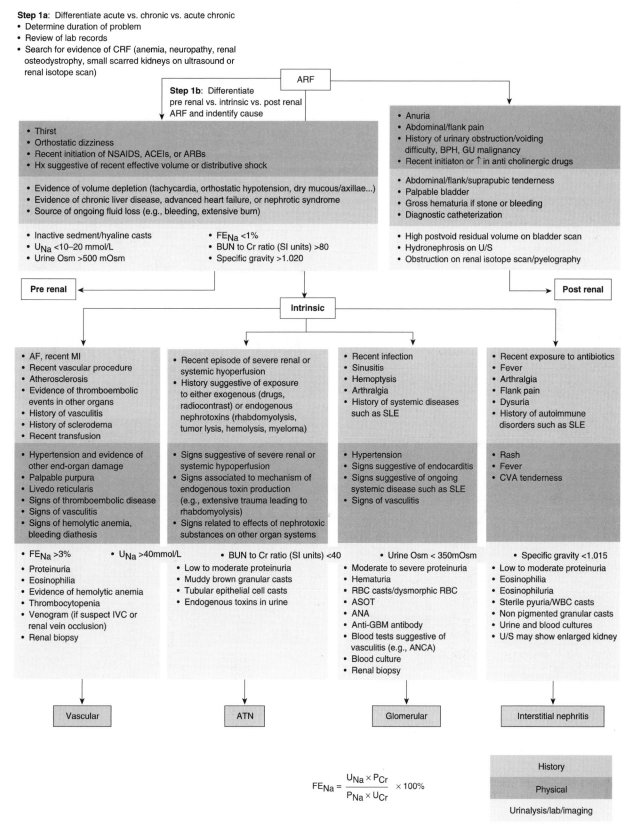

Figure 13.17 Approach to ARF: differentiating types of ARF.

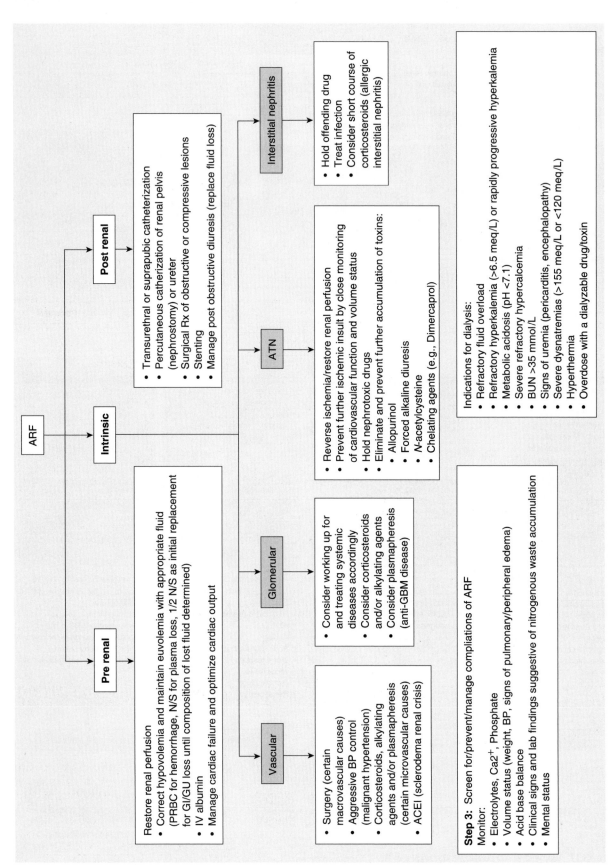

ARF

Pre renal

Intrinsic

Post renal

Restore renal perfusion
- Correct hypovolemia and maintain euvolemia with appropriate fluid (PRBC for hemorrhage, N/S for plasma loss, 1/2 N/S as initial replacement for GI/GU loss until composition of lost fluid determined)
- IV albumin
- Manage cardiac failure and optimize cardiac output

- Transurethral or suprapubic catheterization
- Percutaneous catherization of renal pelvis (nephrostomy) or ureter
- Surgical Rx of obstructive or compressive lesions
- Stenting
- Manage post obstructive diuresis (replace fluid loss)

Vascular

Glomerular

ATN

Interstitial nephritis

- Surgery (certain macrovascular causes)
- Aggressive BP control (malignant hypertension)
- Corticosteroids, alkylating agents and/or plasmapheresis (certain microvascular causes)
- ACEI (scleroderma renal crisis)

- Consider working up for and treating systemic diseases accordingly
- Consider corticosteroids and/or alkylating agents
- Consider plasmapheresis (anti-GBM disease)

- Reverse ischemia/restore renal perfusion
- Prevent further ischemic insult by close monitoring of cardiovascular function and volume status
- Hold nephrotoxic drugs
- Eliminate and prevent further accumulation of toxins:
- Allopurinol
- Forced alkaline diuresis
- N-acetylcysteine
- Chelating agents (e.g., Dimercaprol)

- Hold offending drug
- Treat infection
- Consider short course of corticosteroids (allergic interstitial nephritis)

Step 3: Screen for/prevent/manage compliations of ARF
Monitor:
- Electrolytes, Ca^{2+}, Phosphate
- Volume status (weight, BP, signs of pulmonary/peripheral edema)
- Acid base balance
- Clinical signs and lab findings suggestive of nitrogenous waste accumulation
- Mental status

Indications for dialysis:
- Refractory fluid overload
- Refractory hyperkalemia (>6.5 meq/L) or rapidly progressive hyperkalemia
- Metabolic acidosis (pH <7.1)
- Severe refractory hypercalcemia
- BUN >35 mmol/L
- Signs of uremia (pericarditis, encephalopathy)
- Severe dysnatremias (>155 meq/L or <120 meq/L)
- Hyperthermia
- Overdose with a dialyzable drug/toxin

Figure 13.18 Management of ARF.

356

Table **13.6**	Complications and Initial Management of ARF
ARF Complication	**Initial Management**
Intravascular overload	Salt (1–2 g/d) and water (<1 L/d) restriction Loop diuretics with or without thiazide
Hyponatremia	Free water restriction (both PO and IV)
Hyperkalemia	K^+ restriction Discontinue K^+ supplement and K^+ sparing K^+ diuretics Exchange resins Insulin + glucose Sodium bicarbonate Calcium gluconate (for cardioprotection)
Hyperphosphatemia	Restriction of dietary intake Phosphate binding agents
Hypocalcemia	Calcium replacement (IP or IV)
Hypermagnesemia	Discontinue Mg containing antacids
Hyperuricemia	Provide sufficient calorie intake to avoid catabolism
Metabolic acidosis	Protein restriction (0.6 g/kg/d, rich in essential amino acids)

STEP 2: ELIMINATE OFFENDING AGENT(S)/INITIATE DISEASE-SPECIFIC THERAPIES
See Figure 13.18.

SCREEN FOR/PREVENT/MANAGE COMPLICATIONS OF ARF
- Monitor
  - Electrolytes, Ca^{2+}, phosphate
  - Volume status (weight, BP, signs of pulmonary/peripheral edema)
  - Acid–base balance
  - Clinical signs and lab findings suggestive of nitrogenous waste accumulation
  - Mental status
- Indications for dialysis
  - Refractory fluid overload
  - Refractory hyperkalemia (>6.5 mEq/L) or rapidly progressive hyperkalemia
  - Metabolic acidosis (pH <7.1)
  - Severe refractory hypercalcemia
  - BUN >35 mmol/L
  - Signs of uremia (pericarditis, encephalopathy)
  - Severe dysnatremias (>155 mEq/L or <120 mEq/L)
  - Hyperthermia
  - Overdose with a dialyzable drug/toxin

CLINICAL BOX

Other Complications of ARF

- Anemia
- Leukocytosis
- Bleeding diathesis (2° to uremia-induced platelet dysfunction)
- Progress to CRF
- Uremic syndrome

CHRONIC RENAL FAILURE

DEFINITION
- Evidence of renal damage **or** moderately to severely impaired GFR (<60 mL/min) for at least 3 mo
- CRF = chronic renal disease = CKD (most widely used and accepted terminology)

  Cockcroft-Gault equation:

$$\text{GRF} \sim \text{estimated Cr clearance in mL/min/1.73 m}^2 = \frac{(140 - \text{age}) \times \text{weight in kg}}{P_{Cr} \text{ in } \mu mol/L}$$
$$(\times 1.2 \text{ if male})$$

Table **13.7**	Stages of CKD (NKF KDOQI Clinical Practice Guidelines for CKD)	
Stage	**GFR (mL/min)**	**Note**
1	≥ 90	Normal to ↑ GFR with evidence of kidney damage
2	60–89	Mildly ↓ GFR with evidence of kidney damage
3	30–59	Moderately ↓ GFR
4	15–29	Severely ↓ GFR
5	<15 or dialysis	ESRD or renal failure

MDRD equation:

$$GRF \sim \text{estimated Cr clearance in mL} / \text{min} / 1.73\,m^2 = 175 \times P_{Cr}^{-1.154} \times \text{age}^{-0.203}$$
$$\times\ 0.742 \text{ if female} \times 1.210 \text{ if African American}$$

APPLIED SCIENTIFIC CONCEPTS

RENAL FUNCTIONS

- Maintain consistency of ECF volume (thus regulating BP) and osmolality through handling of NaCl and free water.
- Produce erythropoietin, which stimulates production of RBC by bone marrow.
- Maintain calcium homeostasis through activation of vitamin D and tubular handling of calcium and phosphate under the influence of PTH.
- Maintain electrolyte balance through selective tubular handling.
- Contribute to maintenance of acid–base balance through excretion of H^+ and recovery of $HCO3^-$.

Kidneys compensate for loss of nephrons through hyperfiltration by remaining nephrons mediated through ↑ filtration pressure (thereby ↑ filtration rate) in those nephrons. Progressive renal failure eventually develops as long-term damage occurs due to ↑ excretory burdens and hypertensive injury to surviving nephrons.

CAUSAL CONDITIONS

 C₂LEO Box

- Discuss and respect patient preferences before initiating any treatment.
- Renal replacement therapy: high availability in Canada; lifesaving; but may not benefit every patient to the same extent and not always appropriate to be initiated or continued; treat each case individually.
- One important reason for nonreferral by 1° care physicians to nephrologists for dialysis consideration is patient refusal.
- On the basis of the principle of autonomy and the rights to self-determination, a competent patient has the personal and legal right to refuse or withdraw from dialysis. This right must be respected.
- Voluntary, full and honest informed consent essential in helping patient in end-of-life decision making.

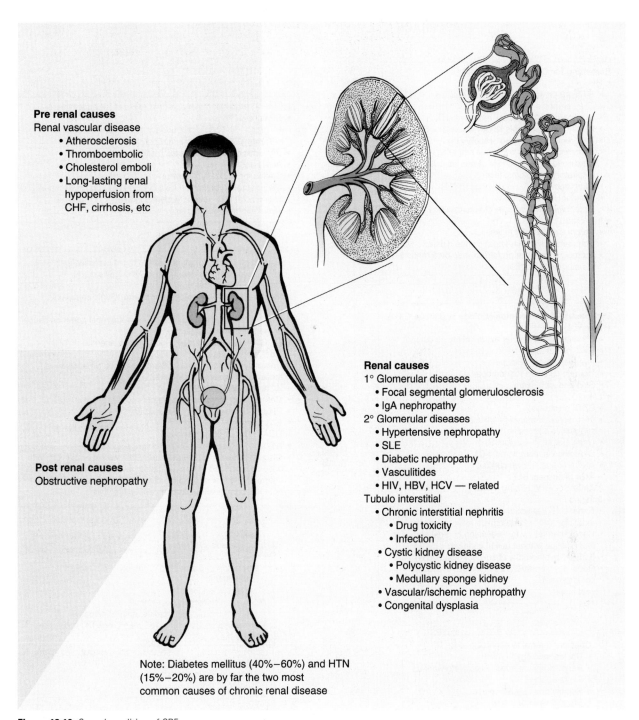

Pre renal causes
Renal vascular disease
- Atherosclerosis
- Thromboembolic
- Cholesterol emboli
- Long-lasting renal hypoperfusion from CHF, cirrhosis, etc

Post renal causes
Obstructive nephropathy

Renal causes
1° Glomerular diseases
- Focal segmental glomerulosclerosis
- IgA nephropathy
2° Glomerular diseases
- Hypertensive nephropathy
- SLE
- Diabetic nephropathy
- Vasculitides
- HIV, HBV, HCV — related
Tubulo interstitial
- Chronic interstitial nephritis
  - Drug toxicity
  - Infection
- Cystic kidney disease
  - Polycystic kidney disease
  - Medullary sponge kidney
- Vascular/ischemic nephropathy
- Congenital dysplasia

Note: Diabetes mellitus (40%–60%) and HTN (15%–20%) are by far the two most common causes of chronic renal disease

Figure 13.19 Causal condition of CRF.

APPROACH

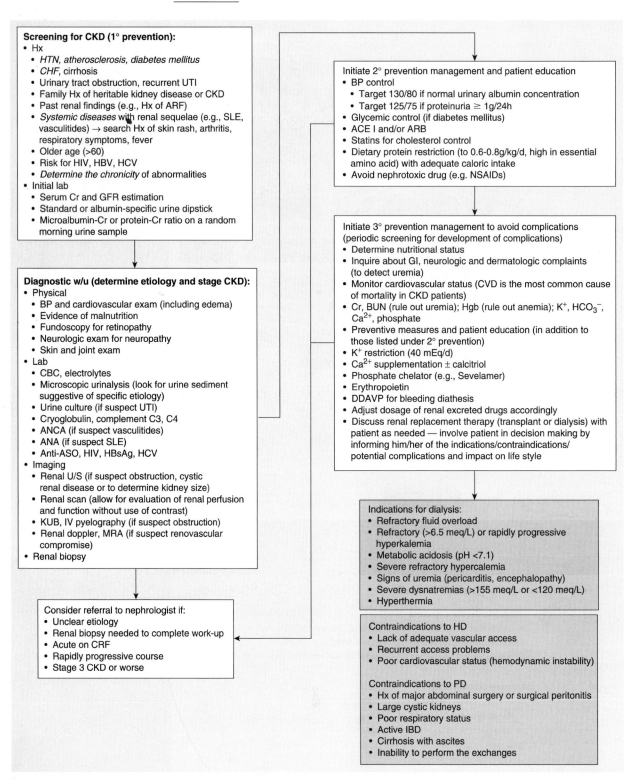

Screening for CKD (1° prevention):
- Hx
  - *HTN, atherosclerosis, diabetes mellitus*
  - *CHF*, cirrhosis
  - Urinary tract obstruction, recurrent UTI
  - Family Hx of heritable kidney disease or CKD
  - Past renal findings (e.g., Hx of ARF)
  - *Systemic diseases* with renal sequelae (e.g., SLE, vasculitides) → search Hx of skin rash, arthritis, respiratory symptoms, fever
  - Older age (>60)
  - Risk for HIV, HBV, HCV
  - *Determine the chronicity* of abnormalities
- Initial lab
  - Serum Cr and GFR estimation
  - Standard or albumin-specific urine dipstick
  - Microalbumin-Cr or protein-Cr ratio on a random morning urine sample

Diagnostic w/u (determine etiology and stage CKD):
- Physical
  - BP and cardiovascular exam (including edema)
  - Evidence of malnutrition
  - Fundoscopy for retinopathy
  - Neurologic exam for neuropathy
  - Skin and joint exam
- Lab
  - CBC, electrolytes
  - Microscopic urinalysis (look for urine sediment suggestive of specific etiology)
  - Urine culture (if suspect UTI)
  - Cryoglobulin, complement C3, C4
  - ANCA (if suspect vasculitides)
  - ANA (if suspect SLE)
  - Anti-ASO, HIV, HBsAg, HCV
- Imaging
  - Renal U/S (if suspect obstruction, cystic renal disease or to determine kidney size)
  - Renal scan (allow for evaluation of renal perfusion and function without use of contrast)
  - KUB, IV pyelography (if suspect obstruction)
  - Renal doppler, MRA (if suspect renovascular compromise)
- Renal biopsy

Consider referral to nephrologist if:
- Unclear etiology
- Renal biopsy needed to complete work-up
- Acute on CRF
- Rapidly progressive course
- Stage 3 CKD or worse

Initiate 2° prevention management and patient education
- BP control
  - Target 130/80 if normal urinary albumin concentration
  - Target 125/75 if proteinuria ≥ 1g/24h
- Glycemic control (if diabetes mellitus)
- ACE I and/or ARB
- Statins for cholesterol control
- Dietary protein restriction (to 0.6-0.8g/kg/d, high in essential amino acid) with adequate caloric intake
- Avoid nephrotoxic drug (e.g. NSAIDs)

Initiate 3° prevention management to avoid complications (periodic screening for development of complications)
- Determine nutritional status
- Inquire about GI, neurologic and dermatologic complaints (to detect uremia)
- Monitor cardiovascular status (CVD is the most common cause of mortality in CKD patients)
- Cr, BUN (rule out uremia); Hgb (rule out anemia); K^+, HCO_3^-, Ca^{2+}, phosphate
- Preventive measures and patient education (in addition to those listed under 2° prevention)
- K^+ restriction (40 mEq/d)
- Ca^{2+} supplementation ± calcitriol
- Phosphate chelator (e.g., Sevelamer)
- Erythropoietin
- DDAVP for bleeding diathesis
- Adjust dosage of renal excreted drugs accordingly
- Discuss renal replacement therapy (transplant or dialysis) with patient as needed — involve patient in decision making by informing him/her of the indications/contraindications/potential complications and impact on life style

Indications for dialysis:
- Refractory fluid overload
- Refractory (>6.5 meq/L) or rapidly progressive hyperkalemia
- Metabolic acidosis (pH <7.1)
- Severe refractory hypercalemia
- Signs of uremia (pericarditis, encephalopathy)
- Severe dysnatremias (>155 meq/L or <120 meq/L)
- Hyperthermia

Contraindications to HD
- Lack of adequate vascular access
- Recurrent access problems
- Poor cardiovascular status (hemodynamic instability)

Contraindications to PD
- Hx of major abdominal surgery or surgical peritonitis
- Large cystic kidneys
- Poor respiratory status
- Active IBD
- Cirrhosis with ascites
- Inability to perform the exchanges

Figure 13.20 Approach to CRF.

CHAPTER 14

Obstetrics and Gynecology

Lamide Oyewumi, Jennifer Lipson, Hisham Khalil, and Andrée Gruslin

DYSMENORRHEA

RATIONALE

- Dysmenorrhea is painful menstruation of uterine origin.
- Affects over 50% of menstruating women to some degree
- Can incapacitate ~10% of women affected for 1 to 3 d/mo
- Most commonly occurs from age 20 to 25
- Single greatest cause of lost working hours and school days among young women

CLINICAL BOX

Dysmenorrhea RFs

1. Presentation at age <30 yr
2. Menarche before age 12
3. Longer cycles/duration of bleeding
4. Irregular or heavy menstrual flow
5. Heavy smoking
6. Nulliparity

CAUSAL CONDITIONS

See Table 14.1.

CLINICAL BOX

Pelvic Pathology

Investigation of pelvic pathology causing dysmenorrhea (2° dysmenorrhea) should be considered if one or more of the following is present:

- **Suspicious** Hx
- Abnormal physical exam
- Failure of NSAID and/or OCP Rx

APPROACH

See Figure 14.1.

Normal Abdo and pelvic exam do not necessarily R/O pathology

CLINICAL BOX

First-line Rx: NSAIDs and/or OCPs

- NSAIDs are effective in up to 70% of women.
- Analgesics may be effective if NSAIDs are contraindicated.
- OCPs can be considered for women who wish to avoid pregnancy.

Table **14.1**	**Classification of Dysmenorrhea**	
	1°	**2°**
Definition	• Menstrual pain **not** caused by an organic disease • No identifiable pelvic pathology • Occurs in ovulatory cycles • Improves in the third decade of reproductive life and after childbirth	• Menstrual pain caused by an organic disease • Associated with pelvic pathology
Onset	• Begins within 6 mo to 2 yr after menarche	• At menarche (during first or second cycles after menarche) or after age 25 • Commonly ages 30–45 yr • Worsens with age (often occurs after years of painless menses)
Etiology	• Pain due to prolonged myometrial uterine contractions and ↓ blood flow to myometrium • These are induced by ↑ PG (PGF$_{2\alpha}$, PGE$_2$) production in the secretory endometrium during ovulatory cycles ("Uterine Angina").	Depends on pelvic pathology: 1. Endometriosis 2. Adenomyosis 3. Uterine leiomyomas (fibroids) 4. Endometrial polyps 5. Nonhormone IUDs 6. PID 7. Ovarian cysts +/− tumors 8. Obstructed outflow tract (i.e., cervical stenosis) 9. Congenital malformations (i.e., bicornuate, septate uterus)
Hx	Pain: • Crampy/colicky • Located in lower Abdo, radiates to lower back, labia, and inner thighs • Starts within 1–4 h of onset of menses; lasts 8–72 h • Is present with every period Other associated Sx (due to PG excess): nausea, vomiting, diarrhea, low backache, headache, dizziness, fatigue	• Pain onset before menses • Other associatedSx: Abdo bloating, pelvic heaviness, back pain • +/− Abnormal bleeding (i.e., premenstrual or IMB, menorrhagia) • +/− Infertility • +/− Dyspareunia • +/− Dyschezia
Physical exam	• Normal external genitalia • Normal pelvic exam (no adnexal tenderness, masses or nodules) • No evidence of vaginal anomalies • May have lower Abdo pain	• May have normal or abnormal pelvic exam.[a] Depends on cause: • Uterine irregularities, cul-de-sac tenderness, or nodularity
Rx	• NSAIDs (if contraindicated, analgesics i.e., acetaminophen) • OCP • Nonpharmacological (i.e., physical exercise, topical heat, high-frequency TENS)	• Little or no response to NSAIDs and/or OCPs • Rx of underlying pathology (i.e., laser ablation or electrocautery of endometriosis)

[a]Normal Abdo and pelvic exam do not necessarily R/O pathology

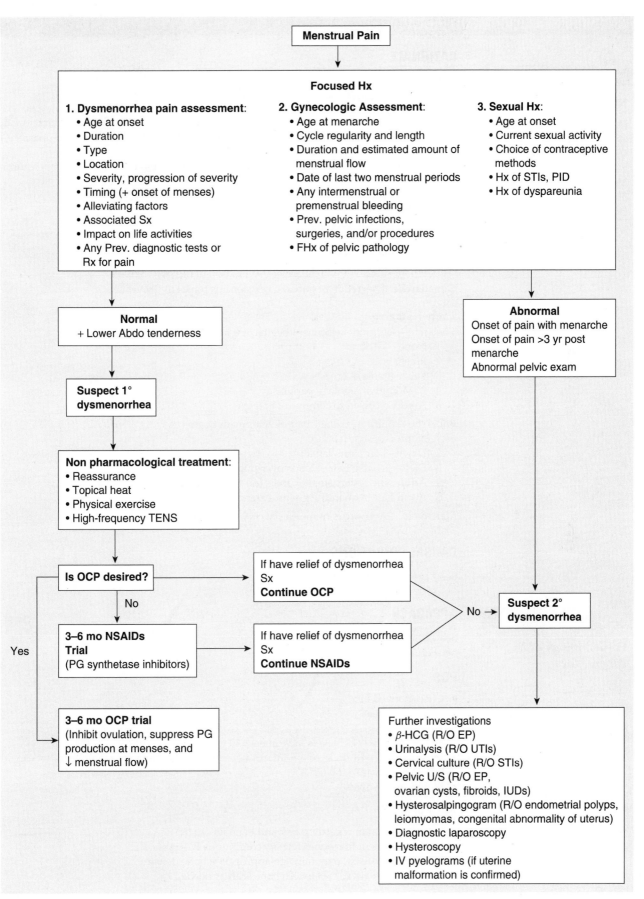

Figure 14.1 Approach to dysmenorrhea.

AMENORRHEA/OLIGOMENORRHEA

Normal Menstruation

Menarche—Avg. age of onset
11 to 13 yr
Menopause—Avg. age of onset
51 yr
Menstruation length—2 to 6 d
Blood loss—20 to 80 mL/cycle
Cycle length—21 to 35 d

RATIONALE

AMENORRHEA

It is the absence or cessation of menstruation.

- **1°**: menstruation that has not started by age 16 in the absence of 2° sexual characteristics (delayed puberty) or menstruation that has not started by age 14 in the presence of normal 2° sexual characteristics
- **2°**: cessation of previously normal menstruation for >6 mo or no menses for >3 normal cycles

OLIGOMENORRHEA

Episodic menstrual bleeding that occurs at intervals of >35 d

STAGES OF PUBERTY: **A G T P M**

Adrenarche: ↑ secretion of adrenal androgens ~2 yr pregonadarche

Gonadarche: ↑ secretion of gonadal sex steroids (onset at ~8 yr)

Tanner Staging

Thelarche—breast development begins at 9 to 11 yr:
1. None
2. Breast bud
3. ↑ Size areola + breasts
4. 2° Mound of areola + papilla
5. Areola recessed to contour of breast

Pubarche —pubic + axillary hair development begins at 11 to 12 yr:
1. None
2. Downy hair along labia
3. Darker/coarse hair extends over pubis
4. Adult type covers smaller areas (no thigh involvement)
5. Adult hair in quantity + type, extends over thighs

Menarche*—Avg. onset of menses at ~13 yr

CAUSAL CONDITIONS

See Table 14.2.

Epidemiology of 2° Amenorrhea

Ovarian causes—40%
Hypothalamic causes—35%
Pituitary disease—19%
Uterine disease—5%
Other—1%

APPROACH

See Table 14.3.
See Figure 14.2 and 14.3.

POF

- Characterized by:
  - Amenorrhea
  - ↓ E
  - ↑ Serum FSH/LH levels in women <40 yr
- Most women with POF retain intermittent ovarian function for many years → can still become pregnant.
- POF ≠ menopause

Rx of POF
- Patient education regarding risk and benefits of HRT
- Replace deficient hormones (cyclic/continuous E + cyclic P)
- HRT to alleviate Sx, maintain age-appropriate bone density
- Yearly F/U of HRT, TSH levels; bone scan as needed

---

*Menarche typically occurs within 2 yr of onset of breast development.

Table **14.2** **DDx of 1° and 2° Amenorrhea**

Body System	1°	2°
Physiologic or pharmaceutical	• Constitutional delay	• Pregnancy • Lactation • Menopause • Drugs (i.e., OCP, danazol phenothiazides, neuroleptics)

Hypothalamus 35% (↓FSH/LH)	• Stress:
	  • Anorexia/bulimia
	  • Nutritional deprivation
	  • Excessive exercise
	  • Emotional stress
	  • Systemic illness
	• Hypothalamic tumor
	• Infiltrate/inflammation/infection of hypothalamus
	• Congenital GnRH deficiency (i.e., Kallmann syndrome)
		• Stress:
		  • Anorexia/bulimia
		  • Nutritional deprivation
		  • Excessive exercise
		  • Emotional stress
		  • Systemic illness
		• Hypothalamic tumor
		• Cushing disease

Pituitary gland 25%	• CNS/pituitary tumor • 1° Hypopituitarism • Hyperprolactinemia	• Sheehan syndrome (postpartum pituitary necrosis after significant PPH) • CNS/pituitary tumor (i.e., prolactinoma)
Thyroid	• Hyper/hypothyroidism	• Hyper/hypothyroidism
Adrenals	• Adrenal tumor—hormone secreting • CAH	• Adrenal tumor—hormone secreting
Ovaries 40%	• PCOS (chronic anovulation) • Androgen insensitivity—XY • Gonadal dysgenesis (Turner syndrome XO)	• Menopause • PCOS (chronic anovulation) • POF • Radiation • Testosterone injections • Chemotherapy
Uterine/outflow tract 5%	• Congenital Müllerian duct abnormalities: • Imperforate hymen • Transverse vaginal septum • Vaginal agenesis (i.e., Mayer-Rokitansky-Kuster-Hauser syndrome)	• Cervical Stenosis • Asherman syndrome* (i.e., Intrauterine adhesions after endometritis, D&C or scarring after delivery

*Most common cause of anatomic amenorrhea

Table **14.3** **Amenorrhea/Oligomenorrhea—Focused Hx and Physical Exam:**

Patient Hx	FHx	Physical Exam
• Menarche • Menstrual Hx • Contraceptive Hx • Sexual Hx • Sources of stress • Diet intake • Exercise Hx, recent weight Δ • Weight—present and 1 yr ago • Growth Hx • Hx of ambiguous genitalia at birth • Drug intake • Exposure to radiation (pelvic, CNS), Prev. pelvic surgeries • Past/current Hx of systemic illness • Anosmia (Kallmann)	• Menarche • Menstrual Hx • Parental height • Parental pubertal Hx • Infertility • Genetic defects • Congenital abnormalities • Endocrinopathies	• Growth chart, BMI • Tanner staging • Thyroid gland exam • Visual acuity • External genitalia (imperforate hymen, atrophic vagina, absence of cervical mucus etc.) • Bimanual exam (enlarged uterus, cystic ovaries etc.) • Signs of abnormal hormone levels (acne, virilization, galactorrhea, hirsutism, etc.) • Dysmorphisms (i.e., Turner—web neck, wide nipples) • Signs of Cushing disease (striae, central obesity, proximal muscle wasting)

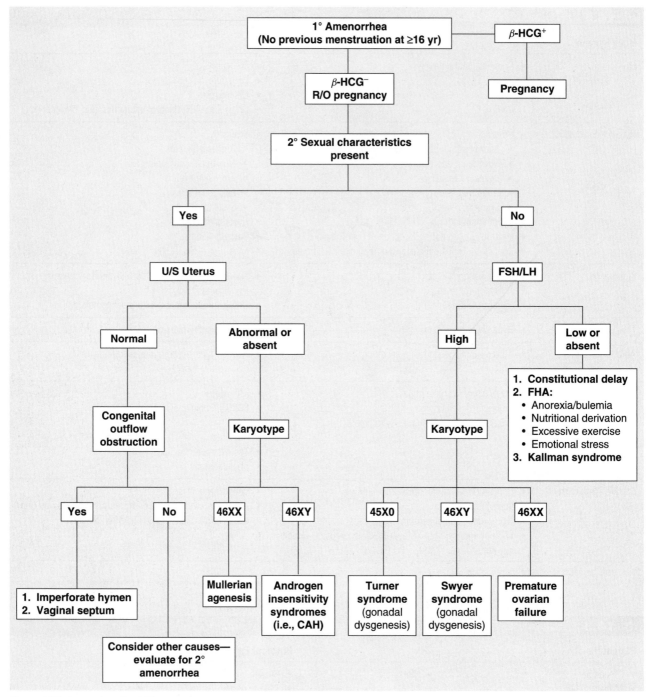

Figure 14.2 Approach to Dx of 1° amenorrhea.

FHA

- Dx of exclusion (must R/O organic disease by imaging)
- Suppression of pulsatile GnRH secretion from hypothalamus → E deficiency

Rx of FHA

- Patient education
- Nutritional counseling regarding ↑ caloric intake
- Ca^{2+} and Vit D supplementation if warranted
- Monitor bone density
- Referral to eating disorder clinics if needed
- Referral to psychologist if needed

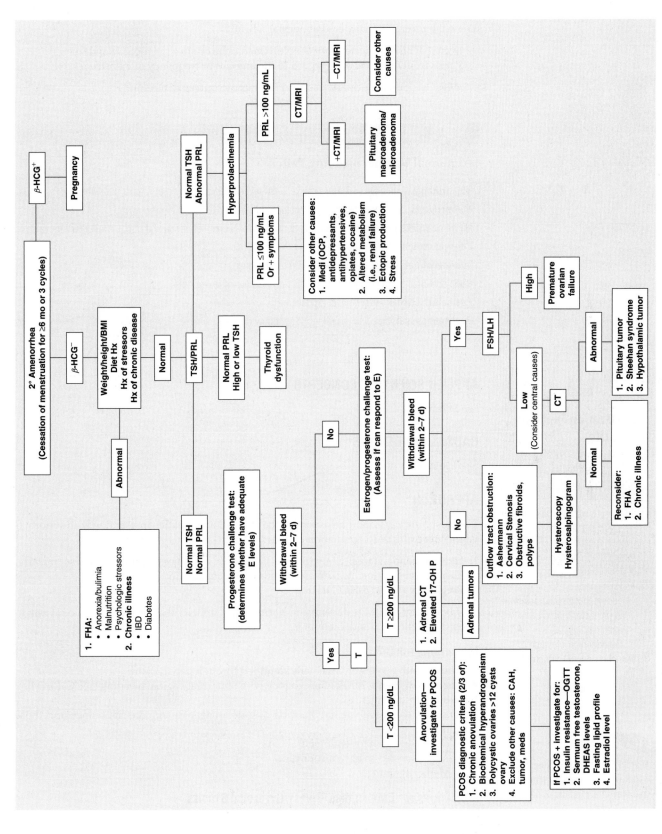

Figure 14.3 Approach to Dx of 2° amenorrhea.

VAGINAL BLEEDING (EXCESSIVE, IRREGULAR, AND ABNORMAL)

DEFINITIONS

Vaginal bleeding is considered abnormal when it:

1. Occurs at an unexpected time—before menarche or after menopause and/or
2. Varies from the norm with regard to the amount or frequency of menstrual flow

> Must exclude the urinary tract and GI tract as sources of bleeding

CLINICAL BOX

Abnormal Vaginal Bleeding Patterns

Menorrhagia: prolonged (>7 d)/excessive (>80 mL) bleeding occurring at regular intervals

Metrorrhagia: bleeding occurring at irregular intervals

Menometrorrhagia: excessive bleeding during normal menstrual period and at other irregular intervals

Polymenorrhea: bleeding occurring at intervals <21 d

Intermenstrual (IMB): bleeding between regular cycles

DVB: abnormal bleeding **not** due to organic disease (Dx of exclusion)

Postcoital: bleeding after vaginal intercourse

Postmenopausal: bleeding occurring >1 yr following menopause

ASC Box

Δs in Ovarian Function during Life

1. Premenopause (~9 to 43 yr): normal menstrual cycle (see Infertility)
2. Perimenopause (~43 to 49 yr): ↓ # ovarian follicles + ↓ FSH sensitivity → ↓ ovarian function → intermittent anovulation
   - P deficiency
   - Unopposed E exposure during anovulation results in unstable, friable endometrium → E breakthrough bleeding.
3. Menopause (~51 yr): chronic anovulatory cycles → E + P deficiency (no CL)

Monthly blood loss >60 mL may result in Fe deficiency anemia and may affect quality of life.

APPLIED SCIENTIFIC CONCEPTS

See Figure 14.4.

CAUSAL CONDITIONS

See Table 14.4.

APPROACH

The most clinically important aspects in the evaluation of a patient presenting with abnormal vaginal bleeding is determination of their:

1. **Hemodynamic status:** vitals (BP, HR), signs/Sx (dizziness, pallor, weakness, malaise, dyspnea on exertion etc.), investigations (CBC, coagulation profile)
2. **Pregnancy status:** β-HCG testing

Hx is helpful but Dx depends on hormonal, cytologic, and/or radiographic investigations. See Figure 14.5 and Table 14.5.

INDICATIONS FOR U/S

- Women with uterine enlargement identified through pelvic exam
- Pregnant women >20 wk of pregnancy with abnormal vaginal bleeding (see C₂LEO Box Liability for negligence)
- Persistent abnormal vaginal bleeding despite a negative endometrial biopsy and those who:
  a. Have a low risk for endometrial CA
  b. Are suspected to have atrophy, or
  c. Medically unfit

INDICATIONS FOR ENDOMETRIAL BIOPSY/CYTOLOGIC STUDIES

- Women >40 yr with abnormal vaginal bleeding or **any** postmenopausal bleeding
- Women at high risk of endometrial CA (>35 yr, nulliparity + Hx of infertility, new onset heavy irregular bleeding, obesity >90 kg, PCOS, FHx endometrial/colon CA, Hx of tamoxifen use)

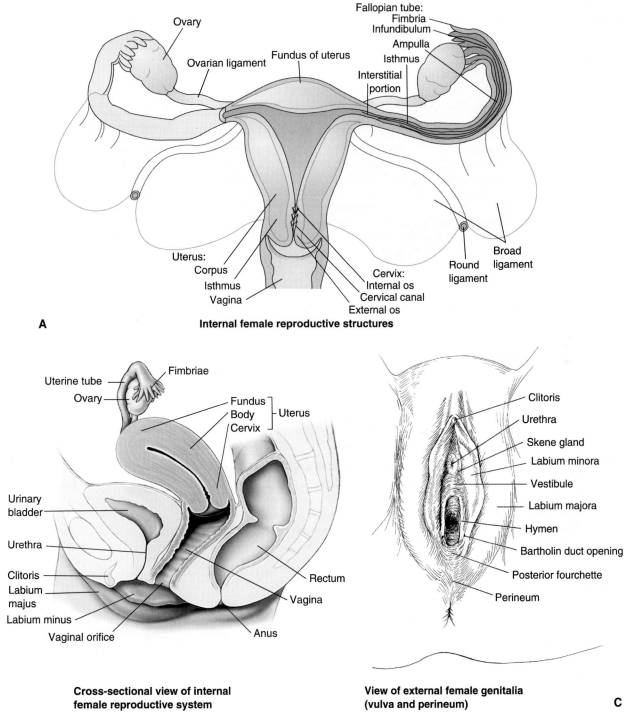

Figure 14.4 Relevant anatomy of the female genital tract.

- Persistent abnormal vaginal bleeding despite a 3-mo course of medical Rx
- Sonohysterography (saline TVS) showing a focal intrauterine pathology (i.e., polyp, submucosal myoma, fibroid etc.)
- Postmenopausal women with TVS showing endometrial thickness >5 mm
- CA screening (i.e., hereditary nonpolyposis colorectal CA)
- F/U of previously diagnosed endometrial hyperplasia or abnormal Pap smear with atypical cells favoring endometrial origin
- Endometrial dating
- Evaluation of infertility

Table **14.4**	DDx of Abnormal Vaginal Bleeding				
Stage in Life	**DDx**				
Premenarchal	1. Precocious puberty 2. Trauma, sexual abuse, foreign body 3. Infection 4. Other: ovarian tumor, urethral prolapsed				
Premenopausal (R/O pregnancy)	**Ovulatory (~90%)**			**Anovulatory (~10%)**	
	Intermenstrual (R/O OCPs, trauma) 1. **Infection:** cervicitis, endometritis, vaginitis, STIs 2. **Benign growths:** cervical/endometrial polyp, fibroids, ectropion 3. **Malignant tumors:** uterine, cervical, vaginal, vulvar, ovarian	**Menorrhagia** 1. **Neoplasms:** Endometrial CA, uterine sarcoma, fibroids, adenomyosis 2. **Coagulopathies** 3. **Other:** endometritis, hypothyroidism	**Age related** 1. Immature HPO axis 2. Menopausal ovarian decline	**Endocrine/metabolic** 1. **Thyroid:** hyper/hypo 2. **Chronic liver or renal disease** 3. **Neoplasms:** prolactinoma, adrenal, ovarian	**Other** 1. PCOS 2. Weight loss 3. Exercise 4. Stress 5. Structural disease
Postmenopausal	**Genital tract disease**		**Systemic disease**	**Drugs**	
	Endometrial CA 1. **Upper:** fallopian tube, ovarian CA 2. **Lower:** uterus/cervix, vagina, vulva, benign/malignant tumor, infection		1. **Coagulation disorders** 2. **Endocrine disorders**: thyroid disease, adrenal tumor, ovarian tumor 3. **Vulva:** Crohn, Behçet, Pemphigus	1. Hormone replacement 2. Contraception 3. Anticoagulants 4. Chemotherapy 5. Steroids	

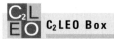

C₂LEO Box

Liability for Negligence
Pelvic exam is contraindicated at >20 wk of pregnancy with bleeding until U/S has excluded placenta previa.

INDICATIONS FOR SPECIALTY CARE REFERRAL IN WOMEN WITH AUB

- Persistent abnormal vaginal bleeding with normal findings through endometrial biopsy/saline infused sonohysterography
- Endometrial pathology—atypia, CA
- Uterine pathology—fibroids, submucosal myoma, polyps
- Endocrine disorders—PCOS, hyper/hypothyroidism, hyperprolactinemia, hypothalamic dysfunction
- Coagulopathies —1° disease, 2° to liver disease or CRF

Table **14.5**	Abnormal Vaginal Bleeding—Focused Hx and Physical Exam
Menstrual Hx	LNMP, precipitating factors, cycle length, pattern, duration, quantity, clots, color
Associated Sx	Pelvic/Abdo pain, weakness etc.
Medical Hx	Coagulopathies, cervicitis, polyps, PID, STIs, PCOS, uterine surgery, Pap tests
Drug Hx	Contraceptives, anticoagulants, HRT
Weight	Δ, diet/exercise Hx
Sexual and pregnancy Hx	Parity, Prev. C/S
FHx	Breast, endometrial, or GI CA Blood dyscrasias Fibroids
Pelvic exam	R/O trauma/sexual abuse, palpable ovarian/uterine mass
DRE	R/O GI bleeding

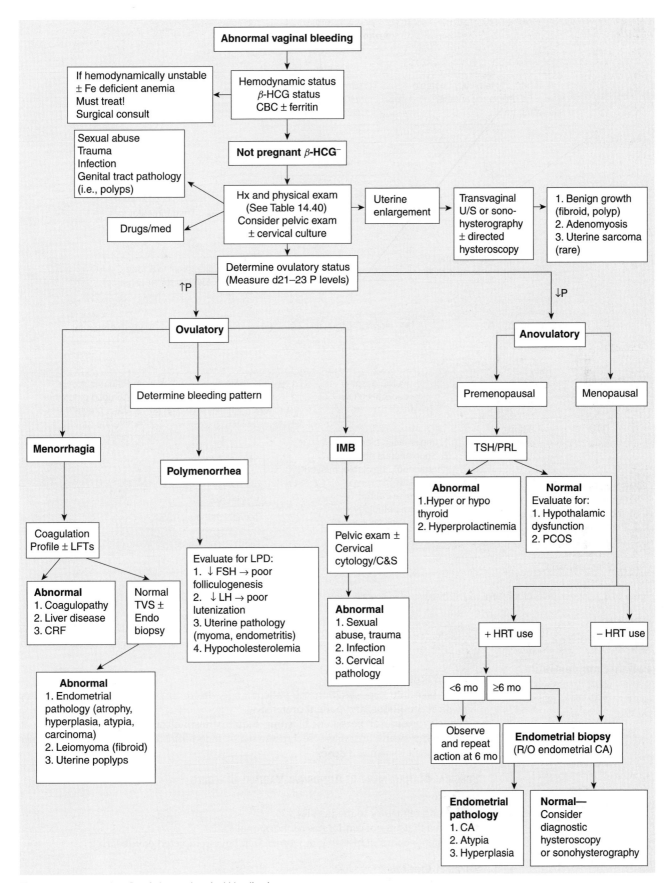

Figure 14.5 Approach to Dx of abnormal vaginal bleeding in nonpregnant women.

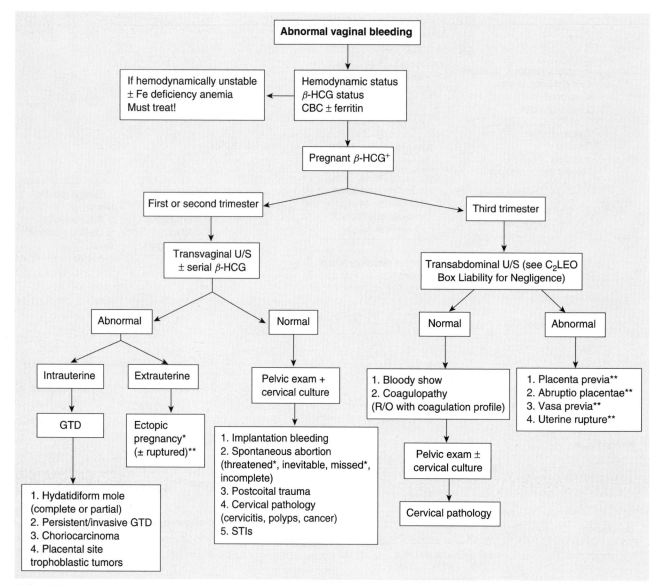

Figure 14.6 Approach to Dx of abnormal vaginal bleeding in pregnant women. **Critical Dx, *emergent Dx.

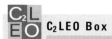 **C₂LEO Box**

Patient Confidentiality

If sexual abuse is suspected as cause of abnormal vaginal bleeding:

- Reporting is at the discretion of the victim unless victim is a child or elder.
- MD must report abuse of children or elders.
- Before collection of samples for evidence, victims should be asked to sign consent forms.
- Samples should be stored securely even if the patient decides against reporting the abuse.

RX

- Depends on the cause
- Must take into consideration the patient's age, desire to preserve fertility, coexisting medical conditions, and patient preference
- Acutely profuse or persistent bleeding requires hospitalization and immediate Rx if: hemodynamically unstable + severe anemia → blood transfusion + 25 mg IV premarin (conjugated E) q4 h × 3 doses

SURGICAL MANAGEMENT OF ABNORMAL VAGINAL BLEEDING

Indications

- Bleeding refractory to medical Rx
- Patients that are not candidates for hormonal Rx
- Persistent abnormal bleeding in women that have completed childbearing

Surgical Options

- Operative hysteroscopy—removal of intrauterine structural abnormalities
- Transcervical endometrial resection or endometrial ablation—Rx resistant abnormal vaginal bleeding

Table **14.6**	**Medical Management of Abnormal Vaginal Bleeding**	
Cause of Abnormal Vaginal Bleeding	**Rx Options**	**Mechanism of Action**
Anovulatory (IMB, LPD)	Low-dose E OCP 30 μg (i.e., containing EE) **Cyclic Progesterone:** 1. Medroxyprogesterone Acetate (**Provera**) 5–10 mg qd ×5–10 d/mo. 2. Norethidrone acetate (**Aygestin**) 2.5–10 mg qd ×5–10 d/mo. 3. Clomiphene citrate (Clomid) 50 mg on cycle d 5–9 (used when pregnancy is desired)	• Cycle regulation • Prevents endometrial hyperplasia • Cycle regulation • Prevent endometrial hyperplasia • SERM → ↑ pituitary FSH secretion → ovulation induction
Ovulatory	**NSAIDs**—start on d 1 of menses ×5 d or until it stops 1. Clomiphene citrate (Clomid) 50 mg on cycles d 5–9 2. Levonorgestrel contraceptive device (IUD) 3. **Antifibrinolytics** (i.e., Tranexamic acid) 1 g q6 h ×4 d of menstrual cycle	• Endometrial PG → ↓ menstrual flow • SERM → ↑ pituitary FSH secretion → ovulation induction • ↓ Menstrual bleeding • Reversible blockade of plasminogen → ↓ menstrual loss

NOTE: See Pregnancy Loss for management and F/U of threatened miscarriage, EP, and GTD.

- Myomectomy or uterine artery embolization—Rx of leiomyomas
- Hysterectomy—Rx of atypical hyperplasia or endometrial CA causing Rx refractory bleeding

PMS

DEFINITION

- **PMS** is the regular monthly experience of physiological, emotional, and behavioral Sx which usually occur before the menstrual cycle and are relieved within a few days of its onset.
- **PMDD** is the most severe form of PMS.
  - These Sx may be severe enough to interfere significantly with work and/or home activities.
- Incidence: PMS affects up to 75% of women with regular menstrual cycles versus PMDD ~3% to 8% of women

Table **14.7**	**Sx Clusters Associated with PMS/PMDD**	
Physical	**Behavioral**	**Emotional**
• Swelling of ankles, hands, and feet • Skin Δs/acne • Insomnia • Nausea/lack of appetite • General malaise and clumsiness • Fatigue, tiredness • Breast tenderness or swelling • Bloating/weight gain • Abdo cramps • ↑ Appetite • Headaches/backaches • Muscle spasms	• Slow thinking • Poor judgment • Sleep disturbances • Difficulty making decisions • Confusion, forgetfulness • ↑ Desire to be alone, ↓ interest in usual activities • Poor concentration	• Low self-esteem • Paranoia • Moodiness, tearfulness • Anger/rage/hostile • Unwanted thoughts • Sadness, depression • Anxious, nervous, panic • Irritability

Table **14.8**	Classification of PMS Spectrum of Disorders
Classification	**Diagnostic Criteria**
PMS	**ICD-10-CM Criteria:** At least 1 of the following affective and somatic syndromes during the 5 d before menses in each of the 3 prior menstrual cycles: • **Affective** → depression, angry outburst, irritability, anxiety, confusion, social withdrawal • **Somatic** → breast tenderness, Abdo bloating, headache, swelling of extremities • Sx are relieved within 4 d of menses onset • Sx present in the absence of any pharmacologic Rx or drug or EtOH use • Sx occur reproducibly during 2 cycles of prospective recording • Patient suffers from identifiable dysfunction in social or economic performance
PMDD	**DSM-IV Criteria:** A. Sx must occur during the week before menses and remit a few days after onset of menses. Five of the following Sx must be present: **≥1 of the following four Sx:** 1. Markedly depressed mood, feelings of hopelessness, self-deprecating thoughts 2. Marked anxiety or tension 3. Affective lability (i.e., angry outbursts) 4. Persistent and marked anger, or **irritability**, or ↑ interpersonal conflicts **Along with any combination of the following Sx:** 1. ↓Interest in usual activities (social withdrawal) 2. Concentration difficulties 3. Marked lack of energy, lethargy, easily fatigued 4. Marked Δ in appetite, overeating, or food cravings 5. Hypersomnia or insomnia 6. Feeling overwhelmed or out of control 7. Other physical Sx (breast tenderness, Abdo bloating, headache, joint/muscle pain B. Sx are absent postmenstrually C. Sx must interfere with work, school, usual activities, or relationships. D. Sx must not, merely be an exacerbation of another disorder. E. Criteria A, B, and C must be confirmed by prospective daily ratings for at least 2 consecutive symptomatic menstrual cycles.

CAUSAL CONDITIONS

- Unknown
- Current theories
  - Complex combination of environmental, metabolic, and behavioral factors produce a "vulnerability" to the hormonal Δs associated with menstruation.
  - 5-HT interfaces with ovarian hormones: ↑ E → ↑ 5-HT versus ↑ Progesterone → ↓ 5HT.

Table **14.9**	Comparison of PMS and PMDD	
	PMS	**PMDD**
Mostly mood Sx	No	Yes
Difficulty conducting day-to-day activities	No	Yes
Timing	Premenstrual phase only	>2 consecutive cycles, occurring in the premenstrual phase
Incidence	Up to 75% of women	3%–8% of women of child bearing age
Severity of Sx	Less severe, primarily physical Sx	More severe, primarily mood Sx

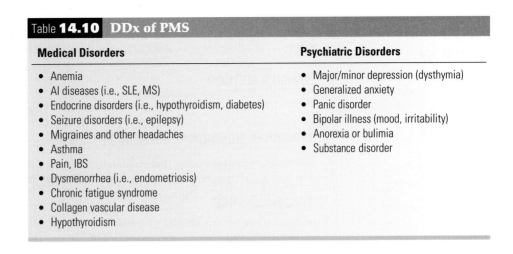

Table **14.10** DDx of PMS	
Medical Disorders	**Psychiatric Disorders**
• Anemia • AI diseases (i.e., SLE, MS) • Endocrine disorders (i.e., hypothyroidism, diabetes) • Seizure disorders (i.e., epilepsy) • Migraines and other headaches • Asthma • Pain, IBS • Dysmenorrhea (i.e., endometriosis) • Chronic fatigue syndrome • Collagen vascular disease • Hypothyroidism	• Major/minor depression (dysthymia) • Generalized anxiety • Panic disorder • Bipolar illness (mood, irritability) • Anorexia or bulimia • Substance disorder

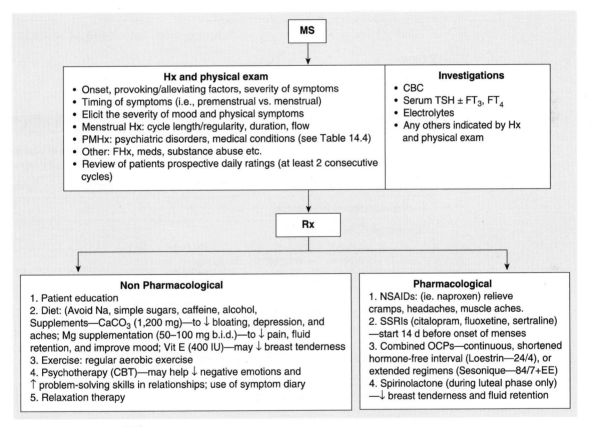

Figure 14.7 Approach to PMS.

Must differentiate between normal premenstrual Sx and other causes of physical and mood Δs (i.e., premenstrual exacerbation of underlying psychiatric disorder)

CONTRACEPTION

DEFINITIONS

- **Contraception** = protection against conception or impregnation
- **Contraceptive effectiveness** depends on
    - i. Inherent effectiveness in preventing pregnancy **and**
    - ii. How consistently and correctly it is used

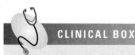

NATURAL FAMILY PLANNING

Controlling fertility without contraceptive device or chemicals

BARRIER METHOD

A mechanical or chemical barrier to sperm entry into upper genital tract (See Table 14.12)

COMBINED HORMONAL CONTRACEPTION

All forms of contraception that contain both E and a P including OCP, TD contraceptive patch, vaginal contraceptive ring, and combined monthly injectable

THE COMBINED OCP

- Monophasic (fixed amount of E and P)
- Biphasic (fixed amount of E, ↑ amount of P in second half of cycle)
- Triphasic (fixed or variable amount of E, P ↑ in 3 equal phases)
- With perfect use = 99.9% effective
- With typical use failure rate ↑ to 3% to 8%
- Effect of body weight on efficacy is controversial (See Tables 14.13, 14.14 and 14.15)

P ONLY

See Table 14.16.

Table **14.11** Natural Family Planning Methods and Effectiveness		
	Percentage of Women with Unintended Pregnancy	
Natural Contraceptive Method	**Perfect Use**	**Typical Use**
Regular unprotected intercourse	85	85
Calendar (periodic abstinence) • Calculate onset and duration of fertile period based on ovulation 12–16 d before menstruation, 5-d sperm survival, and 24-h unfertilized oocyte survival • Avoid intercourse during 8–10 d of cycle	9	
Ovulation method (periodic abstinence) • Monitor volume and quality Δs in mucous. • Mucous becomes clearer and more elastic as ovulation approaches (**spinnbarkeit**) then viscous, opaque and impenetrable to sperm after ovulation	3	

Symptothermal (periodic abstinence)
• Ovulation/cervical mucous method supplemented with calendar method in preovulatory phase and basal body temperature in postovulatory phase
  • Basal body temperature:
    • Following the postovulatory elevation in progesterone, basal body temperature should rise by at least 0.5°
	2	

Postovulation (periodic abstinence) • Reliance on the second infertile phase only	1	
Lactational amenorrhea • Temporary postpartum method of contraception based on hormonal suppression of ovulation in breast-feeding women	2	
Coitus interruptus/withdrawal • Male withdraws penis from vagina before ejaculation	4	27

Table **14.12** **Barrier Methods: Effectiveness and Cautions**

| Barrier Method | Percentage of Women with Unintended Pregnancy | | Mechanism of Action | CIs and Cautions |
	Perfect Use	Typical Use		
Male condom • Latex • Polyurethane • Lambskin • Tactylon	15	2	• Mechanical barrier prevents exchange of fluid/semen and ↓ contact of genital lesions • Prevent pregnancy and STI	• Allergy or sensitivity • [a]No STI protection with lambskin
Female condom • Polyurethane sheath placed in vagina	21	5	• Completely lines vagina completely • Prevents contact between penis and vagina, and trapping sperm • STI prevention similar to male latex condom	• Allergy or sensitivity • Abnormal vaginal anatomy • Inability to insert
Diaphragm • Intravaginal barrier method used with spermicide	16	6	• Physical barrier between sperm and cervix used in conjunction with spermicide • Associated with ↓ cervical neoplasia, dysplasia, gonorrhea, PID and tubal infertility	• Allergy or sensitivity • Large rectocele, cystocele or uterine prolapse (↓ efficacy) • ↑ Risk BV and UTI
Cervical cap • Intravaginal barrier method used with spermicide	32 (**M**) 16 (**N**)	26 (M) 9 (N)	• Silicone cap acts as physical barrier between sperm and cervix used in conjunction with spermicide • Held in place by suction therefore requires snug fitting • Protects against chlamydia and gonorrhea	• Allergy or sensitivity • Vaginal bleeding • Cervical or uterine CA or dysplasia • Current vaginal or cervical infection or PID • Recurrent vaginal, cervical or UTI • <6 wk Postpartum/abortion
Sponge • Intravaginal "one-size-fits-all" barrier method	32 (M) 16 (N)	20 (M) 9 (N)	• 1° Mechanism of action provided by sustained release of spermicide impregnated in sponge • Also absorbs and traps sperm	• Allergy or sensitivity • Abnormal in vaginal anatomy or bleeding • Inability to insert • Hx of TSS or recurrent UTI • Require HIV protection • >6 wk postpartum/abortion
Spermicide	29	18	• Made of surfactants that destroy the sperm cell membrane by altering the lipid layer	• Allergy or sensitivity • [a]Should be used with another contraceptive method

CLINICAL BOX

Facts About the OCP

- The P component is predominantly responsible for the contraceptive effect.
- The most common reason patients discontinue the OCP is abnormal bleeding.
- Irregular bleeding that continues beyond 3 mo must be investigated.
- "Pill breaks" are not necessary and ↑ risk of pregnancy.
- Continuous use of pill is safe.
- If pill free interval >7 d → ↑ risk of ovulation and conception
- After discontinuing the pill, fertility is restored within 1 to 3 mo.
- A pelvic exam is **not** required before prescribing the OCP.
- No routine lab screening is necessary before prescribing the OCP.

Good Candidates for P Only

- CI or sensitivity to E
- >35 y.o. and smoker
- Migraine headaches
- Breast-feeding
- Endometriosis
- Sickle-cell disease
- Anticonvulsant Rx
- Difficulty complying with daily pill (for DMPA)

Pain may be a physiological response to device, but possibility of infection, malposition/perforation or pregnancy should be R/O.

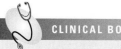

CLINICAL BOX

Risks of DMPA

- Delayed return of fertility— Avg. 9 mo delay before full fertility restored
- ↓BMD—↓ BMD does not induce osteoporosis and appears to be reversible after discontinuing DMPA.

IUD

See Table 14.17.

Table **14.13** CIs to OCP Use	
Absolute CIs	**Relative CIs**
• <6 wk postpartum if breast-feeding • Breast CA (current) • Smoker >35 y.o. (>15 cigarette/d) • Uncontrolled HTN (systolic >160 mm Hg or diastolic >100 mm Hg • Venous thromboembolism (current or Hx) • Ischemic heart disease • Valvular heart disease (PulmHTN, Afib, Hx of SBE) • Diabetes with retinopathy/nephropathy/neuropathy • Migraine headaches with focal neurologic Sx • Severe cirrhosis • Liver tumor (adenoma or hepatoma) • Undiagnosed vaginal bleeding • Known thrombophilia	• Smoker over the age of 35 (<15 cigarette/d) • Adequately controlled HTN • HTN (systolic 140–159 mm Hg, diastolic 90–99 mm Hg) • Migraine headache over the age of 35 • Currently symptomatic gallbladder disease • Mild cirrhosis • Hx of OCP-related cholestasis • Users of medications that may interfere with OCP metabolism

Table **14.14** OCP—Benefits, Side Effects and Risks		
Benefits	**Side Effects**	**Risks**
• Cycle regulation • ↑ BMD • ↓ Dysmenorrhea and moliminal Sx • ↓ Menstrual flow (amenorrhea in 2%–3%) • ↓ Acne and hirsutism	Most resolve in first 3 cycles: • Breast tenderness • Nausea • Irregular bleeding • Chloasma • NO evidence for weight gain and/or mood Δs	• Venous thromboembolism (AR = 1.5/10,000) • Stroke and MI (if EE > 50 μg) • ? ↑ gallbladder disease • Breast CA risk controversial • Cervical CA risk uncertain

Table **14.15** Other Modes of Combined Contraception					
Combined Contraceptives	**Failure Rate Perfect Use (Typical Use)**	**Correct Use**	**CI (Same as OCP plus)**	**Risks/Benefits**	**Side Effects**
• **Patch** (Ortho Evra) • 150 μg Norel—gestromin and 20 μg EE/d • Apply to: buttock, upper outer arm, lower Abdo, upper torso • If patch falls off: reapply new patch • Backup if off >24 h	0.3 (8)	• **Start:** Use backup **unless** start on first d of menses • 1 patch weekly ×3 wk, then 1 wk patch-free wk	↓ Efficacy if body weight >90 kg	Same as OCP	• Breast discomfort (↑ vs. OCP) • Nausea • Spotting • Local skin reaction
• **Vaginal ring** (NuvaRing) • 15 μg EE and 120 mg etonogestrel/d • Effective for up to 4 wk protection	0.3 (6)	• Start: cycle d 1–5 • Left in place ×3 wk, removed for 1 wk • If ring removed >3 h need backup	• Uterovaginal prolapse • Vaginal stenosis (prevent retention of ring)	No studies Assumed to be similar	• Spotting • Headache • Nausea • Breast tenderness • Vaginitis • Leukorrhea

Table **14.16**	P Contraception	
	Injectable P	**Oral P**
Definition	DMPA • 150 mg IM q12 wk • ~2% of Canadian women use DMPA for birth control • Failure rate <0.3%/yr	P-only pill/mini-pill 0.35 mg norethindrone • Failure rate = 0.5% with perfect use (take pill at same time daily) • Failure rate = 5%–10 % with typical use
Mechanism of action	• Inhibits secretion of pituitary gonadotropins → suppress ovulation • ↑ Viscosity of cervical mucous • Induces endometrial atrophy	• Cervical mucus Δ (↓ volume, ↑ viscosity, alter molecular structure → minimal sperm penetration) • May suppress ovulation (40%) and ↓ receptivity of endometrium
Absolute CI	**"PUB"**: • **P**regnancy known or suspected • **U**nexplained vaginal bleeding • **B**reast CA (current)	• Pregnancy (known) • Breast CA (current)
Relative CI	**"ASH"**: • **A**ctive viral hepatitis • **S**evere cirrhosis • **H**epatic adenoma	• Active viral hepatitis • Liver tumors
Side effects	• Menstrual cycle disturbance (spotting or unwanted amenorrhea) • Hormonal (headache, acne, ↓ libido, nausea, breast tenderness) • Weight gain (~2.5 kg after first yr) • Mood (controversial)	• Headache • Irregular bleeding • Bloating • Nausea • Acne • Spotting (most common reason for discontinuing)

Table **14.17**	Comparison of IUD Available for Use	
	Copper IUD	**LNG-IUS**
Description	Has a vertical stem with a silver-cored copper wire wound around	Slow release of levonorgestrel (20 μg/d) from small polyethylene T-shaped frame
Efficacy (Pearl index)	1.26/100WY	0.09/100WY
Failure rate (%)	0.8	0.1
EP rate	0.25/100WY	0.02/100WY
Duration of effect	5 yr	5 yr
Mechanism of action	• Prevention of fertilization through: 1. Foreign body reaction → endometrial Δ causing ↓ sperm transport 2. Direct effect of copper ions on sperm motility (↓ ability to penetrate cervical mucus) 3. ?? Potential to inhibit implantation post fertilization	• Prevention of fertilization through: • Weak foreign body reaction and endometrial decidualization and glandular atrophy • Endometrial E and P receptor suppression • ? thickened cervical mucus as barrier to sperm transport • ? Ovulation inhibition in some women • ?? Potential to inhibit implantation post fertilization
Side effects	• Pelvic pain (~6% of users will discontinue use due to pain) • ↑ Menstrual flow (up to 65%) • Spotting	• Pelvic pain (~6% of users will discontinue use due to pain) • Depression, headache, acne, breast tenderness (maximal in first 3 mo of use) • ↑ Menstrual flow or spotting in first few mo then ↓ bleeding • Functional cysts (~30%)

Table **14.18** CIs of IUD	
Absolute CIs	**Relative CIs**

• Pregnancy
• Current, recurrent or recent (within 3 mo) PID or STI
• Puerperal sepsis
• Immediate postseptic abortion
• Severely distorted uterine cavity
• Unexplained vaginal bleeding
• Cervical or endometrial CA
• Malignant trophoblastic disease
• Copper allergy (for copper IUD)
• Breast CA (For LNG-IUS)
	• RFs for STI or HIV
	• Impaired response to infection
	  • HIV positive
	  • Steroid Rx
	• From 48 h to 4 wk postpartum
	• Ovarian CA
	• Benign GTD

EP

IUD does **not** ↑ risk of EP

However, if pregnancy occurs with IUD in place, ectopic must be R/O

STERILIZATION

Considered a permanent method of contraception for those who wish to remain childless, want no more children, and want an effective method of contraception

1) Tubal ligation: 0.5 % of women experience an unwanted pregnancy in the first year
2) Vasectomy: 0.1 to 0.15% of women experience an unwanted pregnancy in the first year

Indications for EC

• Failure to use a contraceptive
• Condom break/leakage
• Dislodgment of diaphragm or cervical cap
• Two or more missed pills
• Depo-Provera injection over 1 wk late
• Ejaculation on external genitalia
• Mistimed fertility awareness
• Sexual assault (and not using reliable contraceptive method)

Facts About Sterilization

• Vasectomy is a less invasive and more cost-effective procedure than conventional tubal ligation.
• Although vasectomy and tubal ligation are considered safe and effective, complications may occur and failure is possible
• Regret after sterilization is not infrequent.
• Counseling before sterilization should include discussion of alternative methods of contraception, risks, complications, potential for regret, possibility of failure and difficulty, expense and no guarantee of success of reversal if attempted.

EC

• Any method of contraception which is used after intercourse and before potential time of implantation
• Work before implantation therefore **not** abortifacients
• Indications: women wishing to avoid pregnancy and present within 5 d of unprotected or inadequately protected sexual intercourse (IUD may be considered for up to 7 d)
• Mechanism of action: differs between types of EC and timing of initiation but can include interference with follicle maturation, ovulation, cervical mucous consistency, endometrial receptivity, corpus luteum support, fertilization, zygote development, transport and adhesion/implantation.

ECP

Plan B

• Levonorgestrel—only method consisting 2 doses of 750 μg levonorgestrel taken orally 12 h apart
• Only product approved by Health Canada for EC
• May alternatively take levonorgestrel 1.5 mg orally as a single dose

Yuzpe Method

• Oral administration of 2 doses of 100 μg EE and 500 μg levonorgestrel 12 h apart
• "Ovral" tablets are most commonly used to provide these doses.

Facts about EC

• Breast-feeding is not a CI to EC.
• Day of cycle and # episodes of intercourse are **not** relevant to decision for EC.
• Pregnancy test is only required before IUD.
• Only known CI to ECP is pregnancy (because it is not effective).

POSTCOITAL INSERTION OF A COPPER IUD

- Can be placed up to 7 d after intercourse to prevent conception and left in place to provide ongoing contraception

VULVAR ITCH, VAGINAL DISCHARGE, AND SEXUALLY TRANSMITTED ILLNESSES

RATIONALE

- Vaginal complaints are extremely common in 1° care and in gynecology.
- Control of sexually transmitted infections is a major public health concern. Many illnesses are reportable.

APPROACH TO EVALUATION OF VAGINAL COMPLAINTS

Hx

- Menstrual Hx
- Sexual activity
- Presence of IUD
- Progression of Sx
- Antibiotic use
- Hx of diabetes
- Prev. Rx
- Hygienic practices
- Prev. infections
- Dysuria (internal vs. external)
- Vulvar Sx (burning or pruritus)
- Vaginal discharge (consistency, color, odor)
- Pregnancy Hx
- Abdo pain

PHYSICAL EXAM

See Table 14.19.

LAB TESTS

- Vaginal swabs
- Culture of the endocervix for gonorrhea or chlamydia infection
- Pap test
- Urine R&M, C&S
- Vaginal pH (using phenaphthazine paper)—may be altered by lubricating gel, semen, douches, or intravaginal medication.
- CBC, specific blood tests (VDRL, treponemal tests, HSV PCR, HAV, HBV, HIV)

It is imperative to assess any Hx of neoplasia (vulvar/vaginal/cervical/endometrial neoplasia).

CLINICAL BOX

Test for Gonorrhea and Chlamydia

- Sexually active and <25 yr
- In all patients who have a fever, lower Abdo pain, a symptomatic sexual partner,
- a new sexual partner or more than one sexual partner

CLINICAL BOX

Normal Vaginal Discharge

- Physiologic vaginal discharge (1 to 4 mL of fluid daily)
- Discharge may ↑ at times (pregnancy, use of E contraceptives, mid-cycle).
- pH of normal flora is acidic (4.0 to 4.5).
- Normal vaginal discharge ↑ mid-cycle due to ↑ cervical mucus → can be malodorous and can be accompanied by irritative Sx.

CLINICAL BOX

STI RFs

- Prev. STI
- Sexually active <25 yr of age
- Sexual contact with person(s) with a known STI
- A new sexual partner or >2 sexual partners in the past year/serially monogamous patients
- IV drug use
- No contraception or sole use of a nonbarrier method
- Sex workers and their clients
- Street involvement, homelessness
- Victims of sexual assault/abuse
- Anonymous sexual partnering (internet, rave party)
- "Survival sex" (i.e., exchanging sex for money, drugs etc.)
- Unprotected sex, sex with blood exchange

Must consider **sexual abuse** in any child diagnosed with gonorrhea and/or chlamydia after the immediate neonatal period. Suspected or known sexual abuse of children must be **reported** to child protection agencies.

CLINICAL BOX

Coinfections

Test for other STDs including HIV, hepatitis B, and VDRL. Immunize against hepatitis A and B if not already immunized.

CLINICAL BOX

6 mo Repeat Screening of Gonorrhea Indications

Rx failure has occurred previously, patient is a child, compliance is uncertain, there is reexposure of an untreated partner, infection occurs in pregnancy, PID or disseminated gonococcal infection is diagnosed.

CLINICAL BOX

C. trachomatis Repeat Testing

- All individuals with infection 6 mo post-Rx
- Test of cure if: compliance is suboptimal, pregnancy, prepubertal children

Table **14.19**	Physical Exam of Vaginal Complaints
Inspect external genitalia	Edema, excoriations, ulceration, condylomas, discharge on the perineum or introitus
Assessment of inguinal and/or femoral lymph nodes	LAD
Speculum exam	Vaginal discharge, evidence of characteristic lesions (e.g., strawberry cervix of trichomoniasis), presence of cervical discharge
Assess the presence of cervical and upper genital tract inflammation.	Cervical motion tenderness, adnexal tenderness
Assess the presence of systemic Sx.	Fevers, chills, Abdo pain, weight loss
Perform perianal inspection, pharyngeal inspection.	

SEXUALLY TRANSMITTED INFECTIONS

Table **14.20** STIs—Preventative Measures	
1°	**2°**
<ul><li>Identify at-risk individuals: counseling, education and assessment</li><li>Inform patients about signs and Sx of STIs.</li><li>Limit the number of sexual partners.</li><li>Use of barrier contraceptives (i.e., male/female condoms, dental dams)</li><li>HPV vaccine, hepatitis A + B vaccine</li><li>Offer STI screening and testing.</li><li>Assess the presence of violence or abuse.</li></ul>	<ul><li>Use of barrier contraceptives (i.e., male/female condoms, dental dams)</li><li>HPV vaccine, hepatitis A + B vaccine, post exposure immune globulin for hepatitis A</li><li>Detection of infection and Rx</li><li>Partner notification and Rx</li><li>Mandatory reporting of: chlamydia, gonorrhea, chancroid, syphilis, genital herpes, hepatitis B, trichomoniasis (in some jurisdictions), HIV</li></ul>

VULVOVAGINITIS

- Inflammation of the vulva and vagina due to both infectious and noninfectious causes
- Sx of vaginitis are nonspecific → lab findings are required to make a definitive Dx

GONORRHEA AND CHLAMYDIA

See Table 14.23.

Table **14.21** Types of Vaginitis	
Infectious Vaginitis	**Noninfectious Vaginitis**
1. **BV** (40–50% of cases—most common cause of vaginitis in women of reproductive age) 2. Vaginal candidiasis (20%–25% of cases) 3. Trichomoniasis (15%–20% of cases) 4. Other: (less common) <ul><li>Atrophic vaginitis with 2° bacterial infection</li><li>Foreign body with 2° infection</li><li>Desquamative inflammatory vaginitis</li><li>Streptococcal vaginitis (group A)</li><li>Ulcerative vaginitis TSS</li><li>Idiopathic vulvovaginal ulceration related to HIV</li></ul>	1. Atrophic vaginitis 2. Chemical or other irritant 3. Allergic, hypersensitivity and contact dermatitis 4. Other: <ul><li>Traumatic vaginitis</li><li>Postpuerperal atrophic vaginitis</li><li>Desquamative inflammatory vaginitis</li><li>Erosive lichen planus</li><li>Collagen vascular disease, Crohn disease</li><li>Behçet syndrome</li></ul>

Table **14.22**	Dx and Rx of Infectious Vulvovaginitis		
Dx/Causative Agent	**Signs and Sx**	**Diagnostic Criteria**	**Rx Options**
BV • *G. vaginalis* • Bacteroides • Peptostreptococcus • *M. hominis*	Predominant complaint of vaginal odor ↑ Risk with use of an IUD	**Amsel criteria** (3 of 4 of): 1. Thin homogeneous vaginal discharge 2. Clue cells on N/S wet mount or gram stain 3. Positive whiff test on KOH wet mount (presence of characteristically "fishy" [amine] odor) 4. Vaginal pH >4.5	• Metronidazole 500 mg PO b.i.d.×7 d • Metronidazole 250 mg PO t.i.d.×7 d • Clindamycin 300 mg PO t.i.d.×7 d [a]↑ **Risk of preterm birth** (important to treat in pregnancy)
Vaginal candidiasis • *C. albicans* • *C. glabrata* (less common) • Associated with antibiotics use, DM, immunosuppression	• Vulvar/vaginal pruritis • Vulvar erythema, edema, fissures excoriations, external dysuria • Thick flocculent white discharge	1. Normal vaginal pH (4 to 4.5) 2. Hyphae and buds on saline wet mount (yeast) 3. Positive yeast culture from the vagina (many asymptomatic women have vaginal yeast colonization)	• Fluconazole 150 mg PO once • Mycostatin (nystatin) 100,000 U vaginal tablet OD×14 d • Clotrimazole 500 mg tablet p.v.×1 **or** 100 mg tablet p.v. OD×7 d
Vaginal trichomoniasis • [a]*T. vaginalis* • [a]Facilitates HIV transmission, associated with PROM	• Dyspareunia • Vaginal pruritus, vulvovaginal erythema "Strawberry" cervix on exam • Timing: ↑ common during/immediately after menses	1. Trichomonas (motiled flagellum) seen on N/S wetmount 2. High number of PMNs on saline microscopy 3. Positive culture for *T. vaginalis* 4. Vaginal pH 5−6.0	• Metronidazole 2 g PO×1 • Metronidazole 500 mg PO b.i.d.×7 d **Must* treat sexual partners simultaneously to prevent reinfection!
Atrophic vaginitis (postmenopausal)	• Dyspareunia • Vaginal spotting, soreness • Thin vaginal mucosa → erythema, petechiae	1. pH 5.0−7.0 2. ↑ PMNs 3. Replacement of lactobacilli with mixed flora of GN rods	• Topical vaginal E

SYPHILIS

Classically **painless** genital ulcer disease

- The incidence of syphilis has been ↑ nationally over the last 10 y
- Called the **great imitator** as it is associated with a variety of signs and Sx
- Mode of transmission: direct sexual contact with infected lesions, contact with infected blood, vertical transmission (congenital syphilis)
- 1°, 2°, and early latent phases are considered infectious (60% risk of transmission per partner)

SYPHILIS F/U CONSIDERATIONS

- Test for other STDs including HIV, hepatitis B, chlamydia, gonorrhea.
- Genital ulcers should be tested for HSV, chancroid, and/or lymphogranuloma venereum.
- Immunization against hepatitis A and B if not already immunized
- Syphilis is reportable to public health (1°, 2° and early latent): Sexual and perinatal contacts must be tested.

HERPES AND CHANCROID

Classically **painful** genital ulcer diseases

HPV: CONDYLOMA ACUMINATA

Associated with genital warts and lower genital tract CAs

Table 14.23 Dx and Rx of Gonorrhea and Chlamydia

Dx/Causative Agent	Signs and Sx	Diagnostic Criteria	Rx Options
Gonorrhea ↑[a] **N. Gonorrhea** (diplococci)	• Cervicitis, PID • Mucopurulent discharge vagina • Rectal pain and discharge • Dysuria, dyspareunia • Perihepatitis (Fitz-Hugh-Curtis) • Lower Abdo pain • Abnormal vaginal bleeding • Chorioamnionitis/endometritis • Bartholinitis • Conjunctivitis • Pharyngeal infection • Disseminated infection—(arthritis, dermatitis, endocarditis, meningitis)	1. NAAT from endocervical specimens (sensitivity 96%) 2. Gram stain of cervical swab sample 3. Culture from endocervix, pharynx, rectum, conjunctiva Usual incubation period is 2–7 d	• Cefixime 400 mg PO×1[b] • Ciprofloxacin 500 mg PO×1 • Ofloxacin 400 mg PO×1 • Ceftriaxone 125 mg IM×1[b] **plus** Empiric Rx of chlamydia **Mandatory reporting,** Rx/F/U of partners with contact within 60 d of Sx onset
Chlamydia ↑[a] C. trachomatis Serotypes D, E, F, G, H, I, J, K (Obligate intracellular bacteria)	• Majority of cases → asymptomatic • Vaginal discharge • Dysuria, dyspareunia • Lower Abdo pain • Conjunctivitis • Proctitis • Reiter syndrome Incubation period can be up to 6 wk[b]	1. NAAT assay from endocervical, urethral or urinary specimen 2. Throat and/or rectal culture of C. trachomatis[b] Should be done in children OR in circumstances with potential legal implications[b]	Doxycycline 100 mg PO b.i.d.×7 d Azithromycin 1 g PO×1[b] Ofloxacin 300 mg PO b.i.d.×7 d Erythromycin 2 g/d in divided doses×7 d[b] **Mandatory reporting,** Rx/F/U of partners with contact within 60 d of Sx onset

[a] ↑ Over the past decade
[b] Rx options in pregnancy and lactation

Table 14.24 Dx and Rx of Syphilis[a]

Signs and Sx	Incubation Period	Diagnostic Criteria	Rx Options
1°: chancre (genital ulcer), regional LAD Ulcer is classically **painless** 2°: widespread symmetric maculopapular rash (palms and soles), fever, malaise, LAD, mucus lesions, condyloma lata, alopecia, meningitis, headaches, uveitis, retinitis Latent: asymptomatic 3°: aortic aneurysm, AR, coronary artery ostial stenosis Neurosyphilis: asymptomatic to symptomatic with headaches, vertigo, personality Δs, dementia, ataxia Gumma: tissue destruction in any organ. The specific manifestations depend on the site involved.	3–90 d 2 wk–6 mo Early <1 yr Late >1 yr 10–30 yr 2–20 yr 1–46 yr	Dark field microscopy of serous fluid from genital lesions for observation of spirochetes Initial **screening** with nontreponemal antibody tests (VDRL and RPR) If nontreponemal tests positive, retest with treponemal assays FTA-ABS; TP-PA; MHA-TP The treponemal tests remain positive for life, even after successful Rx. CSF samples should be taken in those with neurologic or ophthalmic Sx	**1°,2°, early latent:** • Benzathine Penicillin G 2.4 million units IM×1[b] • Doxycycline 100 mg PO b.i.d.×14 d • Ceftriaxone 1 g IV or IM daily×10 d **Late latent, CVS syphilis and other syphilis not involving CNS:** • Benzathine Penicillin G 2.4 million units IM weekly×3 doses[b] • Doxycycline 100 mg PO b.i.d.×28 d • Ceftriaxone 1 g IV or IM daily×10 d **Neurosyphilis:** • Penicillin G 3–4 million units IV q4 h×10–14 d[b] • Ceftriaxone 2 g IV/IM daily×14 d **Sexual contacts (last 30 d):** • Benzathine Penicillin G 2.4 million units IM×1[b]

[a] ↑ Over the past decade
[b] Rx options in pregnancy and lactation

Table **14.25** Dx and Rx of Herpes and Chancroid			
Dx/Causative Agent	**Signs and Sx**	**Diagnostic Criteria**	**Rx Options**

Herpes
 HSV types 1 and 2
 HSV-1 = oral ulcers
 ↑ HSV-1 genital infection 2° to ↑ oral-genital intercourse
 Must inform sexual partners from the preceding 60 d before Sx
 Asymptomatic shedding of HSV has been demonstrated
	• Painful ulcerating genital lesions (80%)
	 • Atypical presentation (20%) including genital pain, urethritis, cervicitis
	 1° Outbreak:
	 • Painful ulcerative genital lesions
	 • Systemic Sx (fever, myalgias)
	 • LAD
	 • Aseptic meningitis (16%–26%)
	 • Extragenital lesions (10%–28%)
	 2° Outbreak:
	 • 1° Infection → to latent sacral sensory ganglion infection
	 • **Result** = recurrence(s) in tissues innervated by sacral sensory nerves
	 • **Prodromal Sx**: itching, burning, tingling or discomfort
	 • **Triggers:** stress, illness or certain medications
	 • **Clinical presentation:**
	   • ↓ Severity of Sx as vs. 1° infection, ↓ duration
	   • ↓ Extensive genital lesions
	   • Systemic Sx (16%)
	   • Extragenital lesions (8%)
	   • Meningitis (1%)
		• Cultures from HSV lesions (70% sensitive—ulcers, 94% —vesicles)
		 • HSV PCR: 100% specific
		 • Antibody response: early → IgM, followed by IgG
		 • 3–6 wk to seroconversion after 1° outbreak
		 • NAAT assay—vesicle fluid or ulcer swab (~100% sensitivity and specificity)
		 Measures to ↓ transmission
		 1. Counseling (i.e., HSV is not curable, potential for recurrent episodes, sexual transmission, asymptomatic shedding)
		 2. Condom use
		 3. Antiviral Rx to ↓ asymptomatic shedding and recurrent lesions
		 NOTE: Greatest RF for neonatal herpes → new maternal genital HSV-1 or -2 infection without complete maternal immune response by delivery
			Rx of first episode
			 [a]Urinary retention may be an indication for hospitalization
			 Acyclovir 200 mg PO×5daily for 5–10 d
			 Famciclovir 250 mg PO t.i.d.×5 d
			 If severe: IV acyclovir 5 mg/kg over 60 min q8 h until improvement
			 Rx of recurrent episode
			 Acyclovir 200 mg PO×5 daily for 5 d
			 Famciclovir 125 mg PO b.i.d.×5 d
			 Suppressive Rx for nonpregnant patients
			 Acyclovir 200 mg PO t.i.d. to×5 daily for 5 d
			 acyclovir 400 mg b.i.d.
			 Suppressive Rx for pregnant patients
			 Acyclovir 200 mg PO q.i.d.
			 Acyclovir 400 mg PO t.i.d.
			 With either regimen, begin 400 mg PO t.i.d. at 36 wk

Chancroid *H. ducreyi* Known cofactor in HIV transmission	• Small pustule of papules → painful genital ulcers with granulomatous bases • May progress to inguinal ulcers, painful inguinal LAD **NOTE:** 50% of those exposed develop the disease (incubation period 5–14 d)	Culture of *H. ducreyi* Gram stain of GN coccobacilli with "school of fish" pattern Must also R/O *T. Pallidum* or HSV	Ciprofloxacin 500 mg PO×1 Erythromycin 500 mg PO t.i.d.×7 d Azithromycin 1 g PO×1 Ceftriaxone 250 mg IM×1 **Must** empirically treat all individuals with sexual exposure in the last 2 wk from onset

RFs for PID

• STI RFs
• IUDs
• Frequent vaginal douching

Most common causative agents in PID

• *C. trachomatis*
• *N. gonorrhea*
• Other: *E. coli, Peptostreptococcus, G. vaginalis, Prevotella, Bacteroides, Streptococcus, H. influenzae, T. vaginalis, M. genitalium, M. hominis.*

HPV—F/U CONSIDERATIONS

• HPV is not reportable in Canada.
• Once genital warts are healed, routine F/U for cervical CA is recommended.
• Consider sexual abuse in children presenting with genital warts.
• C/S is not indicated unless warts obstruct the birth canal.
• Screen for other STIs.

PID

• Ascending infection of the upper genital tract from the vagina and/or cervix
• Sx range from asymptomatic to severe Sx
• Up to two third of cases go unrecognized
• 10% to 15 % of women of reproductive age will have at least one episode of PID
• PID is the most common infectious cause of lower Abdo pain in women

SIGNS AND SX

• see Clinical Box PID Classic triad
• Dyspareunia
• RUQ pain
• Uterine tenderness
• Dysuria
• Purulent exudates
• Adnexal mass

Table **14.26** Dx and Rx of HPV		
Signs and Sx	**Diagnostic Criteria**	**Rx Options**

• **HPV infection is frequently asymptomatic.**
• HPV lesion: external genital warts (condyloma acuminata)—multifocal cauliflower-like exophytic fronds → +/− pruritus or local discharge
  • On cervix, vagina, or vulva
  • Δ in size and number of warts with pregnancy
• Intraepithelial lesions on Pap smear → cervical involvement (LSIL, HSIL, invasive carcinoma)
• **HIV:** Collaborative care with other specialists is required in patients with HIV due to ↑ risk of cervical CA.
• 90% of patients with external genital warts experience clearance within 2 yr with medical intervention.
	1. **Pap test**
	2. **HPV typing** not indicated for routine Dx/management of visible genital warts
	3. **Colposcopy** if ASCUS, LSIL, HSIL, atypical glandular cells or invasive carcinoma on Pap test **or** positive high-risk HPV subtype twice in the last year
	4. **Anoscopy**: in patients with anal warts due to the risk of anal CA
	5. **Urethroscopy** in patients with extensive urethral warts
	Suspect neoplasia if:
	• Pigmented lesion
	• Bleeding
	• Persistent ulceration
	• Persistent pruritus
	• Recalcitrant lesions
	• Biopsy if lesion suspicious
		No Rx guarantees eradication of HPV.
		Patient applied:
		• Imiquod × 3/wk for up to 16 wk. Cream must be washed off after 6−8 h.
		• Podofilox 0.5%, 0.5 mL q12 h × 3/wk for 6 wk
		Provider-based:
		• Cryotherapy (liquid nitrogen, CO_2)
		• Podophyllin resin 10−25% for 1−4 h, repeated at weekly intervals
		• Bi- or trichloroacetic acid (50%−80% solution)
		• CO_2 laser ablation, excision
		Extensive or resistant lesions:
		• Excision Electroexcision
		• CO_2 laser removal
		Consider cone biopsy of the cervix, loop electrode excision of the transformation zone if indicated.

• 13% of women become infertile after one episode of PID; 55% after three episodes.
• **Infertility** is more common with gonorrhea, and delay of Rx.
• **Fitz-Hugh-Curtis syndrome**: perihepatitis resulting in adhesions between the
• liver capsule and the Abdo wall. Perihepatitis resolves with Rx of PID.

• Vaginal bleeding
• Nausea/vomiting
• ↑ ESR, CRP
• WBC >10,000/mm^3
• Lab confirmation of cervical Dx of chlamydia and/or gonorrhea

CLINICAL BOX

Fitz-Hugh-Curtis Syndrome

Perihepatitis resulting in adhesions between the liver capsule and the Abdo wall. Perihepatitis resolves with Rx of PID.

CLINICAL BOX

Gold Standard Dx

Laparoscopy demonstrating abnormalities consistent with PID including fallopian tube erythema and/or mucopurulent exudates

CLINICAL BOX

PID Classical Triad

1. Lower Abdo pain (+ peritoneal signs)
2. Bilateral adnexal tenderness
3. Cervical motion tenderness or sexual exposure to a person with GC or chlamydia

Rx

Table **14.27** Complications of PID	
Acute complications	• Pelvic peritonitis • Endometritis • Salpingitis • Tubo-ovarian abscess
Chronic complications	• Infertility • chronic pelvic or Abdo pain • pelvic/Abdo adhesions • Fitz-Hugh-Curtis syndrome • EP

Table **14.28**	**Rx Options for PID**
Inpatient Rx	1. Cefotetan IV + doxycycline IV until clinical improvement >24 h then continue doxycycline PO for a total of 14 d
	2. Cefoxitin IV + doxycycline IV/PO until clinical improvement >24 h then continue doxycycline PO for a total of 14 d
	3. Clindamycin IV + gentamicin IV until clinical improvement×24 h then doxycycline PO or clindamycin PO for a total of 14 d
Outpatient Rx	1. Ofloxacin PO×14 d + metronidazole PO b.i.d.×14 d
	2. Levofloxacin PO×14 d + metronidazole PO b.i.d.×14 d
	3. Ceftriaxone IM×1 + doxycycline PO q12 h×14 d
	4. Cefoxitin IM×1 + probenecid PO×1 + Doxycycline PO q12 h×14 d

IUD: The device should not be removed until at least two doses of antibiotic Rx have been administered.

CLINICAL BOX

Criteria for Inpatient Rx

- Pregnancy
- Appendicitis/EP cannot be excluded
- Adolescence/poor compliance
- Inability to follow or tolerate an oral regimen
- If pelvic abscess is suspected
- Patient previously failed to respond to outpatient Rx
- Patient is immunodeficient
- Dx is uncertain (i.e., need for laparoscopy)
- The patient has severe illness (vomiting, fever, pain)
- HIV positive patient
- IUD *in situ*

CERVICAL CANCER SCREENING

RATIONALE

- Carcinoma of the cervix is a preventable disease.
- Female patients visiting their 1° care physicians should follow the provincial screening guidelines for cervical CA.
- Up to 90% of cervical CAs are squamous cell carcinomas. The remainder are adenocarcinomas.
- Rarely, cervical CAs have features of both squamous cell carcinomas and adenocarcinomas (i.e., adenosquamous carcinomas).
- The Pap cytologic test ("Pap test") is the only way to detect abnormal cells on the cervix.
- Cervical CA has a long natural Hx with a long precancerous phase.
- Screening programs ↓ the incidence of invasive disease.
- Only 81% of Ontario women report having had a recent Pap test.

EPIDEMIOLOGY

- Cervical CA is the second most common CA in women <50.
- The median age at Dx of cervical CA is 47 yr.
- The median age at death from cervical CA is 60 yr.
- The 11th most common CA in women and 13th most common CA-related cause of death.
- From 1981 to 2002, the incidence of cervical CA ↓ by ~50% in Ontario, due to Pap smear screening.
- Other causes for abnormal Pap smears, other than the HPV virus, are unknown.

CLINICAL BOX

HPV Subtypes

Low risk: 6, 11, 41, 44

Intermediate risk: 31, 33, 35

High risk: 16, 18, 45, 56

RFs FOR CERVICAL CA

1. HPV infection with high-risk subtype
2. First intercourse at a young age (early coitarche)
3. Multiple sexual partners
4. Cigarette smoking

5. Multiparity
6. Long-term use of OCP
7. Malnutrition or altered immune status
8. Low socioeconomic status
9. High-risk sexual partners (i.e., partners whose Prev. sexual contacts have developed cancerous or precancerous lesions of the cervix)
10. Presence of other STIs

HPV Transmission

- HPV is transmitted sexually and is the most common STI.
- Condoms do not fully protect against transmission of HPV.
- HPV can be transmitted without penetration.

1° Prevention of Cervical CA

- Pap smear: the mainstay of screening for precancerous lesions
- HPV vaccine (See page 391)
- Colposcopy
- Rx of precancerous lesions

HPV

- HPV is one of the most common STIs.
- 75% of Canadians have had one or more HPV infections.
- 95% of squamous cell carcinomas have HPV oncogenic types as do 60% of cervical adenocarcinomas.
- There are 20 HPV types that have been identified as carcinogenic.
- Types **16 and 18** are found most commonly in malignant lesions.

APPROACH

- Pap smears can be obtained by conventional Pap smear or with liquid-based cytology.
- Liquid-based cytology is the preferred method for obtaining cervical cytology.
- The liquid-based cytology screen has been found to be more sensitive and is associated with fewer unsatisfactory specimens.
- The transformation zone undergoes transformation from glandular cells to squamous cells (i.e., metaplasia).
- Areas of active metaplasia are the most susceptible site for infection by HPV, and subsequent development of cervical CA.

POPULATION SCREENING

- Should begin within 3 yr of initiating sexual activity
- Should be conducted annually until three consecutive negative Pap tests
- If these Pap tests are normal → continue screening q2-3 yr.
- Should continue until the age of 69 yr, if there has been adequate screening over the past 10 yr
- If there has been no Pap smear for 5 yr, begin annual Pap tests until three consecutive negative Pap tests, then should continue q2-3yr.
- Discontinue screening at age 70 if >3 normal Pap tests in the last 10 yr.

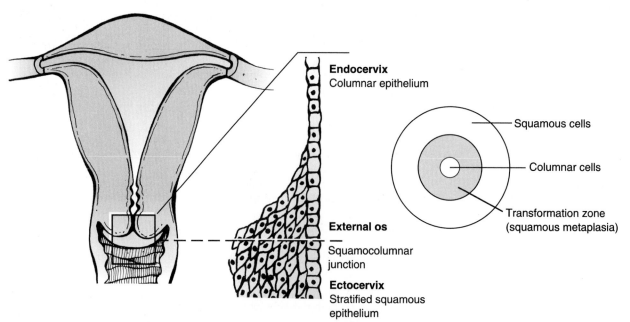

Figure 14.8 How to Obtain a Pap Smear.

Table **14.29** Type of Cervical Pap Smears

Liquid Based Smear	Traditional Pap Smear
1. Specimen is collected by wiping cells from the cervix and endocervix.	1. A wooden spatula is used to wipe cells from the surface of the cervix.
2. The cells are suspended in liquid to remove blood and mucus.	2. A brush is used to wipe cells from the endocervical canal—(may cause bleeding, should be avoided in pregnancy).
• This is the preferred method • Improved Dx of low and high grades SIL • Can be used to identify HPV subtypes	3. These cells are spread onto a slide that is fixed for cytologic exam.

Descriptive convention						
Class system	Class I (normal)	Class II inflammation	Class III Mild dysplasia	Class III Moderate dysplasia	Class IV Severe dysplasia CIS	Class V suggestive of CA or CIS
CIN system	Normal	Inflammatory	CIN I	CIN II	CIN III	Suggestive of CA
Bethesda II system	Within normal limits	a. Without atypia b. With atypia or cellular changes associated with HPV	LSIL	HSIL	HSIL	Squamous cell CA
Bethesda 2001	Negative for intraepithelial lesion or malignancy	ASCUS / ASC–H	LSIL	HSIL	HSIL	Squamous cell CA
Histology						

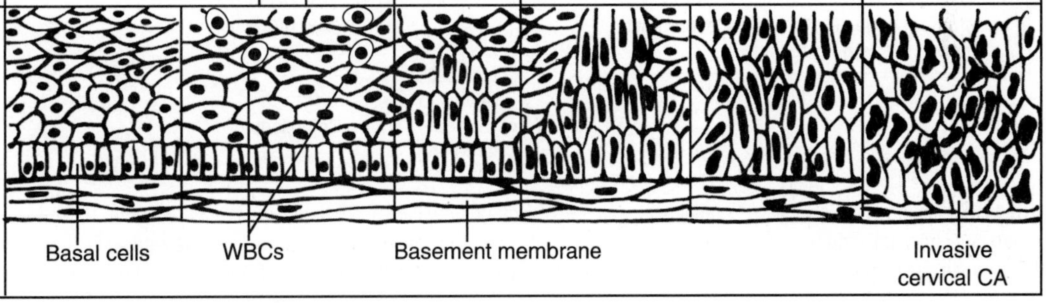

Basal cells   WBCs   Basement membrane   Invasive cervical CA

Figure 14.9 Pap smear descriptive conventions.

Table **14.30** Pap Smear Report Legend

1	Unsatisfactory/inadequate sample
2	Normal
3	Benign atypia (infection, reactive Δs)
4	Epithelial abnormalities:
5	CIN
6	ASCUS
7	ASC-H
8	LSIL
9	HSIL
10	CIS
11	AGUS

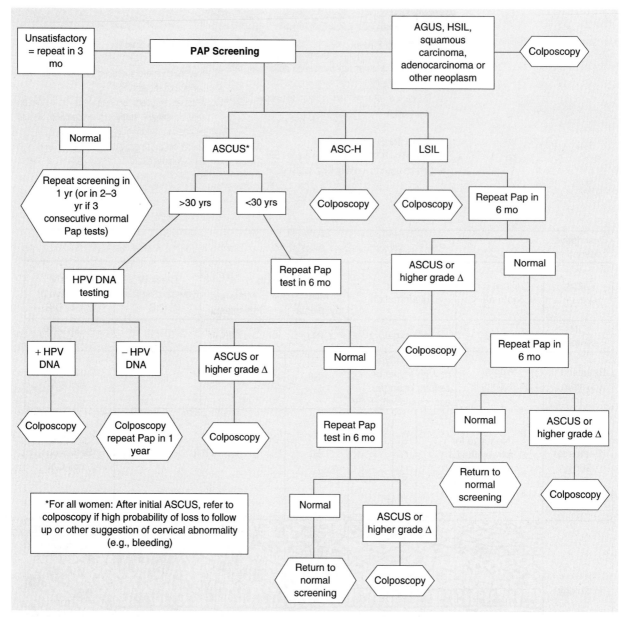

Figure 14.10 Approach to Cervical CA Screening (adapted from Ontario Cervical Cancer Screening Guideline 2005). These are recommended as minimum guidelines adapted from the Ontario Cervical Cancer screening Guideline 2005. Note: For patients with ASCUS who are >30 yr → if HPV DNA testing is not available, repeat cytology in 6 mo is recommended× 2 with colposcopy if ASCUS or higher grade Δ.

SCREENING IN SPECIAL POPULATIONS

- Women with HIV/immunocompromised should receive annual screening.
- Discontinue screening for women who have undergone a total hysterectomy for benign reasons and no Hx of cervical dysplasia or HPV.
- Women who have undergone a subtotal hysterectomy (i.e., cervix intact) should continue routine screening.
- Screening frequency in pregnancy is the same as in nonpregnant women.
- Women who have sex with women should follow the same screening protocol as women who have sex with men.

COLPOSCOPY

- Pap smear carries a false-negative rate of 15% to 40% for invasive CAs.
- Colposcopy provides magnification and illumination of the cervix to:
  - Further assess abnormalities on the cervix
  - Confirm Dx by biopsy

- R/O invasive disease
- F/U after Rx
- Procedure:
  - Magnification to inspect the transformation zone after application of 3% to 5% acetic acid.
  - Biopsies are performed of abnormal appearing epithelium.
  - Colposcopically directed biopsies carry an accuracy of 85% to 95%.
- Endocervical curettage can be performed to R/O dysplasia within the cervical canal.

HPV Vaccine (Gardasil)

- The HPV vaccine protects against HPV types 6, 11, 16 and 18. It is given at zero, 2 mo, and 6 mo intervals.
- It is most effective when given before the onset of sexual activity.
- NACI recommends immunization for:
  1. Women aged 9 to 13 who have not yet become sexually active
  2. Women aged 14 to 26 whether sexually active or not
  3. Women aged 14 to 26 yr who have had Prev. Pap abnormalities, including cervical CA, or have had genital warts or known HPV infection. (They could still benefit from the vaccine as they may not have been infected with the HPV types covered by the vaccine.)
- This position is supported by the interim statement of the SOGC on HPV immunization as well as the American Cancer Society.
- Women who receive the vaccine should continue to get screened regularly for cervical CA since they may still be exposed to or infected with other types of HPV.

Cervical CA

- Peak incidence for cervical CA begins at 45 yr.
- Long precancerous phase with 3 to 5 yr to progress from one grade of dysplasia to the next.
- From the detection of cytologic abnormalities to invasive CA takes 15 to 20 yr.
- Invasive carcinoma of the cervix is usually preceded by a spectrum of preinvasive disease which can be detected by a Pap smear. It usually takes up to 10 yr for abnormal cells to turn into CA.

CLINICAL BOX

Signs and Sx of Cervical CA

- Postcoital/irregular bleeding
- Malodorous, bloody discharge
- Leg edema (advanced disease)
- Deep pelvic pain (advanced disease)
- Sciatica (advanced disease)

Table **14.31** **Staging and Rx of Cervical CA**

Stage	Description	Rx
0	CIS, preinvasive carcinoma No stromal invasion	Localized Rx: cryotherapy, LEEP, laser Rx or conization
I	Invasive carcinoma confined to the cervix	1. Conization for women planning to have children in future
IA	Invasive carcinoma identified microscopically	2. Radical hysterectomy (acceptable for postreproductive age women or if the depth is between 3 and 5 mm)
IA1	Invasion of the stroma <3.0 mm in depth and <7.0 mm horizontal spread	
IA2	Invasion of stroma 3–5 mm in depth and < 7.0 mm horizontal spread	
IB	Clinically visible lesion confined to the cervix or microscopic lesion greater than stage IA2 Subdivided into:	1. Radical hysterectomy and pelvic lymphadenectomy if lesions <4.0 cm • Can spare ovaries 2. Radiotherapy for lesions >4.0 cm.
IB1	Lesions <4.0 cm in size	
IB2	Lesions >4.0 cm in size	
II	Extends beyond the cervix but not onto the pelvic wall +/− upper 2/3 of vagina	1. Radiotherapy 2. +/− Concurrent chemo-radiotherapy
IIA	**No** parametrial involvement	
IIB	Parametrial involvement	
III	Extends to the pelvic wall or involves the lower 1/3 of the vagina	
IIIA	Lower 1/3 of vagina with no involvement of pelvic wall	
IIIB	Lower 1/3 of vagina with extension into pelvic wall or hydronephrosis/nonfunctioning kidney	
IV	Extends beyond true pelvis, or has clinically involved the mucosa of the bladder or rectum	

PELVIC MASS

RATIONALE

- Pelvic masses are common and can be found in females at **any** age (fetal to post-menopausal).
- All pelvic masses should be investigated and diagnosed because early detection may affect outcome.

CAUSAL CONDITIONS

Pelvic masses may originate from gynecologic organs (ovary, fallopian tube, cervix, or uterus) or from other nongynecologic pelvic organs (bowel, bladder, ureters, skeletal muscle, or bone)

Table **14.32** DDx of Pelvic Mass				
Age Group	**DDx**			
	Gynecologic			**Nongynecologic**
	Ovary	**Fallopian Tube**	**Uterus**	

Pre adolescent	1. Benign simple ovarian cysts (i.e., germinal inclusion cyst)
	2. Dermoid cysts (benign cystic teratoma)[a]
	3. Malignant germ cell tumors:
	  • Dysgerminoma
	  • Yolk sac/endodermal sinus tumors
	  • Embryonal carcinoma[a]
	4. Gonadoblastomas (rare)
	5. Paraovarian cysts (rare)
		1. Paratubular cyst
		2. Congenital cysts
		  • Mesonephric
		  • Paramesonephric
			1. Uterine anomaly (bicornuate uterus, uterus didelphy)	1. Pelvic kidney
				2. Distended bladder
				3. Appendiceal abscess

Reproductive	1. Functional ovarian cysts (follicular, corpus luteum, thecal lutein, hemorrhagic)
	2. Polycystic ovaries
	3. Ovarian torsion
	4. Luteoma of pregnancy
	5. Dermoid cyst
	6. Malignant germ cell tumors
	  • Teratoma (solid/cystic)
	  • Choriocarcinoma[a]
	  • Polyembryonal CA[a]
	  • Endodermal sinus/yolk sac (rare)
	7. Gonadoblastomas
	8. Dysgerminomas
		1. EP
		2. Tubo-ovarian abscess/complex
		3. Pelvic adhesions
		4. Hydrosalpinx/pyosalpinx
		5. 1° fallopian tube neoplasm
		6. Inflammatory cysts
		  • Mesonephric
		  • Paramesonephric
			1. Pregnancy
			2. Adenomyoma
			3. Leiomyoma (fibroid)
			4. Hematometria/ Pyometria
			5. Endometrioma/ endometriosis
			6. Endometrial CA (rare)
			7. Leiomyosarcoma (rare)
			8. Imperforate hymen
				1. Distended bladder
				2. Appendiceal abscess
				3. Diverticular disease
				4. 1° CA (rectal, colon, or bladder)
				5. Metastatic CA (breast, colon, lung)
				6. Redundant sigmoid colon
				7. Pelvic kidney

Peri/post menopause (Malignancy until proven otherwise)	**Malignant neoplasms**
	1. **Epithelial cell tumors**
	  • Cystadenocarcinomas (serous or mucinous)
	  • Endometrioid
	2. **Sex cord neoplasms**
	  • Granulosa cell tumor
	  • Sertoli-Leydig cell tumor[a]
	3. **Metastases** (i.e., Krukenberg tumor from GI CA)
	Benign neoplasms (rare)—thecoma or fibromas
		1. Tubo-ovarian abscess
		2. Pelvic adhesions
		3. Hydrosalpinx/pyosalpinx
		4. Inflammatory cysts
		  • Mesonephric
		  • Paramesonephric
		5. 1° fallopian tube neoplasm
			1. Endometrial CA
			2. Leiomyosarcoma (rare)	

[a]**Hormonally active** (can secrete hormones)

APPROACH

The key objectives when investigating a woman with a pelvic mass is determination of:

1. Their pregnancy status (β-HCG testing)
2. Whether the mass is gynecologic versus nongynecologic

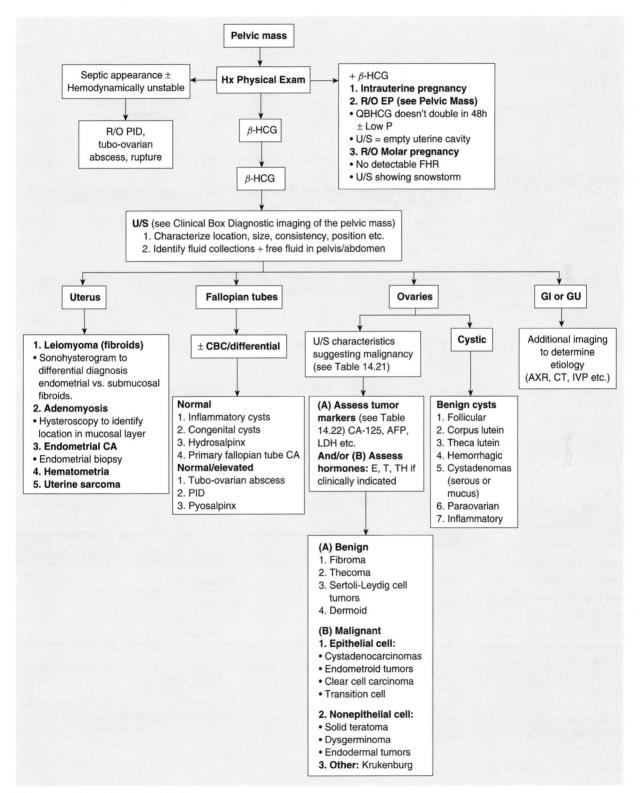

Figure 14.11 Approach to the Dx of pelvic mass.

Table 14.33 Pelvic Mass—Focused Hx

Menstrual Hx	Sexual Hx	OB/GYN Hx	Other

• Menarche
• Cycle length
• Flow duration + heaviness
• Δ in menstrual pattern
• AUB
• PMS
• Menstrual pain
	• # Partners
	• Method(s) of contraception
	• Dyspareunia
		• Hx STIs, vaginitis
		• Hx vaginal discharge
		• Pap smear status
		• GTPAL status
		• Mode of delivery
		• Hx pregnancy complications
			• Characterize any Abdo/ pelvic pain (OPQRST)
			• Medications
			• Past surgical Hx
			• FHx of breast, ovarian,
			• GI, +/− endometrial CA
			• Review of Sx
			  • Weight Δ, energy level
			  • Skin/hair Δ
			  • Breast discharge/pain
			  • Urinary/bowel patterns
			  • Constitutional Sx
			  • GI: early satiety, Abdo fullness

Table 14.34 Pelvic Mass—Focused Physical Exam

Breasts (common site of ovarian metastasis)	• Tanner staging if prepubertal • Tenderness • Masses • Discharge
Abdo	• Organomegaly • Tenderness, guarding, rebound • Ascites

Pelvic ± bimanual Exam	• **External:** Clitoromegaly (>4 mm wide), vagina (color, odor, moistness, rugosity, discharge, mass)
	• **Internal:**
	  • Cervix (discharge, motion tenderness)
	  • Uterus (position, size, shape, mobility, symmetry tenderness, consistency)
	  • Adnexa (size, shape, mobility, tenderness, consistency, location of mass)

Other	• Assess lymph nodes (cervical, supraclavicular and inguinal) • DRE • Rectovaginal exam (assess posterior uterine surface, uterosacral ligaments, parametria, pouch of Douglas and rectum)

CLINICAL BOX

Features Characteristic to Exposure to ↑ Sex Hormone Levels

Features of Androgenization

• Prepubertal age
  • Clitoromegaly (>4 mm wide)
  • Hirsutism
• Reproductive age
  • Hirsutism
  • Acne and/or seborrhea
  • Alopecia
  • Deepening of voice
  • ↑ Muscle bulk

Features of Estrogenization

• Prepubertal age
  • Menarche
  • Advanced tanner staging

Table 14.35 U/S Characteristics of Benign vs. Malignant Ovarian Masses

Characteristics	Benign	Malignant
Patient Age	Reproductive age	Prepubertal Perimenopausal Postmenopausal
Location	Unilateral	Bilateral
Size	<5 cm	>10 cm or >5 cm initially but rapid ↑ (i.e., <6 wk)
Consistency	Cystic	Solid or mixed Multiple and/or thick septae
Shape	Smooth	Irregular Papillary projections
Mobility	Movable	Fixed
Other	No free fluid	↑ Volume of free fluid in pelvis or Abdo (ascites) Note: Doppler flow of the mass showing low resistance

Table **14.36**	Investigation of Pelvic Mass—Lab Markers				
Tumor Marker	**Source**	**Normal Value**	**Abn Value**	**↑↑ Levels Found in**	**Sensitivity**
CA-125 Sensitivity >> Specificity[a]	Glycoprotein produced by fetal coelomic epithelium	<35 U/mL	>200 U/mL	Epithelial cell ovarian tumors (also fibroids, PID endometriosis, cirrhosis adenomyosis, pregnancy, breast/lung/ovarian/colon/fallopian tube CAs, pancreatitis)	• ↑ in ~85% of ovarian CAs • ↑ in ~50% of stage I ovarian CAs • 98% PPV for ovarian CA in post-menopausal women with asymptomatic palpable pelvic masses, CA-125 >65 U/ • Testing for CA-125 in pre-menopausal women not useful because of ↑ # benign causes of its elevation
AFP[a]	Major protein in fetal serum; **not** detectable after birth	<5.4 ng/mL	>500 ng/mL	Germ cell tumors (i.e., endodermal sinus) (also pregnancy, HCC)	• ↑ In ~85% of germ cell tumors • ↑ In ~20% of stage I germ cell tumors
LDH[a]	Enzyme found in almost all body tissues	<250 U/L		Dysgerminomas	• ↑ In some cases of dysgerminomas
hCG[a]	Normally produced by the placenta	<5 mIU/mL	>30 mIU/ mL	Germ cell tumors GTD (i.e., choriocarcinoma) (also pregnancy, marijuana use)	• ↑ In ~80% of germ cell tumors • ↑ In ~20% of stage I germ cell tumors

[a]Not effective screening tool(s) for ovarian CA

CLINICAL BOX

Diagnostic Imaging of Pelvic Masses

1. U/S
   - First choice
   - Delineates mass qualities (cystic vs. solid, size, location)
   - Assess for ascites
   - Safe in pregnancy
2. CT
   - Not good for ovary
   - Assess all other organs, lymph nodes
   - Assess retroperitoneum
3. MRI
   - Identification of soft tissue lesions
   - Safe in pregnancy
   - Does not use radio-opaque contrast agent
4. Other
   - Abdo XR
   - IV pyelogram

3. The anatomic location of the mass (fallopian tube, ovary, or uterus)
4. The characteristics (consistency, size, shape, mobility etc.) of the mass

LAB MARKERS IN DX OF THE PELVIC MASS

Play a crucial role in

1. Detecting disease
2. F/U with respect to Rx and recurrence of disease

CLINICAL BOX

Ovarian Carcinoma—Epithelial Cell Tumors

Epidemiology

- ~80% of ovarian CAs
- Incidence ↑ at age 50 yr up to 80 yr

RFs

- FHx of ovarian CA (5% if one first-degree relative affected; 7% if two)
- Mutations in **BRCA1** (chr17q) and **BRCA2** (chr13q) tumor suppressor genes which account for familial breast ovarian CA
- Excess ovulation (low parity, infertility)
- Lynch II syndrome: familial disposition to endometrial, ovarian, and GU CAs.

Screening

No reliable screening test available

Dx

Surgical staging

Rx

- Surgical debulking, chemotherapy. Follow progress with serum CA-125 levels. If FHx BRCA1 or 2 can recommend prophylactic bilateral oophrectomy when child bearing is complete.

MANAGEMENT

- Depends on the age of patient, size of the mass, U/S features, and tumor markers
- Must take into consideration the patient's age, desire to preserve fertility, and patient preference
- **Any** ovarian mass in a postmenopausal woman is considered CA until proven otherwise.
- **Any** solid ovarian mass in childhood is considered malignant until proven otherwise.

INDICATIONS FOR SPECIALTY CARE REFERRAL IN WOMEN WITH A PELVIC MASS

- Persistent masses (>2 menstrual cycles) in reproductive aged women
- **Any** postmenopausal mass
- **Any** mass with one or more of the following (regardless of if patient is symptomatic): >10 cm, >5 cm with rapid growth, nodular, fixed, solid, presence of ascites, ↑ CA-125 (>200 U/mL premenopause vs. >35 U/mL postmenopause)
- FHx of >1 first-degree relative(s) with ovarian or breast CA
- Suspected abnormal pregnancy, malignancy, and masses requiring surgical intervention

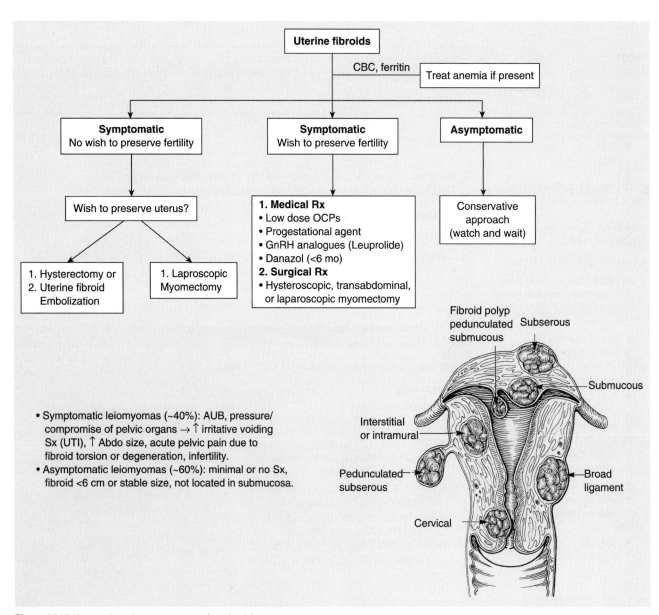

Figure 14.12 Approach to the management of uterine leiomyomas.

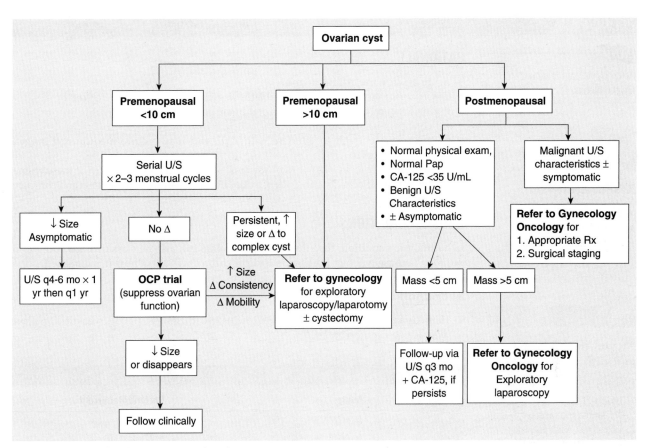

Figure 14.13 Approach to the management of ovarian cysts.

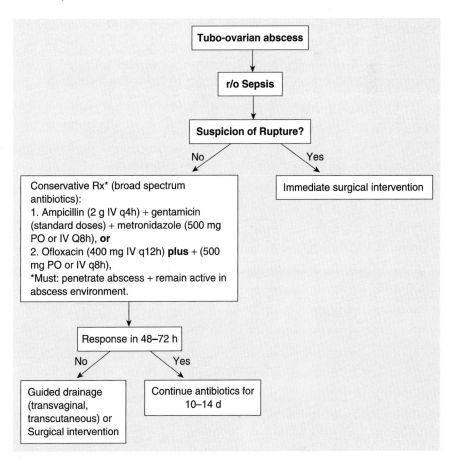

Figure 14.14 Approach to the management of tubo-ovarian abscesses.

PELVIC PAIN

Acute pelvic pain is potentially life threatening.

CLINICAL BOX

RFs for Acute PID

- Age 15 to 25 yr
- Prior Hx PID
- Partner with Hx of urethritis

CLINICAL BOX

Mental Health Issues and CPP

1. ~25% of patients with CPP have a PMHx of sexual/physical abuse.
2. Depression often coexists with CPP (25% to 50%). It is a predictor of:
   - Pain severity
   - Response to Rx

RATIONALE

- Acute pelvic pain: lasting <6 mo
- CPP is one of the most common problems in gynecology. It is characterized by:
  - Pain located below the umbilicus and in the pelvis
  - Pelvic pain lasting >6 mo
  - Pain severe enough to interfere with ADL and may require medical and surgical intervention(s)
- Women Avg. ~2 to 3 visits/yr to physicians' offices with CPP. Only 1/3 of these women are given a specific Dx. The absence of a clear Dx can frustrate both patients and clinicians.

CAUSAL CONDITIONS

In addition to condition, the etiology of pelvic pain can also be classified according to its duration because whether the pain is acute or chronic will affect how it is managed.

APPROACH

1. Hemodynamic status: vitals (BP, HR), signs/Sx (dizziness, pallor, weakness, malaise, dyspnea on exertion etc.)

Table 14.37 DDx of Pelvic Pain

Condition	Acute	Chronic/Recurrent
Gyne	• EP • Aborting pregnancy • Labor/PTL • Molar pregnancy • Abruptio placenta • PID ± adhesions • Ovarian mass/cyst complications (torsion, hemorrhage, rupture) • Degenerating fibroids • Ovulation pain	• Endometriosis • Chronic PID • Adenomyosis • Leiomyomata • Dysmenorrhea • Pelvic adhesions • Dyspareunia • Vulvar vestibulitis • Vulvodynia • Residual ovarian syndrome • Chronic pelvic infection (TB)
GI	• Acute appendicitis • Diverticulitis • Irritable bowel • IBD	• Irritable bowel • IBD • Diverticulitis • Constipation • Hernia • Neoplastic lesions
Urologic	• UTI • Renal calculi	• Chronic UTIs • Interstitial cystitis • Urethral disorders • Bladder neoplasm
MSK	• Levator ani syndrome • Disc disease • Hernia	• Fibromyalgia • Nerve entrapment syndromes • Mechanical low back pain • Disc disease

Systemic	• Sleep disturbance
	• Mental health issues:
	  • Depression, somatization
	  • Abuse (sexual, physical, and/or psychological)
	  • Domestic violence
	  • Substance abuse	

2. Pregnancy status (β-HCG) plus CBC, coagulation profile—if clinically indicated
3. Whether the pain is acute versus chronic. (If acute pelvic pain, may need to stabilize the patient vs. chronic pain, may need to proactively schedule time for complete evaluation and counseling of the patient (can take up to 60 to 90 min.)

MANAGEMENT OF CPP

- Must take into consideration the patients' age; desire to preserve fertility, patient preference, and surgical feasibility.

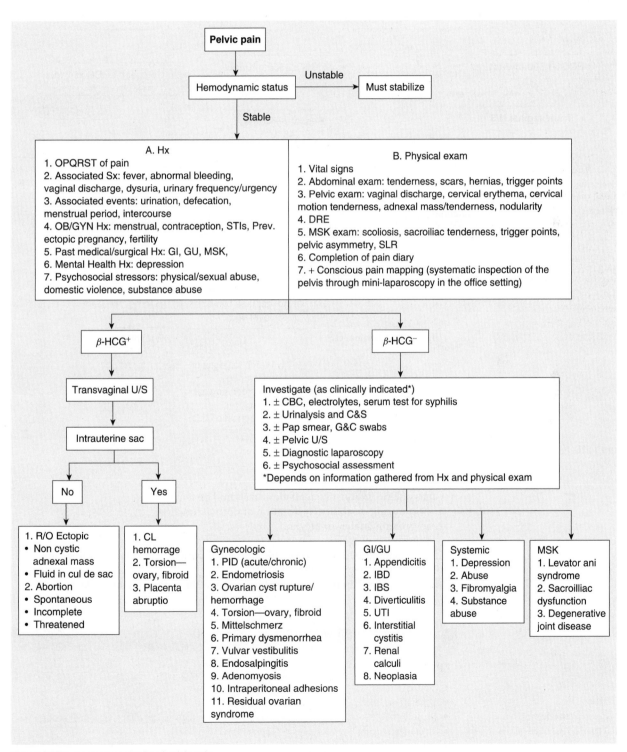

Figure 14.15 Approach to the Dx of pelvic pain.

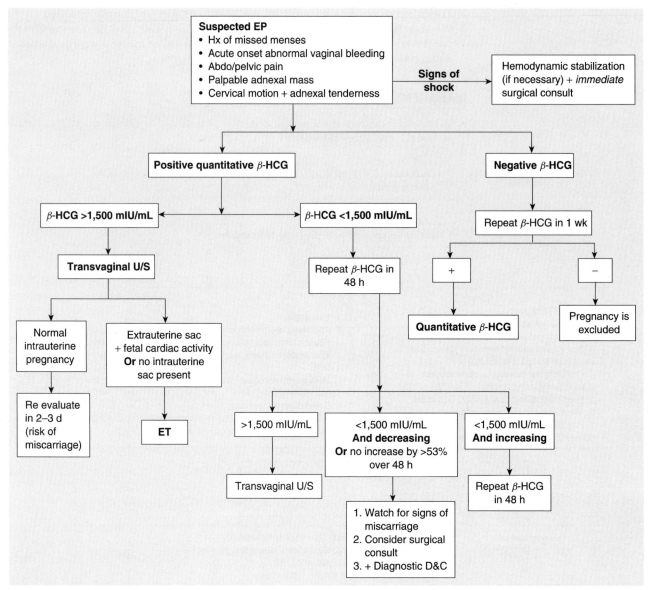

Figure 14.16 Approach to the EP.

- Goals of CPP Rx must be realistic and should be focused on:
  1. Minimizing disability/restoration of normal function,
  2. improving quality of life, and
  3. prevention of relapse.
- CPP Rx should be tailored for the individual patient and often requires simultaneous pharmacologic, psychological, and PT.
- A good relationship between the physician and the patient is essential.

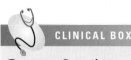

CLINICAL BOX

Common Locations of EP

1. Ampullary: 70%
2. Isthmic: 12%
3. Fimbrial: 11%
4. Ovarian: 3%
5. Others: interstitial/cornual—2%, Abdo—1%, cervical—<1%

CLINICAL BOX

EP RFs

- Prev. EP
- Current/Prev. IUD
- Hx of PID
- Prev. tubal surgery
- *In utero* DES exposure
- Infertility
- Current smoking
- Uterine structure: fibroids, adhesions, abnormal shape, and so on

Table **14.38**	**Management of EP**[a]

Medical	**MTX:**
	• Folic acid antagonist that inhibits DNA synthesis and cell reproduction
	• 86%–94% success rate for Rx of EP
	• **Criteria:**
	  1. Hemodynamically stable
	  2. No active bleeding or signs of hemoperitoneum
	  3. <3.5 cm unruptured mass
	  4. No fetal heart activity
	  5. Noninvasive Dx
	  6. Patient desires future fertility
	  7. Patient is compliant and able to return for F/U care
	  8. No CI to mtx
	• **CI**
	  1. Breast-feeding
	  2. Chronic liver disease (alcoholism, fatty liver etc.)
	  3. Known sensitivity to MTX
	  4. Active disease—lung, blood dyscrasias (i.e., thrombocytopenia, significant anemia)
	  5. Hepatic, renal, or hematologic dysfunction
	• **Dosing:** single IM dose (50 mg/m^2 body surface area) (88.1% success rate); may require a second IM dose
	Monitoring: serial (weekly) β-HCG levels until undetectable

Laparoscopic surgery **or** laparotomy	• **Methods:** linear salpingostomy, linear salpingectomy or segmental resection if tube is salvageable **vs.** salpingectomy if tube requires removal
	• **Indications for laparoscopy:**
	  1. Failed MTX Rx
	  2. Prev. EP in same fallopian tube
	• **CIs to laparoscopy:**
	  1. Hemodynamic instability
	  2. Pelvic adhesions
	  3. Hematoperitoneum
	  4. Pregnancy >4 cm
	• **Indications for laparotomy:**
	  1. Hemodynamic instability
	  2. Prev. EP in same fallopian tube
	  3. Severe pelvic adhesions

[a]If patient if Rh$^-$, MUST give anti-D γ globulin (RhoGAM) before Rx is initiated.

CLINICAL BOX

Laparoscopy and CPP

Role in CPP

- Confirmation of Dx
- Surgical intervention
- Rx
- Patient reassurance

Indications

1. Persistent CPP with no discernable cause after appropriate investigations
2. CPP refractory to pharmacologic Rx

INDICATIONS FOR SPECIALTY CARE REFERRAL IN WOMEN WITH CPP

1. Persistent pain despite a 3 to 6 mo trial of NSAIDs or OCPs
2. Lack of Dx despite appropriate diagnostic investigations
3. Positive result on pregnancy testing (if the family physician is not comfortable managing)

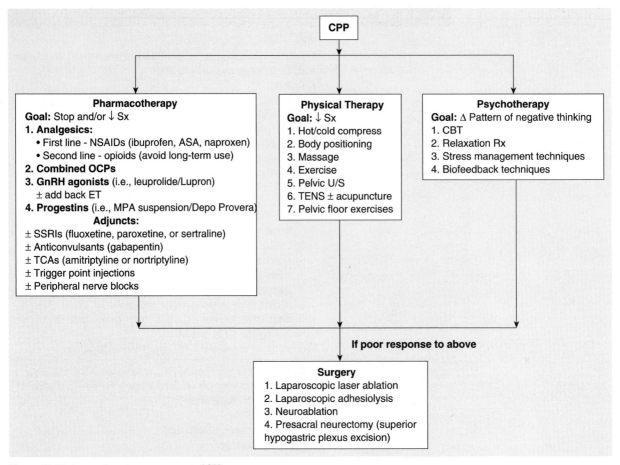

Figure 14.17 Approach to the management of CPP.

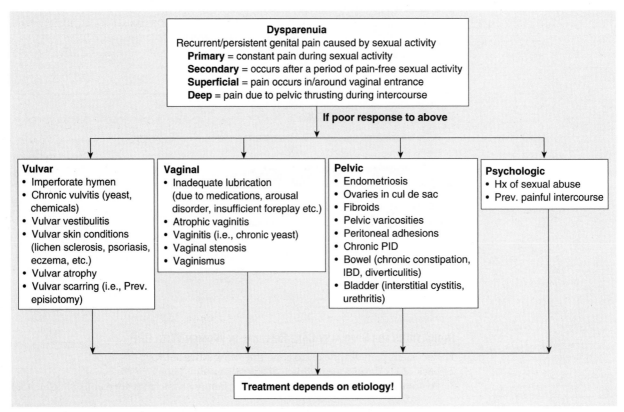

Figure 14.18 Approach to dyspareunia.

PELVIC PROLAPSE/RELAXATION

DEFINITION

- Herniation of one of the pelvic organs (uterus, vaginal apex, bladder, rectum) and its associated vaginal segment from its normal location
- Prolapse is a dynamic condition; regression of prolapse occurs at a similar rate as incidence

APPLIED SCIENTIFIC CONCEPTS

- Pelvic organs are supported by the pelvic floor musculature, fascial supports, and nervous system.
- Prolapse results from site-specific fascial defects cause vaginal segment weakness.
- The muscular pelvic floor is composed of the **levator ani** (combination of puborectalis, pubococcygeus and iliococcygeus) and the **coccygeus muscles** attached to elements of the bony pelvis, coccyx and sacrum.

CAUSAL CONDITIONS

The majority of women with clinically significant prolapse will have at least two RFs:

1. Damage to support
   - Obstetric causes: pregnancy (multiparity), delivery (vacuum/forceps)
   - Surgical causes: hysterectomy
   - E deficiency
   - Chronically ↑ Abdo pressure: obesity, smoking, pulmonary disease (chronic cough), constipation (chronic strain), recreational/occupational activities (weight lifting), ascites
   - Pelvic masses
2. Neuromuscular/connective tissue disorders
3. Genetics

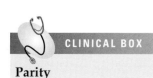

CLINICAL BOX

Parity

Although ↑ parity is a RF for prolapse, nulliparity does not provide absolute protection against prolapse.

CLASSIFYING PROLAPSE

- Many systems for staging prolapse have been described, typically graded on a scale of 0 to 4:
  - 0: No prolapse
  - 1: Halfway to the hymen
  - 2: At the hymen
  - 3: Halfway out of the hymen
  - 4: Total prolapse ("procidentia")
- Standard system approved by the International Continence Society is the POPQ
  - Measures nine locations on the vagina and vulva in centimeters relative to hymen and used to stage 0 to IV
  - More detailed than necessary for clinical care, but used routinely in studies

Table **14.39**	**Types of Female GU Prolapse**
Cystocele	Herniation of the bladder with associated descent of the anterior vaginal segment
Cystourethrocele	A cystocele combined with distal prolapse of the bladder neck ± associated urethral hypermobility
Uterine prolapse	Descent of the uterus and cervix
Vaginal vault prolapse	Descent of the vaginal apex (posthysterectomy) into the lower vagina **or** to the hymenal ring **or** through the vaginal introitus
Rectocele	Herniation of the rectum with associated descent of the posterior vaginal segment

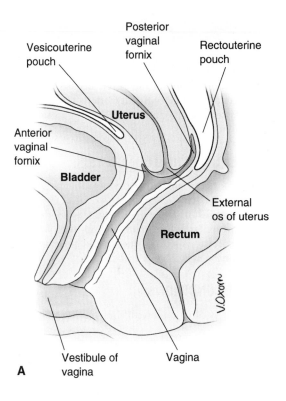

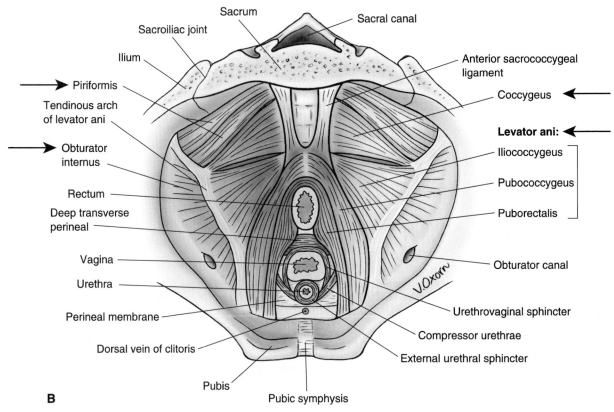

Figure 14.19 Relevant anatomy of female pelvis and pelvic floor.

APPROACH

Table **14.40**	Evaluation of Pelvic Prolapse	
Hx	**Physical Exam**	**Investigations**

• Pelvic pressure/heaviness
• Protrusion of tissue from vagina ("feels like sitting on an egg")
• Inability to wear tampons
• Stress UI (if urethral incompetence)
• Defecatory dysfunction
• Excessive straining
• Incomplete emptying
• Digitation
• ↓ Sexual activity (due to fear/embarrassment/incontinence)
• Vaginal bleeding (due to mucosal irritation)
	• Inspect vulva and vagina for erosions/ulcerations.
	• Examine all aspects of vaginal support:
	  a. In dorsal lithotomy position without pessary
	  b. Using single-bladed speculum to retract anterior/posterior/lateral vaginal walls
	• Standing straining exam to assess maximal prolapsed
	• Digital assessment of pelvic muscle/anal sphincter baseline **and** voluntary contraction tone (strength, duration, symmetry)
	• ±Rectovaginal exam to detect enterocele
		• **No specific tests for prolapse**
		• **Imaging not usually necessary**
		• Biopsy all suspicious persistent vulvovaginal lesions
		• Cystocele evaluation:
		  a. UTI screen
		  b. PVR
		  c. Bladder sensitivity
		• ±Refer to gynecologist for urodynamic testing.

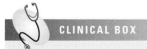

CLINICAL BOX

Variable Sx

Sx are variable depending on the severity and type of prolapse.

MANAGEMENT

OBSERVATION

- Provide information and reassurance
- Appropriate for women whose Sx are not sufficiently bothersome to warrant active intervention
- F/U exams at yearly health maintenance visit or sooner as needed

NONSURGICAL MANAGEMENT

- Sx relief and prevention of worsening prolapse
- Reasonable choice when observation not suitable **but** surgery presents higher-than-acceptable risks or is not wanted by patient

CLINICAL BOX

Occult/Latent Incontinence

Many women with anterior vaginal prolapse are continent either due to a competent urethral sphincter (despite lack of support) **or** an incompetent sphincter kinked by the prolapse, which when repaired results in incontinence known as occult/latest SI.

    Stress UI is not a Sx of prolapse, rather a coincident Sx.

CLINICAL BOX

PVR Normal

There is no consensus on PVR cutoff normal values. If the initial voided volume is >150 mL, a PVR of <100 mL is indicative of appropriate bladder emptying. A PVR of >100 mL indicates impaired bladder emptying which may or may **not** be due to prolapse.

Adjunct Rx for Concomitant Sx

- All patients with defecatory dysfunction should be evaluated from a GI perspective and receive age-appropriate screening for colorectal CA.
- Manage urinary and sexual dysfunction.
- Advise on lifestyle, weight loss, and activity.

Pelvic Floor Muscle Training
- Improving support to pelvic organs with ↑ strength and endurance of pelvic muscles
- **No** evidence for treating or preventing prolapse, but may benefit
- **Is** effective for urinary and fecal incontinence

Pessaries
- Device placed in vagina to provide support +/− fill space
- Support pessaries (the ring) for earlier stages (II and III)
- Space filling pessaries (Gellhorn) for more advanced prolapse
- Ideally changed and rinsed weekly with F/U q3mo
- Lubricants or vaginal E (if atrophy) is often employed with pessaries
- Also useful before surgery to estimate if surgery will provide Sx relief

CLINICAL BOX

Indications for Surgery

- Virtually no indication for surgery in woman with asymptomatic mild prolapse
- **If** advanced prolapse and asymptomatic: must assess efficiency of bladder emptying as at risk for complications of urinary retention (recurrent UTI, urosepsis) and assess exposed vaginal epithelium for erosions at risk for infection (and possibly 2° sepsis).
- More frequent F/U (q3mo) if decided against surgery

CLINICAL BOX

Relative CIs to Pessary

- Inability to comply with pessary maintenance → risk rectovaginal or vesicovaginal fistulae
- Persistent vaginal erosions (consider local E, change size of pessary or potential vaginal neoplasm)

  Note: Depending on setting, pessary may be used to treat persistent erosion.

SURGICAL MANAGEMENT
- An attempt to improve prolapse Sx and concomitant Sx (GI, urinary, and sexual) through techniques to restore normal anatomy **or** obliterate the vagina
- Surgery may combine repairs to anterior vagina, vaginal apex, posterior vagina and perineum, as well as concomitant bladder neck or anal sphincter repair.

UI

See also Chapter 21—Male UI.

DEFINITIONS

Table **14.41**	Types of UI
UI	Involuntary loss of urine when urine loss is not socially or personally acceptable Note: Must be demonstrable to the health care provider
SI	The complaint of involuntary leakage of urine during effort, exertion, sneezing, or coughing
Urodynamic SI	When SI is confirmed during urodynamic testing by identifying leakage from the urethra coincident with ↑ intra-Abdo pressure, but in the absence of bladder contraction
Urge incontinence	Involuntary loss of urine with a strong desire to void Note: Involuntary bladder contractions (detrusor overactivity) are the hallmark of Dx

EPIDEMIOLOGY
- Up to 70% of women living in the community setting and up to 50% of nursing home residents are affected by UI.
- Prevalence of incontinence appears to ↑ gradually during young adult life, has a broad peak around middle age, and then steadily ↑ in the elderly.
- ~1 in 4 women with UI seek medical help.

- Among ambulatory women with incontinence urodynamic SI represents 29% to 75%, detrusor overactivity 7% to 33%, and the remainder are mixed forms.
- Older, noninstitutionalized women generally have more detrusor abnormalities and mixed disorders, and SI is found less often.

CAUSAL CONDITIONS

Table **14.42** DDx of UI in Women		
GU Etiology	**Non-GU Etiology**	**Transient Causes**

• Problem with filling/storing:
  • Urodynamic SI
  • Detrusor overactivity (idiopathic or neurogenic)
  • Mixed types
• Fistula (vesical, ureteral, urethral)
• Congenital (i.e., ectopic ureter)
	• Functional:
	  • Cognitive
	  • Neurologic
	  • Psychological
	  • Physical impairment
	• Environmental
	• Pharmacologic
	• Metabolic
		• UTI/urethritis
		• Atrophic urethritis/vaginitis
		• Drug side effects
		• Pregnancy
		• Delirium
		• ↑ Urine production
		  • Metabolic cause (hyperglycemia, hypercalcemia, diabetes insipidus)
		  • ↑↑↑ fluid intake (psychogenic polydipsia)
		• Volume overload
		• Stool impaction
		• Restricted mobility

Medications Affecting Urinary Function

↑Frequency

- Diuretics
- Caffeine/EtOH

Retention

- Narcotics
- Anticholinergics
- Antidepressants
- Antipsychotics
- α-Agonists
- Ca^{2+}-channel blockers

APPROACH

See Figure 14.20.

Table **14.43** Evaluation of UI in Women		
Hx	**Physical Exam**	**Investigations**

• **Sx:** urgency, frequency, dysuria, nocturia, incomplete emptying, dribbling, pelvic bulge/pressure, medical Hx
• Neurologic Hx (DM, stroke, lumbar disk disease)
• Smoking Hx (COPD)
• **Voiding diary** (3–7 d):
  • Daytime and nocturnal voiding frequency fluid intake (caffeine, EtOH)
  • Incontinence episodes
• Recurrent UTIs GI Hx (incontinence constipation)
• OB/GYN Hx (hysterectomy, vaginal repair, pelvic radiotherapy)
• Medication list
	• **General:** signs of lung disease and ↓ E
	• **Pelvic exam:**
	  • Vulvar or vaginal atrophy
	  • Assess pelvic relaxation
	  • Bimanual exam—R/O gyne pathology
	  • Rectal exam—anal sphincter symmetry, bulk, voluntary contraction
	  • "Cough test"—visualize leakage from urethra at time of cough with full bladder
	• Neurologic exam (S2-4 control micturition):
	  • MSE
	  • Sensation: perineum, sacral dermatomes of lower extremities
	  • Motor: strength and tone of bulbocavernosus muscle, levators, external anal sphincter, and lower extremities
	  • Anal wink
		• PVR
		• U/A (R/O UTI)
		• Consider serum urea, Cr, glucose and Ca^{2+}
		
		Referral to gynecologist or urogynecologist for further testing (i.e., urodynamics, cystoscopy)

MANAGEMENT

See Table 14.44.

Geriatrics

UI has been shown to improve or resolve after removal of fecal impactions in institutionalized geriatric patients.

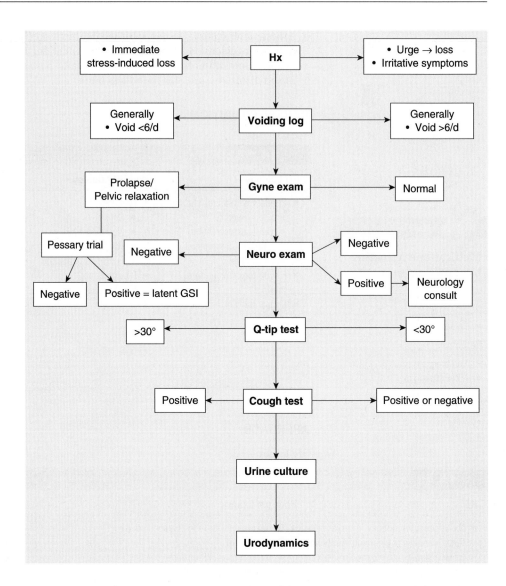

Figure 14.20 Algorithm to assess for SI versus Detrusor Overactivity.

Table **14.44**	Management of UI
Urodynamic SI	**Detrusor Overactivity (Urge Incontinence)**

1. **Behavioral approaches:**
  • **Lifestyle interventions:** weight loss, ↓ caffeine/fluid intake, smoking cessation, Δ activities/exercise, relief of constipation
  • **Pelvic muscle exercises** (aka Kegel): strengthen voluntary urethral sphincter and levator ani muscles; 3 repetitions of 8–10 sustained muscle contractions, 3–4 times weekly; **not** to be done during urination!
2. **Medical management**
  • Some evidence for α-agonists
  • New evidence **against** ET for Rx of SI
3. **Devices** (pessaries and/or urethral inserts)
4. **Surgical management** (refer to urogynecologist)
	1. **Lifestyle modifications:**
	  Caffeine/fluid reduction
	2. **Behavioral approaches**
	  • **"Bladder retraining"** (aka bladder drills or timed voiding): schedule to ↑ interval between voids. **Pelvic muscle exercises** (aka Kegel): **biofeedback**
	3. **Medical management:**
	  • Tricyclic antidepressants, anticholinergic agents, and/or musculotropic drugs
	  • MOA: inhibit contractile activity of the bladder
	4. **Surgical management and devices:** not the usual options

MENOPAUSE

CLINICAL BOX

RFs for Early Menopause

- Smoking (2 yr earlier on Avg.)
- Certain chemotherapy agents
- Radiation
- Hysterectomy
- Epilepsy
- Nulliparity

CLINICAL BOX

RFs for Delayed Menopause

- Obesity
- Multiparity
- EtOH use

CLINICAL BOX

No Proven Effect on Time of Menopause

- OC use
- Age of menarche
- Ethnicity
- Marital status
- Improved nutrition

CLINICAL BOX

Bone Loss

Osteoporosis = BMD >2.5 SD below young adult mean (T-score at or below −2.5)
Osteopenia = BMD between 1 and 2.5 SD below young adult mean (T-score between −1 and −2.5)

RATIONALE

- Occurs with the **FMP** (a discrete point in time)
- Defined retrospectively as 12 consecutive mo of amenorrhea due to loss of ovarian function.

Table **14.45**	Types of Menopause		
	Natural Menopause	**Induced Menopause**	**Premature Menopause**
Definition	Biological process that occurs as part of female aging	Surgical removal of ovaries **or** medical ablation of ovarian function	Occurs at age <2 SDs below mean age of menopause (before age 40 yr)
Causes	Avg. age = 51 yr Avg. woman spends one third of life menopausal	• Iatrogenic • Chemotherapy • Radiation • Oophorectomy	• POF = amenorrhea and persistently high FSH • 40 yr used arbitrarily

PERIODS OF TIME SURROUNDING MENOPAUSE

- **Premenopause:** the entire reproductive period before menopause.
- **Perimenopause:** encompasses the period of time (~2 to 8 yr) characterized by Δs in duration and amount of menstrual flow immediately preceding menopause during and the first year after the FMP
  - **Early:** E normal to ↑, FSH ↑ in normal range
  - **Late:** E ↓ markedly, FSH ↑
- **Postmenopausal:** the period of time following the FMP (regardless of whether menopause was induced or natural)
  - Ovulation ceases → ovaries stop producing estradiol and progesterone but continue to produce testosterone, small amount of E from peripheral conversion (in fat) of adrenal steroids

APPROACH

Table **14.46**	Approach to Dx of Menopausal/Postmenopausal Woman	
Patient Hx	**Pelvic Exam Findings**	**Investigations**
• Menstrual Hx (Δs in volume or duration of flow, date of FMP, abnormal bleeding) • Vaginal Sx (dryness, pruritis, discharge, postcoital bleeding, dyspareunia) • Urinary Sx (dysuria, urgency, ↑ frequency, nocturia) • Vasomotor instability (hot flashes) • Skin/soft tissue Δs • Osteoporosis • Mood and sleep Δs	• Pale, thin, friable vulvo-vaginal epithelium • Vaginal shortening, smooth, narrow walls, loss of rugae • Submucosal petechial hemorrhage • Vaginal wall or uterine prolapse	• ↑ Serum FSH • ↑ Serum LH • ↑ Serum estradiol • ↑ Vaginal pH >6 • Vaginal wall maturation index with ↑ parabasal cells (>20%) • Endometrial biopsy (if abnormal vaginal bleeding) • Osteoporosis RF assessment (bone densitometry as indicated) • Urine R&M, C&S, PVR (if UI)

FEATURES OF MENOPAUSE

See Table 14.47.

Table **14.47**	**Feature of Menopause**
Vasomotor	• Hot flushes are sudden onset of warmth that begin in the chest and progress to face and neck lasting ~4 min. May be associated with chills/sweats. • Maximal prevalence within the first 2 yr of menopause, after which prevalence ↓ • Affects up to 85% of women • Possibly Hypothalamic origin • Can have major impact on quality of life • Management depends on severity
Urogenital atrophy	• The hormone deprived state of menopause results in urogenital aging: • Vulvovaginal Sx: dryness, dyspareunia, thin discharge, pruritus, postcoital bleeding • Urinary Sx: dysuria, urgency, frequency/nocturia, hematuria • Prolapse Sx: pelvic pressure, introital bulge, constipation, incomplete bladder emptying, low back pain
Skeletal Δs	• Progressive reduction in trabecular > cortical bone mass (osteoporosis) • Prevalence of osteoporosis: 6% at age 50, 50% at age 80 • 50 y.o. White female has 40% remaining lifetime risk of fragility # (hip, spine, wrist)
Skin and soft tissue	• Thinning of skin/loss of elasticity, regression in breast size
Sleep difficulties	• Hallmark of menopause transition including insomnia (sleep onset and sleep maintenance) and sleep apnea
Psychological	Mood disturbance, anxiety, cognitive difficulties (likely 2° to hot flush/trouble sleeping)
Hormonal	↑ FSH and LH

CLINICAL BOX

Health Hazards of Menopause

- Osteoporosis is the main health risk of perimenopause.
- Heart disease is the main cause of death in post-menopausal women.
- All vaginal bleeding that occurs 12 mo after amenorrhea is considered post-menopausal bleeding and requires investigation.

MANAGEMENT

CLINICAL BOX

Rx Triad

1. Behavioral modifications
2. Nonhormonal medications
3. HRT
   - **Oral** most effective Rx for severe hot flushes, first-line Rx for women with osteopenia and early menopause (<45 yr), and for prevention of osteoporosis or #
   - Benefits must outweigh the risks of HRT.
   - Reasonable choice in the absence of CI
   - **Intravaginal E:** first-line Rx for isolated urogenital Sx
   - **Nonhormonal Rx** are a reasonable choice for women with CI or concerns about HRT.

VASOMOTOR SX (85% TO 95% RESOLVE WITHIN 5 YR)

- **Reassurance and lifestyle Δs:** cool fan, dress in layers, quit smoking, exercise, weight loss if overweight, avoid hot food and EtOH
- **Alternative medicine:** lack evidence of long-term safety/efficacy for black cohash, dietary soy, phytoestrogens clover, Vit E, kava, evening primrose oil, Chinese herbs
- **Nonhormonal Rx:** venlafaxine/SSRIs, gabapentin, clonidine, bellergal
- **Nonestrogenic hormonal Rx:** Ps
- **Systemic HRT:** ET, EPT

UROGENITAL SX (GENERALLY WORSENS WITH AGE)

- Reassurance, patient education and smoking cessation
- Vaginal moisturizer (polycarbophil gel/Replens)
- Local ET: intravaginal E is the Rx of choice for isolated vaginal Sx (e.g., Vagifem)
  - At recommended dose/frequency do not need to add P
- Systemic HRT

CLINICAL BOX

RFs for Osteoporosis

- Age >65 yr
- Vertebral compression #
- >40 yr with fragility #
- Low BMD
- FHx osteoporotic # (especially maternal hip #)
- POF
- Systemic steroid use >3 mo
- Malabsorption, falls, hyperparathyroidism

CLINICAL BOX

Indication for Spine XR in Postmenopausal Women

- Historic height loss >6 cm
- Prospective height loss >2 cm (↑ kyphosis)
- Acute, incapacitating back pain: to R/O vertebral #

R

Do not prescribe unopposed E to a woman with an intact uterus.

Do not prescribe P alone in patient with breast CA.

Do not prescribe for the specific purpose of preventing CHD.

Osteoporosis (Generally Worsens with Age)

- **Patient education:** exercise, healthy diet, and smoking cessation
- Osteoporosis RF assessment
- **Vit D (800 IU/d) and Ca^{2+} supplementation (1 g/d):** recommended as mandatory adjunct to other pharmacological Rx to maintain bone and prevent accelerated bone loss
- **Bisphosphonates (alendronate, risedronate):** efficacious in ↓ #
- **SERMs):** efficacious in prevention and Rx of osteoporosis
- **Calcitonin:** approved for Rx **not** prevention of osteoporosis
- **E:** ↓ bone resorption, ↑ intestinal Ca^{2+} absorption, ↓ renal Ca^{2+} excretion

CLINICAL BOX

CIs to HRT

CIs to ET: CULT

Cancer (breast or uterine)

Undiagnosed vaginal bleeding

Liver disease (acute)

Thromboembolic disease (active)

CI to PT: PUB

Pregnancy

Undiagnosed vaginal bleeding

Breast CA

Relative CI

Strong FHx breast CA

Atypical hyperplasia of the breast, fibroids

Migraines

↑ TGs

Active gallbladder disease

HRT

A thorough assessment of **individualized** risks and benefits is required.

Valid Indications Include

- Moderate to severe menopausal Sx
- Prevention of osteoporosis, #

Risks and Benefits

Initial support for the use of HRT to prevent CVD, osteoporotic #, colon CA, and dementia was based on **observational studies** and is now being contradicted by RCTs such as the following:

- **WHI:** designed to evaluate the long-term benefits and risks of E and combination HRT in postmenopausal women (1° prevention)
- **The HERS:** first large RCT of continuous E-progesterone for 2° prevention of CAD in postmenopausal women

Modes of Hormone Delivery (Cyclic or Continuous)

1. **E (ET):** oral/TD/vaginal (TD preferred if ↑ TG, ↓ sex drive)
2. **Progesterone (PT):** Oral/TD/IM/intrauterine (Recommend lowest dose for shortest possible time required to treat Sx.)
   - Low-dose OC may be prescribed for relief of hot flashes and contraceptive benefit in perimenopause.

Table **14.48** Duration of HRT in Rx of Menopause	
Short-Term Use (<5 yr):	**Longer-Term Use (>5 yr):**
• Appropriate for relieving moderate to severe Sx of menopause if no CI • Avoided or considered second line in those with CHD	• Consider risk of breast CA with extended use. • Good candidates: individuals with documented or high risk for osteoporosis/osteopenia and no CI • Poor candidates: personal Hx of CHD/CVD, breast biopsy with atypia or CA, first-degree relative with breast CA, BRCA1, BRCA2

Table **14.49**	Definite Risks and Benefits of HRT	
Type of HRT	**Benefits**	**Risks**

All types	**Menopausal Sx:** >70%–80% improvement
	Osteoporosis:
	• Prevention of bone loss, #
	• First-line preventative Rx in postmenopausal women with:
	    a. Low BMD
	    b. Early onset menopause (<45 yr)
	• **Note**: Risks may outweigh the benefits if used **only** for prevention of postmenopausal osteoporosis.
	• Second-line Rx for postmenopausal women with osteoporosis
		See HRT specific risks.

ET and EPT	Same as above	**Stroke:** ET and EPT ↑ risk of stroke in healthy postmenopausal women
ET only	Same as above **plus** **Osteoporosis:** ↑ BMD, ↓ risk of nonvertebral #	**Endometrial** CA: • ↑ Risk of endometrial CA (unopposed ET). (**Note**: Risk ↓ with addition of progesterone).
EPT only	Same as above **plus** **Osteoporosis:** ↑ BMD, ↓ vertebral, hip and other # **Colon** CA: ↓ risk	**VTE:** • ↑ Risk of VTE in women with CAD or healthy postmenopausal women **CAD:** • No benefit for prevention of CAD • ↑ Risk of second CV event in the first yr of Rx only • ↑ The risk of CAD in healthy postmenopausal women **Breast CA:** • ↑ Risk of incident breast CA after 5 yr of use • This ↑ risk is felt to return to normal 5 yr after stopping HRT.

[a]Based on findings from WHI and/or HERS studies

PROBABLE RISKS
- Gallbladder disease:
- Observational studies and RCTs reveal 1.5 to 2.0 fold ↑ in gallbladder disease associated with HRT (HERS 2° outcome)

POSSIBLE RISKS/BENEFITS
Ovarian CA
- Observational studies reveal a small ↑ risk with ET
- Small, nonsignificant ↑ risk of ovarian CA with EPT (WHI)

Cognition
- **WHIMS** showed that E alone does not protect women (>65) from normal ↓ in cognitive function when compared to placebo.
- ↓ Cognition, memory, and mood may be 2° to vasomotor Sx (hot flashes, sweats, and difficulty sleeping); therefore, improvement on HRT may be 2° to improvement of vasomotor Sx.
- Evidence supporting role of HRT in preservation of cognitive function in healthy postmenopausal women **or** for Rx of Alzheimer disease is weak or absent.

FEMALE INFERTILITY

See also Chapter 21—Male Infertility.

RATIONALE
- In women there is a significant age-related ↓ in fertility and ↑ in spontaneous miscarriage largely attributable to progressive follicular depletion and ↑ incidence of abnormalities of aging oocytes.
- Must investigate both partners to identify the cause of infertility and then tailor the Rx accordingly

- Infertility affects ~15% of couples.
- Female-associated factors account for ~50% of infertility problems.
- Male-associated factors contribute significantly to infertility in up to ~35% of couples.
- ~10% to 15% of couples will have "unexplained infertility" (cause is uncertain).

Table **14.50**	**Definitions of Infertility**
Infertility	Inability to conceive after 1 yr of regular intercourse **without** contraception
Fecundability	Probability that a single cycle will result in **pregnancy** (20%–25%)
Fecundity	Probability that a single cycle will result in a **live birth**

ASC Box

Menstrual Cycle

Menstrual phase: 1 to 4 d

Follicular phase: 5 to 13 d

Ovulation: 14 d

Luteal phase: 15 to 28 d

 C₂LEO Box

Physicians Approach in Infertility
- Discuss in a nonjudgmental manner.
- Full disclosure to patients (make certain patients have full access to relevant information) → ensures informed consent.
- Identify if certain options lie outside your moral boundaries and refer to another MD if appropriate.
- Consult with appropriate hospital ethics committees or boards.
- Protect the patients' right to freedom of moral choice.

CLINICAL BOX

RFs for Tubal Infertility

- Hx of PID
- Hx of tubal or pelvic surgery
- Hx of endometriosis
- Prev. EP
- *In utero* DES exposure
- Hx of septic abortion

CAUSAL CONDITIONS

Table **14.51**	**DDx of Female Factor Infertility**		
Mechanism	**DDx**		
Ovulatory dysfunction (15%–20%)	• Hypothalamic (FHA, hypothalamic disorder 2° to stress, poor diet, or excessive exercise) • Pituitary (prolactinoma, medication-induced, hypopituitarism) • PCOS • POF • LPD (poor folliculogenesis, premature corpus luteum degeneration, ↓ uterine response to progesterone) • Systemic disease (thyroid dysfunction) • Reproductive aging		
Outflow tract abnormality (25%–35%)	**Uterine factors (<5%)** • Infection (chronic endometritis) • Fibroids • Agenesis • Malformations • Congenital anomalies (uterine septum, bicornuate uterus) • Asherman syndrome	**Cervical factors (5%)** • Acidic cervical mucus • Antisperm antibodies • Structural defects (Prev. LEEP, cone biopsy, cryo/laser Rx)	**Tubal factors (20%–30%)** • **PID** • Tubal occlusion (Prev. ectopic) • Tubal adhesions (Prev. surgery, endometriosis)
Other (40%–45%)	• Endometriosis • Multifactorial • Unexplained		

CLINICAL BOX

Lifestyle Factors Associated with ↑ Infertility

- Obesity
- Smoking
- EtOH use
- Marijuana use
- Cocaine use

CLINICAL BOX

Evaluation of Couples Infertility Factor

- Sexual dysfunction issues (dyspareunia, impotence etc.)
- Frequency of intercourse
- Timing of intercourse
- Use of lubricants

APPROACH TO INFERTILITY

1. Evaluate her male partner for male infertility factor (**Chapter 21—Male Infertility**).
2. Determine whether her cycles are ovulatory.
3. Identify factors that ↑ risk of tubal infertility.

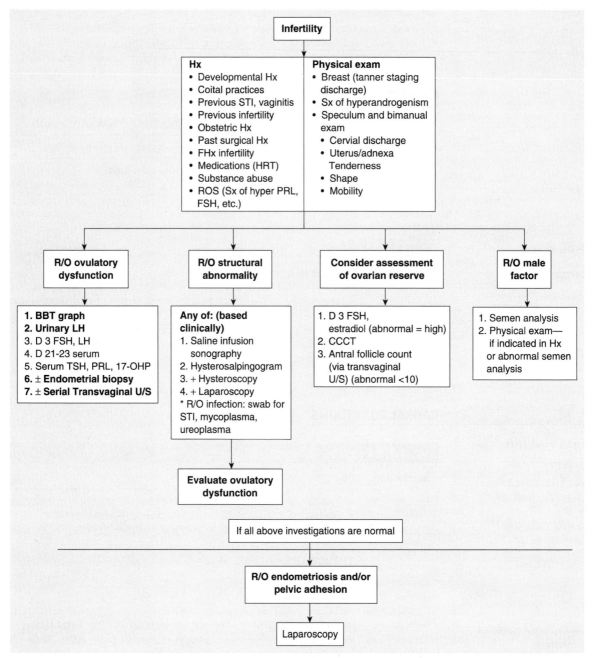

Figure 14.21 Approach to infertility. Ovarian reserve: the size and quality of the remaining ovarian follicular pool intended to predict future fecundability or provide prognostic information regarding likelihood of successful Rx.

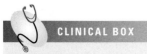

CLINICAL BOX

Prognosis

The majority of spontaneous pregnancies will occur within 3 yr, after this the prognosis for success without Rx is relatively poor.

4. Examine her for signs of endocrinopathy + gynecologic disease.
5. Evaluate couple's infertility factor.

MANAGEMENT

EVALUATION OF INFERTILITY SHOULD BE OFFERED TO

- All couples that have failed to conceive after ≥1 year of unprotected intercourse
- All women >35 yr*
- Women with irregular or infrequent menses*
- Women with a Hx of PID or endometriosis*
- Men with known or suspected poor semen quality*

---

* A year of infertility is not a prerequisite in these individuals

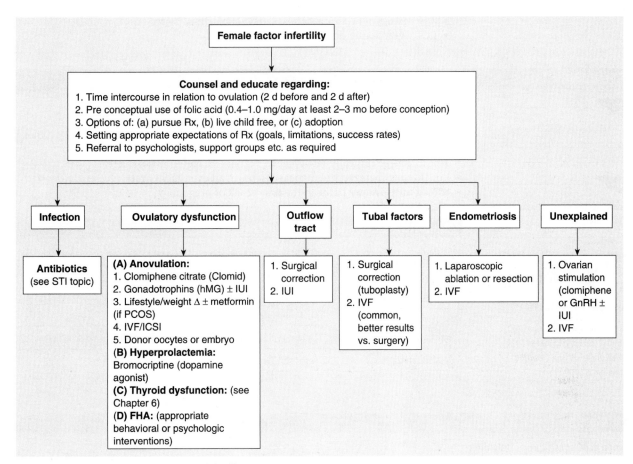

Figure 14.22 Management of female factor infertility.

INDICATIONS FOR SPECIALTY CARE REFERRAL IN COUPLES PRESENTING WITH FEMALE

Factor infertility (gynecologist and/or reproductive endocrinology and infertility specialist):

- Female with abnormal d 3 FSH and/or estradiol
- Female with abnormal HSG due to:
    a. Bilateral proximal fallopian tube occlusion
    b. No patency or abnormal distal fallopian tube or
    c. Abnormal intrauterine cavities
- Women with laparoscopy showing severe pelvic adhesions.
- Women in whom pregnancy fails to occur after surgical Rx of endometriosis
- Couples desiring IVF and/or other advanced reproductive technologies

THERAPEUTIC OPTIONS FOR COUPLES WITH INFERTILITY

- Counseling and education
- Rx of ovulatory dysfunction, if it exists
- Consider surgical management of tubal disease, if it exists.
- Management of male factor infertility (therapeutic donor insemination, IVF, ICSI; Chapter 21—Male Infertility).

IVF

- Rx of choice for severe tubal disease, and severe sperm defects
- ↑ Incidence in congenital malformations in children born as a result of IVF (natural 4.2% vs. IVF 9.0%)
- Indications:
    - Severe tubal disease
    - Advanced stage endometriosis
    - Severe male factor
    - Multifactor infertility

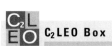 **C₂LEO Box**

Controversial and Ethical Issues in Infertility
- Surrogacy
- Donor eggs
- Therapeutic donor insemination in same sex couples
- Preimplantation genetic testing
- Multiple gestation pregnancies
- Other advanced reproductive technologies

- Age related or otherwise unexplained subfertility
- POF (with young donor egg)

PREGNANCY LOSS

EP must always be R/O when assessing patients for miscarriage.

The Rh status must always be determined.

CLINICAL BOX

Retained Products

Following Rx of a miscarriage, consider a F/U U/S to confirm the absence of any retained products of conception.

RATIONALE

- Miscarriage (i.e., spontaneous abortion) is one of the most common clinical problems in gynecology.
- 10% to 20% of clinically recognized pregnancies end in miscarriage.
- Loss of unrecognized pregnancies occurs at an even higher rate.
- 80% of miscarriages occur in the first 12 wk of pregnancy

Table **14.52**	**Definition of Pregnancy Loss**
Stillbirth	Death that occurs following 20 wk gestation or weighing more than 500 g
Abortion	Termination of pregnancy before viability
Miscarriage	Pregnancy which ends spontaneously before the fetus reaching 500 g or 20 wk gestation
Embryonic miscarriage	Embryo with a crown-rump length >5 mm without cardiac activity
Fetal miscarriage	Fetus of 10 to 20 wk size, without cardiac activity

Table **14.53**	**Types of Miscarriage**	
Types of Miscarriage	**Definition**	**Rx**
Missed abortion	• Death of the fetus occurring *in utero* with retention of the pregnancy • Anembryonic pregnancy: a type of missed abortion characterized by a gestational sac with no fetal pole	• D&C • Misoprostol • Expectant management
Complete abortion	• Spontaneous expulsion of all fetal and placental tissue before 20 wk of gestation	• Ensure hemodynamic stability • Supportive
Incomplete abortion	• Incomplete expulsion of the products of conception before 20 wk of gestation	• D&C • Misoprostol
Threatened abortion	• Bleeding occurring during the first 20 wk of gestation without the passage of tissue or cervical dilation • In the presence of fetal cardiac activity, a high proportion of pregnancies continue. • [a]Occurs in 30%−40% of all pregnancies	• Watchful waiting
Inevitable abortion	• Bleeding ± ROM accompanied by cramping and dilation of the cervix • Gestational tissue may be seen through the internal os	• D&C • Misoprostol
Septic abortion	• Infection of retained products of conception by *S. aureus*, GN bacilli, or gram-positive cocci • Infection can cause peritonitis and sepsis.	• IV Antibiotics • D&C
Recurrent abortion	• >3 spontaneous first trimester losses	• D&C • Misoprostol • Work-up for recurrent abortion (see Table 14.54)

CLINICAL BOX

Trisomies

The most frequent trisomies in clinical miscarriage are 16, 22, 21, 15, and 13.

RFs FOR PREGNANCY LOSS

- GA (↑ risk with earlier age)
- Advanced maternal age
- Prev. miscarriage
- Smoking
- EtOH
- Cocaine use

- >1 alcoholic drink/d
- Caffeine (>375 mg of caffeine)

    Please see diagnostic algorithm in Vaginal Bleeding

ETIOLOGY OF SPONTANEOUS ABORTION
- Blighted or anembryonic pregnancy
- Chromosomal anomalies (50%)
- Teratogen exposure (e.g., maternal diabetes, mercury)
- Trauma (e.g., amniocentesis)
- Uterine factors (e.g., uterine septum, submucosal fibroids)
- Maternal infection/disease
- Maternal endocrinopathies (e.g., LPD, hypothyroidism)
- Thrombophilia
- Unexplained

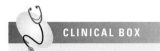

CLINICAL BOX

Prevalence

Threatened abortion may occur in up to 30% of pregnancies.

Above 40 yr of age, the miscarriage rate is estimated at 45%.

RECURRENT PREGNANCY LOSS

DEFINITION
- Recurrent pregnancy loss is defined as three or more first trimester miscarriages. Recurrent pregnancy loss affects 5% of couples attempting to conceive.

Table 14.54 Lab Investigations for Recurrent Miscarriage "TIE GAME"

Factor	Diagnostic Test	Rx
1. **T**hrombophilic: • Inherited coagulopathy leading to thrombosis of the intervillous space and spiral arteries	• Factor V Leiden mutation • Prothrombin gene mutation • Homocysteine level • Protein C activity • Protein S activity • Antithrombin activity	• Heparin—LMWH or unfractionated • Folic acid
2. **I**mmunologic	• Lupus anticoagulant • Anticardiolipin antibody (IgG/IgM) • B$_2$-glycoprotein-1 (IgG/IgM) • Antiphospholipid antibodies	• ASA • Heparin
3. **E**ndocrine • DM • Thyroid dysfunction • Hyperprolactinemia • LPD • PCOS	• Fasting insulin and glucose • TSH (hypothyroidism) • PRL • Midluteal progesterone/endometrial biopsy (See Infertility chapter)	• Metformin, insulin, hypoglycemic diet • Levothyroxine • Bromocriptine, cabergoline • Progesterone
4. **G**enetic/chromosomal	• Cytogenetic analysis of both partners • (e.g., balanced reciprocal translocation)	• Genetic counseling • Donor gametes • Preimplantation genetic Dx
5. **A**natomic • Septate uterus • Leiomyomas • Cervical incompetence • Intrauterine synechiae (i.e., Asherman syndrome) • Intrauterine septum	• Hysteroscopy • HSG	• Adhesionolysis • Hysteroscopic metroplasty • (i.e., uterine septum resection)
6. **M**icrobiologic • Listeria monocytogenes • Toxoplasma gondii • Cytomegalovirus • 1° Genital herpes	• Cervical/vaginal cultures • Endometrial biopsy	• Antibiotics identified pathogens
7. **E**nvironmental/toxicologic	• Review tobacco, ethanol, caffeine use. • Review exposure to toxins and chemicals.	• Eliminate consumption or exposure.

Close monitoring of the psychosocial well-being of patients with recurrent pregnancy loss is essential because these patients are susceptible to depression, anxiety, and heightened anger.

CLINICAL BOX

TIE GAME

Thrombophilic

Immunologic

Endocrine

Genetic

Anatomic

Microbiologic

Environmental

- In 2/3 of couples with recurrent pregnancy loss, one or more factors will be identified as being responsible.
- Infertility or advancing maternal age may prompt investigation for recurrent pregnancy loss after two miscarriages.

EVALUATION OF RECURRENT PREGNANCY LOSS

Hx

- Estimated gestation of each miscarriage (by U/S, LNMP, embryopathology if available)
- Features of rheumatic diseases
- Hx of infertility
- Sx of hypothyroidism or prolactinoma
- Toxicologic Hx (including tobacco, EtOH and caffeine use)
- Hx of lupus
- Hx of thrombosis

CLINICAL BOX

Luteal Phase Deficiency

Defined as a midluteal progesterone of <10 ng/mL resulting in a delay in the histological development of the endometrium. This may be treated with supplemental progesterone.

STILLBIRTH

Table **14.55** Stillbirth—Definitions	
Fetal mortality rate	Number of stillbirths per 1,000 total births
Infant mortality rate	Number of deaths of live-born babies in the first year of life per 1,000 live births
Fetal mortality rate in Canada	4.5 per 1000 total births in 2000
Etiology	The definitive cause of fetal death is unrecognized in >25% of cases. However, numerous investigations are recommended following a stillbirth

Table **14.56** Investigating a Stillbirth	

Maternal investigations	• CBC
	• Blood group and antibody screen
	• HbA1c
	• Kleihauer-Betke test
	• TORCH infection serology: toxoplasma, rubella, cytomegalovirus, herpes virus, parvovirus B19
	• Karyotype of both parents
	• Hgb electrophoresis (possible thalassemia)
	• Antiplatelet antibodies (possible alloimmune thrombocytopenia)
	• DIC screening (INR, PTT, fibrinogen)
	• Thrombophilia screen 6 to 8 wk after delivery (as protein levels normally ↓ during pregnancy):
	  • Antithrombin
	  • Protein C and protein S deficiency
	  • Factor V Leiden
	  • Factor II mutation
	  • MTHFR mutation
	  • Hyperhomocysteinemia
	  • Lupus anticoagulant
	  • Anticardiolipin antibodies.

Table **14.56**	*(continued)*
Fetal	• Autopsy (can aid in determining a cause of death; ~25% of cases, no cause of death can be identified) • Karyotype • Cytogenetic studies (if have evidence of congenital malformation, IUGR, hydrops, ambiguous genitalia, or dysmorphic features)

Placental	• Careful exam of the placenta:
	  • Chorionicity of the placenta
	  • Thrombosis of the cord?/true knot in the cord?
	  • Visible abruption, placental infarcts
	  • Placental vascular malformations (vasa previa)
	  • Signs of chorioamnionitis
	• Bacterial culture of chorion (GBS, Listeria, *E. coli*)

Table **14.57**	RFs for stillbirth		
Maternal RFs		**FHx**	**Fetal Conditions**

• Extremes of maternal age—nulliparity
• Maternal smoking during pregnancy
• High prepregnancy weight
• Prior fetal loss
• Inadequate prenatal care
• Lower SES
• Reproductive tract infections
• Abdo trauma
• Maternal medical disorders:
  • Thromboembolic disorders
  • DM
  • Hypertensive disorders
  • Thrombophilia
  • AI diseases
  • Epilepsy
  • Severe anemia
  • Severe maternal heart disease
  • Cholestasis of pregnancy
		• Hx of recurrent spontaneous abortions
		• VTE and/or PE
		• Prev. child born with a congenital anomaly, abnormal karyotype or syndrome
		• Child with documented developmental delay
		• Consanguinity
			• Congenital anomaly
			• Fetal infection (TORCH)
			• Fetal growth restriction
			• Prev. fetal demise
			• Massive placental abruption
			• Maternal-fetal hemorrhage
			• Rh alloimmunization
			• Multiple gestation

CLINICAL BOX

Grief Management

- It is imperative to consider the emotional consequences of stillbirth on patients and their families.
- Patients should be referred to support services (social worker, psychologist, and psychiatrist if needed).
- Following investigations for stillbirth, information about the cause of death should be provided to the family in a timely manner.

INDUCED ABORTION

C₂LEO Box

Physician Obligations

Health professionals are not required to perform abortions, but have a duty to share all information and options with their patients, and make appropriate arrangements.

Termination of pregnancy that is performed electively due to fetal anomalies, maternal illness, or because of unwanted pregnancy.

EPIDEMIOLOGY

- 46 Million women have abortions each year.
- The World Health Organization estimates that half of these are performed unsafely (particularly in third world settings).
- For legal abortions, the risk of death is 1 in 100,000.

PSYCHOSOCIAL CONSIDERATIONS OF INDUCED ABORTION

Abortion may provoke a number of emotions in patients, including relief, guilt, and sadness or depression. It is important to explore these issues with patients. Referral to a mental health professional may be warranted.

Table **14.58** Methods of Abortion		
	Method	**Mechanism**
Firsttrimester abortion	Vacuum curettage	1. Cervical dilatation using metal dilators ± vaginal misoprostol before procedure. 2. A plastic vacuum canula is placed in the uterus through the cervix and the products of conception are aspirated. 3. Performed under general of local anaesthesia, or with conscious sedation.
	Misoprostol	Analogue of PGE_1 Vaginal administration of 800 μg×2 (24 h apart) produces complete abortion in 91% of pregnancies up to 56 d of amenorrhea.
	Mifepristone + misoprostol	Mifepristone (RU486) = progesterone antagonist 1. When given with misoprostol, mifepristone is highly effective (96%) up to 49 d of amenorrhea.
Second-trimester abortion (>13 wk)	D&E	1. Prepare cervix with laminaria (hygroscopic dilator which expands as it absorbs moisture) ± misoprostol to dilate cervix. 2. A vacuum cannula is used to extract the fetus and placenta under general anaesthetic.
	Labor induction	1. Misoprostol administered vaginally may induce labor—400 μg administered vaginally q6 h (highly effective) 2. Dinoprostone (a PGE_2 analogue) may also be used
	Oxytocin	Oxytocin may be used from 17 to 24 wk of pregnancy.

R/O pregnancy and Rh factor in all terminations.

Uterine rupture: A few case reports have been reported in patients given misoprostol who have had a Prev. C/S.

COMPLICATIONS OF ABORTION

SIDE EFFECTS AND COMPLICATIONS OF MISOPROSTOL

- Fever
- Nausea/vomiting
- Diarrhea
- Retained products of conception
- Bleeding
- Uterine rupture:

COMPLICATIONS OF D&C/D&E

- Bleeding
- Uterine perforation
- Endometritis
- Retained products of conception

ANTEPARTUM CARE

RATIONALE

- The purpose of **antepartum care** is to help achieve as good a maternal and infant outcome as possible.
- Goals of antepartum care:
  a) Ongoing risk assessment
  b) Define health status of mom and fetus.
  c) Promote healthy behavior through lifestyle modification and screening.
- Both psychosocial issues and biological issues need to be addressed.
- Antepartum care helps to ↓ prenatal and maternal mortality rates.

APPLIED SCIENTIFIC CONCEPTS

See Table 14.59.

Table **14.59** Physiological Δs Associated with Pregnancy	
Organ System	**Physiological Δ**
CV	• Hyperdynamic circulation → ↑ CO, ↑ HR, ↑ SV • ↓ Mean arterial BP (lowest at 24 wk) • BP affected by position (i.e., supine hypotension) due to ↓ venous return and ↑ venous P due to compression of IVC + pelvic veins by uterus • ↓ PVR due to P induced vasodilation • ↓ Venous return and ↑ venous P due to compression of IVC + pelvic veins by uterus
Hematologic	• Hemodilution (↑↑ plasma volume relative to ↑RBCs) → apparent ↓ Hgb and Hct • ↑ WBC but ↓ function leads to improvement of AI disease • ↓ # Platelets → gestational thrombocytopenia • Hypercoagulable state → ↑ risk DVT, PE
Respiratory	• Level of diaphragm rises and ↑ intercoastal angle • ↑ O_2 requirements • ↓ TLC, FRC, RV • ↑ RR
Breasts (preparation for lactation support)	• Breast tenderness, tingling (P induced) • ↑ Breast size, enlargement of nipples • ↑ Vascularity/blood flow to breast • ↑ Cuboidal alveolar cell and ductal (E induced) • ↑ Synthesis of milk components—casein, lactalbumin, FA (P and PRL induced) • Initiation of secretory activity due to PRL and hPL (expression of colostrum (thick glossy, protein rich fluid) from second trimester onward + first 30 h after delivery • Inhibition of full lactation due to high E + P levels during pregnancy
Skin	• ↑ Pigmentation (chloasma—under eyes, areola, linea alba—anterior Abdo wall) → due to ↑ secretion of pituitary MSH • Stretch marks—striae gravidarum (Abdo wall, lateral thighs, breasts) → due to ↑GC
GI	• ↓ Tone and motility of stomach, small/large intestines → constipation • ↑ GERD Sx due to ↑ intra-Abdo pressure and ↓ LES tone • ↑ Gallstones • Hemorrhoids
Renal	• ↑ GFR, (↑ renal blood flow) • ↑ Urinary frequency • ↑ UTI risk due to ↑ urine stasis + ↑ glucose content of urine • ↓ Bladder tone, ↑ ureter and renal pelvis dilation (P induced smooth muscle relaxation)
Endocrine	• ↑ Size and vascularity of pituitary, thyroid glands • ↑ PRL, oxytocin, ↑ ACTH, ↑ GC secretion vs. normal TSH, ↑ TH, ↑BMR • Suppressed GH but replaced by hPL
Uterine (Δ size, shape, consistency, + position)	• ↑ Size uterine fundus through hypertrophy of stroma • Δ from pear shape to globula R/O void shape in second and third trimester → expansion of uterine cavity from 4 mL in nonpregnant state to 4,000 mL at full term • Hypertrophy of blood vessels supplying uterus → dilation of arteries, ↑ blood flow

APPROACH

Key objectives:

• Develop an appropriate relationship and rapport.
• Counsel about pregnancy before conception, if possible.
• Determine whether the patient is pregnant and estimate the date of confinement—EDC.
• Educate the patient regarding physiological Δs associated with pregnancy.

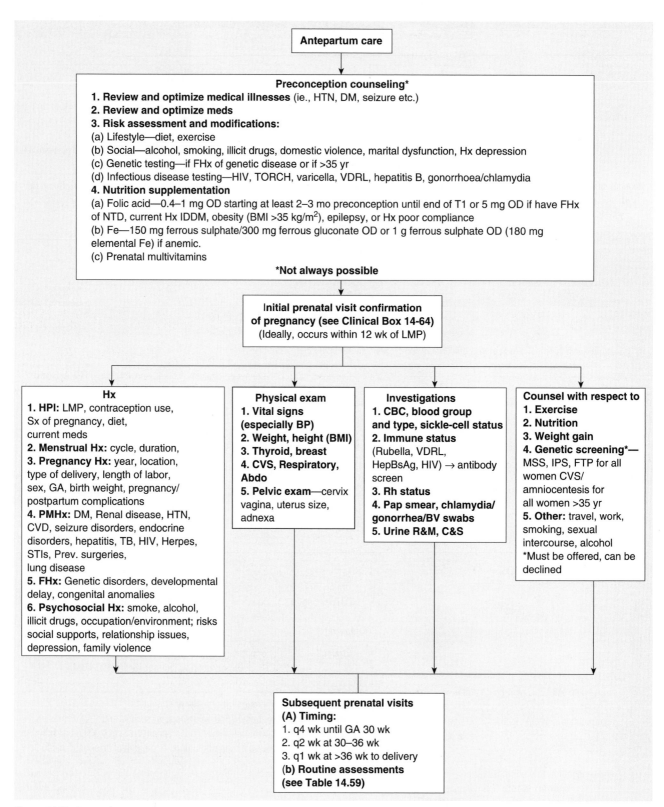

Figure 14.23 Approach to antepartum care.

GTPAL

Gravida (G): total # pregnancies (current, abortions, miscarriages, ectopic)

Parity (TPAL):

T = # term infants delivered (37–40 + wk).

P = # premature infants delivered (20–36 wk).

A = # abortions (induced, or spontaneous loss of intrauterine pregnancy before fetus viability—<20 wk + <500 g

L = # living children

Estimating Date of Confinement

EDC

- First d of LMP
- Naegele rule = LMP + 7 d − 3 mo (for 28 d menstrual cycle)
- Date of conception
- Date of positive pregnancy test
- U/S findings
- Size of uterus (SFH)-12 wk at symphysis, 20 wk at umbilicus

Factors That Can △ EDC

- Hx of irregular menstrual cycle
- Unknown LMP

Table **14.60**	**Routine Antenatal Assessments According to GA**
GA (wk)	**Antenatal Routines**
8–12	• Dating U/S → measure of crown-rump length; margin of error ± 3 d
10–12	• CVS
11–14	• FTS → measures (1) NTUS, (2) β-HCG, + (3) PAPP-A; provides risk estimate for Trisomy 21. If + CVS or amnio should be offered. • IPS part 1 (NTUS + PAPP-A)
11–13	• NTUS → measures AFV behind neck of fetus; early screen for congenital anomalies i.e., Trisomy 21 measures "thickness of neck"
14–20 to term	• FMs (quickening)
15–18	• IPS Part 2 (MSS markers)
15–20	• MSS (triple screen for Trisomy 21, 18, and open NTD) → measures (1) MSAFP, (2) β-HCG, + (3) unconjugated E (E3/estriol) • Amniocentesis if indicated.
18–20	• U/S for (a) anatomy and growth of fetus; margin of error +/− 7 d; (b) placental position; (c) AFV

24–28	• Screen for Gestational Diabetes (GDM)—50 g oral glucose challenge test
	  • Plasma glucose <7.8 mmol/L → normal
	  • One of following = IGT vs. >2 of following = GDM:
	    • Fasting plasma glucose > 5.3 mmol/L
	    • Plasma glucose >10.3 (50 g OGTT) → GDM
	    • Plasma glucose > 7.8–<10.3 mmol/L (50 g OGTT) → do 2 h 75 g OGTT
	    • 1 h plasma glucose (75 g OGTT) > 10.6 mmol/L
	    • 2 h plasma glucose (75 g OGTT) > 8.9 mmol/L

28	• Repeat CBC (Hg, Hct) • Check Rh—antibody titers • RhoGAM (RhIgG) for all Rh⁻ women (see Intrapartum care topic).
35–37	• Vaginal and anorectal culture for GBS.
Every visit	• Hx: Estimate GA, Hx of present pregnancy, vaginal bleeding/leaking, Abdo cramping. • Weight of mother (steadily ↑ ~25–35 lbs throughout pregnancy) • Maternal BP (normal <140/80 mm Hg) • FHR using doppler U/S (normal = 110–160 bpm) • FMs → noticed by 18–20 wk in primigravida vs. 14–16 wk in multigravida • Leopold maneuvers for lie, position, and presentation of the fetus (especially important toward the end of third trimester for delivery) • Size of uterus (SFH)—at 12 wk—symphysis, 20 wk—umbilicus, 36 wk—xiphoid process • Urine glucose and protein (diabetes, kidney disease) • Additional U/S done if medically indicated

CLINICAL BOX

Confirmation of Pregnancy

β-HCG

Peptide hormone produced by trophoblast cells; maintains the CL of pregnancy

Detected in serum 10 d and urine 10 to14 d post conception.

Serum β-HCG concentration is ~10 IU at time of missed menses, 100,000 IU at 10 wk, and 10,000 IU at term.

Transvaginal U/S

Visible gestational sac at 5 wk (β-HCG >1,500 to 3,000 IU), fetal pole at 6 wk, and fetal heart beat by 7 wk

Transabdominal U/S

Intrauterine pregnancy visible by 6 to 8 wk (HCG >6,500 IU)

CLINICAL BOX

Leopold Maneuvers

A series of 4 Abdo palpitations of the gravid uterus used to determine fetal lie, presentation, and position

1. First maneuver determines what part of the fetus occupies the fundus.
   - Head = round, hard, and ballotable versus buttocks = irregular
2. Second maneuver determines which the side the fetal back lies on.
   - Spine = long, linear, and firm versus extremities = multiple mobile small parts
3. Third maneuver determines the presenting part of the fetus.
   - Vertex (head) = round, firm ballotable versus breech (sacrum) = irregular and nodular
4. Fourth maneuver determines the position of the fetal head by palpating the cephalic prominence.
   - Flexed versus extended = occiput felt on same side as spine

MANAGEMENT OF THE PREGNANT PATIENT

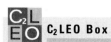 **C₂LEO Box**

Truth Telling
- The physical demands of mother's employment should be considered and disclosed to the patient, especially to women at high risk for preterm delivery.
- High cumulative work fatigue scores as the strongest (OR 1.63) work-related RF for PTL

 C₂LEO Box

Consent to Investigation or Rx
- Provide all women who wish to become pregnant with clinically indicated immunizations, at least 3 mo before conception
- If at high risk for hepatitis A or pneumococcal infection should be immunized
- Vaccines may be given during pregnancy if:
  - Have ↑ risk exposure to infection
  - Infection is hazardous to mom or fetus
  - Immunizing agent not likely to cause harm
- Inactivated virus vaccines, toxoids, and immune globulin = safe in pregnancy → delay administration until T2

CLINICAL BOX

Types of Prenatal Screening Tests

1. **FTS** = measures NTUS + PAPP-A + β-HCG
   - Estimates the risk for Trisomy 21; ~85% sensitivity when combined with age
2. **MSS** = measures MSAFP + β-HCG + unconjugated E
   - Estimates the risk for NTD, Trisomy 21, Trisomy 18
     a. **NTD** → ↑ MSAFP ~80% to 90% sensitivity
     b. **Trisomy 21** → ↓ MSAFP, ↑ β-HCG, ↓ unconjugated E ~65% sensitive
     c. **Trisomy 18** → ↓ MSAFP, ↓ β-HCG, ↓ unconjugated E ~80% sensitive
   - **IPS** = combines MSS markers + NTUS + PAPP-A
     - Estimates the risk for Trisomy 21, 18, and NTD

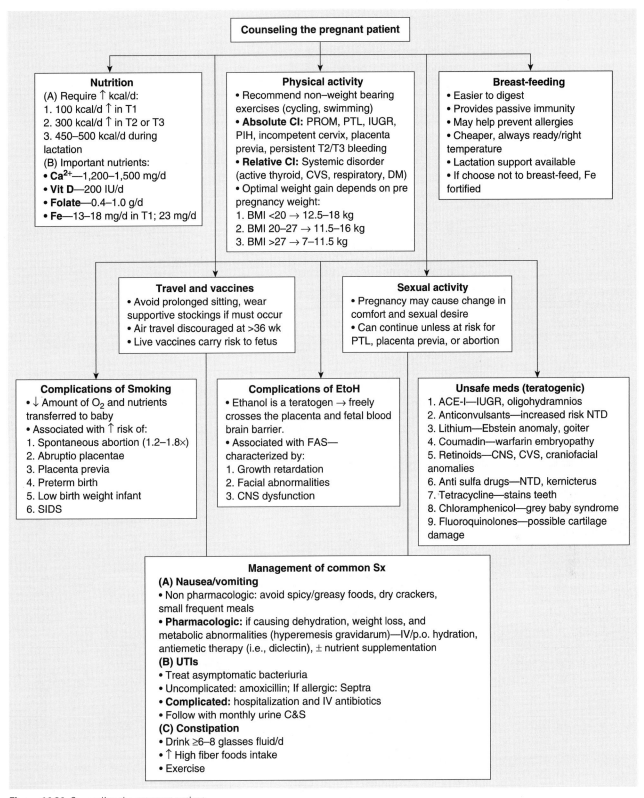

Counseling the pregnant patient

Nutrition
(A) Require ↑ kcal/d:
1. 100 kcal/d ↑ in T1
2. 300 kcal/d ↑ in T2 or T3
3. 450–500 kcal/d during lactation
(B) Important nutrients:
• **Ca^{2+}**—1,200–1,500 mg/d
• **Vit D**—200 IU/d
• **Folate**—0.4–1.0 g/d
• **Fe**—13–18 mg/d in T1; 23 mg/d

Physical activity
• Recommend non–weight bearing exercises (cycling, swimming)
• **Absolute CI:** PROM, PTL, IUGR, PIH, incompetent cervix, placenta previa, persistent T2/T3 bleeding
• **Relative CI:** Systemic disorder (active thyroid, CVS, respiratory, DM)
• Optimal weight gain depends on pre pregnancy weight:
1. BMI <20 → 12.5–18 kg
2. BMI 20–27 → 11.5–16 kg
3. BMI >27 → 7–11.5 kg

Breast-feeding
• Easier to digest
• Provides passive immunity
• May help prevent allergies
• Cheaper, always ready/right temperature
• Lactation support available
• If choose not to breast-feed, Fe fortified

Travel and vaccines
• Avoid prolonged sitting, wear supportive stockings if must occur
• Air travel discouraged at >36 wk
• Live vaccines carry risk to fetus

Sexual activity
• Pregnancy may cause change in comfort and sexual desire
• Can continue unless at risk for PTL, placenta previa, or abortion

Complications of Smoking
• ↓ Amount of O$_2$ and nutrients transferred to baby
• Associated with ↑ risk of:
1. Spontaneous abortion (1.2–1.8×)
2. Abruptio placentae
3. Placenta previa
4. Preterm birth
5. Low birth weight infant
6. SIDS

Complications of EtoH
• Ethanol is a teratogen → freely crosses the placenta and fetal blood brain barrier.
• Associated with FAS— characterized by:
1. Growth retardation
2. Facial abnormalities
3. CNS dysfunction

Unsafe meds (teratogenic)
1. ACE-I—IUGR, oligohydramnios
2. Anticonvulsants—increased risk NTD
3. Lithium—Ebstein anomaly, goiter
4. Coumadin—warfarin embryopathy
5. Retinoids—CNS, CVS, craniofacial anomalies
6. Anti sulfa drugs—NTD, kernicterus
7. Tetracycline—stains teeth
8. Chloramphenicol—grey baby syndrome
9. Fluoroquinolones—possible cartilage damage

Management of common Sx
(A) Nausea/vomiting
• Non pharmacologic: avoid spicy/greasy foods, dry crackers, small frequent meals
• **Pharmacologic:** if causing dehydration, weight loss, and metabolic abnormalities (hyperemesis gravidarum)—IV/p.o. hydration, antiemetic therapy (i.e., diclectin), ± nutrient supplementation
(B) UTIs
• Treat asymptomatic bacteriuria
• Uncomplicated: amoxicillin; If allergic: Septra
• **Complicated:** hospitalization and IV antibiotics
• Follow with monthly urine C&S
(C) Constipation
• Drink ≥6–8 glasses fluid/d
• ↑ High fiber foods intake
• Exercise

Figure 14.24 Counseling the pregnant patient.

CLINICAL BOX

Signs and Sx of Pregnancy

Appear once hCG has reached sufficient levels ~3 to 4 wk post conception:

Sx

1. Amenorrhea
2. Nausea/vomiting
3. ↑ Urinary frequency
4. ↑ Fatigue/lassitude
5. Breast tenderness/heaviness
6. Constipation
7. Lower Abdo cramps
8. Backaches/headaches

Signs

1. Uterine enlargement
2. Chadwick sign—blue cervix/vagina at 6 wk
3. Goodell sign—soft cervix at 4 to 6 wk
4. Hegar sign—soft cervical isthmus at 6 to 8 wk

INDICATIONS FOR SPECIALTY CARE

Table **14.61** Indications for Specialty Care Referral in Prenatal Women

Maternal Factors	Current Pregnancy Complications	Past Pregnancy Hx
• Diabetes • Chronic HTN • Obesity (BMI >35) • Severe psychosocial issues • FHx genetic disease or congenital anomalies • Other significant FHx: DVT/PE, recurrent pregnancy loss • Significant tobacco, EtOH, drug use • Significant medical illness (heart failure, renal disease, HIV)	• Gestational HTN • Placenta previa (± bleeding) • Ongoing antepartum hemorrhage • High order multiple gestation (> triplets) • PPROM • PTL • Rh or atypical blood group sensitization (i.e., C, E) • Hydramnios (poly or oligo) • Fetal malposition (breech, transverse at 36 wk) • Postdates >41 wk • Anemia not responding to Fe + Hgb <100 g/L • Fetal congenital anomaly	• PTL <36 wk • Still birth or neonatal death • IUGR, <10th %, reverse flow Doppler • Cervical incompetence • Prev. uterine surgery

CLINICAL BOX

Indications for Prenatal Dx

1. Maternal age >35 yr
2. Teratogen exposure
3. Abnormal U/S
4. Abnormal prenatal screen
5. PMHx or FHx genetic disease, chromosomal anomalies, recurrent pregnancy loss, consanguinity

Types

1. **CVS** = biopsy of placental tissue
2. **Amniocentesis** = U/S guided transabdominal extraction of amniotic fluid

 C₂LEO Box

Patients Rights

- Failure to offer prenatal screening throughout pregnancy may violate the patient's rights.
- Failure to counsel a pregnant woman >35 yr about prenatal Dx may violate the patient's rights.
- Genetic testing has ethical implications to the mother and fetus, therefore counseling must be nondirected and not restricted to those open to abortion.
- Women must not be pressured into prenatal Dx if the only realistic options are abortion, selective conception, or childlessness.
- Reproductive decisions must not be coerced based on test results

ANTEPARTUM COMPLICATIONS

Table **14.62** Initial Management of Antepartum Complications

Antepartum Complications	Initial Management
Discrepancy in SFH—smaller than expected	• **Identify causal factors:** incorrect dates, small mother, inadequate weight gain, multiple gestation, maternal illness (DM type 1, SLE, pulmonary disease, renal disease, cyanotic heart disease, HTN—gestational or chronic), placenta abnormalities, teratogen exposure, TORCH infection, congenital anomalies • **Modify controllable factors:** smoking, EtOH/ substance abuse, proper nutrition, Rx of maternal illness • **Fetal surveillance:** serial NST/BPP, daily FM counts, SFH measurements; +/– U/S assessment of fetal growth, umbilical artery Doppler • **Consider amniocentesis if** IUGR diagnosed at <32 wk GA, IUGR severe < third percentile • **Counsel regarding** complications of IUGR → hypoglycemia • **IUGR <34 wk GA:** bed rest, fetal surveillance, ensure adequate nutrition • **IUGR >37 wk GA:** immediate delivery • **IUGR 34–37 wk GA:** Deliver if no fetal growth documented.
Discrepancy in SFH—larger than expected	• **Identify causal factors:** incorrect dates, maternal obesity, GDM, postdates • **Modify controllable factors:** Rx of GDM • **Fetal surveillance:** serial NST/BPP, daily FM counts, SFH measurements, umbilical artery Doppler • **Counsel regarding** complications of macrosomia → ↑ risk of (a) FTP in labor (due to CPD), (b) shoulder dystocia (c) possibility of C/S
Post dates (see Clinical Box Postdates pregnancy)	• **Expectant management** (GA 40–41 wk): fetal surveillance; evidence does not support labor induction or C/S unless have RF for morbidity (see Box 8) • **Labor induction** (GA >41 wk): if no CIs to vaginal delivery
↓ FMs	• **Identify causal factors:** maternal anxiety, maternal medications (i.e., sedatives), fetal sleep/inactivity, fetal distress, abruptio placenta, ruptured uterus, fetal death • **Modify controllable factors:** medications, EtOH abuse • **Fetal surveillance:** NST/BPP, daily FM counts (expect >10 in 12 h), SFH measurements, U/S assessment of fetal growth and to R/O fetal death
Elevated BP	see **Obstetric Complications**
PTL	See **Obstetric Complications**
Diabetes	See **Obstetric Complications**
Bleeding in first, second, or third trimester	See **Abnormal Vaginal Bleeding**

CLINICAL BOX

Discrepancy in SFH

1. Incorrect dates
2. IUGR
   • Infant weight <10th percentile for GA
   • SFH >2 cm behind GA
3. Macrosomia
   • Infant weight >90th percentile GA or >4 kg
   • SFH >2 cm ahead of GA

CLINICAL BOX

Postdates Pregnancy

Pregnancy >42 wk GA
Etiology

• Idiopathic (majority)
• Anencephaly (rare)
• Placental sulfatase deficiency (rare)

At ↑ Risk for

• Macrosomia
• Postmaturity syndrome
• Oligohydramnios
• Meconium aspiration

• Asphyxia
• Intrauterine infection
• Placental insufficiency
• Fetal distress
• Dystocia

RF for Morbidity

• DM
• HTN
• IUGR
• Multiple gestation
• Abruptio placenta

CLINICAL BOX

Prevention of RhD Isoimmunization

RhD Isoimmunization leads to:

a. Fetal/neonatal hemolytic anemia +/− hyperbilirubinemia 25% to 30% and/or
b. Hydrops fetalis 25%

The amount of Rh D+ blood required to cause isoimmunization is small (<0.1 mL).

Causes of Isoimmunization

1. Fetomaternal hemorrhage at delivery, Prev. EP, or Prev. abortion
2. Spontaneous antenatal fetomaternal hemorrhage
3. Invasive procedures during pregnancy (i.e., cerclage, amniocentesis)

Prophylaxis for All Rh⁻ Women
Administration of one prophylactic dose (300 μg) of RhoGAM (↓ rate of developing antibodies to Rh Ag)

1. At 28 wk unless the father of the baby is known to be Rh⁻
2. Within 72 h of delivery of an Rh⁺ infant
3. Post first trimester pregnancy loss
4. Post invasive procedures (i.e., CVS, amnio, fetal blood sampling)
5. Rh⁻ patient with Prev. threatened abortion, second/third trimester bleeding, external cephalic version, or Abdo trauma

C₂LEO Box

Legal Liability for Negligence
- Failure to act on abnormal prenatal screening results may be considered a cause of harm.
- Failure to recognize Rh isoimmunization in a pregnant woman may be considered a cause of harm → due to failure to meet the standard of care.

INTRAPARTUM AND POSTPARTUM CARE

RATIONALE

- **Intrapartum care** is the care of the mother and fetus during labor.
- **Postpartum (Puerperium) care** is the care of the mother and fetus during the 6 wk period following birth. During this period, the reproductive tract returns to its normal nonpregnant state.
- **Labor** is the process by which products of conception are delivered from the uterus by **progressive** cervical **effacement** and **dilatation** in the presence of regular uterine contractions.
- **Braxton Hicks** contractions: irregular contractions, **not** associated with any cervical Δs or descent of fetus
  - Approximately 85% of pregnant women will undergo spontaneous labor between 37 and 42 wk GA.
  - Approximately 15% of pregnant women will undergo labor between (a) 20 to 36 wk GA (**preterm**) or (b) >42 wk GA (**post-term**).

APPLIED SCIENTIFIC CONCEPTS

ENDOCRINOLOGY OF PARTURITION

Table **14.63**	**Four Distinct Physiological Phases of Myometrial Activity in Pregnancy**
Phase	**Mechanism(s)**
0. Myometrial inhibition	• During pregnancy, uterus remains quiescent because **inhibitors** active • Putative inhibitors = progesterone, prostacyclin, relaxin, NO, placenta CRH
1. Myometrial activation	• Occurs as term approaches • Uterus activated in response to **uterotropins** (i.e., E) • **Result**: (a) uterus become primed; (b) have development of regular, rhythmic contractions
2. Stimulatory	• Stimulation of primed uterus by uterotonic agonists (i.e., Oxytocin, PGE₂, PGF₂α).
3. Involution	• Occurs after delivery • Mediated by oxytocin

Table **14.64**	**Factors Promoting Labor**
Factor	**Mechanism of Action**
1. Fetal	• Activation of fetal HPA axis → ↑ cortisol which acts on placenta → ↑ E production → ↑ E:Progesterone ratio • **Result**: (a) ↑ PGF_α release; (b) ↑ myometrial response to oxytocin; (c) ↑ contractions
2. Maternal	• Activation of maternal HPA axis → possible activation of fetal HPA • Oxytocin → ↑ PG receptors, ↑ Oxytocin receptors, and ↑ gap junctions in uterine myometrium
3. Myometrial	• ↑ Free intracellular Ca^{2+} → contraction of uterine myocyte cells • Possible mechano-transduction through stretching or shortening

Regulation of the myometrial activity of the uterus relies on fetal and maternal paracrine/autocrine factors, as well as intrinsic factors within myometrial cells. This is because the uterus is **not** densely innervated.

PATHOGENESIS OF PRETERM BIRTH

Table **14.65**	**1° Pathogenic Processes Leading to Preterm Delivery and Birth**	
Pathogenic Process	**RFs**	**Postulated Mechanism(s)**

1. Premature activation of the maternal or fetal HPA axis	• Fetal stress:
	  • Placenta insufficiency
	  • Placental pathology
	• Maternal stress:
	  • Domestic violence
	  • Depression, anxiety
	  • Other life events
		1. ↑ CRH → ↑ maternal and fetal adrenal cortisol → ↑ PG production
		2. ↑ Fetal adrenal DHEAS production → ↑ placental E production

2. Inflammation/infection (chorioamnionitis, decidual)	• GU infection (i.e., asymptomatic bacteriuria, pyelonephritis) • BV • STI • Pneumonia • Peritonitis • Periodontal disease	1. ↑Maternal and fetal cytokines → ↑ PG → ↑ uterine contractions 2. Maternal proteases and cytokines → breakdown fetal membranes and cervix

3. Decidual hemorrhage	• Placenta abruption	• Release of decidual tissue factor
		• Initiation of coagulation cascade and thrombin production →
		  • Cervical ripening
		  • PPROM
		  • Uterine contractions

4. Pathologic uterine distension	• Polyhydramnios (AFI >25 cm)
	• Multiple gestation
	• Structural uterine abnormality (i.e., bicornuate, unicornuate)
		• Mechanical stretching →
		  • ↑ Myometrial gap junctions
		  • Activation of oxytocin receptors
		  • ↑ PG synthesis

STAGES OF LABOR

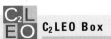 **C₂LEO Box**

Physician's Legal Liability for Negligence
Failure to recognize RFs for group B Streptococcal infection in a pregnant woman.

Table **14.66**	Stages of Labor		
Stage	Definition	Avg. Duration	
		Nulliparous	**Multiparous**
First	Interval between onset of labor to full cervical dilation (10 cm) Divided into two phases:	~10 h	~8 h
	a. Latent phase: begins with onset of regular uterine contractions with slow cervical dilation up to ~3–4 cm	~6.5 h Prolonged >20 h	~4.5 h Prolonged >14 h
	b. Active phase: ↑ rate of cervical dilation to maximum, regular contractions, and descent of fetus	Cervical dilation 1.2 cm/h Fetal descent >1 cm/h	Cervical dilation 1.5 cm/h Fetal descent >2 cm/h
Second	Interval between full cervical dilation and delivery of infant	~50 min Prolonged (no epidural) >2 h	~20 min Prolonged(no epidural) >1 h
Third	Interval between delivery of infant and delivery of placenta	~10 minProlonged if >30 min	
Fourth	Interval from delivery of placenta through to the resolution of physiologic Δs of pregnancy	6 wk	

Sterile speculum and vaginal exams are contraindicated in known or suspected cases of placenta previa.

Cervical exams should be kept to the minimum needed to detect abnormalities in labor progression.

CLINICAL BOX

The Vaginal Exam in the Management of Labor

A sterile vaginal exam is done to determine cervical dilation and effacement as well as the position and station of the fetus.

1. **Dilation** is the estimated measure of the diameter of the internal cervical os.
2. **Effacement** is the shortening and thinning of the cervix expressed as length (cm) or a percentage (0% = no reduction vs. 100% = minimal palpable cervix).
3. **Position** is the position of the presenting part of fetus relative to the maternal pelvis. Most commonly OA, but can also be OP, or OT.
4. **Station** is the estimated distance (cm) of the leading presenting part relative to the ischial spines.

At the level of the spines = 0 (engaged) versus centimeters below (+1 to +5) and centimeters above (−1 to −5).

Indications for Vaginal Exams in Labor

- On admission (if no suspicion/Dx of placenta previa)
- q2-4 h in first stage and q1 h in second stage
- At ROM to evaluate for cord prolapse
- Before intrapartum administration of analgesia
- When the patient feels the urge to push (to determine if cervix is fully dilated)
- To evaluate cause of ↓ FHR (R/O cord prolapse or uterine rupture)

THE CARDINAL MOVEMENTS OF LABOR

Sequence of movements, involving Δs in position of the fetal head, that enables the fetus to successfully negotiate the pelvis during labor.

1. **Engagement**—Widest diameter of the fetal head (biparietal diameter) enters the maternal pelvis below the plane of the pelvic inlet.
2. **Descent**—downward passage of the presenting part through to the pelvic floor. Greatest rate is during the second stage of labor.
3. Passive **flexion** of the fetal occiput permits the smallest diameter of the fetal head (suboccipitobregmatic ~9.5 cm) to be presented for optimal passage through the pelvis.
4. **Internal rotation**—rotation of the occiput from its original position toward the symphysis pubis (OA) or toward the sacrum (OP). This enables the AP diameter of the fetal head to line up with the AP diameter of the pelvic outlet.
5. **Extension**—delivery of the fetal head by extension and rotation of the occiput around the symphysis.
6. **Restitution and external rotation**—with the fetus' head free of resistance, it untwists causing the occiput and spine to line in the same plane

CLINICAL BOX

Signs of Placental Separation

1. Contraction and rise of the uterus
2. Cord lengthening
3. Gush of blood

7. **Expulsion**—delivery of the anterior shoulder under the symphysis pubis followed by quick expulsion of the rest of the body

FETAL MONITORING IN LABOR

- Goal is to reduce perinatal/neonatal mortality and morbidity by early detection of fetal decompensation.
- Achieved by assessment of FHR through fetal CTG, which allows for simultaneously measures of uterine contractions and FHR

1. **IA**
   - **Indications:** Healthy women with no RFs for adverse perinatal outcomes.
   - **Frequency of IA = for 1 full min after contraction:** q1 h during latent phase, q15-30 min in active phase, and q5 min in second stage of labor
2. **Continuous EFM**
   - **Indications:** (a) nonreassuring auscultation, (b) pregnancies at risk of adverse perinatal outcomes (i.e., meconium in amniotic fluid—sign of fetal distress, vaginal bleeding, GDM, prolonged ROM >24 h, abnormal vitals etc.), (c) induced, augmented, or prolonged labor
   - Can be done externally through Doppler or internally through a fetal scalp electrode
   - Use of EFM is not associated with a significant improvement in neonatal well-being and has been shown to ↑ rates of medical intervention (i.e., C/S, operative vaginal deliveries).

↓ or absent FHR variability is due to (a) persistent hypoxia leading to acidosis, (b) fetal sleep (c) Medications—that is, narcotics, sedatives, β-blockers, (d) prematurity, and (e) fetal tachycardia. Must investigate if lasts >40 min!

CLINICAL BOX

Management of an Atypical or Abnormal FHR Tracing

1. Recheck the tracing
2. Call for backup
3. Change maternal position to LLDP—relieves compression of IVC by the gravid uterus
4. Provide fetus O₂ by 100% O₂ mask to mother
5. Stop augmentation of labor—↓ hyperstimulation
6. Fetal scalp stimulation
7. R/O causes of uteroplacental deficiency (i.e., correct any maternal hypotension—IVFs, ephedrine)
8. Amniotomy
9. Fetal scalp electrode
10. Measurement of fetal scalp blood pH—(pH ≥7.25 = normal, pH ≤7.20 = fetal acidosis)
11. +/− Amnioinfusion—protects cord from compression

Table **14.67** **Classification of EFM Tracings during Labor**

FHR	Normal (Previously "Reassuring")	Abnormal (Previously "Nonreassuring")	Abnormal (Previously "Nonreassuring")
Baseline (indicator of fetal status)	110–160 bpm	1. Bradycardia 100–110 bpm 2. Tachycardia >160 for >30 min or <80 min 3. ↑ Baseline	1. Bradycardia <100 bpm 2. Tachycardia >160 for <80 min 3. Erratic baseline
Variability Characteristic of FHR due to effect of vagus nerve on heart: 1. **Minimal**: <5 bpm 2. **Moderate**: 6–25 bpm (Physiologic = acceptable fetal acid base status) 3. **Marked**: >25 bpm	• 6–25 bpm • <5 bpm for <40 min	<5 bpm for 40–80 min	• <5 bpm for >80 min • >25 bpm for >10 min • Sinusoidal
Accelerations	1. ↑ >15 bpm for >15 s (>34 wk GA) 2. ↑ >10 bpm for >10 s (<32 wk GA) 3. Spontaneous 4. Present with fetal scalp stimulation	Absent with fetal scalp stimulation	Usually absent (if present, does not change classification of tracing)
Decelerations (see Table 14.68)	1. None 2. Occasional early deceleration 3. Occasional uncomplicated variable decelerations	1. >3 uncomplicated variable decelerations 2. Occasional late decelerations 3. Single prolonged decelerations >2 min but <3 min	1. >3 complicated variable decelerations 2. Late decelerations >50% of contractions 3. Single prolonged deceleration >3 min but <10 min
Management	• Continue EFM • Can interrupt EFM for <30 min if mother and fetus stable +/− oxytocin infusion rate stable	• Intrauterine resuscitation • Determine cause/duration • Perform fetal scalp stimulation +/− fetal blood sampling if >34 wk GA • Evaluate total clinical picture (GA, EFW, stage of labor etc.) • Close ongoing fetal surveillance	• Intrauterine resuscitation • Determine cause • Perform fetal blood sampling if >34 wk GA • Evaluate total clinical picture (GA, EFW, stage of labor etc.) • Immediate operative deliver/transfer

CLINICAL BOX

Epidural or Spinal Considerations

CIs

1. Patient refusal
2. Untreated coagulopathy
3. Skin infection of lumbar area
4. Refractory hypotension/hypovolemia
5. Active neurologic disease
6. Septicemia

Risks

1. Infection
2. Maternal hypotension
3. Neurologic complications: spinal headache, back pain, nerve palsies
4. Toxic drug reaction
5. Rare neurologic disease

Table **14.68**	Types of Decelerations Seen in Labor	
Deceleration	**Cause**	**Description**
1. Early	**Head compression** → vagal slowing of heart	• Seen in active phase of labor • Uniform shape • FHR: gradual ↓ and return to baseline • Coincides with contraction

2. Variable	**Cord compression**	• Variable shape, onset, duration
		• FHR: abrupt drop and return to baseline
		• Most common deceleration seen in labor
		• **Complicated**:
		  • Deceleration to <70 bpm
		  • >60 bpm below baseline
		  • Lasts >60 s long

3. Late	**Uteroplacental deficiency** due to: (a) maternal hypotension, (b) uterine hyperstimulation, or (c) placental dysfunction **Result** = hypoxia +/− acidosis of fetus	• Uniform shape • Gradual ↓ • Late onset (starts at end of contraction) • Can cause change in baseline or ↓ variability

Table **14.69**	Medications for Pain Relief in Labor
Medication	**Description**
Entonox	• A mixture of nitrous oxide gas and O_2 administered through a mask • Patient can control how much gas is inhaled. • Can continue its use right up to the moment of giving birth • Effects **not** passed on to the fetus
Narcotics	• Options: nalbuphine (Nubain) 5–10 mg SC or IV q2-3 h, meperidine (Demerol) 25–50 mg IV q1-2 h • Avoid if their peak action will not have diminished by the time of delivery • Can cause respiratory depression in the neonate, reverse with narcan 0.01 mg/kg
Regional anaesthesia	• Loss of pain sensation occurs below T8/T10 with varying degrees of motor blockade. • Must hydrate the patient with dextrose free isotonic IV fluid before initiation of epidural

INDUCTION OF LABOR

Occurs when the benefits of delivery to either the mother or fetus outweigh the benefits of continuing the pregnancy.

CLINICAL BOX

Cervical Ripening

• Done to promote softening, effacement and dilation of the cervix in preparation for induction
• Also ↑ sensitivity of uterus to oxytocin
  1. **Pharmacologic:** (a) Intravaginal PGE_2 insert (Cervadil) containing 10 mg dinoprostone. Slow, controlled release of medication **and** can be removed if hyperstimulation occurs. (b) Intravaginal PGE_2 gel (Prostin) containing 0.5 mg dinoprostone which is injected into cervical canal q6 h× 3 doses.
  2. **Mechanical:** 24 French Foley balloon with 30 mL bulb, laminaria (osmotic dilator), or hydroscopic dilators

Table **14.70**	Induction of Labor		
Requirements	1. **Favorable** cervix (short/soft/thin, open internal os)—(see clinical box Cervical Ripening) 2. Normal "reassuring" fetal CTG 3. Cephalic/vertex presentation 4. Access to proper fetal monitoring		
Indications	Maternal factors	Fetal factors	Combined factors
	• PIH • Renal or pulmonary disease • Diabetes	• Intrauterine death (IUD), • Severe IUGR • Distress (as indicated by CTG, U/S etc.)	• PROM • Alloimmunization • Post-term pregnancy ($>$42 wk GA), • Chorioamnionitis.
CIs	• Unstable status • Prev. classical/ T-incision of uterus • Abnormal pelvis structure • ↑↑↑ CPD • Active genital herpes • Invasive cervical CA	• Distress • Malpresentation (transverse, breech) • Preterm (immature lungs)	• Placenta previa • Cord compression • Vasa previa
Methods	1. **Artificial ROM** (amniotomy)—stimulates PG synthesis and secretion 2. **Oxytocin** (Pitocin)—Use minimum dose needed to achieve cervical dilation of ∼1 cm/h in active phase.		
Side effects	• Need for C/S (fail to achieve vaginal delivery) • Uterine hyperstimulation (reversible ↓/stop rate of oxytocin infusion or with β-adrenergic agent) • Uterine rupture • Uterine atony +/− PPH • Hypotension—if IV oxytocin is rapidly infused • Hypovolemia +/− hyponatremia with prolonged use (oxytocin acts as an antidiuretic)		

ABNORMAL LABOR

- **Dystocia**—the abnormally slow progress of labor **or** failure of labor to progress
- Diagnosed when have a failure of:
  a. Cervical dilation in the active phase of the first stage → demonstrated by $>$4 h of $<$0.5 cm/h dilation
  b. Fetal head descent in the second stage, despite $>$1 h of active pushing

  Three possible causes for FTP are as follows:

1. **Power** → inefficient uterine action (hypotonic, uncoordinated, difficulty pushing by mother)
2. **Passenger** → fetal position (i.e., OP), size, and presence of anomalies (i.e., hydrocephalus)
3. **Passage** → pelvic structure (i.e., CPD), maternal soft tissue factors (i.e., full bladder)

Table **14.71**	Disorders Leading to Dystocia in Labor		
Disorder	**Definition**	**Etiology**	**Management**
Arrest of dilation	Cervical dilation stops for $>$2 h in the active phase.	Inefficient uterine action	• Appropriate assessment of progress in labor
Arrest of descent	Fetal descent fails to progress for $>$1 h during second stage.	**CPD** (especially if uterine contractions are adequate)	• Appropriate intervention when necessary:
Protraction of dilation	Slow rate of cervical dilation (i.e., $<$1.2 cm primigravida vs. $<$1.5 multigravida)	Inefficient uterine action	• Analgesia • Rest
Protraction of descent	Slow rate of fetal descent during second stage ($<$1 cm primigravida vs. 2.0 multigravida)	**CPD**	• Ambulation • Amniotomy • Oxytocin augmentation
Prolonged latent phase	$>$20 h in primigravida and $>$14 h in multigravida	Due to **improper** Dx of early labor	• Fetal health assessment

CLINICAL BOX

Augmentation of Labor

- Promotes adequate uterine contractions when spontaneous labor fails to progress:
  a. Slow progression through latent phase (inadequate cervical dilation) **or**
  b. Protraction and/or arrest disorders of labor **or**
  c. Hypotonic uterine contraction pattern
- IV infusion of oxytocin run at 0.5 to 4 mIU/min IV with incremental ↑ of 1 to 2 mIU/min q20-30 min.
- Reassess progression of labor once at dose of 20 mIU/min

Indications for Augmentation of Labor

- Rupture of fetal membranes
- Absence of meconium fluid
- Singleton fetus in vertex position
- Normal FHR pattern (no evidence of fetal distress)

> Oxytocin is used for both **induction** and **augmentation** of labor.

OPERATIVE DELIVERIES

Table **14.72**	Types of Operative Deliveries		
	Definition	**Indications**	**Complications**
Vacuum extraction	Operative vaginal delivery Suction/traction instrument used to deliver the fetus	1. Abnormal or Atypical EFM tracing 2. Prolonged second stage 3. Impaired pushing by mother (exhaustion, ↑↑↑ analgesia)	Neonatal injury • Soft tissue trauma • Hemorrhage—subglial, subaponeurotic • Maternal perineal, vaginal lacerations • Bladder/uterus/pelvic nerve damage • Infection • PPH
Forceps	• Operative vaginal delivery • Classified according to level + position of the fetal head in the birth canal at the time the forceps are applied • Types: low/outlet forceps, mid forceps, and high forceps		
C/S	Low transverse incision (most common)	1. Maternal → active herpetic lesions, maternal illness (PIH, GDM, invasive cervical CA) 2. Fetal → distress, malpresentation, cord prolapsed 3. Combined→ FTP, placenta abruption/previa	• Anesthesia • Hemorrhage • Infection • Injury to bladder, bowel, uterus • ↑ Recovery time/stay in hospital

> There is no benefit to **routine** episiotomy at normal deliveries.

EPISIOTOMY
- Incision of the vaginal opening through the perineal body at the time of delivery
- Done to facilitate vaginal delivery when indicated

SHOULDER DYSTOCIA
- **Life-threatening emergency**
- Impaction of the anterior shoulder behind the pubic bone after delivery of the head
- Results in the "turtle sign" = retraction of the delivered fetal head against the bottom of the symphysis pubis

RFs
1. **Maternal:** obesity, pelvic abnormality, GDM, postdates pregnancy, Prev. shoulder dystocia
2. **Fetal:** macrosomia
3. **Labor:** prolonged active phase of first stage, prolonged second stage of labor, assisted vaginal delivery (i.e., forceps)

Table **14.73**	**Episiotomies**

Types	1. **Median (Midline)**—incision through the central tendon of the perineal body
	   Advantage = easy repair and improved healing
	2. **Mediolateral**—incision through the levator ani bulbocavernosus, and superficial transverse perineal muscles
	   Advantage = ↓ likely to extend into anal sphincter and rectum.

Indications	• Delivery with a high risk of perineal laceration • Soft tissue dystocia • Immediate delivery of compromised fetus • Instrumental delivery
Possible complications	• Infection • Hematoma • Fistula formation—rectovaginal • Fecal incontinence • Median → likely to extend into anal musculature/rectal mucosa • Mediolateral → ↑ scar tissue, ↑ blood loss, ↑ pain, ↑ difficult to repair, dyspareunia sequelae

COMPLICATIONS

1. **Maternal:** PPH, symphyseal separation or diathesis, third or fourth degree
2. lacerations, uterine rupture
3. **Fetal:** hypoxia +/− permanent neurologic damage, brachial plexus injury, clavicular, or humerus #, death

---

CLINICAL BOX

Active Management of Third Stage of Labor

Done to help reduce the risk of uterine atony and ↓ postpartum blood loss. Oxytocin is the ideal uterotonic agent due to its (a) short t1/2 ~2 to 3 min, (b) minimal side effects, and (c) usability in all women.

1. Administration of 10 U oxytocin IM, within 1 min of delivery
2. Early cord clamping
3. Controlled cord traction

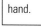

Never apply cord traction (pull) without counter traction (push) above the pubic bone with one hand.

An Rh⁻ mother should receive 300 μg of Rhlg within 72 h of delivery if her fetus is Rh⁺ **even** if she received her antepartum dose.

POSTPARTUM (PUERPERIUM) CARE

• Early postpartum care involves monitoring of maternal vital signs, pain management, and surveillance for complications.
• Education regarding maternal self-care and appropriate activities is key during this time period (See Table 14.74).

OBSTETRIC COMPLICATIONS

See also Chapter 3—Pregnancy-Associated HTN.

RATIONALE

• Virtually any maternal medical or surgical condition can complicate the course of a pregnancy and/or be affected by the pregnancy.
• Conditions arising in pregnancy can have adverse effects on the mother and/or the fetus. For example, babies born prematurely account for >50% of perinatal morbidity and mortality.
• ~5% of women will describe bleeding of some extent during pregnancy, and in some patients the bleeding will endanger the mother.

Table **14.74**	Common Postpartum Complications	
Complication	**Definition**	**Initial Management**

PPH	• Excessive blood loss in the postpartum period
	• Can be seen as:
	  a. Estimated blood loss >500 ml for vaginal delivery or >1,000 mL for C/S, **or**
	  b. Any amount of blood loss that threatens a woman's hemodynamic stability, **or**
	  c. A 10% ↓ in Hct between admission and the postpartum period
	• Types:
	  1. **1°/early PPH** occurs within the first 24 h after delivery
	  2. **2°/late PPH** occurs >24 h after delivery
		1. **Resuscitation**: large bore IVs ± IVFs, O₂ using mask, cross and type 4 units pRBC, monitor vital signs (BP, HR, SaO₂, RR)
		2. **Assess Etiology**: "4 Ts"
		  a. **Tone**—assess uterine atony
		  b. **Tissue**—explore uterus for retained placental tissue or blood clots
		  c. **Trauma**—explore the lower genital tract for lacerations
		  d. **Thrombin**—review if patient has Hx of coagulopathy (vWD, ASA use, DIC, ITP, etc.)
		3. **Investigations**: CBC, coagulation profile
		4. **Directed Rx**: based on findings of assessment

Postpartum fever	• Fever >38° C on > 2 occasions at least 4 h apart, after the first 24 h postpartum
	• DDx:
	  a. Breast engorgement, mastitis (*S. aureus*)
	  b. Atelactasis, pneumonia
	  c. Wound infection—C/S or episiotomy site (polymicrobial)
	  d. Endomyometritis
	  e. Thrombophlebitis, DVT
		Investigations ordered depend on clinical Sx

Postpartum blues	• Commonly occurs in >80% of new mothers • Usually begins between postpartum d 3 and 10 • Due to adjustment to baby and hormonal Δs	• Self-limited • No need for psychiatric medications • Supportive care

Postpartum depression	• Depression occurring in a woman within 6 mo of childbirth
	• RFs:
	  a. Stressful life circumstances
	  b. Personal or FHx depression
	  c. Poor social supports
	  d. Colicky infant
		• Antidepressants
		• Psychotherapy
		• Supportive care

CAUSAL CONDITIONS

Table **14.75**	DDx of Obstetric Complications
Etiology	**DDx**
Preexisting maternal conditions	• Late maternal age • HTN • Diabetes • Cardiac disease • Chronic renal disease • Other (thrombosis, SLE, drug use)
Maternal conditions arising in pregnancy	• Pregnancy-induced HTN • Gestational diabetes • Gestational thrombocytopenia • Thrombosis • Viral infections (TORCH, rubella, varicella, HIV) • Other (drug use, physical/emotional abuse/trauma)
Fetal conditions	• Large for GA/small for GA • Structural abnormality of fetus/ABO • Alloimmune disease (Rh isoimmunization)
Complications inherent to pregnancy	• Antepartum hemorrhage • PTL • Preterm PROM

GENERAL APPROACH

The most clinically important aspects in the evaluation of a pregnant patient at risk for obstetric complications are as follows (see Antepartum care for details):

1. Identification of RFs at the initial prenatal visit (antenatal Hx and physical exam are very important)
2. Appropriate fetal and maternal surveillance during pregnancy including uterine height (SFH), measurement amniotic fluid, BPP, and so on
3. Identification of patients in need of specialty care referral
4. Implement a "preventative/improving outcome of pregnancy" program for all pregnant women (i.e., smoking cessation counseling, folic acid/prenatal Vits, gestational diabetes and HTN screening, determination of Rh status etc.).

DIABETES IN PREGNANCY

Poorly controlled blood sugar levels during pregnancy are associated with an ↑ risk of polyhydramnios, fetal macrosomia, preeclampsia, operative delivery, birth trauma, and neonatal hypoglycemia.

CLASSIFICATION OF DIABETES IN PREGNANCY

1. **Pre-GDM** (type 1 or 2)
2. **GDM** (onset of DM during pregnancy)
   - GDM is usually diagnosed in the late gestation (i.e., T2 pregnancy)
   - If diagnosed before 24 wk GA is likely undiagnosed pre-GDM type 2

RFs for GDM

1. Prev. Hx of GDM or glucose intolerance
2. FHx of diabetes
3. Prev. macrosomia (>4,000 g)
4. Prev. unexplained stillbirth
5. Prev. neonatal hypoglycemia, hypocalcemia, or hyperbilirubinemia
6. Advanced maternal age
7. Obesity
8. Repeated glycosuria in pregnancy
9. Polyhydramnios
10. Suspected macrosomia

Pre-GDM

↓

Preconception counseling:
1. Attempt to achieve euglycemic control before conception (HgA1c ≤7%)
2. Ophthalmology consult
3. ECG if >35 yr and a smoker
4. Renal function evaluation (24 h urine for CrCl)
5. Initiate preconceptual folic acid for prevention of NTD (5 mg/d at least 3 mo before conception)
6. Dietician consult

↓

Management:
(A) Strict glycemic control:
1. Diet and exercise
2. Insulin → continue on pre pregnancy regimen and increase as indicated by blood work
- Metformin and Lantus not currently approved for use in pregnancy
(B) Fetal surveillance:
1. T1: dating U/S and FTS
2. T2 MSS, fetal echo at 19–22 wk GA
3. T3: U/S for (a) EFW at 28–30 wk, then at 34–36 wk GA; (b) (d) FM counts (10 movements in 12 h period)
(C) Delivery:
1. Recommend delivery by 39–40 wk
2. If EFW > 4.5 kg → C/S recommended
3. Intrapartum: serial plasma glucose measurements q 1 h
- During active labor, insulin to keep plasma glucose in rage of 3.5–6 mmol/L ± IV 5% dextrose infusion to manage hypoglycemia
(D) Postpartum:
1. Insulin requirements post delivery → monitor plasma glucose q 6h
2. No insulin required postpartum until plasma glucose >8 mmol/L → restart at 1/3–1/2 antepartum dose

Figure 14.25 Pregestational diabetes—preconceptual planning.

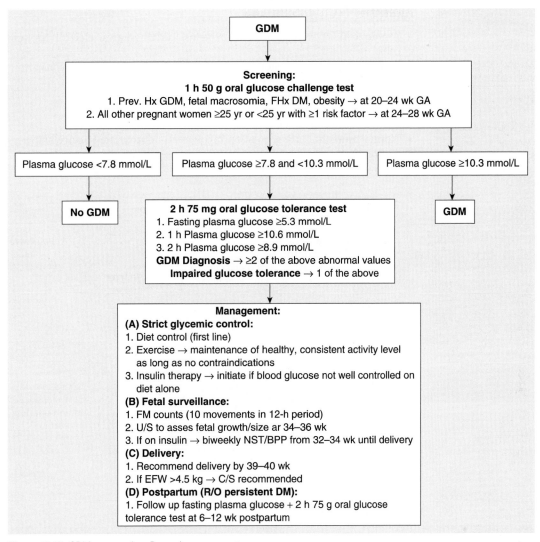

Figure 14.26 GDM—screening, Dx, and management.

Table **14.76**	Complications due to DM in Pregnancy

Maternal	Fetal

A. **Obstetric:**
   • Preeclampsia
   • ↑ Risk of C/S
   • ↑ Risk of birth trauma
   • ↑ Risk spontaneous abortion
   • ↑ Risk stillbirth
B. **Metabolic:** ↑ risk of
   • DKA
   • Severe hypoglycemia
C. **Worsening microvascular disease:**
   • CAD
   • Retinopathy
   • HTN
   • Nephropathy
   • Neuropathy
   • Retinopathy
D. **Postpartum**
   • ↑ Risk infection
	A. **Growth:**
	   • Macrosomia
	   • IUGR
	   • IUFD
	B. ↑ **Risk of structural malformations:**
	   • Congenital heart defects
	   • NTD
	C. **Neonatal sequelae:**
	   • RDS
	   • Hypoglycemia
	   • Hyperbilirubinemia/jaundice
	   • Hypocalcemia

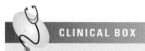

Assessing AFV

1. **AFI**—measurement and summation of deepest pocket in 4 quadrants
2. Verification of **2×2 cm pocket**—U/S survey to verify presence of >1 2× 2 cm pocket

AMNIOTIC FLUID DISORDERS

- Amniotic fluid is composed of proteins, carbohydrates, electrolytes, and fetal skin cells.
- Amniotic fluid is essential for proper fetal development as it functions to:
  1. Cushion the fetus from external injury
  2. Ensure proper MSK development
  3. Develop the fetal lungs and GI system
  4. Maintain a constant temperature
- Normal amniotic fluid regulation involves an appropriate balance between production and removal.

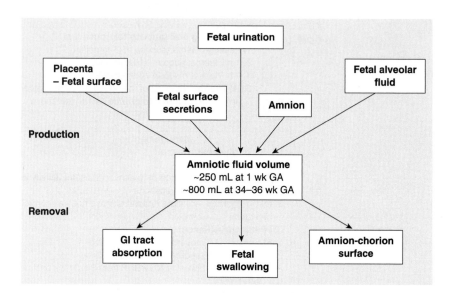

Figure 14.27 Physiology of amniotic fluid regulation.

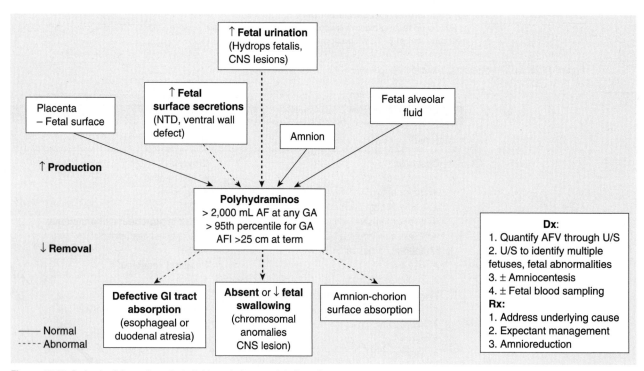

Figure 14.28 Pathophysiology of amniotic fluid regulation—polyhydramnios.

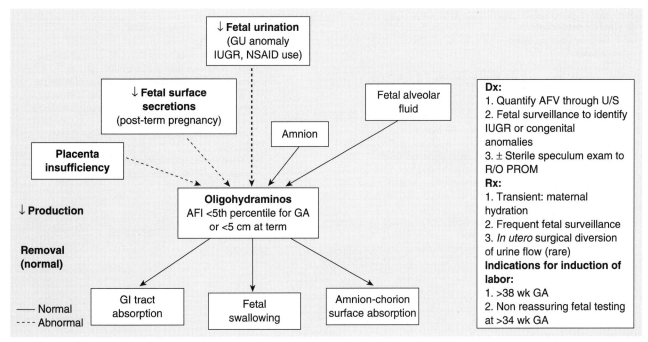

Figure 14.29 Pathophysiology of amniotic fluid regulation—oligohydramnios.

- Amniotic fluid disorders occur when amniotic fluid is too low (oligohydramnios) or too high (polyhydramnios)

PTL

- **PTL** is labor (regular contractions causing a cervical Δ) occurring between 20-37 wk GA.
- Occurs in ~9% to 11% of all pregnancies.
- Very preterm birth occurs at <32 wk and extreme preterm birth occurs at <28 wk GA.
- Preterm birth is the leading cause of infant mortality. See Figure 14.30.

> **CLINICAL BOX**
>
> ### Sx of PTL
>
> Pregnant women should be counseled with regard to the Sx of PTL
>
> - >1 or more of regular uterine contractions
> - Pelvic pressure, vaginal bleeding
> - Δ in vaginal discharge
> - Low back pain
> - Cramping

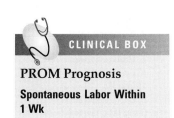

> **CLINICAL BOX**
>
> ### PROM Prognosis
>
> **Spontaneous Labor Within 1 Wk**
>
> - ~50% of women <26 wk GA
> - ~85% of women 28 to 34 wk GA
>
> **Complications**
>
> - Chorioamnionitis
> - Cord prolapse
> - Premature delivery
> - Limb contracture

PROM

- **PROM** is the spontaneous rupture of the amnion and chorion before the onset of labor.
- **Latency period**: time between ROM and onset of labor
- PROM occurs in ~10% of all pregnancies and is responsible for ~30% of all preterm deliveries. See Figure 14.31.

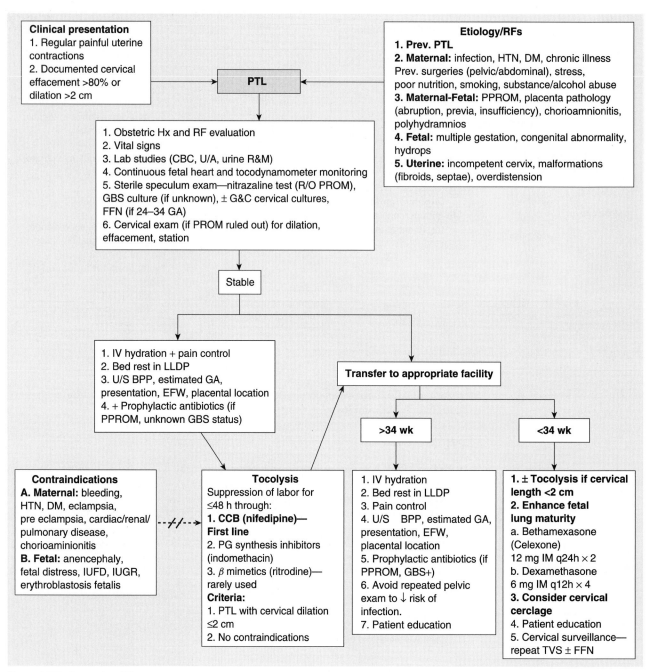

Figure 14.30 Approach to PTL.

Table **14.77**	**Ruptured Membranes—Definitions**
PROM	ROM before labor at any GA
Prolonged PROM	>24 h between ROM and labor onset
Preterm ROM	ROM before 37 wk GA
Preterm PROM (PPROM)	ROM before 37 wk GA and before onset of labor

Table **14.78** **PROM RFs**		
Maternal	**Fetal**	**Other**
• Infection (UTI, STI, cervicitis, vaginitis, intrauterine) • Prev. Hx or FHx of PTL or PPROM • Cervical insufficiency • Trauma	• Fetal malformations • Multiple gestations • Polyhydramnios	• Smoking • Trauma • Amniocentesis • Low SES, poor nutrition

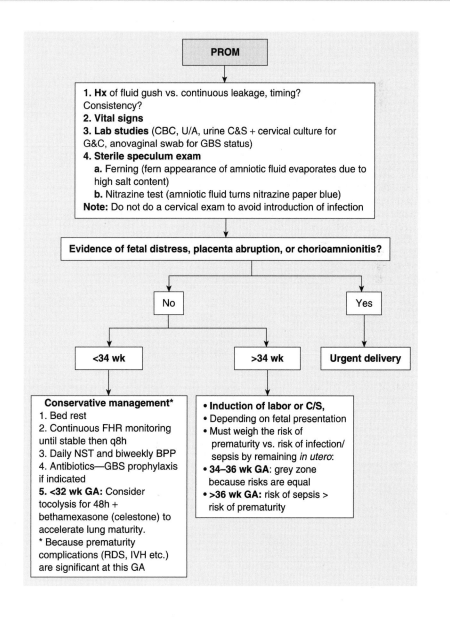

Figure 14.31 Approach to PROM.

CONTRAINDICATIONS TO **FFN** TESTING

1. Vaginal bleeding
2. Hx of intercourse or vaginal exam within the last 24 h
3. PROM

PREVENTION OF **PTL**

1. Identification of at-risk pregnancies
2. Reduce RFs
3. Good prenatal care
4. Rx of systemic maternal infections (i.e., UTI etc.)

Oncology

Lilly Teng, Dr. Leora Horn, and Dr. Natasha B. Leighl

BREAST LUMP/SCREENING

DEFINITION

- Breast lumps are common, generally associated with benign breast disease
- Must always be pursued to diagnosis or resolution due to risk of BRCA

APPLIED SCIENTIFIC CONCEPTS

BREAST ANATOMY

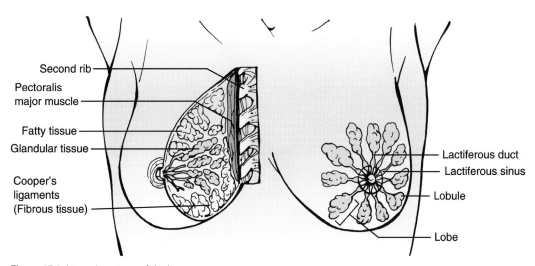

Second rib

Pectoralis major muscle

Fatty tissue

Glandular tissue

Cooper's ligaments (Fibrous tissue)

Lactiferous duct

Lactiferous sinus

Lobule

Lobe

Figure 15.1 Internal anatomy of the breast.

Regular mammography screening has been shown to reduce BRCA mortality in women aged 50 to 69 and in those with a positive family history of BRCA.

CAUSAL CONDITIONS

See Figure 15.2.
See Table 15.1.

APPROACH

HISTORY

See Figure 15.3.

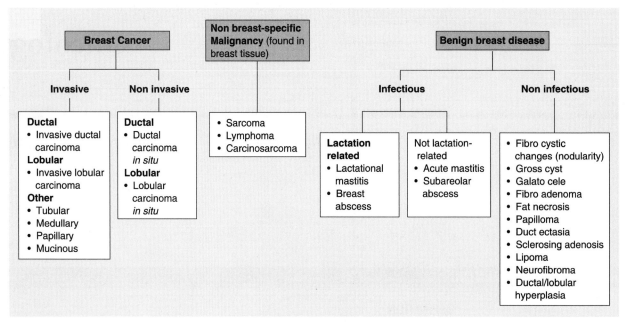

Figure 15.2 Breast Lump: causal conditions.

Table **15.1** **BRCA Screening**		
Mammography (± Clinical Exam)	**Breast Self-Exam**	**Genetic Testing for BRCA 1 or 2 Gene**[a]

40– 49 y.o.
• No evidence to include or exclude screening exam as it has not been consistently shown to reduce mortality
50–69 y.o.
• Every 1–2 yr
Positive family history in 1st degree relative
• Every 1–2 yr starting 10 yr before youngest age of presentation
	• No clear evidence of benefit in reduction of BRCA mortality	**Ashkenazi Jewish women**
		• Any 1st degree relative **or** two 2nd degree relatives from the same side of the family, with BRCA or ovarian cancer
		All other women
		• Patient age <35 at diagnosis of BRCA
		• Patient or 1st degree relative with both BRCA and ovarian cancer regardless of age at diagnosis
		• Patient or 1st degree relative with bilateral BRCA
		• Patient with strong family history of BRCA and/or ovarian cancer
		  • Two 1st degree relatives, one age <50 at diagnosis **or** three 1st degree relatives regardless of age at diagnosis
		  • Combination of two or more 1st or 2nd degree relatives with ovarian cancer regardless of age at diagnosis
		• History of BRCA in male relative

[a]Guidelines from U.S. Preventive Services Task Force. Genetic risk assessment and BRCA mutation testing for breast and ovarian cancer susceptibility: Recommendation statement. *Ann Internal med* 2005;143:355.

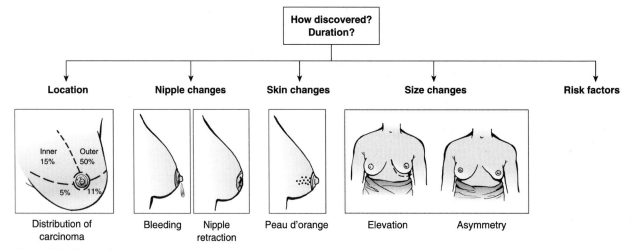

Figure 15.3 History of a breast lump.

Risk Factors for BRCA

- Age (>50)
- Female
- Prior history of breast or ovarian cancer
- Prior breast biopsy (regardless of pathology)
- Prior radiation therapy at site
- Family history of breast or ovarian cancer in 1st/2nd degree relatives

- History of prolonged hormone exposure
  - Nulliparity
  - First pregnancy >30 y.o.
  - Menarche <12 y.o.
  - Menopause >55 y.o.
  - HRT >5 yr
  - Obesity
- Excessive alcohol intake

PHYSICAL EXAM

Inspection

Breasts—4 S's
- **S**ize
- **S**ymmetry
- **S**hape
- **S**kin changes

Nipples—6 S's
- **S**ize
- **S**ymmetry
- **S**hape
- **S**kin changes
- **S**pontaneous secretions
- **S**upernumerary nipples

Palpation

Breast

Lymph nodes

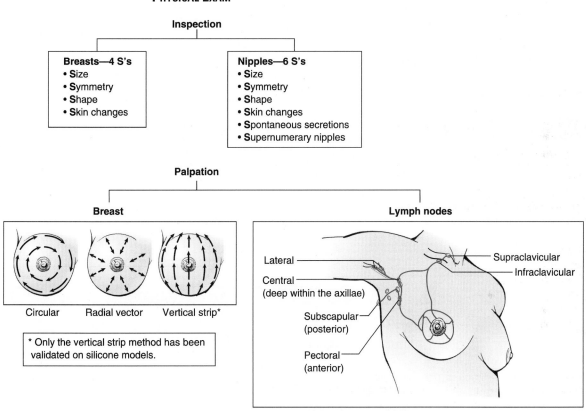

Circular   Radial vector   Vertical strip*

* Only the vertical strip method has been validated on silicone models.

Lateral
Central (deep within the axillae)
Subscapular (posterior)
Pectoral (anterior)
Supraclavicular
Infraclavicular

Figure 15.4 Physical exam of breast lump.

Characteristics of Cancerous Lesions

Location	Unilateral
Number	Solitary
Size	≥2 cm[a]
Borders	Irregular
Consistency	Firm/hard
Mobility	Immovable[a]
Change with menses	No change

[a]A lesion that is <2 cm or movable may still be cancerous.

INVESTIGATION

Table **15.2**	Investigation of Breast Lump		
Modality	**Indications**	**Use**	**Interpretation**
Mammography	• Any woman with a breast lump	• Search for other lesions that are clinically occult • Evaluate lump	Features suggesting malignancy • Increased density • Irregular margins • Spiculation • Accompanying clustered irregular microcalcifications
U/S	• Any woman with a breast lump	• Differentiate between simple or complex cystic or solid lumps	• Risk for cancer is low if lesion is a simple cyst • Complex cystic or solid lumps require further investigation
FNAB	• Complex cyst or solid lump found on U/S	• Collect samples for cytology	• Fluid obtained without blood unlikely to be cancer • If fluid is bloody, send for cytology • If no fluid, aspirate cells for cytology
Core needle biopsy	• Atypical or suspicious FNAB	• Collect samples for histology • Allows staining for ER, PR, and Her2/neu where indicated	• Can differentiate between atypical hyperplasia and ductal carcinoma *in situ* from invasive disease
MRI[a]	• Any women for whom mammogram and U/S results are inconclusive	• Detection of breast lump • Further characterization of mass detected on screening for BRCA	Features suggesting malignancy • Increased density • Irregular margins • Spiculation • Rim pattern of enhancement • Wash-out of signal intensity

[a]Limited availability for evaluation of breast lump in some areas.

Investigation for a suspicious breast lump consists of a combination of appropriate imaging and progressively more invasive biopsies as deemed necessary.

CLINICAL BOX

Triple Diagnosis

Refers to diagnosing palpable breast lumps, with concurrent use of

1. Physical exam
2. Mammography
3. Skilled FNAB

Very few BRCAs are missed using triple diagnosis.

MANAGEMENT

Table **15.3**	Indications for Adjuvant Therapy

Indications for Adjuvant Therapy		
Radiotherapy • After lumpectomy • After mastectomy in stage IIIB disease • With axillary node involvement	**Hormonal** • Almost all patients with tumor size >1 cm, ER/PR positive following surgery • Premenopausal: tamoxifen, or ovarian ablation, or ovarian ablation and aromatase inhibitor (anastrazole, letrozole) • Postmenopausal: tamoxifen, or aromatase inhibitor	**Chemotherapy** • Depends on tumor size, number of involved lymph nodes, and patient performance status • Most patients with stage II or III disease • Stage I disease with Her2-neu positive tumor • Trastuzumab (Herceptin) should be used in all Her2-neu overexpressing tumors

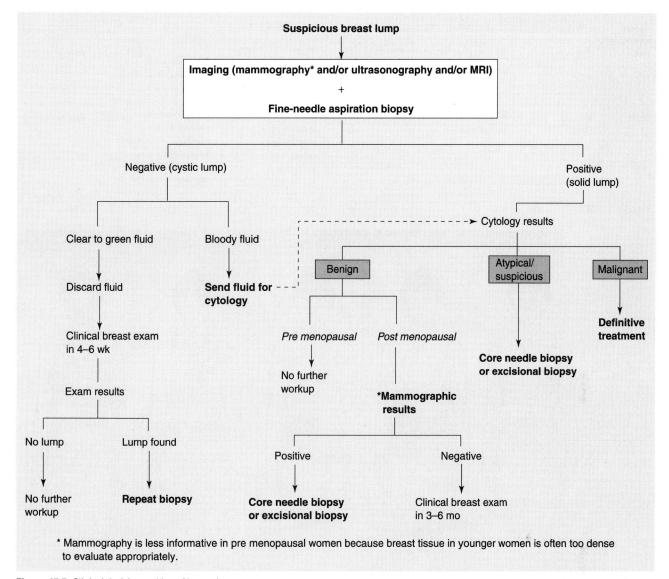

Figure 15.5 Clinical decision-making of breast lump.

ONCOLOGIC EMERGENCIES

See Table 15.4.

C₂LEO

DOCTOR–PATIENT RELATIONSHIP

- The physician will place the best interest of the patient first.
- Establish a relationship of trust between physician and patient.
- Follow through on undertakings made to the patient, in good faith.

ROLE OF THE PRIMARY CARE PHYSICIAN

- Appropriate and prompt evaluation and delivery of appropriate therapies for breast lumps is essential to relieve extreme anxiety experienced by patients.
- Primary care physician may initiate work-up with radiographic imaging and biopsy referrals.
- Primary care physician must be advocate for patient throughout course of evaluation: learn about proficiency of local consultants.
- Follow patient carefully.
- Provide support and thorough communication at every point of process until resolution.

Treatment for BRCA consists of surgery and a combination of radiotherapy, hormonal therapy, and chemotherapy individualized to the disease condition and treatment goals of the patient.

Stage	0	I	IIA		IIB		IIIA		IIIB	IV
Tumor	**Tis** (*in situ*)	**T1** (≤ 2 cm)	**T1**	**T2** (≥ 2 cm ≤ 5 cm)	**T2**	**T3** (≥ 5 cm)	**T1-2**	**T2**	**T4** (any size with extension to chest wall or skin)	**Any T**
Node	No (none)	No	**N1** (ipsilateral axillary)		**N1**	**N0**	**N2** (ipsilateral axillary and/ or internal mammary)	**N1-2**	**N3** (ipsilateral axillary and/or internal mammary and/or infra-clavicular and/or supraclavicular)	**Any N**
Metastasis	M0 (none)	M0	M0		M0	M0	M0	M0	M0	**M1**

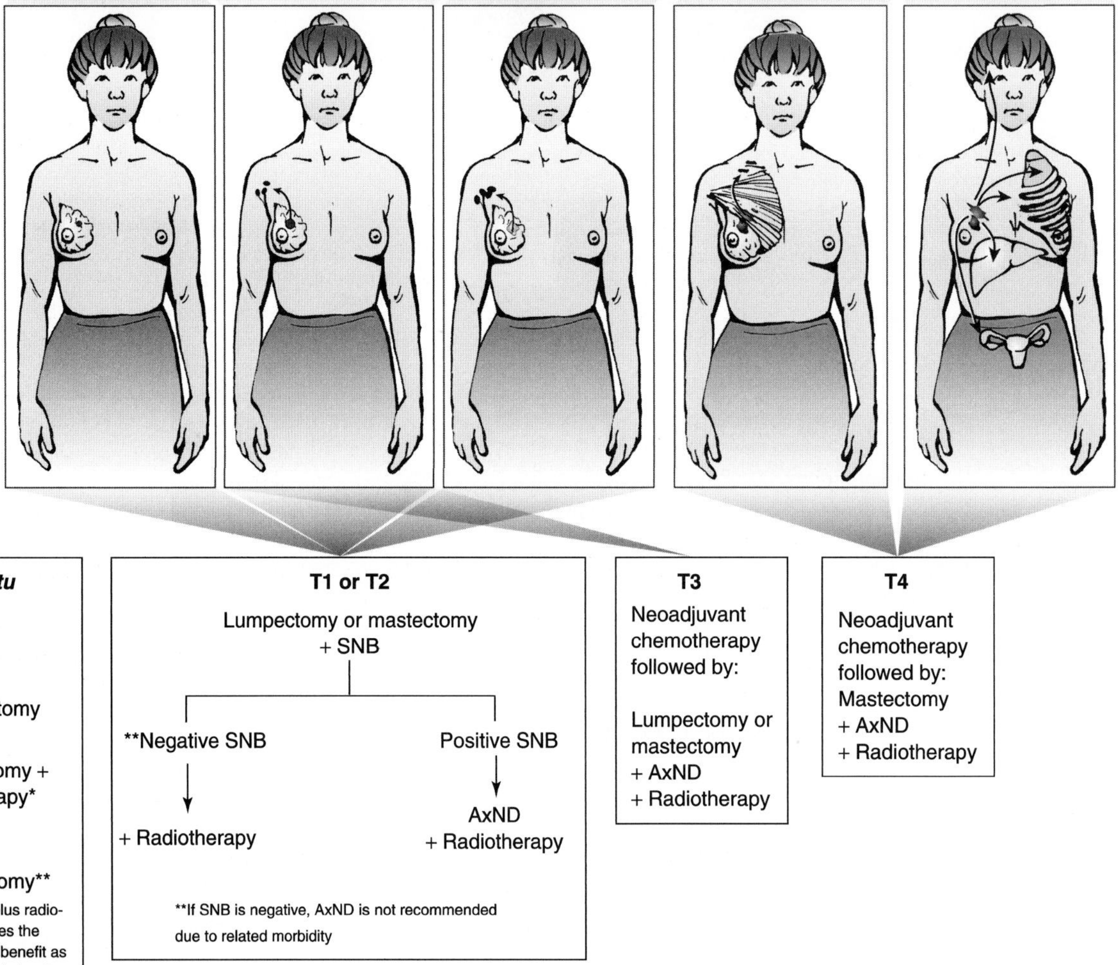

In situ
↓
Lumpectomy
Or
Lumpectomy + radiotherapy*
Or
Mastectomy**

*Lumpectomy plus radio-therapy achieves the same survival benefit as mastectomy with *in situ* and stage I & II disease

**If patient undergoes mastectomy, radiation therapy is not required

T1 or T2
Lumpectomy or mastectomy + SNB

**Negative SNB   Positive SNB

↓   ↓

+ Radiotherapy   AxND + Radiotherapy

**If SNB is negative, AxND is not recommended due to related morbidity

T3
Neoadjuvant chemotherapy followed by:

Lumpectomy or mastectomy + AxND + Radiotherapy

T4
Neoadjuvant chemotherapy followed by: Mastectomy + AxND + Radiotherapy

Figure 15.6 Breast cancer staging and management.

CLINICAL BOX

Staging

BRCA staging requires removal of the primary tumor and ipsilateral axillary lymph node dissection.

- If tumors are >5 cm and axillary lymph nodes are positive, additional staging tests (chest x-ray, bone scan, CT abdomen) are required.
  - Smaller tumors with negative axillary lymph nodes do not mandate additional staging tests unless symptoms of metastatic involvement are present.

Table **15.4**	Oncologic Emergencies (not Specific to BRCA)
Oncologic Emergency	**Description**
Metabolic	
Tumor lysis syndrome	• Triad of hyperuricemia, hyperkalemia, hyperphosphatemia • Results from rapid release of intracellular contents of tumor cells into bloodstream • Hyperkalemia is the most life-threatening problem
Hypercalcemia of malignancy	• Disorder of calcium metabolism due to alterations in the pathways of calcium regulation involving PTH, calcitonin, and $(1,25[OH]_2$ vitamin D) • Patients are invariably dehydrated
Neurologic	
Strokes and seizures	• Both hemorrhagic and thrombotic subtypes of strokes • Occur in both patients with and those without cerebral metastases
Mechanical	
SVC syndrome	• Cough; dyspnea; dysphagia; swelling and discoloration of the neck, face, or upper extremities; and possibly vocal cord paralysis and Horner syndrome • Results from an increase in central venous pressure caused by vena caval obstruction
Spinal cord compression	• Symptoms include pain, weakness, sensory deficits, autonomic dysfunction • Results from spinal cord being compressed by tumor • Not immediately life-threatening unless involving level C3 or above, but may lead to profound, permanent morbidity
Treatment-related	
Extravasation of chemotherapeutic drugs	• Leakage of chemotherapeutic drugs into the skin, leading to pain, redness, swelling, and possibly necrosis • Typically results from infusion therapy
Neutropenic fever	• Neutrophil count <0.5 × 10(9)/L (500/mm³), or <1.0 × 10(9)/L and expected to decline below <0.5 soon • Fever defined as single temperature of 38.3°C (101.0°F) or a temperature of 38.0°C (100.4°F) or higher lasting over 1 hr

MUSCULOSKELETAL MASS

DEFINITION

- Most masses of MSK system are caused by benign soft tissue neoplasms or tumor-like conditions.
- Malignant lesions are less frequent.

CAUSAL CONDITIONS

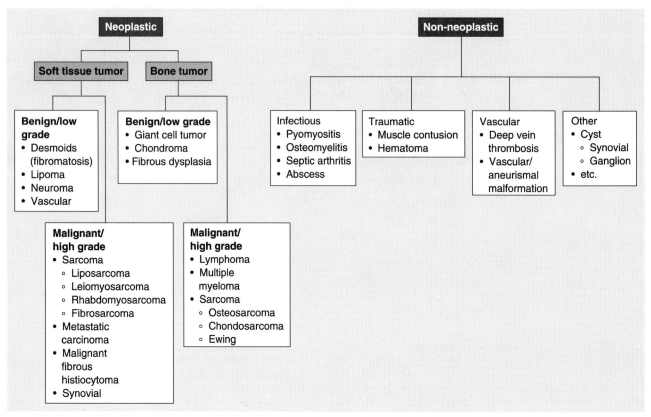

Figure 15.7 MSK lump/mass: causal conditions.

APPROACH

HISTORY

Table **15.5**	History of Musculoskeletal Mass
Question to Ask	**Relevance**
Age	• Rhabdomyosarcomas—most common soft tissue sarcomas in children
Location	• Thigh/buttock/groin region—most common site of soft tissue sarcoma
Duration and course	• Long-standing nonenlarging mass—most likely benign • New, enlarging mass—more likely malignant

Pain	• Most often painless
	• Local pain and swelling from larger masses associated with:
	  • Primary bone tumors
	  • Pyomyositis
	  • Septic arthritis
	  • Osteomyelitis
	  • DVT
	  • Muscle contusion
	  • Abscess

Table **15.5** *(continued)*	
Question to Ask	**Relevance**

Neurologic symptoms	• Large soft-tissue sarcomas **or** smaller benign peripheral nerve sheath tumors (ganglion cysts) may cause
	  • Pain
	  • Paresthesia
	  • Weakness
	  • Decreased sensation
	  • Muscle wasting

Systemic symptoms	• Malignant neoplasms or infections may cause
	  • Fever
	  • Chills
	  • Night sweats

Fluctuation in size	• Associated with benign causes (e.g., synovial cyst or hemangioma)
History of trauma	• May be associated with • Muscle contusion • Hematoma • Infection • DVT • Osteomyelitis • Septic arthritis
Risk factors for infectious lesions	• Muscle injury • Injection drug users • HIV/Immunocompromised • Diabetic • Systemic infection (that seeds a joint)
History of radiation	• Associated with malignant neoplasms
History of prior tumors/cancer	• Lung cancer, renal cancer—propensity for soft tissue metastases • Malignancy—increased risk of DVT
Personal or family history associated with soft-tissue sarcoma	• Type I (peripheral) neurofibromatosis • Gardner syndrome (variant of familial adenomatous polyposis, characterized by GI polyps, multiple osteomas, skin and soft tissue tumors) • Maffucci syndrome (genetic disorder characterized by benign enlargement of cartilage, bone deformities, and hemangiomas)

R

Malignant MSK lesions are more likely to be new and enlarging, cause systemic symptoms, and are associated with a history of radiation, personal tumors/cancers, and family history of tumors/cancers.

PHYSICAL EXAM

Table **15.6** **Physical Exam of Musculoskeletal Mass**	
Cause of Mass/Lump	**Clinical Characteristic**
Malignant/infectious	• Lymphadenopathy at local lymph nodes

Soft tissue sarcoma	• Size most predictive of metastatic propensity
	  • Size >**5 cm or deep to the fascia**—most likely malignant
	  • Size <**25 mm**—metastases unlikely
	• May be associated with
	  • Fever
	  • Sweats
	  • Weight loss

(Continued)

Table **15.6** *(continued)*	
Cause of Mass/Lump	**Clinical Characteristic**
Benign soft tissue tumor	• Most soft tissue masses • <5 cm **and** superficial • Lipoma—most common in adults • Hemangiomas—most common in children
Synovial cyst	• Transilluminates if superficial in location • Fluctuation in size independent of activity • Tense but indentable on palpation

Hemangioma	• Fluctuation in size depending on activity
	  • Enlarges with exercise (mass becomes engorged with blood)
	  • Shrinks/completely abates with rest
	• Compressible on palpation
	• Vascular ectasia in overlying skin

Vascular aneurysm/malformation	• Audible bruit • Palpable trill
Hematoma	• Accompanied by subcutaneous ecchymosis • Hematoma-like lesions without ecchymosis should be considered a tumor until proved otherwise (malignant tumors—e.g., extraskeletal osteosarcoma—may masquerade as hematomas)
Muscle contusion	• Local muscle pain, swelling • Limited joint ROM near the injury, weakness/stiffness in injured muscle • May be accompanied by subcutaneous ecchymosis
Abscess	• Superficial, erythematous, rapidly enlarging, swollen, warm, tender • May be deep • Fever
Pyomyositis	• Crampy local muscle pain • Swelling • Low grade fever • May appear toxic in later stages
DVT	• May feel palpable cord (reflecting a thrombosed vein) • Ipsilateral edema • Warmth • Superficial venous dilation • Pain and tenderness • Tenderness on deep palpation of calf muscles
Osteomyelitis/septic arthritis	• Bone pain, tenderness, warmth, swelling • Pain occurs with or without movement of joint • Decreased range of motion in joint • Fever, rigors

CLINICAL BOX

DVT risk factors: Virchow's triad
1. Hemostasis (period of immobility)
2. Hypercoagulability
3. Endothelial damage (inflammation)

MANAGEMENT

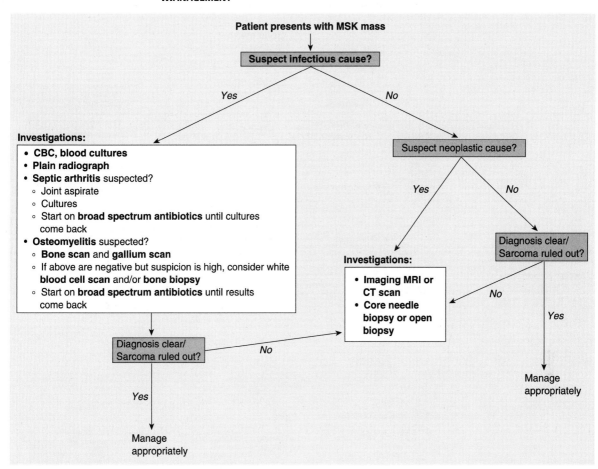

Figure 15.8 Approach to musculoskeletal lump/mass.

LYMPHADENOPATHY

DEFINITION

- Countless potential causes of peripheral lymphadenopathy
- May be benign finding or may be associated with illness
- May be primary or secondary manifestation of illness

APPLIED SCIENTIFIC CONCEPTS

THE IMMUNE SYSTEM

- Main function of immune system is protecting body from foreign organisms.
- Key strategy consists of distinguishing self from non-self followed by elimination of non-self.

Table **15.7** Branches of the Immune System	
Natural Immunity	**Adaptive Immunity**
• Nonspecific defence barriers (e.g., skin, stomach acidity), molecules (e.g., complements, cytokines) and cells (e.g., macrophages, mast cells)	• Highly specific defence molecules (antibodies) and cells (lymphocytes) • Consists of humoral response (antibodies) and cell-mediated response (T cells)

Adaptive Immunity

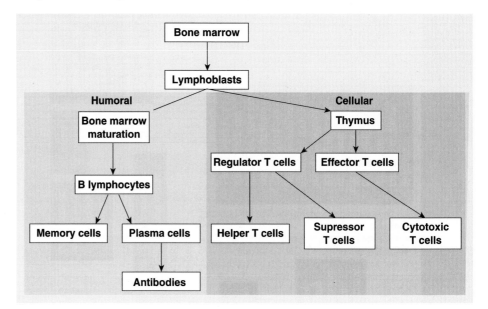

Figure 15.9 Differentiation of B and T cell.

(From Smeltzer SC, Bare BG. *Textbook of Medical-Surgical Nursing*, 9th ed. Philadelphia: Lippincott Williams & Wilkins; 2000.)

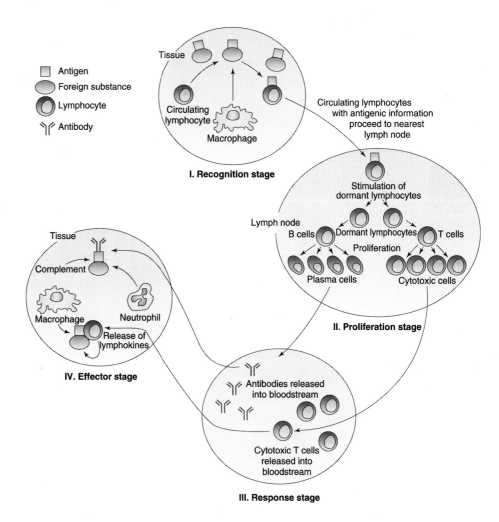

Figure 15.10 Activation of adaptive immunity consists of four stages. Recognition stage: antigens are recognized by circulating lymphocytes and macrophages. Proliferation stage: dormant lymphocytes proliferate and differentiate into cytotoxic (killer) T cells or B cells responsible for formation and release of antibodies. Response stage: cytotoxic T cells and B cells perform cellular and humoral functions, respectively. Effector stage: Antigens are destroyed or neutralized through the action of antibodies, complement, macrophages, and cytotoxic T cells.

(From Smeltzer SC, Bare BG. *Textbook of Medical-Surgical Nursing*, 9th ed. Philadelphia: Lippincott Williams & Wilkins; 2000.)

CLINICAL BOX

Lymph Node Function

- Storage/proliferation of B and T cells
- Antibody production
- Nonspecific filtration by macrophages

THE LYMPHATIC SYSTEM

- Part of the circulatory system
- Includes lymphatic vessels, lymph nodes, lymphoid tissue, lymph organs (e.g., spleen).
- Right lymphatic duct drains
  - Right side of the head and neck;
  - Right upper limb and pectoral region;
  - Right half of the thoracic cavity
- Thoracic duct drains the rest

CAUSAL CONDITIONS

- Generalized lymphadenopathy: involving more than one region
- Regional lymphadenopathy: involving only one region (e.g., neck or axilla)

GENERALIZED LYMPHADENOPATHY

Table 15.8 Generalized Lymphadenopathy

Infectious Causes	Inflammatory Diseases	Malignant Diseases	Other
Viral • EBV • CMV • Hepatitis • Measles • Rubella • HIV • Varicella • Herpes simplex Bacterial • Brucellosis • TB • Streptococci • Atypical mycobacterium • Syphilis Fungal • Histoplasmosis • Coccidioidomycosis Parasitic • Toxoplasmosis • Leishmaniasis • Filariasis • Trypanosomiasis	Collagen-vascular disease • Rheumatoid arthritis • Lupus (SLE) • Dermatomyostasis • Sjögren syndrome • Vasculitis • Mixed connective tissue disease • Serum sickness • Drug hypersensitivity • See list in History • Sarcoidosis	Lymphoma • Hodgkin disease • Non-Hodgkin disease • Acute or chronic lymphocytic leukemia • Hairy cell leukemia • Amyloidosis	Other • Hyperthyroidism • Castleman disease • Sarcoid familial Mediterranean fever • Lipid storage disease (Gaucher, Niemann-pick)

Supraclavicular lymphadenopathy is especially concerning for malignancies.

LOCALIZED LYMPHADENOPATHY

See Figure 15.11.

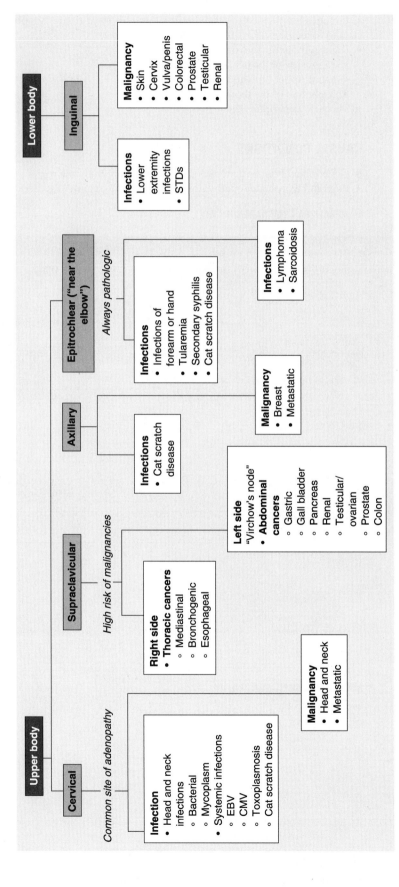

Figure 15.11 Localized lymphadenopathy.

APPROACH

HISTORY

Table **15.9** History of Lymphadenopathy					
Exposure	**Constitutional Symptoms**	**Medications**		**High Risk Behavior**	**Age**
• Cat (cat scratch disease) • Undercooked meat, fish, unpasteurized cheese (toxoplasmosis) • Tick bite (Lyme disease) • Travel • Occupation • Smoking history	• Fever, night sweats, weight loss (TB, lymphoma, other malignancies, immunologic disease)	• Allopurinol • Atenolol • Captopril • Carbamazepine • Cephalosporins • Gold • Hydralazine	• Penicillin • Phenytoin • Primidone • Pyrimethamine • Quinidine • Sulfonamides • Sulindac	• Multiple partner/ unprotected sex • Recreational drug use	• Age <50 more likely to be a benign cause

History of medication usage is very pertinent in the assessment of lymphadenopathy.

PHYSICAL EXAM

Splenomegaly in the context of lymphadenopathy implies systemic involvement.

Table **15.10** Physical Exam of Lymphadenopathy				
Location	**Size**	**Consistency**	**Fixation**	**Tenderness**
• Regional • Generalized	• Size >1 cm	• Hard • Firm • Rubbery • Soft	• Freely mobile in subcutaneous space • Fixed in adjacent tissue	• Tender • Nontender

Table **15.11** Splenomegaly		
Infectious	**Malignant**	**Immunologic**
• Infectious mononucleosis • Toxoplasmosis • Cat-scratch disease	• Lymphoma • Chronic lymphocytic leukemia • Acute leukemia	• Lupus

CLINICAL BOX

Nodal Characteristics

Lymphoma	**Metastatic**
• Large • Symmetric • Rubbery • Firm • Mobile • Nontender	• Hard • Fixed • Nontender

Unless a malignant cause is suspected, it is entirely appropriate to wait 2 to 4 wk before commencing invasive investigation.

INVESTIGATIONS

If cause of lymphadenopathy is not obvious from history and physical, further workup may be warranted (see below).

MANAGEMENT

See Figure 15.12.

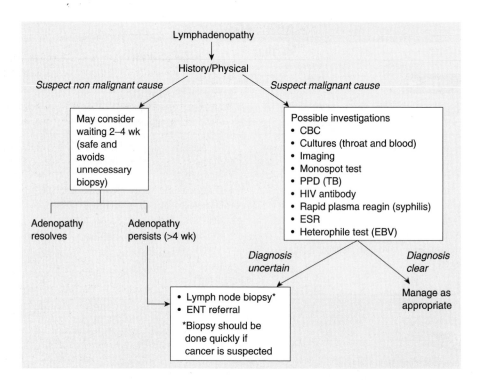

Figure 15.12 Approach to lymphadenopathy.

MEDIASTINAL MASS/HILAR ADENOPATHY

DEFINITION

- Mediastinum contains all structures in chest except lungs and pleurae.
- Extends superiorly from superior thoracic inlet to diaphragm inferiorly, and anteriorly from sternum and costal cartilages to bodies of thoracic vertebrae posteriorly
- Bound laterally by pleural cavities
- Evaluation of mediastinal mass guided by anatomy of mediastinum

APPLIED SCIENTIFIC CONCEPTS

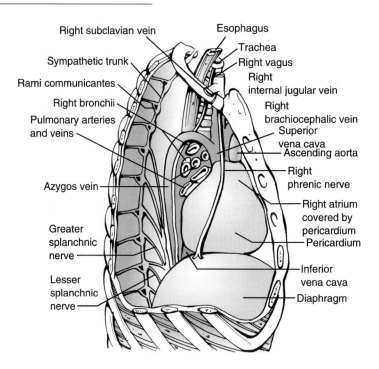

Figure 15.13 Anatomy of mediastinum.

CAUSAL CONDITIONS

Table 15.12 Anatomy of Mediastinum

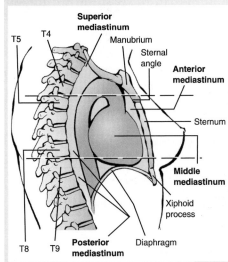

	Content/Organ	Disease
Extends from superior thoracic inlet to horizontal plane passing through sternal angle and inferior vertebrae of T4	• Thymus • Esophagus, trachea • Great vessels of heart	• Thymoma • Thymic cyst • Esophageal tumor • Aneurysm
Extends from sternum to anterior border of pericardium or pericardial sac 60% of masses are malignant	• Thymus • Esophagus, trachea • Thyroid (abnormal) • Pericardium, extra pericardial aorta and branches, great veins • Connective tissue • Other	• Thymoma • Thymic cyst • Esophageal tumor • Intrathoracic goiter • Aberrant thyroid • Parathyroid adenoma • Aneurysm • Pericardial cyst • Epicardial fat pad • Lipoma • Liposarcoma • Lymphangioma • Hemangioma • Malignant fibrous histiocytoma • Extraosseous osteogenic sarcoma • Diaphragmatic hernia • Primary teratoma • Carcinoid tumor
Bounded by pericardium anteriorly, the posterior pericardial reflection, the diaphragm, and the thoracic inlet • Clinically most important • 30% of masses are malignant	• Thyroid (abnormal) • Heart, pericardium, proximal great vessels • Main bronchi • Other	• Intrathoracic goiter • Aberrant thyroid • Parathyroid adenoma • Aneurysm • Pericardial cyst • Bronchogenic cyst • Bronchogenic tumor • Diaphragmatic hernia • Metastatic teratoma
Extends from posterior pericardium and diaphragm to posterior border of inferior eight thoracic vertebral bodies • 16% of masses are malignant	• Esophagus • Thoracic duct • Vagus nerve, sympathetic chain • Pericardium • Other	• Esophageal tumor • Thoracic duct cyst • Neurogenic tumor • Aneurysm • Diaphragmatic tumor • Metastatic teratoma • Enteric cysts • Bronchogenic tumor

---

The anatomic location (superior, anterior, middle, or posterior mediastinum) is very important in guiding the assessment of mediastinal masses.

CLINICAL BOX

The 6 Ts of an Anterior Mediastinal Mass*

- Thymoma
- Thyroid mass (intrathoracic goiter, aberrant thyroid)
- Teratoma
- "Terrible" lymphoma
- Thoracic aortic aneurysm
- Tumors (parathyroid, esophageal, connective tissue)

*Masses in the anterior compartment are more likely to be malignant than those found in the other compartments

Masses that can occupy any inferior mediastinal compartment:

- Lymphadenopathy
- Sarcoma
- Lymphoma
- Granulomatous disease

APPROACH

HISTORY AND PHYSICAL EXAM

Table **15.13** Physical Exam of Mediastinal Mass	
Sign or Symptom	**Cause**
Recurrent pulmonary infection	Airway compression
Cough, shortness of breath	Airway compression
Hemoptysis	Airway compression Invasion of tumor into a vessel
Dysphagia	Esophageal compression If esophageal cancer, due to narrowing of lumen
Paralysis	Spinal column involvement
Hoarseness	Recurrent laryngeal nerve involvement
Elevated hemi-diaphragm	Phrenic nerve involvement
Horner syndrome (ptosis, miosis, anhydrosis)—see Figure 15.1	Sympathetic ganglion involvement
SVC syndrome (dyspnea, trunk or extremity swelling, facial swelling, cough, orthopnea, headache, nasal stuffiness, light-headedness)	SVC involvement (gradual, insidious compression/obstruction of the SVC)
Fever, chills, or night sweats	Lymphoma Large mass
Pain	Compression of surrounding structures Inflammatory reaction
Gynecomastia	Germ cell tumor (teratoma)
Hypertension	Neuroblastoma Thyroid disorder
Hypercalcemia symptoms (stones, bones, moans and groans)	Parathyroid adenoma
Thyrotoxicosis	Thyroid disorder
Cushing's (moon facies, central obesity, striae, buffalo hump, etc.)—see Figure 15.2	Carcinoid

Systemic Diseases

Some mediastinal masses are associated with systemic diseases.

- **Thymoma**
  - Myasthenia gravis
  - Immune deficiency
  - Red cell aplastic anemia
- **Intrathoracic goiter**
  - Thyrotoxicosis
  - Parathyroid adenoma
  - Hyperparathyroidism

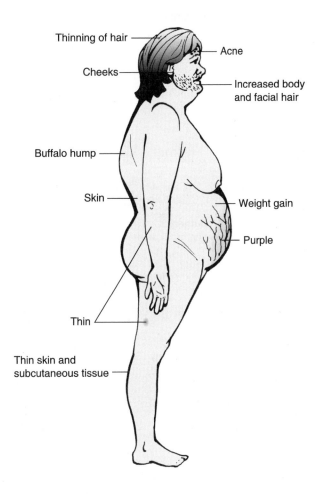

Thinning of hair

Acne

Cheeks

Increased body
and facial hair

Buffalo hump

Skin

Weight gain

Purple

Thin

Thin skin and
subcutaneous tissue

Figure 15.14 Cushing syndrome.

INVESTIGATIONS

Table **15.14**	**Investigation of Mediastinal Mass**
Investigation	**Use**
Chest radiograph	All mediastinal masses
CT scan with contrast	Indicated whenever a mediastinal mass is detected on plain film Helps define location, morphology, density, mass multiplicity, relation to vascular structures
MRI	Usually adds little additional information to CT with contrast Specifically indicated in the assessment of neurogenic tumors
U/S	Differentiates cystic from solid masses and their relation to surrounding structures Especially helpful in evaluation of structures close to the heart and pericardium
Radionuclide scanning	I-123 thyroid scanning for intrathoracic thyroid Gallium scanning for lymphoma Sestamibi scanning for parathyroid adenoma
Thyroid function studies	Intrathoracic goiter (TSH may be high or low)
Thyroid immune globulin	Thyroid cancer
Serum calcium, magnesium, phosphate, PTH.	Parathyroid adenoma (elevated calcium, low phosphate, elevated intact PTH)
PTHrP	PTHrP secreting tumor cells (most commonly lung cancer)
AFP and/or β-HCG	AFP is elevated in nonseminomatous germ cell tumors (if elevated in a pure seminoma, indicates element of nonseminoma in the tumor) β-HCG can be elevated in seminoma or nonseminoma Should be obtained in all males with a mediastinal mass

MANAGEMENT

- Clinical overview of middle and posterior mediastinal tumors

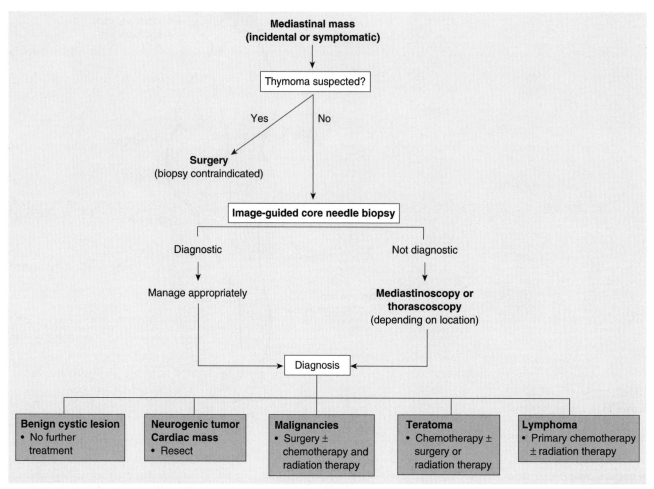

Figure 15.15 Approach to mediastinal mass.

Ophthalmology

*Kaylyn Kit Man Wong, Dr. Radha P. Kohly, Dr. Rajeev H. Muni,
and Dr. Wai-Ching Lam*

DIPLOPIA

DEFINITION

Double vision: visual perception of two images from a single object, leading to blurred vision

C₂LEO Box

Statutory Requirements and Negligence

- Physicians who diagnose diplopia are required to advise both the patient and/or the motor vehicles branch (provincial statutes vary) that driving is not permitted unless the diplopia is reversed.
- If a motor vehicle accident occurs, the physician who diagnosed diplopia may be legally liable if both the patient and/or the motor vehicles branch (provincial statutes vary) were not advised that driving is not permitted (until the diplopia is reversed, if possible).

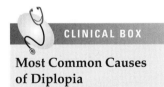

CLINICAL BOX

Most Common Causes of Diplopia

Monocular: cataract

Binocular: thyroid eye disease

Table **16.1**	**Classification of Diplopia**	
Type	**Manifestation**	**Cause**
Monocular	Diplopia disappears when affected eye is covered	Structural (benign) or functional (rare retinal or cerebral lesions)
Binocular	Diplopia disappears when **either** eye is covered, may be intermittent or constant	Ocular misalignment due to lesion anywhere along pathway from peripheral EOMs to central nuclei that drive them

MONOCULAR DIPLOPIA

Table **16.2**	**Common Causes of Monocular Diplopia**
Cornea	Opacity, scarring, keratoconus
Lens	Refractive: astigmatism, dislocated lens Opacity: cataract (most common cause)
Vitreous	Opacity
Other (rare)	Extra pupillary openings, retinal disease

BINOCULAR DIPLOPIA

- Vertical, horizontal, or oblique
- Comitant: misalignment same in all directions of gaze
- Incomitant: misalignment different in different directions of gaze

Table 16.3 Common Causes of Binocular Diplopia

EOMs (restriction, entrapment, or tethering)	Thyroid eye disease (i.e., Graves ophthalmopathy) Orbital cellulitis Orbital inflammation Orbital tumor: primary, secondary to invasion into orbit or metastatic Blow-out fracture of orbital floor (affecting maxillary bone and posterior medial floor, with prolapse into maxillary sinus)	Most common Ocular emerg Orbital inflammatory pseudotumor Ocular emerg if muscle entrapment
Neuromuscular junction	Myasthenia gravis	Affects all EOMs including lids, sparing pupillary and ciliary muscles
CN dysfunction	Nerve palsy: see below INO	Brainstem disease involving the medial longitudinal fasciculus
Nuclear	Nuclear pathology (tumor, vascular, MS, trauma)	

Table 16.4 Differentiating Nerve Palsies

#1 Findings	#2 Findings	Affected eye.	#3 Findings	Head tilt to minimize diplopia
• Diplopia worse when looking to one side and better on the other side • Eyes seem crossed	• Ptosis • Presence of any of the following: poor inward turning (adduction), impaired elevation, or depression of eye • +/− Enlarged pupil (ocular emerg R/O aneurysm)	Impaired adduction, elevation (down and out position)	• Head tilt • Diplopia mainly vertical • Worst when looking down and to one side	More diplopia when look down and left Less diplopia when look down and right
Sixth nerve palsy	Third nerve palsy		Fourth nerve palsy	
Etiologies include ischemia, diabetes, tumor, or any cause of increased ICP, trauma	Etiologies include ischemia, diabetes, aneurysm, tumor, trauma		Etiologies include ischemia, diabetes, trauma	

Common Conditions Requiring Immediate Action
Help **I** **C**an't **S**ee **A** **T**hing!
Hemorrhage, increased **I**CP, **C**ompressive mass lesion, **S**troke, suspected **A**neurysm, orbital **T**rauma or fractures

Figure 16.1 Eye movement and EOMs.

APPLIED SCIENTIFIC CONCEPTS

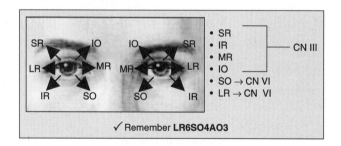

Table 16.5 Causes of Muscle Fatigue and Paralysis

Motor	CNS	PNS	Neuromuscular Junction	Muscle Fiber
Muscle weakness	Partial interruption of communication between cerebral cortex and upper motor neurons	• Partial loss of myelination • Ischemia to lower motor neuron	• Partial obstruction of receptors • Myasthenia gravis	Loss of muscle contraction due to electrolyte imbalances (i.e., hypo or hyperkalemia)
Muscle paralysis	Complete interruption of communication between cerebral cortex and upper motor neurons (i.e., spinal cord injury)	• Severe demyelination (Guillain-Barré syndrome) • Complete loss of lower motor neuron (i.e., poliomyelitis, amyotrophic lateral sclerosis)	• Complete obstruction of receptors • Botulism	• Severe electrolyte imbalances • Inherited deficiencies of muscular structural proteins

Table 16.6 Hx of Diplopia

Inquiry	Outcome or Response	Interpretation or Possible Cause
Onset of diplopia	Sudden onset	Indicates acute processes (i.e., ischemia)
	Gradual with steady worsening	Indicates long-standing conditions (i.e., tumor, inflammation)
Direction of image separation? Does head tilt improve diplopia?	• Vertical, horizontal, or oblique separation • Worse with head tilt generally indicates fourth nerve palsy	May point to palsy of a specific EOM
In which direction of gaze is double vision worst? i.e., in which direction of gaze are the images farthest apart?	Diplopia worst in the **same** gaze direction as the field of action of an EOM	Indicates muscle paresis/nerve paralysis
	Diplopia worst in the gaze direction **opposite** to the field of action of an EOM	Indicates muscle restriction
Was there pain or headache associated with the diplopia? When was the onset of the pain or headache?	Generalized headache or pain in temple area	Intracranial problem but always remember GCA
	Sudden onset of an extremely severe headache (thunderclap headache)	Suggest intracranial aneurysm
	Pain on eye movement	Demyelination, myositis, myopathy or orbital lesion
Does diplopia change as the day goes on?	Worsens later in the day	Myasthenia gravis
Neurologic symptoms	Presence of other neurologic symptoms	Intracranial pathology

Table 16.7 Physical Signs Associated with Diplopia

Feature	Interpretation
Head tilt	Typically CN IV palsy
Dilated pupil	R/O compression of CN III (posterior communicating artery aneurysm, tumor, can also see with ischemia)
Ptosis	CN III palsy or myasthenia gravis
Lid retraction	Graves ophthalmopathy
Proptosis	Graves ophthalmopathy, orbital mass or inflammation
Conjunctival or episcleral injection	Orbital space-occupying lesion, cavernous sinus disease (i.e., cavernous carotid fistula)
Abnormal gait, coordination, speech	Neurologic involvement

PARASYMPATHETIC PATHWAY OF PUPIL CONSTRICTION

- Parasympathetic nerves run along CN III and mediate pupillary constriction by innervating the sphincter pupillae muscle.
- Also involved as efferent limb of pupillary light reflex.
- Compression of CN III first manifests as a delayed pupillary response to light on the ipsilateral side.

GCA is an ocular emerg that must be R/O.

APPROACH TO DIPLOPIA

CLINICAL BOX

Imaging Investigations in Diplopia

- CT scan is best for detecting fractures and Graves ophthalmopathy.
  - Good to differentiate Graves ophthalmopathy (infiltrative lesion) from other conditions
- MRI is best for detecting orbitocranial junction or intracranial lesions including space-occupying masses, trauma, aneurysm, ischemia, and demyelination.
  - Can also detect small brainstem lesions affecting the medial longitudinal fasciculus (e.g., INO)
- Cerebral angiography is best for detecting aneurysms and ischemic lesions.

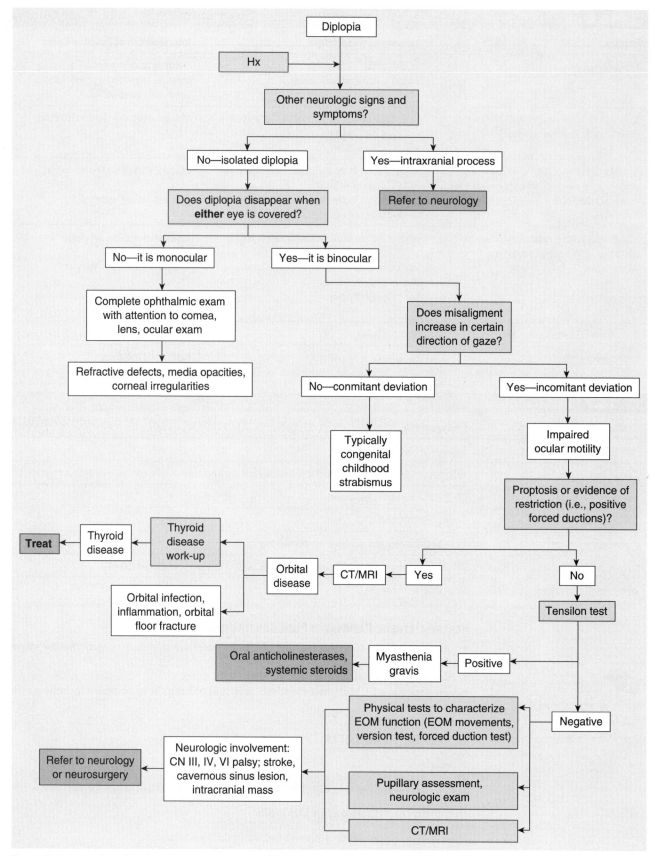

Figure 16.2 Approach to diplopia.

Table **16.8**	**Key Indications for Investigations**
Investigation	**Indications**

CT scan of orbits and head (if suspect orbital pathology always ask for fine cuts of orbit e.g., 1 mm)	• Complicated fractures, head trauma
	• Orbital tumors and mass lesions
	• Muscle restriction with uncertain diagnosis
	• All third nerve palsies if:
	  • 50 yr or younger (unless have known diabetes or HTN)
	  • Pupillary involvement
	  • >3 mo with no improvement
	  • Additional CN or neurologic abnormality
	• Presence of aberrant regeneration

MRI of orbits	• Suspected orbitocranial or intracranial lesion • Suspected tumors or masses • Any CN palsy with other abnormality or severe pain • Hx of cancer presenting with a nerve palsy • All children with acquired palsy • Adults with a nerve palsy without vasculopathy risk factors • Unresolved CN palsy or new abnormality
Cerebral angiography	• Any case of suspected aneurysm • Those 10 yr and older with third nerve palsy and pupil involvement, and where MRI and/or CT scan is normal or shows a possible aneurysm

RED EYE

Commonest Causes of Red Eye: CIF

Conjunctivitis (allergic or viral), **I**ritis, **F**oreign body

Red Eye in Need of Urgent Attention

AACG, infectious keratitis, and endophthalmitis are ocular emerg that need to be seen urgently.

Hyphema and iritis should be seen within 24 h.

Referral if no improvement after 24 to 48 h of care by primary physician: **c**ontact lens overwear (with no indication of corneal ulcer) and corneal abrasions.

RATIONALE

Very common ocular symptom; identify less common causes that may be sight-threatening

CAUSAL CONDITIONS

ASC Box

Common Infectious Pathogens in Various Conditions

Blepharitis	
Anterior	Staphylococcus or seborrheic or mixed
Posterior	Meibomian seborrhea or meibominitis
Orbital cellulitis	
Bacterial	*H. influenzae, Strep pneumo, S. aureus, S. pyogenes*
Fungal	Phycomycetes (mucormycosis) and aspergillosis
Conjunctivitis	
Bacterial	*S. aureus, Strep pneumo, H. influenza*
Viral	Adenovirus, HSV
Chlamydial	
Allergic	Atopic, vermal, or seasonal
Keratitis	
Bacterial	*P. aeruginosa, S. aureus, S. epidermidis, N. gonorrhea, H. influenzae*
Viral	HSV, Herpes zoster
Fungal	Aspergillus spp., Candida spp.
Protozoan	Acanthamoeba

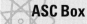 **ASC Box**

Ocular Anatomy

Sinuses and cellulitis
Orbit is surrounded by paranasal sinuses: frontal (superiorly), maxillary (inferiorly), ethmoid (medially). Infection or tumor may spread from the sinuses, particularly **ethmoid** sinus, to the orbit causing orbital cellulitis or globe displacement with diplopia.

Acute chamber angle
AACG: Peripheral iris reduces anterior chamber angle and blocks trabecular meshwork, preventing aqueous fluid from leaving anterior chamber leading to higher IOP.
Uveitis: Inflammation of iris and ciliary body and exudation of blood cells and proteins into anterior chamber blocks and anterior chamber angle and trabecular meshwork leading to higher IOP.

Table **16.9**	**Common Causes of Red Eye**	
Orbits	Preseptal cellulitis	Bacterial infection of superficial periorbital tissues and eyelid, globe spared, normal EOM, normal pupils; can progress to orbital cellulitis
	Orbital cellulitis[a]	Bacterial infection, globe involved; if not treated can progress to cavernous sinus thrombosis or meningitis
Lid and lashes	Blepharitis	Inflammation of eyelid margin
	Hordeolum	Blocked, infected eyelid gland
	Chalazion	Blocked meibomian gland
Conjunctiva and sclera	Conjunctivitis	**Commonest** cause of red eye— bacterial, viral, chlamydial, allergic
	SCH[a]	Common, bleeding under conjunctiva, spontaneous resolution; if 360° of SCH associated with trauma, R/O globe rupture
	Episcleritis	Common, usually idiopathic, self-limited
	Scleritis	Often associated with systemic autoimmune disease
	Pingueculum /pterygium	Degenerative changes in conjunctiva causing raised lesions
	Foreign body	Relevant Hx, may have corneal abrasion
Cornea	Infectious keratitis[a] (HSV, bacterial ulcer)	Fluorescein staining for epithelial dendrite, chalky white lesion through which cannot see iris detail with overlying fluorescein staining indicates ulcer
	Foreign body	Relevant Hx, foreign body in cornea
	Abrasions	Relevant Hx, fluorescein staining
	Contact lens use	Common with overwear, poor cleaning, sensitivity to lens solutions
Anterior chamber and iris	AACG[a]	Painful eye, IOP >30 mm Hg, mid-dilated pupil, diffuse conjunctival injection
	Anterior uveitis	Inflammation of iris and/or ciliary body
		Present with "**PRP**": **P**ain, **R**edness, and **P**hotophobia
		WBCs and flare (protein) in anterior chamber. Several etiologies including trauma, secondary to corneal pathology, infections (toxoplasmosis), or autoimmune diseases (JIA, ankylosing spondylitis, sarcoidosis, etc.)
	Hypopyon[a] (collection of WBCs)	Severe iritis with layering of WBCs inferiorly in anterior chamber. Assume endophthalmitis (if recent surgery) or infectious keratitis if corneal ulcer present
	Hyphema (collection of RBCs)	Assess IOP and R/O globe rupture
Always R/O globe rupture	Globe rupture (R/O intraocular foreign body)	360° SCH, peaked pupil, full thickness corneal or scleral laceration with prolapsed choroids (dark tissue), or decreased IOP in setting of trauma then R/O **global rupture**[a]. Imaging by CT, X-ray, MRI (contraindicated if metal intraocular foreign body object suspected)
Lacrimal system	Nasolacrimal duct obstruction	Persistent tearing, discharge, crusting, recurrent conjunctivitis

[a]Ocular emerg

APPROACH

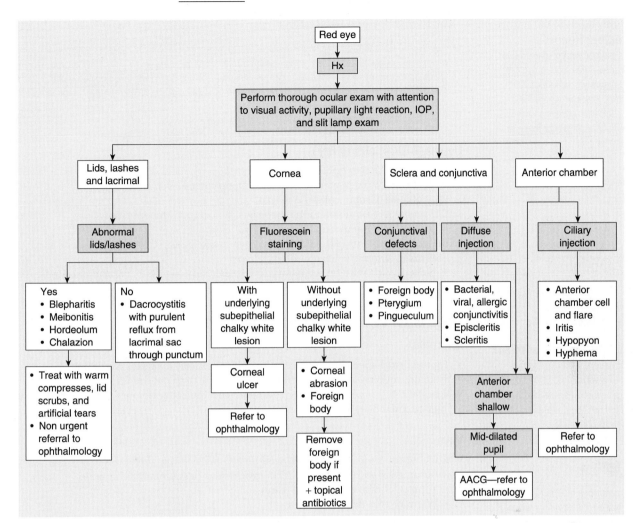

Figure 16.3 Approach to the red eye.

ASC Box

Association between Systemic Conditions and Eye Redness

Immune mechanisms
- Deposition of immune complexes → complement activation and inflammation
- Autoantibodies produced by B cells → complement activation and inflammation
- Autoreactive T cells → activate inflammatory cells, B cells
- Molecular mimicry → antibodies produced against infectious organisms recognize self-antigens → attack host tissues

Pharmacologic Rx in systemic diseases
- Goal: to prevent inflammation
- Anti-inflammatory—NSAIDs (inhibit cyclo-oxygenase and prostaglandin production and inflammation)
- Immunomodulatory agents—azathioprine, methotrexate, cyclosporine (suppress immune responses)
- Biologic agents—anti-TNF antibodies, TNF soluble receptors (to block inflammatory effects of TNF, a major inflammatory cytokine)

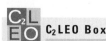

Legal Aspects of Medical Records

In a patient with ocular trauma, document pre-existing eye disease, safety precautions that were in place or ignored at the location where trauma occurred, condition at presentation, and initial Rx given.

Key Investigations for Red Eye

- For corneal infiltrates or conjunctivitis suspected bacterial (including gonococcal) or chlamydial conjunctivitis and corneal ulcers, need to do stat gram stain and cultures.
- Work-up for uveitis, after initial episode, includes HLA-B27 (R/O ankylosing spondylitis), CXR (R/O TB and sarcoidosis), angiotensin-converting enzyme (R/O sarcoidosis), VDRL/FTA-ABS (syphilis), and PPD.

UVEITIS (7 QUESTIONS TO ASK)

1. Rash (herpes zoster ophthalmicus, syphilis)
2. Arthritis or low back pain (ankylosing spondylitis, Reiter, psoriasis, JIA)
3. GI problems (Crohn, colitis, Whipple)
4. GU problems (tubulointerstitial nephritis, IgA glomerulonephritis)
5. Mouth and genital ulcers (Behçet)
6. Breathing problems (TB, sarcoidosis)
7. Trauma (traumatic iritis, microhyphema)
    - Note: uveitis may be secondary to corneal pathology (i.e., corneal abrasions, ulcers, and HSV keratitis)

TREATMENT OF COMMON CAUSES OF RED EYE

BACTERIAL

- Topical broad-spectrum antibiotic (e.g., ciprofloxacin) for faster resolution
- Systemic antibiotics (e.g., erythromycin) if severe or in children
- If suspect *N. gonorrhea* infection: systemic and topical antibiotics, and refer to ophthalmology immediately

VIRAL

- Adenovirus: Hx of red eye followed by second eye involvement 3 to 5 d later, contact with someone with red eyes, URTI, preauricular or submandibular node
    - Topical lubrication (artificial tears)
    - Warm or cold lid compresses
    - Hygiene: wash hands often, use separate soap, towels, and so on because viral conjunctivitis (i.e., adenovirus) is highly contagious
    - Refer to ophthalmology in 2 wk if confident of adenovirus conjunctivitis
- Herpes simplex
    - If corneal dendrites, treat with topical antivirals (refer to ophthalmology)
    - Never prescribe topical steroids without consulting ophthalmology

CHLAMYDIAL

- Swabs for stat gram stain and C&S
- Empiric Rx with systemic antibiotics
- Refer to ophthalmology

ALLERGIC

- Conservative
    - Remove allergens, cold compresses, minimize trauma (rubbing, contact lenses)
- Topical Rx
    - Antihistamine, mast cell stabilizer, NSAIDs, steroids, immunosuppressants (cyclosporine)
- Systemic Rx (if severe)
    - Antihistamine, steroid

RX OF FOREIGN BODY—DEPENDS ON LOCATION AND EXTENT

Conjunctival/Scleral

- Remove foreign body if visible
- Topical broad-spectrum antibiotic

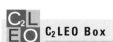

Contact Tracing with STI

In a patient with eye redness from chlamydial or gonococcal conjunctivitis, the sexual partners of the patient require identification and Rx.

N. gonorrhea may perforate cornea and is an ocular emerg requiring immediate referral.

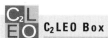

Negligence

In a patient with eye redness that is painful and associated with diminished or loss of vision, any uncertainty should lead to early, prompt referral to a specialist (i.e., worsening of herpes simplex keratitis with topical steroids may lead to physician civil liability).

Corneal

- R/O corneal perforation by exam
- Perform Seidel test (moisten fluorescein strip with Alcaine and paint over cornea under cobalt blue light; if see leakage of aqueous diluting the fluorescence then Seidel positive indicating globe rupture, if no leakage then Seidel negative)
- Remove foreign body with needle; but if object is deep, nonpenetrating, unexposed, noncentral and an inert material then observe
- Topical antibiotics
- Patch or bandage contact lens if needed (never patch contact lens wearers, increased risk for bacterial keratitis)

Intraorbital

- Minimize further damage by avoiding pressure or movement of the foreign body
- Refer to ophthalmology
- If small inert object and absence of ocular or optic nerve injury → prophylactic systemic antibiotics
- Prophylactic tetanus booster if needed
- Surgically remove foreign object (by oculoplastic surgeon) if:
  - Fistula formation
  - Evidence of infection
  - Optic nerve involvement
  - Intolerable or large foreign body
  - Easily removable foreign body

PUPIL ABNORMALITIES

DEFINITION

Anisocoria: condition in which the pupils differ in size by >2 mm

APPLIED SCIENTIFIC CONCEPTS

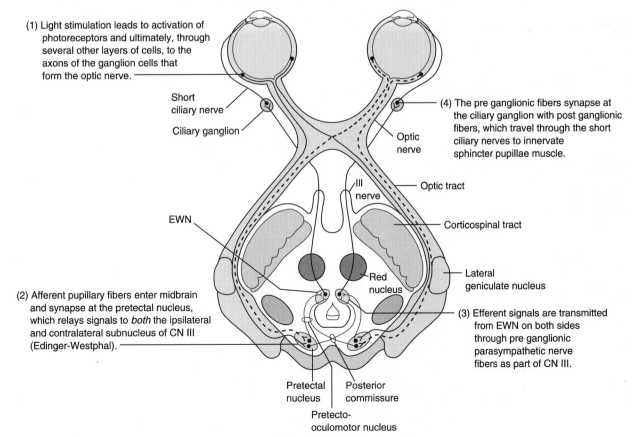

(1) Light stimulation leads to activation of photoreceptors and ultimately, through several other layers of cells, to the axons of the ganglion cells that form the optic nerve.

Short ciliary nerve

Ciliary ganglion

(4) The pre ganglionic fibers synapse at the ciliary ganglion with post ganglionic fibers, which travel through the short ciliary nerves to innervate sphincter pupillae muscle.

Optic nerve

III nerve

Optic tract

EWN

Corticospinal tract

Red nucleus

Lateral geniculate nucleus

(2) Afferent pupillary fibers enter midbrain and synapse at the pretectal nucleus, which relays signals to *both* the ipsilateral and contralateral subnucleus of CN III (Edinger-Westphal).

(3) Efferent signals are transmitted from EWN on both sides through pre ganglionic parasympathetic nerve fibers as part of CN III.

Pretectal nucleus

Posterior commissure

Pretecto-oculomotor nucleus

Figure 16.4 Mechanism of pupillary constriction—afferent signals received in one eye cause efferent pupillary constriction in both eyes (direct and consensual responses).

Table **16.10** **12 CN Function and Assessment**

Sensory Fibers		Motor Fibers
Smell	I—olfactory Test smell using familiar nonirritating stimulants	
Vision Afferent limb of pupillary light reflex	II —optic Visual acuity—Snellen chart Visual fields by confrontation Pupillary light reflex Fundoscopy	
	III—oculomotor (III, IV, VI tested together) (see III) Inspect for ptosis, pupil size and shape, eye position and alignment, primary position nystagmus Ocular movements (smooth pursuit), nystagmus, saccadic eye movements Accommodation reflex Pupillary light reflex Swinging flashlight test—relative afferent pupillary defect	EOMs (SR, IR, MR, IO) Eye opening—levator palpebrae muscle Efferent limb reflex— sphincter pupillae muscle Accommodation reflex—ciliary muscle
	IV—trochlear (see III)	SO muscle
Sensation in the face, scalp, sinuses, nasal, and oropharyngeal cavities (V1, V2, V3) Afferent limb of corneal (V1) and jaw jerk (V2) reflex	V —trigeminal Inspect for temporal wasting and jaw opening deviation to the affected side Test of light touch, pain, and temperature sensation in the V1, V2, V3 distributions Corneal reflex Test muscles of mastication—palpate temporalis and masseter during teeth clench, resist jaw opening by upward pressure, resist lateral jaw movement Jaw jerk reflex	Muscle of mastication
	VI—abducens (III)	LR muscle
Taste from anterior 2/3 tongue Sensation from pinna and external auditory canal	VII—facial Inspect for facial asymmetry, flattened nasolabial fold, widened palpebral fissure, drooping mouth, involuntary facial movement Test muscles of facial expression—resistance against raising eyebrows, eye opening, showing teeth, puffing cheeks, showing bottom teeth Corneal reflex Taste in anterior 2/3 tongue	Efferent limb of corneal reflex Secretion of all glands in head except parotid Muscle of facial expression
Hearing— cochlea Balance— semicircular canals	VIII—vestibulocochlear Hearing—whisper test for auditory acuity, Rinne test for bone and air conduction, weber test for sound lateralization Vestibular function—observe for gaze nystagmus	
Taste from posterior 1/3 tongue Sensation of inner surface of tympanic membrane and upper pharynx	IX—glossopharyngeal (IX and X tested together) Palatal elevation and symmetry—uvula deviates to normal side Gag reflex—can be normal to have absent reflex Swallowing Phonation Taste at posterior 1/3 tongue	Swallowing and phonation —pharyngeal muscles Secretion of parotid gland
Sensation from posterior meninges, lower pharynx, larynx, thoracic and abdominal viscera	X —vagus (see IX)	Swallowing and phonation —pharyngeal and laryngeal muscles Secretion of thoracic and abdominal viscera
	XI —accessory Inspect for atrophy, asymmetry, and fasciculations in neck and shoulder Test sternocleidomastoid—patient turns head to side with and without resistance Test trapezius—patient shrugs shoulders with and without resistance	Sternocleidomastoid muscle Upper fibers of trapezius muscle
	XII —hypoglossal Inspect for atrophy, asymmetry, fasciculations in tongue Deviation to affected side Test muscles of tongue—lateral movement against resistance	Muscle of tongue

RAPD

DIFFERENTIAL DIAGNOSIS FOR RAPD

- All asymmetric optic nerve lesions: glaucoma, arteritic (GCA) and nonarteritic ischemic optic neuropathies, infiltrative, inflammatory or compressive lesions, radiation neuropathy, demyelination, and so on.
- Optic tract lesion
- Large retinal detachment, ischemic CRVO

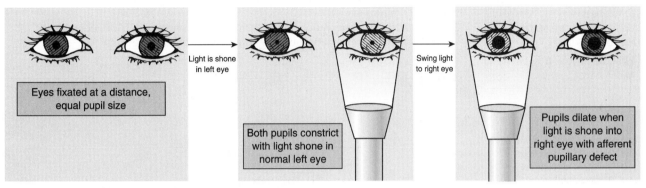

Figure 16.5 RAPD in right eye using a swinging flashlight test.

OTHER PUPILLARY ABNORMALITIES: LIGHT-NEAR DISSOCIATION

Pupils do not constrict to light but constrict as part of triad (of convergence, accommodation, and constriction) to near stimulus. As shown in Figure 16.4, the EWN sends out parasympathetic fibers that travel along CN III and synapse at the ciliary ganglion. There are two subtypes of efferent parasympathetic fibers: (a) pupillomotor fibers (~3%) that enter the dorsal EWN and ultimately innervate the iris sphincter and (b) accommodative fibers (~97%) that enter the ventral EWN and innervate the ciliary muscle. Both enter the eye through the short posterior ciliary nerves.

DIFFERENTIAL FOR LIGHT-NEAR DISSOCIATION

Argyll Robertson Pupils (Neurosyphillis)
- Small irregular pupils
- Affects pretectal light fibers that enter dorsal side of EWN, sparing fibers for near response (accommodation) that enter EWN more ventrally; therefore pupils do not constrict to light but they do constrict when fixating at near stimulus = light-near dissociation.
- Investigations: VDRL, FTA-ABS, CSF analysis

Dorsal Midbrain Syndrome (Also Known as Parinaud Syndrome)
- Lesion affects fibers that enter dorsal side of EWN, sparing more ventral fibers responsible for near response.
- Etiology depends on age (infancy—congenital aqueductal stenosis; 10 to 20s—pinealoma; 20s—trauma; 30s—brainstem AVM; 40s—MS; 50+—basilar artery infarct).
- Includes other ocular findings such as upgaze palsy, lid retraction, and convergence retraction nystagmus.

TONIC PUPILS

- Lesion of ciliary ganglion or short ciliary nerve affecting axons destined for ciliary muscle but aberrantly generated to iris sphincter.

- Three categories:
  1. Local: sarcoidosis, herpes zoster, orbital tumor, trauma or surgery
  2. Neuropathic (diabetes, alcoholism, Guillain-Barré, familial dysautonomia)
  3. Adie tonic pupils
     - Young (20 to 50s), female (70%)
     - Unilateral in 80% of cases, but becomes bilateral at 4%/yr
     - Pupil dilated initially and becomes smaller with time
     - Lesion in ciliary ganglion or short ciliary nerves
     - Poor response to light stimulus with sectoral ("vermiform") palsy of iris, slow and tonic redilation after constriction to near stimulus, paresis of accommodation (may need bifocals)
     - Cholinergic denervation supersensitivity (respond to 0.125% pilocarpine)
     - Usually asymptomatic, but may complain of difficulty reading

Horner Syndrome

Acute Horner syndrome needs to be worked up ASAP to R/O life-threatening causes! (chronic Horner is less urgent.)

PAM triad: **P**tosis, **A**nhydrosis, **M**iosis

APPROACH

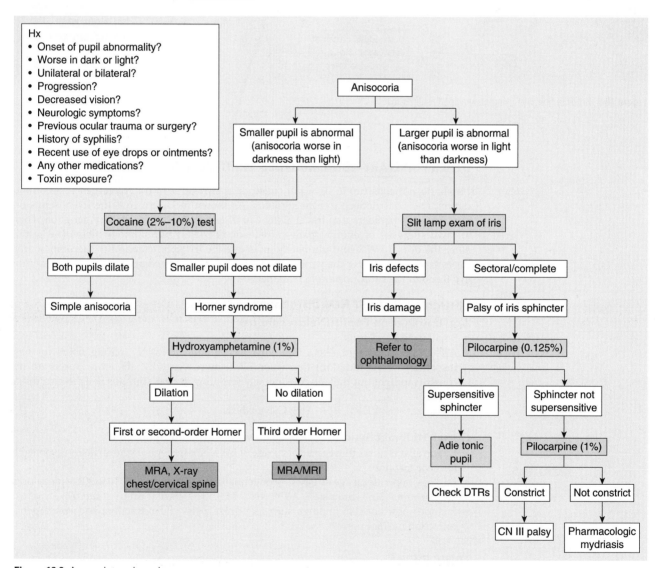

Figure 16.6 Approach to anisocoria.

Table **16.11** Neurologic Causes of Abnormal Pupil			
	Causal Condition	**Main Signs and Symptoms**	**Notes**
Impaired pupil dilatation— **more anisocoria in dark**	Horner syndrome • Loss of sympathetic innervation • Central (first order), pre- (second order), or post- (third order) ganglionic lesion	• Ptosis, anhydrosis, miosis • Poor dilatation of affected pupil, greater impairment in dim light	• Many causes depending on location of lesion • First order: tumor, vascular, MS, trauma (MRI) • Second order: pancoast tumor, bony metastases, cervical fracture (X-ray of chest and cervical spine) • Third order: R/O carotid dissection, cavernous sinus lesion, neck compression, basal skull fracture (MRA, MRI)

Impaired pupil constriction— **more anisocoria in light**	CN III palsy	• Ptosis, impaired EOMs, diplopia
		• Differential diagnosis for CN III includes:
		  • Ischemic (typically pupil-sparing) common secondary to DM, HTN, etc.
		  • Orbit apex pathology
		  • Cavernous sinus tumor, hemorrhage, mass
		  • Subarachnoid space: PCA aneurysm or less common basilar artery aneurysm
		  • Tentorial edge: supratentorial space-occupying lesion causing downward displacement and herniation of uncus with compression of third nerve; dilated fixed pupil (**Hutchinson pupil**) may be first sign
		  • Fascicular or nuclear (midbrain lesion)
		• See Table 16.4
			• Pupil is unreactive to weak cholinergic agents, but constricts to regular-strength miotic drops

STRABISMUS AND/OR AMBLYOPIA

DEFINITION

AMBLYOPIA

- Decreased vision in an anatomically normal eye due to abnormal binocular interaction or form deprivation
- Causes include media opacities (usually U/L), refractive error (U/L [unilateral, lower] or B/L [bilateral, lower]), or misalignment of eyes (usually U/L, causing suppression of one retinal image).
- Earlier Rx correlates with better visual outcomes, therefore patching or refractive correction best when administered at earliest age possible.

STRABISMUS

- Misalignment of eyes
- Often due to disorders of EOMs
- May be congenital or acquired, horizontal or vertical, comitant (deviation same in all directions) or incomitant (deviation varies in different directions)
- Strabismus can lead to amblyopia, and vice versa

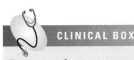

CLINICAL BOX

Beware of Pseudostrabismus!

Apparent ocular misalignment due to shape of eyelids or epicanthal folds

Table 16.12 Descriptions of Ocular Misalignment

Phoria

- Eyes aligned under normal binocular vision

Affected eye

- Become misaligned when binocular fusion is broken

Covered eye; in absence of binocular vision, eye deviates

Horizontal deviation

Esotropia
Affected eye inward

Vertical deviation

Hypertropia
Affected eye upward

Tropia

- Eyes constantly deviated due to ocular misalignment
- Uncorrected by fusion mechanism (i.e., binocular vision)

Affected eye is misaligned even in binocular vision

Exotropia
Affected eye outward

Hypotropia
Affected eye downward

APPROACH

Divergence insufficiency:

- Esodeviation, in adults, is greater at distance than near.
- Can be primary or secondary to head trauma or pontine tumors; clinical exam usually distinguishes whether divergence insufficiency is primary or secondary.
- Do a CT scan of the head or MRI to R/O an intracranial mass lesion.

CLINICAL BOX

Amblyopia

Even in severe cases, amblyopia is rarely associated with a significant RAPD.

Rx

- Always correct for any refractive errors.
- For patients with strabismus and amblyopia, a trial of patching is usually attempted to correct amblyopia; the earlier the Rx, the better the visual prognosis.
- Muscle surgery is usually performed after prolonged patching and the clinician feels that maximum visual recovery has been achieved.

Table **16.13** Causal Conditions of Strabismus and/or Amblyopia

Horizontal Strabismus

Esotropia most common				Exotropia intermittent (2 y.o.) or constant		
Congenital	Accommodative	Nonaccommodative	Incomitant	Congenital	Acquired	Convergence insufficiency
• Presents by 6 mo • FHx • Early surgery	• High refractive error or increased amount of convergence for each unit of accommodation	• Sensory deprivation • Divergence insufficiency • Postsurgical	• Sixth nerve palsy • MR restriction (thyroid, orbital fracture)	Rare	Children ≥5 y.o.	• Female preference • Rare <10 y.o. • Rx: orthoptic exercises, bilateral MR resection (if severe)

Vertical Strabismus

- Typically incomitant
- Usually due to abnormal overactions or underactions of the SO and IO muscles, paresis or contracture of one or more of these muscles (including superior and inferior recti) or mechanical restriction in vertical movement
- Differential diagnosis:
  - Overaction of SO
  - Overaction of IO
  - SO muscle palsy (U/L or B/L)
  - Brown syndrome: restriction of elevation in adduction due to local trauma in trochlear area or systemic inflammatory conditions (congenital or acquired)
  - IO muscle palsy—rare
  - CN III palsy
  - Orbital floor fractures
  - Congenital fibrosis syndrome
  - Thyroid ophthalmopathy
    - Myasthenia gravis

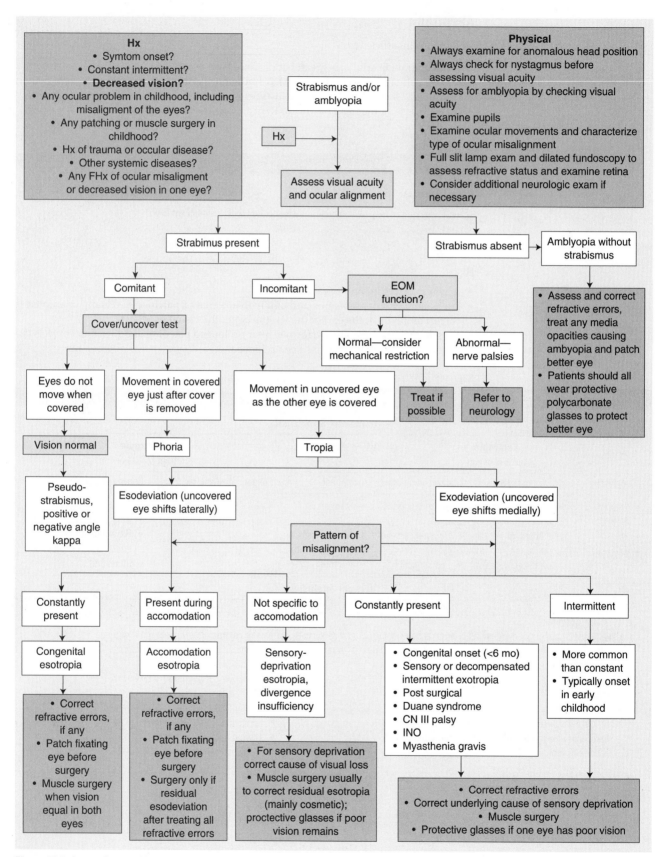

Figure 16.7 Approach to strabismus and amblyopia.

Table **16.14**	Tests for Strabismus		
Test	**Purpose**	**Procedure**	**Interpretation**
Monocular cover-uncover test	To detect presence of tropia and to differentiate a phoria from a tropia	• Cover one eye and watch for any movement in uncovered eye • Then remove cover and watch for any movement of initially covered eye	• Movement of uncovered eye indicates the presence of a tropia • Movement of the eye as it is uncovered indicates a phoria that becomes manifest when binocular fusion is interrupted
Alternate cover test	To detect presence of phoria and tropia; does not differentiate between phoria and tropia	• Same as cover/uncover test except that cover is alternated from one eye to the other • One eye is covered for a few seconds and then cover is quickly moved to the other eye, back and forth between the two eyes • Movement of uncovered eye is observed between alternations	• Uncovered eye moving to target signals the presence of ocular misalignment (which may be a phoria or a tropia)
Hirschberg test	To assess if eyes are aligned	• Shine penlight from a distance to point equidistant between the two eyes • See if light refracted from cornea is symmetrically situated with respect to eyes	Corneal reflex within pupils / Corneal reflex / Corneal reflex Asymmetry of light reflex indicates a positive test and presence of ocular misalignment

VISUAL DISTURBANCES/LOSS

Visual Disturbances

Acute vision loss, especially if associated with RAPD, indicates a serious problem and requires urgent referral to ophthalmology!

CLINICAL BOX

Common Causes of Chronic Visual Loss

The big 4: **C**ataract, **D**iabetic **R**etinopathy, chronic **G**laucoma, **M**acular **D**egeneration. (Call **DR**. G**rumpy M.D.**)

FEATURES ASSOCIATED WITH DECREASED VISION

• Duration of visual loss: transient <24 h, persistent >24 h
• Rapidity of onset: acute (minutes to days), chronic (weeks to months)
• Presence of pain
• Distribution: unilateral or bilateral

    Occasionally, monocular visual loss due to a chronic etiology remains undetected until the unaffected eye is covered.
    See Figure 16.8.
    See Tables 16.15 and 16.16.

CLINICAL BOX

Clinical Correlates of Visual Defects

Bitemporal hemianopsia: **P**ituitary adenoma, suprasellar **M**eningioma, **C**raniopharyngioma, and **A**neurysm of internal carotid artery are four most common lesions affecting optic chiasm (**CAMP**).

APPROACH

Table **16.15**	Common Causes of Acute Visual Disturbance
Diagnosis	**Common Signs**
AACG[a]	Microcystic edema, mid-dilated pupil, high IOP, shallow chamber
Total hyphema	Entire anterior chamber filled with blood
Subluxed lens	Lens subluxed into anterior or posterior chamber
Retinal detachment[a]	May be precipitated by new onset floaters and flashes of light (lasting seconds and more obvious in darkness) Undulating retina detached from RPE, may see retinal tear Ocular emerg: if decreased central vision <24 h or field defect progressing
Acute macular lesion	Drusen + hemorrhage for AMD, hemorrhage if macroaneurysm
Anterior ischemic optic neuropathy[a]	Disc swelling with hemorrhage +/− RAPD Note: if suspect arteritic ischemic optic neuropathy then Ocular emerg: do stat ESR, CRP and platelets and refer to ophthalmology
Migraine	Flashing lights (lasting minutes to hours), decreased vision that returns
TIA	Decreased vision "like curtain" coming over eye, lasting <24 h
Occipital infarct/hemorrhage	Field defect respecting vertical midline
Vitreous hemorrhage	Complete or partial vision loss, hemorrhage evident on fundoscopy (see in hemorrhagic vitreous detachments, severe AMD, macroaneurysms and in diabetics with proliferative retinopathy)
CRVO	Blood and thunder fundus (extensive hemorrhage and cotton wool spots)
CRAO	Cherry red spot because edematous retina but underlying choroid is seen through the macula where there is less retinal tissue
Blunt trauma	Corneal abrasion or laceration, hyphema, globe rupture, lens dislocation, vitreous hemorrhage, choroidal rupture, traumatic optic neuropathy
Penetrating trauma	Globe perforation, intraocular foreign body, optic nerve injury
Other	Corneal ulcer, chemical splash, increased IOP, endophthalmitis[a] (ocular emerg if Hx of recent surgery)

[a]Ocular emerg

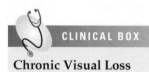

CLINICAL BOX

Chronic Visual Loss

Chronic visual loss is usually painless! In elderly, chronic visual loss may be binocular but asymmetrical. If normal physical exam including visual fields, color vision and pupils, consider long-standing childhood amblyopia, particularly if patient has anisometropia.

Table **16.16**	Some Conditions Causing Chronic Visual Disturbance	
Anterior segment	Corneal	Dystrophy, scarring, edema
	Lens	**Cataract:** age-related, trauma, steroid-induced
	Glaucoma	**Primary or secondary glaucoma**
Retinal	Diabetes	**Diabetic retinopathy,** macular edema
	Tumor	Melanoma (may have melanoma of iris, ciliary body, and/or choroid), hemangioma
	Macular	**AMD**, dystrophy
Optic nerve	Optic chiasm	Pituitary adenoma
	Optic nerve	Compressive optic neuropathy: intracranial masses, thyroid disease
	Toxic/ nutritional	Nutritional deficiencies (B_1, B_6 and B_{12}, folate), tobacco-alcohol amblyopia, methanol, amiodarone, chloroquine, hydroxychloroquine, digitalis
	Hereditary	Leber optic neuropathy, dominant optic atrophy, recessive optic atrophy

* Most common in bold.

Visual Acuity and Field Testing

Always conduct testing with best corrected vision (e.g., with corrective glasses).

Test both distance vision (Snellen chart) and near vision (pocket vision chart).

If Snellen chart cannot be read at 3 ft, test ability of patient to (in the following order): count fingers, see hand motion, or perceive light perception. Record farthest distance the task can be completed.

Test visual field by confrontation; the exact areas of defect may give clue to site of lesion.

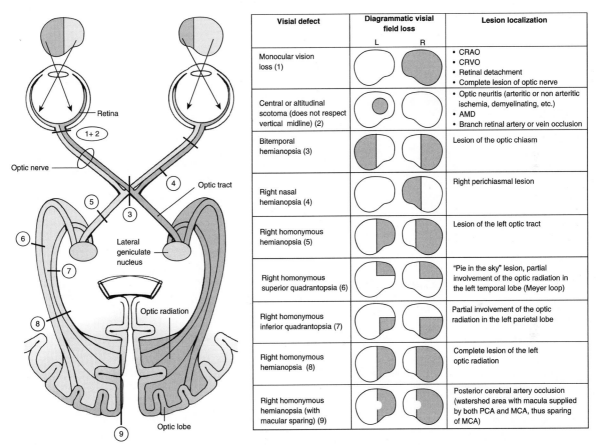

Visial defect	Diagrammatic visial field loss		Lesion localization
	L	R	
Monocular vision loss (1)			• CRAO • CRVO • Retinal detachment • Complete lesion of optic nerve
Central or altitudinal scotoma (does not respect vertical midline) (2)			• Optic neuritis (arteritic or non arteritic ischemia, demyelinating, etc.) • AMD • Branch retinal artery or vein occlusion
Bitemporal hemianopsia (3)			Lesion of the optic chiasm
Right nasal hemianopsia (4)			Right perichiasmal lesion
Right homonymous hemianopsia (5)			Lesion of the left optic tract
Right homonymous superior quadrantopsia (6)			"Pie in the sky" lesion, partial involvement of the optic radiation in the left temporal lobe (Meyer loop)
Right homonymous inferior quadrantopsia (7)			Partial involvement of the optic radiation in the left parietal lobe
Right homonymous hemianopsia (8)			Complete lesion of the left optic radiation
Right homonymous hemianopsia (with macular sparing) (9)			Posterior cerebral artery occlusion (watershed area with macula supplied by both PCA and MCA, thus sparing of MCA)

Figure 16.8 Normal visual pathway (A to G) and visual defects associated with lesions along the visual pathway: **A:** Light from nasal visual field simulate photoreceptors of temporal retina, and vice versa. **B:** Photoreceptors synapse with and transmit signals to bipolar cells, then to retinal ganglion cells. Ganglion cell axons converge into optic nerve. **Each optic nerve carries signals from one eye. C:** The two optic nerves join into optic chiasm. **D:** Fibers from nasal halves of retina decussate, and join temporal fibers from contralateral eye to form optic tracts. **The left and right optic tracts carry signals from left and right halves of the visual field, respectively. E:** Each optic tract synapses with lateral geniculate body on the same side (some fibers that are involved in light reflex go to pretectal nucleus [**see Figure 16.6**]). **F:** From lateral geniculate bodies, signals are transmitted through the geniculocalcarine tract. **Fibers that carry signals from upper visual fields fan out and go to the Meyer loop and lateral part of the geniculocalcarine tract. G:** Signals go to occipital (calcarine) cortex, specialized for sense of vision, on the same side of hemisphere as geniculate bodies.

Table **16.17**	**Fluorescein Angiography Indications**
Dm	• Distinguish between nonischemic vs. ischemic diabetic maculopathy • Detect and localize macular edema for laser Rx
Renal vein occlusion	• Assess capillary bed in fovea, extension of capillary nonperfusion, and degree of macular edema due to venous occlusion • Distinguish collateral vessels from neovascularization
AMD	• Assess the type of subretinal neovascularization and possibility for laser Rx
Other (depending on condition or suspicion)	• Identify subretinal neovascular membrane • Detect abnormal blood vessels • Detect breakdown of RPE tight junction • Support diagnosis of certain retinal conditions

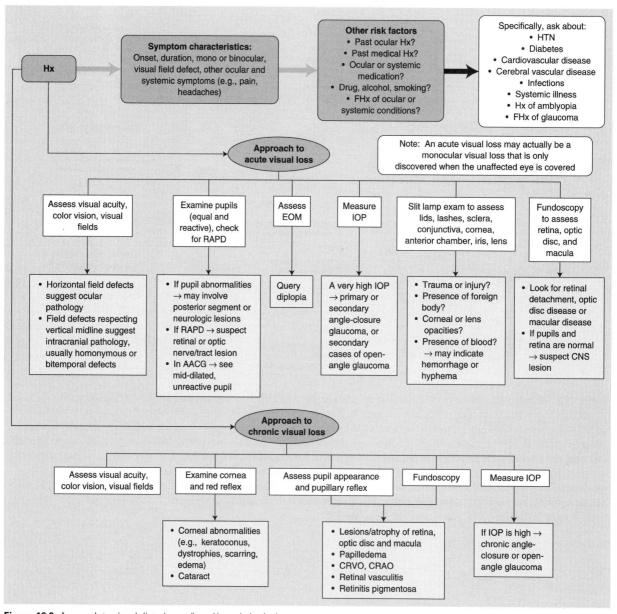

Figure 16.9 Approach to visual disturbance/loss: Hx and physical.

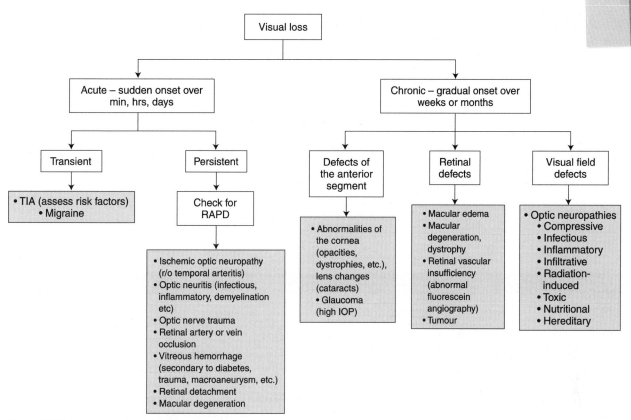

Figure 16.10 Approach to visual disturbance/loss.

INVESTIGATIONS

FLUORESCEIN ANGIOGRAPHY

- To study blood flow in retina and choroid
- Sodium fluorescein: orange-red colour with a peak absorption of 465 to 490 nm and an emission peak of 520 to 530 nm
- In the intravascular space: ~70% to 80% of sodium fluorescein bound to plasma proteins
- IVFA: injecting a bolus of fluorescein dye into a peripheral vein (typically antecubital vein); dye first enters the choroidal circulation then the retinal circulation
- Fundus photos of the circulation of the fluorescein through the choroid and retinal vasculature are taken by illuminating the fundus with a blue light (peak absorption of fluorescein), thereby exciting sodium fluorescein molecules to a higher energy state. These molecules then return to their resting state and release a longer wavelength of yellow-green light. The photographic film detects only the yellow-green light.
- Retinal blood endothelium normally impermeable to dye due to tight junctions
- Any leakage from retinal vessels is abnormal (See Table 16.17 and Figure 16.9)

CHAPTER 17

Orthopedics and Rheumatology

Niloofar Dehghan, Dr. Stephen Kingwell, Dr. Robert J. Feibel,
Michelle L. Catton, Dr. Stephane Michel Gauthier,
and Dr. C. Douglas Smith

FRACTURES

DEFINITION

- **Dislocation**—complete loss of contact between the articular surfaces of a joint.
- **Subluxation**—incomplete dislocation, results in a nonconcentric joint surface.
- **Reduction**—a maneuver whereby a fracture or dislocation is returned to anatomic alignment.
- **Nonunion**—failure of the bony edges to unite (hypertrophic, atrophic).
- **Malunion**—healing of the bony fragments in a faulty position → causing an imperfect alignment, deformity, or rotation.

APPLIED SCIENTIFIC CONCEPTS

FRACTURES HEAL IN FIVE OVERLAPPING STAGES

1. Hematoma—fracture and soft tissue bleeding.
2. Inflammatory—hematopoietic cells secrete growth factors; fibroblasts, mesenchymal cells, osteoprogenitor cells at fracture site.
3. Callus—osteoblasts and osteoclasts appear. Bridging (soft) callus forms within weeks, is later replaced by woven bone (hard callus).
4. Consolidation—woven bone replaced by stronger lamellar bone, fracture is solidly united, can carry normal loads.
5. Remodeling—thicker lamellar bone where the stress is higher (Wolff's law), may take months to years.

RATE OF FRACTURE HEALING DEPENDS ON

- **Biological factors:** Blood supply, age, comorbidities, nutritional status, neurovascular function, hormones, growth factors, cigarette smoke, local pathologic conditions, type of bone affected, extent of bone loss.
- **Mechanical factors:** Soft tissue attachments, stability, anatomic location, level of energy imparted, extent of bone loss.

COMPLICATIONS

- **Local:** Hemorrhage, neurologic compromise, infection, compartment syndrome, malunion, nonunion, post-traumatic arthritis, osteonecrosis, osteomyelitis, heterotopic ossification
- **Systemic:** DVT, PE, fat embolism syndrome, ARDS

CAUSAL CONDITIONS

TYPES OF FRACTURES

- Closed fracture: overlying skin is intact.

- Open fracture: skin is punctured, susceptible to infection.
  1. <1 cm: Low risk of infection (cefazolin/ancef)
  2. 1–10 cm: No flap/skin graft needed, moderate risk of infection (Ancef + aminoglycoside)
  3. >10 cm, extensive muscle/bone/soft tissue injury: High risk of infection (Ancef + aminoglycoside + anaerobic coverage) (a) no flap needed, (b) needs muscle flap, and (c) needs revascularization, risk of amputation.
- Stress fracture: microfractures that coalesce, due to repetitive stresses. Common in tibia, fibula, metatarsals, especially in athletes.
- Pathological fracture: in weakened bone under normal stress.

FRACTURE PATTERNS

- Transverse—perpendicular line produced by bending, direct force.
- Compression—crush injury, cancellous architecture of bone collapses. Usually in the elderly (especially vertebral bodies, calcaneus).
- Avulsion—detachment of bony fragment from where tendon/ligament attaches to bone.
- Greenstick—fracture on one side and a plastic deformation on the other side of the bone, not a complete break. Occurs in children only.
- Intra-articular—epiphyseal fracture that extends through the joint line. Use Salter-Harris classification for pediatric considerations.

DISPLACEMENT

- Describes how fracture fragments have moved from their original location (distal fragment as reference). Usually described in terms of apposition (medial, lateral, shortened, lengthened), angulation (with respect to its apex), and rotation.

CLINICAL BOX

Causes of Pathologic Fractures

- **Generalized bone disease:** Paget, metabolic bone disease (osteoporosis, hyperparathyroidism, osteomalacia), EtOH, poor diet
- **Local disease:** Bone cyst, chronic infection
- **Malignancy:** Metastasis, sarcoma, multiple myeloma

APPROACH

HISTORY

- One time traumatic event or repetitive strain
- Pain, neurologic symptoms: weakness, numbness, tingling
- Other medical conditions: cancers, osteoporosis, Paget disease
- Use of EtOH or steroids

CLINICAL BOX

Fractures: Causal Conditions

- Normal bone + abnormal force = **traumatic fracture**
- Abnormal bone + normal force = **pathologic fracture**
- Normal bone + repetitive force = **stress fracture**

CLINICAL BOX

Describing a Fracture

- Location
- Fracture pattern (can be more than 1)
- Open versus closed
- Displacement
- Angulation

CLINICAL BOX

Malignancies that Metastasize to Bone

- Breast, lung, prostate, kidney, thyroid

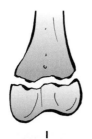 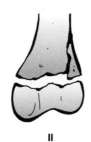 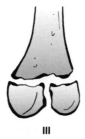 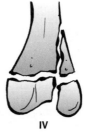 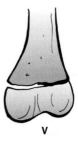

I = Physis
II = **M**etaphysis
III = **E**piphysis
IV = **ME** (Metaphysis + Epiphysis) **M+E = ME**
V = Crush

Figure 17.1 Slater-Harris classification.

PHYSICAL EXAM

- Evaluate the fracture and entire area from at least one joint above and one joint below the injury, repeat following fracture reduction
- Inspection: integrity of soft tissue (open vs. closed fracture), deformity, swelling, bruising, cyanosis, pallor
- Palpate the compartments assessing for compartment syndrome
- ROM: active and passive in joints distal to the injury
- Neurologic complications: motor and sensory integrity proximal and distal to the fracture site. Evaluate each nerve individually.
- Vascular complications: presence and strength of pulses distal to the fracture site. Check for capillary refill and skin temperature.

Compartment Syndrome

- First symptom—pain out of proportion to the injury
- First signs—loss of muscle function, and later pain with passive stretch
- Pulselessness, paresthesia, pallor, paralysis, pain are **late** signs and apply to vascular injury
- Use intracompartmental pressure readings for obtunded patients
- Treatment: early recognition and fasciotomy

CLINICAL BOX

X-ray

- Minimum two views
- Joints above + below
- Before + after reduction

CLINICAL BOX

Investigations for Pathologic Fractures

- Serum Ca^{2+} phosphate, alkaline phosphate, PTH, TSH, T3/T4
- Serum protein electrophoresis
- Bone density
- Bone scan
- Bone biopsy

INVESTIGATIONS

- X-ray—mandatory for suspected fractures.
- CT—intra-articular fractures, life-threatening soft tissue injury
- MRI—occult fractures, injury within the bone (swelling or bruising)
- Bone scan—suspected pathologic fracture

CLINICAL BOX

Principles of Fracture Treatment

- Obtain reduction
- Maintain reduction
- Early mobilization
- Pain management

CLINICAL BOX

Complications of Casting

- Compartment syndrome
- Soft tissue/skin injury
- Pressure sores
- Chaffing/pruritus
- Swelling
- Muscle atrophy

TREATMENT

Traumatic Fractures

- Observation and follow-up—certain fracture locations do not need reduction/splinting (rib fractures, isolated mid-shaft fibula).
- Closed reduction:
  - In a simple closed fracture, where good reduction and union of the bone fragments can be achieved.
  - Reduction, immobilization (tape, sling, splint, cast, external fixation), follow-up (assess healing, complications).
- Open reduction
- Internal fixation via IM nail or plate and screws

Stress Fractures

- Avoidance of the painful activity, immobilization if pain at rest
- Surgical treatment in rare cases of nonunion, fracture propagation, long-term disability

Pathologic Fractures

- Usually reduction, immobilization (depends on underlying disease)
- Internal fixation in generalized bone disease and metastatic lesions

Salter-Harris Fractures

- Salter-Harris I, II—closed reduction + cast (heals well)
- Salter-Harris III, IV—ORIF (may develop growth deformities)
- Salter-Harris V—no specific treatment (high risk of growth arrest)

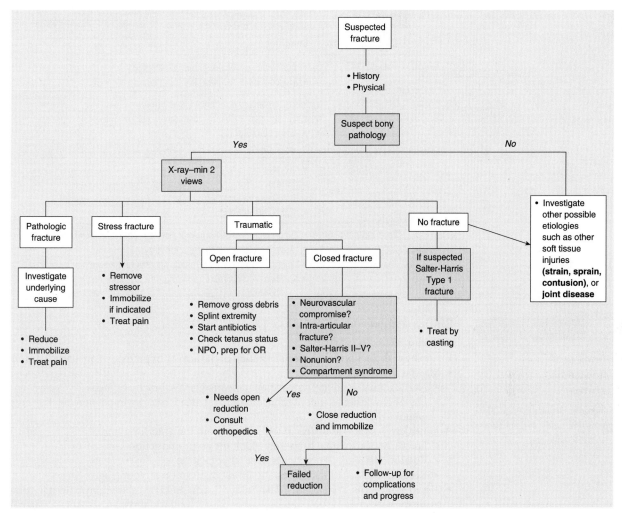

Figure 17.2 Approach to suspected fracture.

PAIN: SHOULDER

DEFINITION

- The shoulder girdle is composed of three bones (clavicle, scapula, proximal humerus), and four articulations: SC, AC, GH, scapulothoracic.
- The GH joint is the main articulation, referred to as the **shoulder joint**. It is an extremely mobile joint → less stable, more susceptible to injury
- The rotator cuff muscles (subscapularis, supraspinatus, infraspinatus, teres minor) attach to the head of humerus and stabilize the GH joint
- All the nerves of the upper limbs arise from the brachial plexus. Injury to the plexus or the peripheral nerves can present as shoulder pain

CAUSAL CONDITIONS

CLINICAL BOX

Referred Pain

- Referred pain (less common): poorly localized, full ROM without pain.

CLINICAL BOX

Intrinsic Shoulder Pathology

- Pain caused by specific movement, weakness, stiffness, instability

Table **17.1**	**Shoulder Pain: Causal Conditions**
Cause of Pain	**Conditions**
Trauma	• Fractures—clavicle, humerus, scapula • Dislocation—AC joint, GH joint
GH	• Frozen shoulder (adhesive capsulitis) • GH arthritis—OA, RA, crystalline • GH instability • SLAP lesion
Periarticular	• AC arthritis • Rotator cuff injury—impingement, tendinopathy, tear • Biceps tendinopathy/rupture • Subacromial bursitis
Referred pain	• Neurologic—disk herniation/stenosis, brachial plexus injury • Abdo—splenic injury, hepatobiliary • Thoracic—apical lung tumor, upper lobe pneumonia • Cardiac—Myocardial ischemia (left shoulder only)

CLINICAL BOX

Patients with Dislocations or Fractures

Patients with dislocations or fractures will rarely attempt to re-enact the maneuver.

GH DISLOCATION

Anterior 85%

- Etiology: abduction and external rotation of the arm or hyperextension, usually traumatic
- May be associated with:
  - Nerve injury—axillary, musculocutaneous nerves; brachial plexus
  - Hill-Sachs lesion—indentation of humeral head due to impaction on the anterior glenoid rim
  - Bankart lesion—avulsion of the labrum from the anterior glenoid
  - Fractures of proximal humerus—look for on prereduction x-ray
  - Rotator cuff tears—in patients over 50 yr (>50%)
  - Recurrent dislocations—specially if first dislocation at young age
- Signs/symptoms: "squared off shoulder," arm held in abduction/internal rotation, humeral head may be palpable. ± Nerve injury: axillary nerve → weakness, paresthesia of lateral deltoid. Musculocutaneous nerve → weak biceps, lateral forearm paresthesia.
- Treatment:
  - Sedation, muscle relaxant, longitudinal traction. Repeat x-ray and neurovascular exam postreduction.
  - Sling for 3 wk, rehab to strengthen external rotators and abductors.
  - Older patients require shorter immobilization time to prevent stiffness.
  - Surgery considered for recurrent instability.

Posterior 15%

- Etiology: high-energy force when arm in adduction and internal rotation. May associated with Es (**E**pilepsy, **E**tOH, **E**lectrical shock, **E**ncephalitis).
- Signs/symptoms: flattening of anterior shoulder, prominent coracoid, arm held in adduction/internal rotation, limited abduction/external rotation.
- Treatment: Same as anterior dislocations; however, reduction under general anesthesia with inferior traction.

CLAVICLE FRACTURE

- Etiology: Fall on outstretched hand or shoulder. Middle-third injury more common than distal or proximal.
- Signs/symptoms: deformity, pain with ROM, ± nerve injury
- Treatment: proximal and middle fractures → sling 2–3 wk, rehab to ↑ROM and strengthening. Distal third → if unstable may need ORIF.

AC LIGAMENT SPRAIN

(AC separation)

- Tear of AC ligament, usually from direct fall on shoulder.
- Grading based on ligaments disrupted (1°–3°, common), and displacement of clavicle (4°–6°, rare).

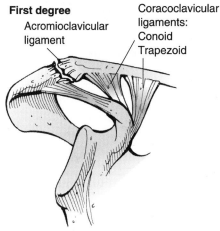
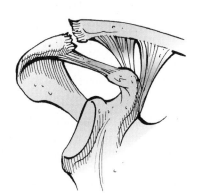
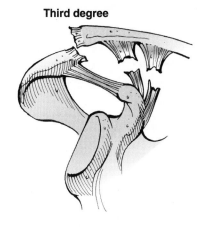

First degree
Acromioclavicular ligament

Coracoclavicular ligaments:
Conoid
Trapezoid

Second degree

Third degree

Figure 17.3 AC separation.

- Signs/symptoms: focal tenderness over AC joint, palpable step-off deformity in 2°–3°, patient may hold the arm close to chest and resist ROM.
- Treatment: 1°, 2° → sling 1 wk, then rehab to ↑ROM and strength. 3°→ controversial, 4°–6° → ORIF in young/active patient.

ROTATOR CUFF IMPINGEMENT

- Compression of the rotator cuff tendons (and the subacromial bursa) between the acromion and the humeral head → related to narrowing of supraspinatus outlet or muscular dysfunction/capsular tightness
- Signs/symptoms: shoulder pain with overhead activities, painful arc (60 degrees to 120 degrees), positive impingement tests (Neer, Hawkins), atrophy of muscles around the joint in chronic cases.
- Risk factors: acromial morphology, rotator cuff dysfunction, repetitive overhead activities
- Treatment: NSAIDs, physiotherapy, subacromial decompression

ROTATOR CUFF TENDINOPATHY

- Degeneration of rotator cuff tendons (especially supraspinatus), may lead to rotator cuff tears. Aggravated by repetitive overhead activity (abduction, external rotation)
- Signs/symptoms: pain along lateral deltoid with overhead activity (reaching, pulling), positive painful arc test, ↑ pain when sleeping on affected side
- Treatment: NSAIDs, steroid injection

ROTATOR CUFF TEAR

- Supraspinatus most common in patients over age 40 with chronic impingement or tendonitis, with/without trauma (fall on outstretched arm or directly on the shoulder, heavy pushing/pulling).
- Signs/symptoms: anterolateral pain, night pain, shoulder weakness (unable to reach overhead), popping/catching of shoulder with movement, positive drop arm test (in complete tear).
- Treatment: acutely → heat, exercise, local anesthetic injections. After 3 wk → young/active patients—surgical repair, elderly/sedentary—conservative treatment.

BICEPS TENDON INJURY

- Biceps tendinopathy: irritation of the long head of biceps from repetitive lifting/reaching overhead. Often associated with other shoulder pathology.
- Biceps rupture: rupture of long head of biceps tendon, from degenerative changes.
- Signs/symptoms: anterior pain with flexion/lifting/reaching overhead, weakness, positive Speed's tests. Biceps tears also have deformity "Popeye sign"; function is preserved since short head of biceps and coracobrachialis are main elbow flexors.
- Treatment: conservative, surgical repair only in distal biceps ruptures.

CLINICAL BOX

Posterior Shoulder Pain

Posterior shoulder pain is not very common. It is usually from rotator cuff tendinopathy or referred pain from the cervical spine.

CLINICAL BOX

Shoulder Pain—Causal Conditions and Presentations

- Rotator cuff tendinopathy/ impingement → pain with overhead activity
- Rotator cuff tear → weakness + pain
- Frozen shoulder → ↓ROM

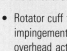

CLINICAL BOX

SLAP Lesion

SLAP lesion = tear of labrum at the point of biceps tendon attachment → labrum and biceps tendon tear.

Conditions that Can Lead to Adhesive Capsulitis

- Rotator cuff injury (most common)
- Diabetes
- Use of sling
- Stroke
- Axillary surgery

AC Osteoarthritis

Grinding/popping sensation when reaching overhead or across the chest.

Testing External Rotation and Abduction

Put hands behind neck: Tests external rotation and abduction.

Testing Internal Rotation and Adduction

Put hands behind back: Tests internal rotation and adduction.

ADHESIVE CAPSULITIS/FROZEN SHOULDER

- Reversible GH stiffness, due to pain, disability, lack of use/mobility
- Signs/symptoms: stiffness, ↓ROM (external rotation > abduction > internal rotation) unable to reach up, put on clothes, ± pain with movement/direct pressure
- Predictable stages (freezing, frozen, thawing)
- Treatment: NSAIDs, local heat, physiotherapy to ↑ROM and prevent further stiffening (not helpful in freezing phase), ± injection of local anesthetic or corticosteroids. Arthroscopic release if non-Op unsuccessful

GH OA

- OA of the GH joint is uncommon, usually caused from previous trauma (dislocation or fracture of the humeral neck/head)
- Signs/symptoms: chronic and progressively worsening stiffness and pain (especially with abduction and external rotation)
- Treatment: NSAIDs, physiotherapy to ↑ROM, steroid injections, definitive treatment is shoulder replacement

SUBCAPSULAR/SCAPULOTHORACIC BURSITIS

- Owing to pressure/friction between the scapula and adjacent second/third ribs.
- Signs/symptoms: localized pain in the back, audible pop with shoulder shrugging. Patients usually have poor muscle development and posture.
- Treatment: conservative, ± steroid injections, physiotherapy.

APPROACH

HISTORY

- Pain: location (specific or generalized), quality, specific movements that bring on the pain, acute or chronic (2 wk)
- History of trauma, weakness, paresthesia
- Other medical conditions: neurologic, cardiac, abdominal, respiratory (referred pain)
- Previous history of OA, gout, RA, rotator cuff injury, biceps tendon injury

PHYSICAL EXAM

- Examine all four articulations and associated bones, compare both sides
- Inspection: asymmetry, deformity, muscle atrophy, bruising
- Palpation: SC joint, clavicle, AC joint, acromion, subacromial space, greater/lesser tuberosities, bicipital groove, spine of scapula, cervical spine → looking for point tenderness, step deformities
- ROM: passive then active. Normal ROM—flexion 180°, ext 45°, abduction 180°, internal rotation 90°, external rotation 90°
- Special tests: shoulder instability → anterior/posterior apprehension test, sulcus test. Biceps pathology → Speed test. Rotator cuff impingement → painful arc test. Rotator cuff tear → drop arm test.

INVESTIGATIONS

- X-ray—AP, lateral, transcapular (Mercedes Benz sign), axillary
- U/S—if suspicious of joint fluid, detect rotator cuff tears
- CT—in case of a complex fracture
- MRI—rotator cuff tears, labral tears (SLAP or Bankart)
- Arthroscopy—assess extent of damage from OA, rotator cuff/labral tears

PAIN: ELBOW

DEFINITION

- Flexion/ext occurs at the ulnar–humeral joint (biceps and triceps muscles). Supination/pronation occurs at the radiohumeral and proximal radioulnar articulations (biceps, supinator and pronator teres muscles).
- The medial epicondyle is the tendinous origin of the flexor muscles, and the lateral epicondyle is the origin of extensor muscles.
- Ulnar nerve runs in cubital tunnel, median nerve runs anterior to elbow joint.

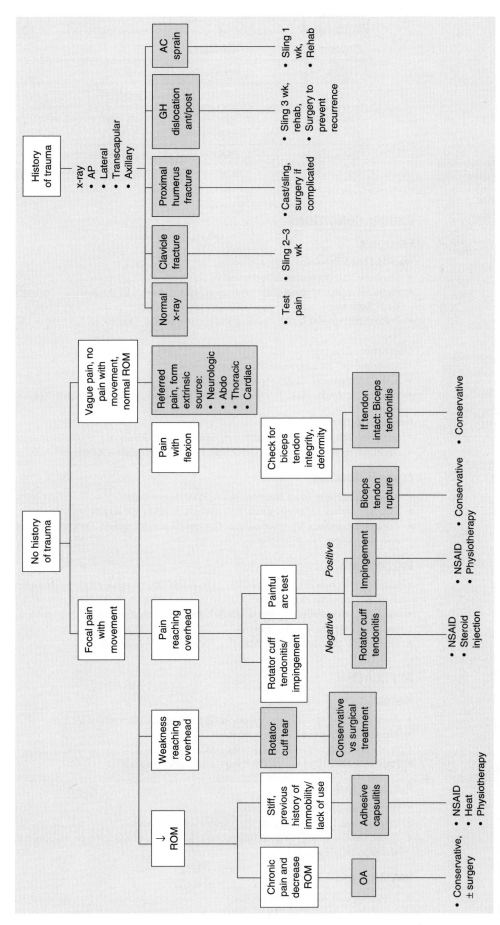

Figure 17.4 Approach to patient complaining of shoulder pain.

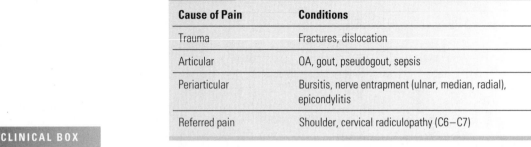

Table **17.2**	Elbow Pain: Causal Conditions
Cause of Pain	**Conditions**
Trauma	Fractures, dislocation
Articular	OA, gout, pseudogout, sepsis
Periarticular	Bursitis, nerve entrapment (ulnar, median, radial), epicondylitis
Referred pain	Shoulder, cervical radiculopathy (C6–C7)

CLINICAL BOX

Paresthesias in the Ulnar Aspect of the Hand

Any process that distends the elbow joint tends to impinge upon the ulnar nerve → causing paresthesias in the ulnar aspect of the hand.

CLINICAL BOX

Olecranon Bursitis

Olecranon bursitis can be due to sepsis, gout, trauma.

CAUSAL CONDITIONS

FRACTURES

Radial Head Fracture
- Etiology: fall on outstretched hand
- Signs/symptoms: pain with pronation/supination, ↓ROM, anterior/posterior fat pad on x-ray (sail sign)
- Treatment: undisplaced → sling 1 wk, early ROM. Displaced/↓ROM→ ORIF

Olecranon Fracture
- Etiology: fall on elbow, avulsion by triceps
- Signs/symptoms: unable to extend elbow
- Treatment: undisplaced → above elbow cast 2 wk, early ROM. Displaced → ORIF

Supracondylar Fracture
- Etiology: fall on outstretched hand, usually in children
- **Treatment:** undisplaced → reduce and cast. Displaced → ORIF

ELBOW DISLOCATION
- Etiology: usually from trauma: MVA, sporting events
- Complications: stiffness, intra-articular loose bodies, early onset OA
- Treatment: reduce by traction and flexion. Posterior splint 2 wk in 90 degrees of flexion and pronation

EPICONDYLITIS
- Lateral epicondylitis (tennis elbow): localized lateral epicondyle pain, aggravated by use of wrist/forearm extensors
- Medial epicondylitis (golfer's elbow): localized medial epicondyle pain, aggravated by use of the wrist/forearm flexors
- Treatment: physiotherapy, NSAIDs, local injections, bracing

APPROACH

HISTORY
- Pain: position, quality, radiation, severity, timing, alleviating factors
- Mechanism of injury, history of trauma
- Associated paresthesia, weakness, ↓ROM
- Previous history of elbow fractures, gout/pseudogout

PHYSICAL EXAM
- Inspection: swelling, deformities
- Palpate: joint, olecranon, medial/lateral epicondyles
- ROM: flexion/ext (0 degree full ext to 135 degrees of flexion), pronation/supination (full arc 170–180 degrees)

INVESTIGATIONS
- X-ray: Obtain at least two views

PAIN: WRIST AND HAND

DEFINITION

- Bones: eight carpals, five metacarpals, three phalanges (proximal, middle, distal) in each finger, two phalanges in the thumb.
- Joints: MP, PIP, DIP. The thumb has only an IP joint.
- Nerves:
  - Ulnar: sensory→ fifth and half of fourth digits, motor→ intrinsic hand muscles (other than two radial lumbricals and some of thenar muscles)
  - Median: sensory → palmar aspect of first three-and-a-half digits, motor → thenar muscles (specifically abductor pollicis brevis), two radial lumbricals.
  - Radial: sensory → dorsum of the hand.

Table **17.3**	Wrist and Hand Pain: Causal Conditions	
Location	**Cause of Pain**	**Conditions**
Wrist	Trauma	Fractures, dislocation
	Repetitive use	Carpal tunnel, de Quervain tenosynovitis, dorsal ganglion, radiocarpal arthritis
Hand	Trauma	Fractures, dislocations
	Repetitive use	Arthritis (OA, RA), carpal tunnel, Dupuytren contracture
	Vascular	Embolus, Raynaud, thoracic outlet

CAUSAL CONDITIONS

FRACTURES

Scaphoid Fracture

- Etiology: fall on outstretched hand.
- Signs/symptoms: pain in anatomic snuff box (over scaphoid tubercle), pain with ROM. May not see the fracture initially on x-ray.
- Complications: nonunion, AVN. Blood supply is distal to proximal → high incidence of AVN with fracture of the proximal third.
- Treatment: x-ray is negative but a high suspicion → cast, repeat x-ray in 2 wk. Undisplaced → cast for 8 wk, examine weekly to assess healing. Displaced →ORIF.

Colles Fracture

(most common wrist fracture)

- Fracture of distal radius, with a specific set of radiographic findings
- Etiology: fall on outstretched hand, at risk with osteoporosis
- Signs/symptoms: dinner fork deformity, swelling, ecchymosis, may have neurovascular deficits (carpal tunnel)
- Treatment: undisplaced → cast in neutral position 6–8 wk. Displaced → reduce, cast 6–8 wk. If unable to reduce to a good position → ORIF

CARPAL TUNNEL SYNDROME

- Etiology: Type of nerve entrapment syndrome → compression of the median nerve in the carpal tunnel.
- Signs/symptoms: Pain/paresthesia (night) in the thumb, second, third, and half of fourth digits, palmar branch of median nerve spared. Thenar atrophy, weak abductor pollicis brevis. ↓Two-point discrimination, positive Tinel's, Phalen's, and carpal compression tests.
- Treatment: NSAIDs, splinting, steroid injections. Final treatment is surgical release of transverse carpal ligament.

CLINICAL BOX

Complications of Wrist Fracture

Wrist fractures may lead to complications such as stiffness, weakness, OA.

CLINICAL BOX

Night Stick Fracture

Isolated fracture of the ulna.

CLINICAL BOX

Galeazzi Fracture

Fracture of the distal radius, as well as distal radioulnar joint injury.

CLINICAL BOX

Conditions Associated with Carpal Tunnel Syndrome

Occupation, RA, pregnancy, obesity, hypothyroidism, diabetes, ESRD

DUPUYTREN'S CONTRACTURE

- Fibrous nodules in the palmar fascia, creates contractures → flexion of fingers at the MP joint and PIP
- Etiology: genetic, repetitive use, common in white males over age 50
- Signs/symptoms: painless, stiffness, ↓ext of digits (usually fourth and fifth)
- Treatment: stretching, corticosteroid injections, if persistent surgical release of the palmar fascia

TRIGGER FINGER/FLEXOR TENOSYNOVITIS

- Irritation or inflammation of flexor tendon sheath of thumb/finger
- Etiology: repetitive use, direct pressure
- Signs/symptoms: pain, snapping, finger locking in flexion, lack of smooth motion with ROM
- Treatment: immobilization, corticosteroid injection, if unsuccessful surgical release of involved tendon

APPROACH

HISTORY

- Pain: position, quality, radiation, severity, timing, alleviating factors
- Mechanism of injury, history of trauma
- Associated paresthesia, weakness, ↓ROM
- Presence of other associated/related medical illnesses

PHYSICAL EXAM

- Inspection: look for deformities, contractures, nodules, inflamed joints
- Palpation: joints, bones, soft tissues, ROM: of wrist, digits
- Special tests: Tinel's sign, Phalen's test → suggests carpal tunnel syndrome
- Neurovascular exam: motor and sensory exam of ulnar, median, radial nerves

INVESTIGATIONS

- X-ray: obtain at least two views
- Bone scan: if high suspicion of fracture, but negative x-ray imaging

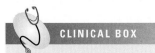

CLINICAL BOX

Sites of OA in the Hand/Wrist

DIP, PIP, First CMC

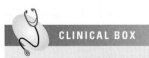

CLINICAL BOX

Sites of RA in the Hand/Wrist

PIP, MCP, wrist

PAIN: HIP

DEFINITION

- The hip joint is formed by the articulation of the femoral head with the acetabulum (made of ilium, ischium, pubis).
- Blood supply to the head and neck of the femur is from the medial femoral circumflex artery (branch of common femoral artery).
- Main muscles: **Abductors**—gluteus medius and gluteus minimus. **Extensors**—gluteus maximus, hamstrings. **Flexors**—iliopsoas

CAUSAL CONDITIONS

See Table 17.4.

HIP DISLOCATIONS

- Associated with trauma → may have associated fractured of acetabulum, fractured femoral head, nerve injury; may occur following total hip arthroplasty
- 80% are posterior: leg shortened, adducted, internally rotated, flexed
- 20% are anterior: externally rotated, abducted, flexed, sometimes see bulge of femoral head
- Complications: can develop post-traumatic OA, AVN
- Treatment: reduction under general anesthesia, treat other associated injuries; if due to total hip arthroplasty, educate the patient regarding unstable positions (e.g., crossing the legs); can make the joint more stable by changing the components of the artificial hip

CLINICAL BOX

Location of Hip Pain

- **Anterior** hip/groin pain is usually due to hip join pathology.
- **Lateral or posterior/gluteal** pain is usually **not** due to hip joint pathology.

Hip Pain: Causal Conditions

Trochanteric bursitis, osteoarthritis, and fractures of the femoral neck are the most common conditions leading to hip pain

Location of Pain	Conditions
Table 17.4	**Hip Pain: Causal Conditions**
Articular	• Arthritis: OA, inflammatory, septic • Hip/pelvic trauma • AVN • Aortoiliac vascular occlusive disease
Periarticular	• Pelvic fractures • Trochanteric bursitis • Metastatic bone cancer • Lateral femoral cutaneous nerve entrapment/meralgia paresthetica
Referred pain	• GI (inguinal hernia, abdominal disease) • Lumbar radiculopathy

Think of fractures if:

• History of trauma, fall, osteopenia, previous pathologic fractures, past history of cancers

HIP FRACTURES

• Bimodal distribution: low-energy trauma (elderly, osteoporosis) versus high-energy trauma (young patients); lack of trauma suggests pathologic fracture (malignancy or severe osteoporosis)
• Signs/symptoms: pain, inability to weight bear, shortened and externally rotated limb.
• Types
  • Femoral neck/subcapital fractures
    • Leads to AVN or nonunion due to disruption of the blood flow to the femoral head
    • Treatment: if undisplaced or young patient (even if displaced) → ORIF; if displaced or older patient → partial hip replacement, or total hip replacement if preexisting OA of the fractured hip or a very active patient
  • Intertrochanteric fractures: very low risk of AVN
• Treatment: obtain good reduction, internal fixation with dynamic hip screw

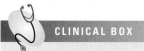

A pelvic ring fracture is an orthopedic emergency.

PELVIC FRACTURES

• Pelvic ring disruption—from high-energy trauma (MVA, fall from height). There are usually two injuries to the pelvic ring. Can be stable or unstable.
  • Stable: minor disruption of the SI joint, may sometimes be treated nonoperatively.
  • Unstable: SI joint disruption → deformity and instability of the pelvis. Difficult to manage. **Significant associated injuries**: life-threatening hemorrhage, bladder/urethral injury, neurologic injuries. Is an orthopedic emergency, needs ORIF or external fixation.
• Acetabular fractures—also from high-energy trauma (MVA, fall). Can be difficult to treat if complicated fracture. Can lead to hemorrhage, post-traumatic OA later in life. Requires ORIF.
• Sacrum/coccyx fractures—from fall, direct blow, or associated with pelvic ring disruption.
• Stability depends on injury pattern (see Figure 17.5).

X-ray Findings in OA

Joint space narrowing, subchondral sclerosis, cyst formation, marginal osteophyte formation

OSTEOARTHRITIS

See Polyarthritis section.

• 1° OA—in older patients (>50 yr old), due to degenerative changes. 2° OA—can occur in younger patients (in their 30s) with history of trauma or pediatric hip condition.
• Signs/symptoms: ↓ ROM (↓flexion, ↓abduction, ↓internal rotation), morning stiffness <30 min, positive Trendelenburg sign, activity-related pain better with rest. Severe OA may result in constant pain and/or night pain.
• Treatment: NSAIDs, analgesia, intra-articular cortisone injection, walking aids (cane in contralateral hand). May eventually need hip replacement.

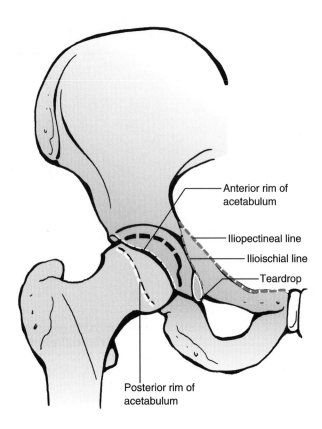

Figure 17.5 Pelvic fractures on x-ray.

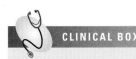

Think of AVN if history of:

• EtOH abuse, steroid use, sickle cell, previous hip fracture treated with internal fixation

Septic joint is an orthopedic emergency; it requires urgent irrigation and debridement and IV antibiotics.

AVN (OSTEONECROSIS/ASEPTIC NECROSIS/ISCHEMIC NECROSIS)

• Compromise of the bone vasculature → death of bone and marrow cells → mechanical failure. Joint destruction within 3–5 yr if left untreated.
• Risk factors: over 90% attributed to excess EtOH use and use of corticosteroids. Other risk factors include previous femoral neck fracture, sickle cell, hemoglobinopathies, thrombophilia.
• Diagnosis should be considered in patients with acute onset groin pain and risk factors.
• Treatment: determined by amount of collapse of the femoral head. May eventually need hip arthroplasty.

TROCHANTERIC BURSITIS

• Inflammation of the trochanteric bursa from ↑ pressure/friction, due to gait abnormalities (from lumbosacral spine stiffness, leg length discrepancy, knee arthritis, ankle sprain).
• Symptoms: point tenderness over trochanteric bursa, pain when sleeping on affected side.
• Treatment: conservative—rest, ice, NSAIDs. Can inject with cortisone and a small amount of local anesthetic to confirm the diagnosis.

APPROACH

HISTORY

• Ask about pain: position, quality, radiation, severity, timing, alleviating factors
• History of trauma/fall, constitutional symptoms, osteoporosis, use of EtOH or steroids, previous hip fractures, joint prosthesis (can become infected or loose)

PHYSICAL EXAM

• Vitals: fever, signs of sepsis
• Inspection: swelling, atrophy, abnormal limb position (excess rotation), leg length discrepancy
• Palpation: deformities, focal tenderness, crepitus

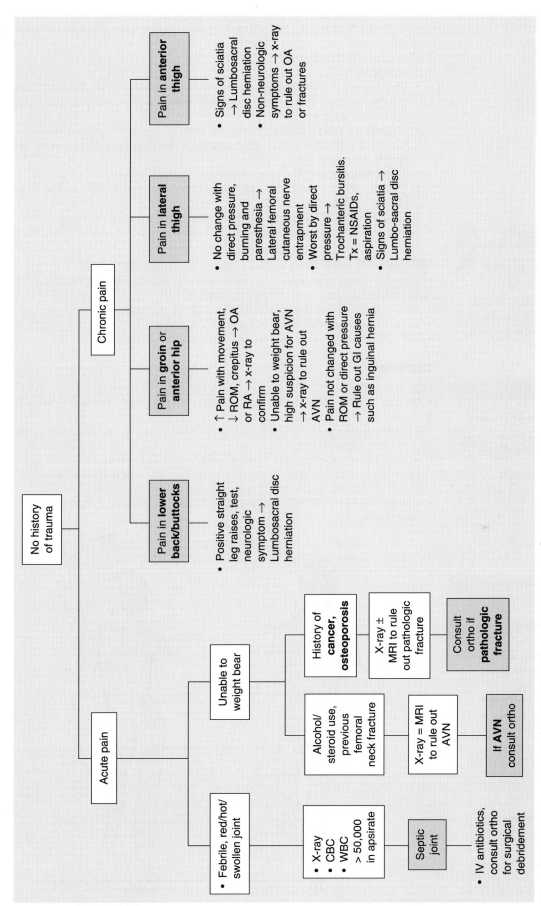

Figure 17.6 Approach to patient with hip pain with no history of trauma.

- ROM: make sure the pelvis is stable when testing ROM. Normal ROM: flexion = 130, ext = 30, abduction = 45, adduction = 30, internal rotation = 30–40, external rotation = 60–70
- Gait: presence of limp, pain
- Special tests:
  - **Thomas**—Both hips are flexed maximally to eliminate lumbar lordosis. Then one hip is fully extended. If this hip cannot fully extend → Positive test, flexion contracture exists (e.g., in OA).
  - **Straight leg raise**—Passively raise the affected leg off the ground while keeping the leg straight. Positive test, if reproduction of shooting pain down the leg between 30 and 70 degrees of flexion.
  - **Trendelenburg** (see Pediatric section and Figure 17.7 below)
  - **FABER**—**F**lex, **a**bduct, and **e**xternally **r**otate the hip. Positive test is when pain is elicited → SI joint tenderness
- Neurological exam: Dermatomes, myotomes, reflexes
- Abdominal exam if indicated, urogenital and rectal exam in case of pelvic fractures

INVESTIGATIONS

- X-ray: AP, lateral hip. Judet views (obturator oblique, iliac oblique) for acetabular fracture and inlet and outlet views for pelvic fractures.
- MRI: if suspect bony metastasis, AVN, occult hip fracture
- CT: can also be used to assess in hip fractures
- CBC, blood culture, joint aspiration—if septic joint suspected

TREATMENT

Hip Arthroplasty

- Used in patients with severe hip joint pathology: OA, AVN, femoral neck fractures
- Two types:
  - Partial replacement: only femoral neck and head are replaced. Can be converted to a total hip replacement.
  - Total hip replacement: the femoral head/neck and the articular surface of the acetabulum are replaced. Wear of the acetabular liner can lead to local osteolysis and failure of the implants, necessitating revision surgery after 10–15 yr.
- Complications: infection, loosening, dislocation, nerve and vascular injury, thromboembolic disease (DVT and PE).

CLINICAL BOX

AVN and Occult Hip Fracture

AVN and occult hip fracture can have normal x-rays, use MRI if high suspicion (100% sensitivity)

CLINICAL BOX

Conservative Treatment of MSK Injuries —PRICE

- **P**ain control (NSAIDs)
- **R**est
- **I**ce
- **C**ompression
- **E**levation

CLINICAL BOX

DVT prophylaxis is needed in:

- Hip fractures—start after admission, stop at least 12 h before surgery
- Pelvic or acetabular trauma
- Post-Op (total hip/knee replacement) 21/7 days, respectively

  Use low-molecular-weight heparin

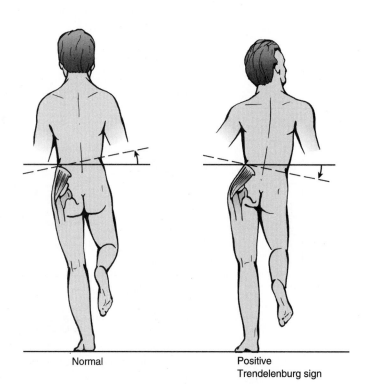

Normal

Positive Trendelenburg sign

Figure 17.7 Trendelenburg test. Inability to maintain the pelvis horizontally when standing on the affected leg—pelvis falls on the opposite side. It is due to weakness of the hip abductors on the affected side.

PAIN: KNEE

Valgus versus Varus

- Va**L**gus force = causes a **L**ateral displacement of the limb distally
- Varus force = causes a medial displacement of the limb distally

DEFINITION

- The knee is a hinge joint formed by the femoral condyles and the tibial plateaus. It is divided into three compartments: medial tibiofemoral, lateral tibiofemoral, patello-femoral.
- The knee has a medial and a lateral meniscus. The meniscus is a fibrocartilage pad between the bony surfaces, which has shock absorbing properties and adds stability.
- The main ligaments of the knee are the ACL, PCL, MCL, and LCL.
- Muscles of the knee: ext by quadriceps muscles, flexion by hamstrings.

CAUSAL CONDITIONS

OA

See Monoarthritis section.

- Owing to age-related wear and tear, medial compartment > lateral compartment. May have history of injury or previous surgery (meniscectomy).
- Treatment: Rest, NSAIDs, walking aids, bracing, shoe orthotics. Cortisone injections can be used twice/year (will relieve pain symptoms for a few months). Definitive treatment is a knee replacement: partial, or total.

LIGAMENT SPRAINS

- Collateral ligaments
  - MCL—common, from valgus force
  - LCL—less common, from trauma/direct varus force
  - Signs/symptoms—swelling, tenderness on affected side, joint laxity
- Cruciate ligaments:
  - ACL—Usually caused by direct trauma in males, indirect trauma in females (hyper-extension, pivoting maneuver). Can lead to hemarthrosis, knee giving out, instability.
  - PCL—from trauma displacing the tibia posteriorly on the femur (e.g., hitting the dashboard of a car with a flexed knee).
  - Signs/symptoms: audible "pop" heard at time of injury, immediate effusion, pain, joint laxity.

Classification of Ligament Sprains

- **1st degree**—irritation/inflammation, but intact
- **2nd degree**—partially torn, laxity but can feel an end point
- **3rd degree**—completely torn, lax, no end point

ACL Tear

Sudden knee pain following a pivoting maneuver, along with audible "pop," immediate swelling and knee instability → ACL tear

Table **17.5**	**Knee Pain: Causal Conditions**
Cause	**Etiology**
Trauma	• Fractures (tibial plateau, distal femur, patella) • Meniscal tears • Ligament injury • Soft tissue, contusion
Repetitive stress	• Bursitis • Patella-femoral syndrome • Patellar tendonitis • Iliotibial band syndrome
Inflammatory	• Gout • RA • Pseudogout
Degenerative	• OA
Infectious	• Septic joint
Referred pain	• Lumbar radiculopathy • SI joint • Hip joint

- Diagnosis: with physical exam findings, can confirm with MRI
- Treatment: grades 1–2 conservative treatment, immobilization, and strengthening. If complete, tear may need surgical repair or reconstruction.

MENISCAL TEAR

- Mechanism of injury: in young patients from twisting the knee with the foot fixed on the ground → joint tenderness, effusion, locking, premature OA. In older patients the tears are due to wear and tear.
- Medial meniscal injury is more common than the lateral meniscus, and it is also associated with ACL and MCL tears.
- Signs/symptoms: clicking, locking, knee instability, positive McMurray's test, positive Appley's maneuver, joint-line tenderness (most sensitive physical exam finding).
- Diagnosis: clinical findings, MRI, knee arthroscopy.
- Treatment: conservative treatment, arthroscopic repair, or partial meniscectomy.

FRACTURES

- History of fall/trauma or repetitive stress
- Fracture of the tibial plateaus—focal tenderness over the tibial plateau involved. Will usually require ORIF.
- Fracture of the patella—focal tenderness over the patella. If minimally displaced can be treated conservatively with immobilization. If displaced >2 mm, ruptured hamstrings or comminuted will need ORIF.

PATELLAR DISLOCATION

- Most dislocations are laterally. Patients often have anatomic predisposition (Q-angle, shallow trochlea)
- Signs/symptoms: Pain, effusion, swelling, knee is held in flexion
- Treatment: Usually reduce spontaneously. If not will require closed reduction under procedural sedation, and gently bringing the knee into ext. If complicated or associated with fractures may need open reduction.

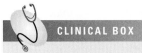

CLINICAL BOX

Acute Traumatic Hemarthrosis

Causes of acute traumatic hemarthrosis in the knee: ACL tear, peripheral meniscus tear, osteochondral fracture

IT BAND SYNDROME

- Pain with movement of the IT band over the lateral femoral condyle. Almost always in runners: due to excessive running, running on uneven surfaces, inappropriate shoe wear, leg length discrepancy.
- Signs/symptoms: focal tendered on the lateral side (where the IT band courses over the lateral femoral condyle), ± snapping sound.
- Treatment: NSAIDs, steroid injections, stretching and strengthening of the IT band, proper footwear, run on level surfaces.

PATELLA-FEMORAL SYNDROME

- Family of conditions: chondromalacia patella (softening of the patellar articular cartilage), patellar subluxation (uneven tracking of patella in the femoral groove), patella alta (high riding patella), patellofemoral arthritis.
- Pain at the patellofemoral joint due to trauma or repetitive irritation. Self-limited, in patients <45 yr old, mostly women.
- Signs/symptoms: Anterior knee pain, worst with flexion of the knee/stair climbing, presence of grinding/clicking.
- Treatment: NSAIDs, isometric quadriceps strengthening. Rarely surgical intervention.

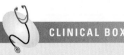

CLINICAL BOX

Night Pain

Constant, night pain suggests inflammatory or neoplastic process

BURSITIS

- The most common bursa affected are anserine and prepatellar bursas:
  - Anserine—on the medial side, 6 cm below the joint line. Usually accompanies medial compartment OA.
  - Prepatellar/housemaid's knee—largest bursa of the knee, between the patella and skin. Usually due to trauma/repetitive kneeling.
- Signs/symptoms: Both present with focal tenderness over the area, pain at rest or with motion, ↓ROM, ± swelling/erythema/warmth.
- Treatment: Conservative treatment. If very large can aspirate to relieve pain symptoms, but may enlarge again.

Joint Effusion

Generalized swelling + impaired bending

Acute Ligament Injury

Acute ligament injury will be accompanied by joint effusion/swelling → may limit ROM and ability to assess the joint (may even see ↓ROM vs. joint laxity).

In these cases treat the patient conservatively, and re-evaluate in 1–2 wk time when the swelling has decreased.

Septic Joint Aspiration Analysis

- WBC >50,000 (less if infected total joint arthroplasty)
- Presence of RBC
- ± Presence of bacteria

Infection can coexist with crystalline arthropathy

BAKER'S CYST

- Consequence of chronic knee effusion due to joint disease (OA, RA, etc.), which then forms a cyst at the posterior aspect of the knee joint.
- Signs/symptoms: fullness behind the knee, fluid-filled mass palpable in the popliteal fossa.
- Treatment: treat the underlying cause.

APPROACH

See Figure 17.8.

HISTORY

- Pain: position, quality, radiation, severity, timing, alleviating factors.
- Swelling, locking, clicking, grinding, popping, snapping, instability, ↓ROM, limp, fever, chills
- Other joints involved: rule out polyarthropathies.
- History of trauma/twisting the knee, history of IV drug use, history of sexually transmitted infections, presence of prosthesis → can all lead to septic joint, osteomyelitis.

PHYSICAL EXAM

- Vitals, fever, signs of sepsis
- Examine both knees and compare the two sides
- Inspection: redness, swelling, deformity, atrophy, valgus/varus knee, gait abnormalities
- Palpation: palpate along the joint line, patella, and behind the knee. Look for pain, joint effusion, warmth, deformities, feel for crepitus/clicking/locking, baker's cyst
- ROM—Normal ROM: flexion = 130 degrees, ext = 0 degrees
- Special tests:
  - ACL: anterior drawer test, Lachman's test
  - PCL: posterior drawer test, posterior sag test
  - MCL/LCL: valgus/varus stress tests
  - Meniscal tears: McMurray's test, Appley's test
  - Effusions: patellar tap, milking the effusion
- Neurologic exam: sensory, motor power, reflexes, gait
- Examine hips and ankle joints

INVESTIGATIONS

- X-ray—AP, lateral, skyline (if patellar fracture, patellofemoral OA)
- MRI—for meniscus and ligament injury
- CT—for complicated fractures requiring ORIF
- Arthroscopy—assess the extent of damage in OA, meniscal tears
- Joint aspiration—if suspect septic joint, gout, pseudogout
- CBC, blood culture ESR, CRP—if suspect septic joint, osteomyelitis
- ANA and ESR (if suspect RA)

PAIN: LEG, FOOT, ANKLE

DEFINITION

- Ankle joint (mortise)—articulation of the talus with the tibia and fibula. Movements: dorsi flexion, plantar flexion. Subtalar joint—articulation of the talus with the calcaneus. Movements: inversion and eversion.
- The ankle has four main ligaments: Medially—Deltoid ligament. Laterally—anterior talofibular, posterior talofibular, calcaneofibular ligaments.

CAUSAL CONDITIONS

See Table 17.6.

TIBIAL FRACTURES

- Most common fractured long bone, from trauma
- Signs/symptoms: pain, deformity, may be open or closed, ± neurovascular changes, ± compartment syndrome

Leg Pain: Common Causes

Venous insufficiency and arterial insufficiency are common causes of leg pain.

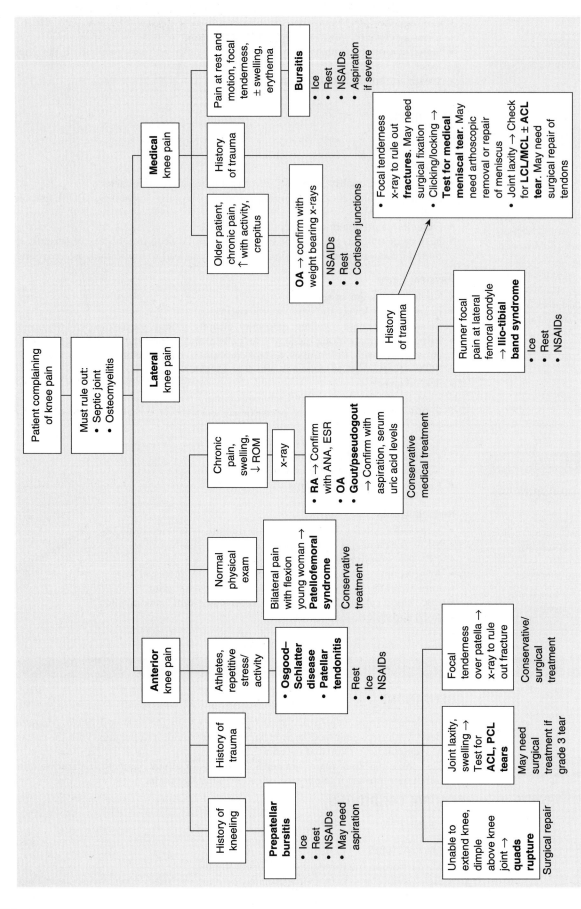

Figure 17.8 Approach to knee pain.

Table **17.6**	Leg, Foot, and Ankle Pain: Causal Conditions	
Location	**Etiology**	
Leg	• DVT • Muscle strain • Fractures	• Arterial insufficiency • Venous insufficiency
Ankle	• Ligament sprain • Fracture	• Tendinopathy (tib post) • Achilles tendinopathy/rupture
Foot	• Periostitis • Fractures • Plantar fasciitis	• Gout • Bunions/hallux valgus

- Treatment:
  - Tibial diaphysis: If nondisplaced → a long leg cast for 6 wk. If displaced or comminuted → ORIF with IM nail
  - Tibial metaphysic: ORIF with plate and screws

ANKLE FRACTURE

- Fracture of the tibia and fibula at the malleolar level or more proximal, ± disruption of the syndesmosis/talofibular ligament
- Mechanism of injury: usually rotational
- Signs/symptoms: open or closed fracture, focal bony tenderness of the malleoli, swelling, unstable ankle, associated with ligamentous injuries
- Treatment: if undisplaced → cast. If displaced/open/avulsion of medial malleolus/involving the joint → ORIF

LIGAMENT SPRAIN

- Lateral ligaments—more common
  - Mechanism of injury: Inversion of the ankle while plantar flexed → swelling and tenderness, ecchymosis

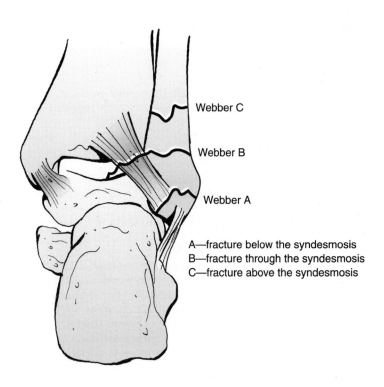

Figure 17.9 Webber classification of ankle fractures.

- Deltoid ligament (less common)
  - Mechanism of injury: eversion of the ankle
  - Requires higher force than the lateral ligaments → may be associated with medial malleolus fractures
- Signs/symptoms: pain, swelling, ecchymosis, positive ankle drawer test. Patient may be predisposed to recurrent sprains
- Treatment—Grade 1: conservative; Grade 2: ankle wrap, RICE (rest, ice, compression, elevation), physiotherapy; Grade 3: cast 4–6 wk, physiotherapy, ± surgical intervention. Recurrent instability may require ligament reconstruction

ACHILLES TENDINOPATHY/RUPTURE

- Usually due to degenerative changes of the tendon in patients over 40 yr. Sudden contraction of the gastrocnemius muscle in jumping or running, can lead to rupture of the tendon (eccentric contraction).
- Signs/symptoms: can see and feel a gap deformity, patient is unable to plantar flex, unable to walk on tiptoes, positive Thompson test.
- Treatment: conservative or surgical approximation of the tendon ends, timing of mobilization is controversial.

METATARSAL FRACTURES

- Mechanism of injury: can be stress fractures (e.g., in runners, commonly the second, third, fifth), avulsion fracture (fifth), or from direct trauma (first)
- Signs/symptoms: focal tenderness over the fractured area
- Determine need for x-ray based on Ottawa foot rules
- Look for associated injury to tarsometatarsal joints (Lisfranc)
- Treatment: first, fourth, fifth metatarsals: if none displaced → below the knee cast 6 wk. If displaced → ORIF. Second, third metatarsals: are not mobile unlike the others. Therefore, no need for immobilization. Treat the pain.

PLANTAR FASCIITIS

- Inflammation and microtears of the plantar fascia due to repetitive strain
- Common in athletes, patients with diabetes, arthritis
- Signs/symptoms: morning stiffness, pain with dorsi flexion, or palpation of calcaneal origin
- Treatment: conservative, counter force taping, stretching, surgical release of fascia if severe

BUNIONS/HALLUX VALGUS

- Common, genetically predisposed, associated with inappropriate footwear
- Signs/symptoms: valgus/lateral deviation of the big toe, with prominence of the first metatarsal head, it is usually bilateral. Usually painless, unless inflammation or 2° OA present
- Treatment: supportive measures. Comfortable shoe wear, wide shoes, use of padding. Surgical osteotomy is the only corrective measure

APPROACH

HISTORY

- Pain—position, quality, radiation, severity, timing, alleviating factors, associated with activity or at rest. Able to weight bear or not
- History of trauma, repetitive stress; risk factors for arterial/venous insufficiency, DVT; previous history of OA, RA, gout, pseudogout

PHYSICAL EXAM

- Separate exam of hindfoot, midfoot, forefoot
- Inspection—deformities, bruising, gait, signs of arterial/venous insufficiency, footwear. Always examine in weight-bearing and non–weight-bearing position
- Palpation: ankle joint (heat, swelling, pain), measure calves and thighs in case of DVT, palpation of peripheral arteries
- ROM of the ankle joint: dorsi flexion 20 degrees, plantar flexion 45 degrees, inversion 20 degrees, eversion 30 degrees
- Special tests: anterior drawer, Thompson (squeeze calf, see plantar flexion of foot)

CLINICAL BOX

March Fracture

Midshaft fracture of second/third metatarsal

CLINICAL BOX

Jones Fracture

Midshaft fracture of fifth metatarsal.

CLINICAL BOX

Gout

Hot, swollen, erythematous first metatarsophalangeal joint is the hallmark of gout.

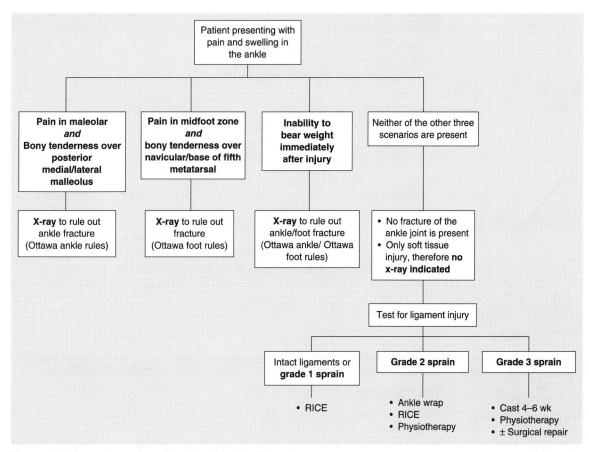

Figure 17.10 Approach to patient with ankle pain and swelling.

INVESTIGATIONS

- X-ray—only if indicated by the Ottawa ankle/foot rules. AP, lateral, mortise view (15 degrees of ankle internal rotation)
- CT—gain further information on complicated fractures before ORIF
- MRI—ligament injury, osteochondral fractures, tendinopathy
- Joint aspiration—for diagnosis of septic joint, gout, pseudogout
- Doppler and angiography—for DVT, arterial/venous insufficiency

CHILD WITH PAIN AND LIMP

DEFINITION

- Limp: uneven or jerky walk, due to pain, weakness, or deformity.
- Usually due to benign conditions, but may be life or limb threatening.
- Epidemiology: ~2/1,000, M > F, pain in hip > knee > leg

CAUSAL CONDITIONS

CLINICAL BOX

Two Common Types of Limps

- **Antalgic gait** = Short stance when walking, caused by pain in the weight-bearing extremity. Most common cause of limp.
- **Trendelenburg gait** = Downward pelvic tilt during swing phase, due to weakness or spasm in the contralateral gluteus medius muscle.

Table **17.7**	**Child with Limp/Pain: Causal Conditions**
Causes	**Conditions**
General causes	Trauma—fractures, dislocations Infectious—septic arthritis, osteomyelitis Inflammatory—juvenile rheumatoid arthritis, reactive arthritis Hematologic—leukemia, sickle cell, hemophillia Neoplastic—ewing sarcoma, osteosarcoma, osteochondroma Metabolic—rickets Soft tissue—contusions, bursitis, cellulitis Other—growing pains, muscular dystrophy, child abuse
Anatomic causes	Brain/spine—meningitis, cerebral palsy, discitis, spinal epidural abscess Hip—Legg–Calvé–Perthes, slipped capital femoral epiphysis, DDH, transient synovitis Knee—Osgood–Schlatter disease, patella dislocation, meniscus injury, patellofemoral syndrome Leg/foot—leg length discrepancy, poor foot wear

APPROACH

CLINICAL BOX

Radiography

Initial radiographs maybe normal in: stress fractures, Salter-Harris type I, septic arthritis, early osteomyelitis

CLINICAL BOX

Be aware of referred pain.
Knee pain can be attributed to a hip pathology.

HISTORY

- Limp and pain → duration, quality, what makes them better or worst
- History of trauma → think of fractures, soft tissue injuries
- Constitutional symptoms → think of malignancies
- Fever, red, hot swollen joint → septic joint, transient synovitis of the hip
- Endocrine dysfunction → slipped capital femoral epiphysis
- Morning stiffness → juvenile RA
- Back pain → think discitis, meningitis, vertebral osteomyelitis
- Recent viral/streptococcal infection → think postinfectious arthritis
- New or ↑ sports and activity → think stress fractures
- Current and past medical conditions
- Family history of connective tissue diseases, sickle cell
- Child abuse

CLINICAL BOX

Growing Pains

Night time, poorly localized pain in lower limbs (mostly shins), in kids 2–12 yr old.

Always think of and rule out child abuse.

PHYSICAL EXAM

- Vitals: look for signs of sepsis
- MSK exam (lower extremities, spine → joints, soft tissue, bones)
  - Inspection—deformities, joint effusions, redness, asymmetry
  - Palpation—location of pain (joint or soft tissue), bony deformities
  - ROM: active and passive
  - Special tests: Trendelenburg test, Barlow, Ortolani
  - Measure leg length discrepancy (>1.25 cm), assess gait
- Neurologic exam: CNS, PNS, strength, reflexes, myotomes, dermatomes
- Full physical exam

INVESTIGATIONS

- X-ray imaging—First-line imaging in a child with limp.
- U/S—DDH in <3 mo, small joint effusions, guided joint aspiration
- CT/MRI—In special cases: osteomyelitis, spine pathologies, malignancy
- Blood work—WBC, ESR, C-reactive protein
- Synovial fluid analysis—For inflammatory and infectious conditions

Table **17.8**	Approach to Child with Limp/Pain					
Condition	**Age**	**Pathophysiology**	**Risk Factors**	**Signs/Symptoms**	**Investigations**	**Treatment**
Hip etiology: Legg–Calvé–Perthes	• 4–10 yr • M:F = 4:1	• Idiopathic AVN of proximal femoral epiphysis • Bilateral (10%–15%), never presents at same stage • Chronic	• Male • Family history	• Trendelenburg limp and sign • Pain—hip, anterior thigh • ↓ Internal rotation • ↓ Abduction • ↓ Flexion • Chronic presentation	• X-ray • Can be negative early on • Later collapsed femoral head	• No definite treatment, goals: ↓ pain, ↑ROM, containment of femoral head • Physiotherapy, brace, NSAIDs • Pelvic, femoral osteotomy
Slipped capital femoral epiphysis	• Adolescents • M:F=1.5:1	• Type 1 Salter-Harris: slippage through growth plate • Acute or chronic • Stable or unstable • Bilateral 25%	• Over weight • Obesity • Hypothyroid • Family history	• Antalgic or Trendelenburg limp • Pain in hip ± knee • ↓ Hip internal rotation • Obligate external rotation of hip with flexion	X-ray (AP, frog view)	Hip pinning in situ (without attempt at reduction)
DDH (Congenital dislocation of the Hip)	• 0–4 yr • M:F=1:5	• Femoral head may move in and out of acetabulum in the neonate • Continuum from dislocated hip to acetabular dysplasia	• Family history • Breech • First born • Female • Oligohydramnios • ↑ Birth weight	• Short leg (Galeazzi test) • Trendelenburg limp • ↓ Abduction of affected hip • Extra skin folds on the affected side • Uni/bilateral	• Ortolani test • Barlow test • Trendelenburg test • U/S (<3 mo) • X-ray (>3 mo old)	• <6 mo—Pavlik harness • 6–18 mo reduce + hip spica • >18 mo open reduction/osteotomy
Infections Septic arthritis	• Any age	• Infection of joint through hematogenous or direct spread • Hip and knee most common	• IV drug use • Unprotected sex • Active TB	• Fever, ill looking, • ++pain, • Will not walk • Joint effusion, warmth	• ESR >20,↑ WBC • X-ray (joint effusion) • Synovial fluid analysis	• IV antibiotics • Analgesia • Irrigation and debridement • Surgical emergency
Osteomyelitis	• 0–5 yr	• Infection of bone • Hematogenous spread, local invasion, or direct trauma to the area	• Immune compromised • Sickle cell • Open fractures	• Fever • ↓ ROM • Pain and swelling over metaphysis	• ESR >20,↑ WBC • ↑ CRP • X-ray • MRI/CT • Bone scan	• IV antibiotics • Aspiration • Irrigation + debridement
Benign conditions Transient synovitis	• 3–8 yr • M:F = 2:1	• No clear precipitant, may be related to viral illness or trauma • Most common cause of nontraumatic hip pain in children		• Pain • ↓ ROM • Antalgic gait ± low fever • Unilateral • Self-limited	• Rule out hip infection (WBC, ESR, CRP ± aspiration) • Diagnosis of exclusion	• NSAIDs
Osgood–Schlatter disease	• Teens	• Traction apophysitis of tibial tubercle apophysis → apophysis becomes fragmented	• Athletes • Family history • Trauma	• Anterior knee pain, ↑ with activity • Prominence of tibial tuberosity • Soft tissue swelling • Uni/bilateral	• Clinical diagnosis • X-ray to rule out other conditions	• NSAIDs • Ice • May need to stop sporting activity

PAIN: NECK AND UPPER BACK

APPLIED SCIENTIFIC CONCEPTS

- The spine is made of 33 vertebrae: 7 cervical, 12 thoracic, 5 lumbar, 5 sacral, and 4 coccygeal.
- Atlanto-occipital joint is between occiput and C1 → main ROM is flexion and extension.
- Atlantoaxial joint is between C1 and C2 → main ROM is rotational
- C4-7 is the site of greatest wear and tear, may affect nerve roots C5, C6, C7 which pass through them → cervical radiculopathy

CAUSAL CONDITIONS

Muscle spasm/strain—Pain, stiffness, tightness in upper back and shoulders, acute, without neurologic deficits

WHIPLASH

- Abrupt flexion/ext movement to the cervical spine. Often multiple structures can be injured including soft tissues, spinal nerve, intervertebral disk, posterior longitudinal ligament, facet joints, or other osseous structures.
- Signs/symptoms: severe pain, spasm, loss of ROM in the neck, and occipital headache.
- Investigations: MRI, CT, x-ray, or bone scan imaging may be normal.

CERVICAL RADICULOPATHY

- Spinal nerve root dysfunction. Owing to many different conditions, but >70% are due to degenerative changes in the spine
- Signs/symptoms: weakness in the associated muscles, sensory changes, ↓ reflexes
- Treatment: treat the underlying cause, conservative treatment

APPROACH

INVESTIGATIONS

- X-ray—indications based on Canadian C-Spine Rules
- CT—indicated if neurologic findings present
- MRI—indications same as CT, also good for disc herniation, tumors, infections, spinal cord pathology
- EMG—Good for peripheral nerve entrapment syndromes

MANAGEMENT

- Conservative medical management for degenerative disc disease: posture modification, cervical collar, physical therapy, local pain relief, drugs, trigger point injections

Table **17.9** Causal Conditions: Neck/Upper Back Pain	
Cause of Pain	**Conditions**
Muscular	• Muscle spasm/strain (from poor posture) • Whiplash • Myofascial pain syndromes
Cervical spine pathology	• Spinal stenosis • Degenerative arthritis • Cervical spondylosis • Disc herniation (C5-6, C6-7, C7-T1) • Systemic diseases (RA, PMR) • Metastatic bone cancer • Infectious (osteomyelitis, soft tissue) • Malignancy
Referred pain	• Angina pectoralis • Meningitis

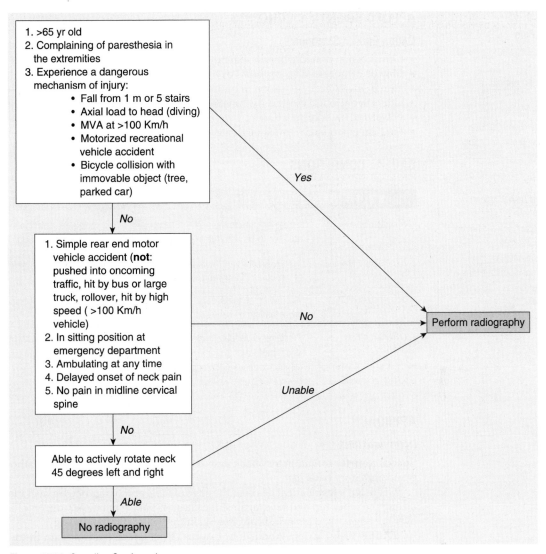

Figure 17.11 Canadian C-spine rules.

- If pain is not correlated with neuroanatomic pathways, consider myofascial pain or fibromyalgia

PAIN: LOWER BACK

DEFINITION

- 10%–15% of adults experience an episode of mild to moderate low back pain each year
- 90% of these patients recover but 10% go on to suffer from chronic pain
- **Mechanical:** Stiffness following prolonged inactivity, present for minutes not hours. Symptoms worse with activity, better with rest.
- **Inflammatory:** Worse with rest and relieved with activity, severe morning stiffness lasting for hours. Typical symptomology of seronegative. spondyloarthropathies (AS, **see Polyarthritis**).
- **Discogenic/radicular:** Back pain associated with pain or paresthesias in the legs (sciatica) and along the distribution of the compromised nerve. Pain is worse with sitting, better with standing or lying down. Described as burning, shooting, or electrical.
- **Pathologic:** Constant pain, not alleviated by rest or exercise. May be associated with constitutional features. Consider malignancy, infection, or referred pain from visceral organs (AAA, GI, GU, renal colic).

Low Back Pain

- Acute onset localized spine pain
- Pain waking patient up at night
- History of cancer
- Unexplained weight loss
- Immunosuppression (infection risk)
- Fever
- Trauma
- Bladder or bowel incontinence
- Urinary retention (with overflow incontinence)
- Saddle anesthesia
- Loss of anal sphincter tone
- Motor weakness in lower extremities
- Point vertebral tenderness

APPLIED SCIENTIFIC CONCEPTS

CAUDA EQUINA SYNDROME

- Compression of nerve bundle extending from the bottom of the spinal cord.
- May be compressed by ruptured or herniated disk, tumor, or abscess.
- Pain in lower back, sensation in buttocks, thighs, bladder, and rectum reduced.
- Other symptoms: erectile dysfunction, urinary retention, loss of ankle reflex, loss of bowel and bladder function.
- Surgical emergency—must be treated immediately!

CAUSAL CONDITIONS

Table **17.10**	Disorders of the Spine
Spondylolysis	Stress fracture in the pars interarticularis of the vertebrae; common in young athletes (gymnasts/wrestlers) and caused by hyperextension/rotation
Spondylolisthesis	Complete bilateral fracture of the pars interarticularis causing anterior slippage of vertebrae (Scotty dog sign on x-ray)
Spinal stenosis	Narrowing of spinal canal—most often attributed to osteoarthritis; may be accompanied by bony spurs
Disk herniation	Pressure on vertebral disk by adjacent vertebrae (i.e., lifting a heavy object) can cause rupture of disk and nucleus propulsus bulging; the bulge can compress, irritate, or damage the adjacent spinal nerve root

APPROACH

INVESTIGATIONS

Special tests for inflammatory back pain (HLA-B27): see Polyarthritis for pathophysiology of inflammatory back pain

Gaenslen's test: Patient lies near the edge of table and hangs one leg over the side while flexing the other hip and knee against the chest. If pain ↑ in buttock region of leg hanging over the edge of the table, indicative of SI joint inflammation/pathology.

FABER test: **F**lexion, **A**bduction, **E**xternal **R**otation at the hip. Pain in the buttock is suggestive of SI joint inflammation.

Modified Schober's test: Evaluates the degree of movement in the lumbar spine with forward flexion. Make the patient stand in upright position with back exposed. Mark the skin 10 cm above the dimples of Venus, then ask the patient to flex forward to touch their toes (ext at knees). An ↑ of <4 cm between the mark and the dimples of Venus suggest spine immobility (i.e., AS).

Chest expansion: A limitation in chest expansion of 2 cm or less when measuring around the chest at nipple level is pathognomonic for spondylitis.

Table **17.11**	Physical Exam of the Lumbar Spine
Gait and Posture	**Examine for Structural or Functional Scoliosis**
ROM	Pain on forward flexion suggests mechanical cause while pain on ext suggests spinal stenosis
Palpation of spine and paraspinal muscles	Point tenderness over one vertebrae suggests infection or fracture
Heel-to-toe walking	A patient unable to heel-to-toe walk may have cauda equina syndrome 2° to multiple nerve root involvement
Straight leg raise	Pain between 30 and 60 degrees is suggestive of nerve root irritation; pain on crossed straight leg raise is suggestive of disc herniation
Neurologic testing	Weakness of dorsiflexion at first MTP and ankle suggest L4/L5 radiculopathy; sensory testing of medial (L4), dorsal (L5), and lateral (S1) areas of foot can be helpful in determining nerve root compression
Femoral stretch	Patient lies prone while hip is extended and knee flexed; pain indicates lumbar nerve root irritation

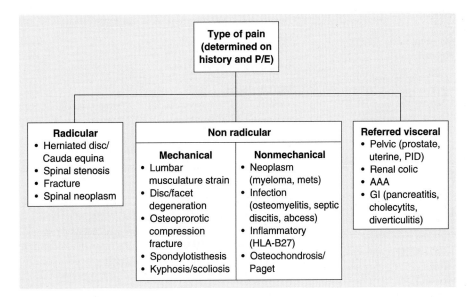

Figure 17.12 Approach to low back pain.

Occiput-to-wall distance: The patient stands with their back to the wall and heels touching the baseboard. Measure the distance between the occiput and the wall—it should be zero. Serial measurements are helpful in evaluating disease progression.

MANAGEMENT OF ACUTE MECHANICAL LOW BACK PAIN

Most episodes of pain resolve in 1–2 wk. Even with no treatment, 80%–90% of episodes resolve within 6 wk.

- Avoidance of activities which stress the spine (i.e., heavy lifting)
- Bed rest should not last for more than 2 d
- NSAIDs or muscle relaxants for pain
- Heat or cold massage, acupuncture, support garments
- Physiotherapy for accessory muscle strengthening

Proper posture, avoidance of standing or sitting in one position for long periods of time, sleeping on a firm mattress, and learning to lift properly can all reduce the rate of recurrence of low back pain.

SPINE COMPRESSION/OSTEOPOROSIS

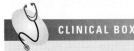

CLINICAL BOX

Risk Factors for Fracture

- Dementia
- Advanced age
- Maternal history of hip fracture
- Female
- Caucasian
- Current smoking
- Body weight <127 lbs
- Early menopause

DEFINITION

SPINAL COMPRESSION

- Compression fractures of the vertebral bodies can be anterior (wedge deformity), posterior (crush deformity), or central (biconcave).
- 90% of spine fractures in the elderly are attributable to osteoporosis.
- Most are asymptomatic.

OSTEOPOROSIS

- 40%–50% of white women older than 50 yr will suffer an osteoporotic hip fracture.
- Most common fracture sites are hip, spine, and radius.
- Mortality rate ↑ by 12%–20% in the year after a fracture due to complications of immobilization.

APPLIED SCIENTIFIC CONCEPTS

MEASURING BONE DENSITY: DEXA SCAN

Peak bone mass is attained by age 20–30 then remains relatively stable until menopause. A 2%–3% ↓ in bone mass occurs for 5 yr after menopause.

A combination of BMD measurements at the hip, spine, and radius (lowest value at these sites) provides the T-score. T-score = number of standard deviations from the mean

T-Score

- 2.5 to −1: Normal
- −1 to −2.5: Osteopenia
- <2.5: Osteoporosis

2° Causes of ↓ Bone Mass

- Gonadal deficiency
- Lifelong Ca^{2+} deficiency
- Chronic EtOH and/or nicotine use
- Immobilization
- Medications (glucocorticoids, anticonvulsants, excessive thyroid supplementation)
- Endocrine disorders (hyperparathyroid, hyperthyroid, hypercortisolism)

for young adult women. Z-score = individual score based on age, race, and sex matched controls.

CAUSAL CONDITIONS

OSTEOPOROSIS

- Skeletal disease marked by architectural deterioration of bone and ↓ bone mass
- Owing to normal age-related changes in bone remodeling causing net bone loss as bone resorption outpaces bone formation
- Genetic factors are major determinants of peak skeletal mass and density

Pathology: ↓ volume of mineralized bone and number of trabeculae, cortical thinning, ↓ bone strength.

Glucocorticoid osteoporosis: use of steroids like prednisone is the most common cause of 2° osteoporosis. They induce osteoblast and osteocyte apoptosis, resulting in ↓ bone formation and healing. Three months of prednisone treatment is sufficient to ↑ lifelong fracture risk, although risk falls after discontinuation. Consider adding Ca^{2+}, Vit D, and a bisphosphonate when prescribing prednisone.

APPROACH

SPINAL COMPRESSION

Signs and Symptoms
- Chronic back pain
- Loss of height
- Kyphosis (stooping posture)
- Disability
- Restrictive lung disease
- Tooth loss
- ↑ Occiput-to-wall distance
- Abdominal distention
- Early satiety and constipation

Differential Diagnosis
- Osteoporosis (1° or 2°)
- Spinal neoplasm
- Osteomalacia (bone pain)
- Rickets
- Paget's disease

Management
- Normal center of gravity is anterior to the spine, but fractures cause angular deformity which shifts it forward
- Added stress on adjacent vertebrae ↑ the risk of more compression fractures
- Paraspinal muscle fatigue, imbalance, and gait disturbances result from the shifted orientation leading to an ↑ risk of future falls and a 4.5-fold ↑ risk of hip fracture
- Treatment strategies:
  - Pain control—opioids, anti-inflammatories
  - Physiotherapy—to strengthen adjacent muscles
  - Surgical options: **vertebroplasty** (injection of bone filler into compressed vertebrae), **balloon kyphoplasty** (insertion of balloon into vertebrae)

OSTEOPOROSIS

Management
- Reduce likelihood of falls by treating predisposing comorbidities, reducing use of unnecessary sedatives, and adjusting the home environment (no throw rugs, good lighting, balance bars)

Smoking cessation

Ca^{2+} and Vit D replacement

Calcitonin nasal sprays

Bisphosphonates (inhibit function and lifespan of osteoclasts)

PTH, SERMs

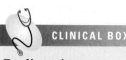

Predisposing Comorbidities

- Dementia
- Gait disorders
- ↓ Vision
- ↓ Muscle mass
- EtOH addiction

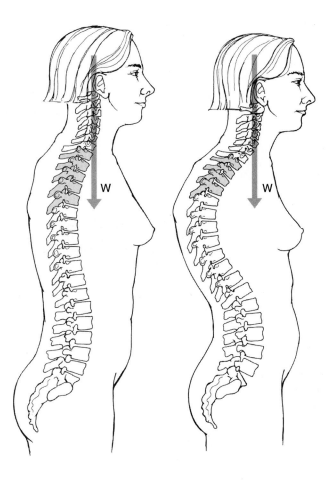

Figure 17.13 Center of gravity of the spine. Normal center of gravity is anterior to the spine. In spinal fracture the angular deformity shifts the center of gravity even farther forward. Normal center of gravity is anterior to the spine. In spinal fracture the angular deformity shifts the center of gravity even further forward.

MONOARTICULAR JOINT PAIN

DEFINITION

MONOARTHRITIS

- Inflammation of a single joint
- Presents with both pain and swelling
- Various causes
- Infection can cause rapid destruction and prolonged morbidity if left untreated even for a few days, must be ruled out early

DESCRIBING ARTHRITIS

- **Arthritis versus Periarticular disease:** Warmth, swelling, and tenderness surrounding the joint coupled with painful ROM in all planes suggest articular disease. Retention of normal joint motion or pain limited to one movement and one location suggest soft tissue disorders such as bursitis, cellulitis, or tendonitis.
- **Acute versus Chronic:** Acute monoarthritis presents as a rapidly swelling joint with severe pain and restricted ROM within minutes to days. The patient can usually pinpoint the exact onset of symptoms. Chronic, or subacute, monoarthritis has a more insidious onset that lasts from weeks to months.
- **Mono versus Polyarticular:** Systemic diseases may present as monoarticular arthritis. Rheumatoid arthritis, SLE, arthritis of IBD, psoriatic arthritis, and reactive arthritis can all begin as inflammation in one joint. Evaluating patients for underlying systemic diseases can lead to early diagnosis of a systemic etiology. Monoarthritis can progress from one joint to few joints (oligo) then to many joints (poly). See Joint Pain—polyarticular.

CAUSAL CONDITIONS

Table **17.12** Acute Monoarthritis

Mechanism	Risk Factors	Pathophysiology	Signs and Symptoms	Diagnostics	Treatment
Infection	Immune compromise Parenteral drug use Extremity wounds Recent surgery Prosthetic joint GI cancers STI	Hematogenous spread, infection in bone or soft tissue, or direct inoculation during trauma, injection, or surgery; bacterial, viral, mycobacterial, or fungal	Heat, swelling, erythema, and painful ROM of the infected joint; may have fever and/or chills	Joint aspiration and synovial fluid anaylsis; 50–100,000 WBC/mm^3 = bacteria, 10–30,000/mm^3 = fungal or mycobacterial	Empiric systemic antibiotics and specific therapy postculture; drainage of purulent fluid from the joint is also indicated
Crystal arthropathy (gout or CPDD)	History of prior gout Renal insufficiency Diuretic use HTN Obesity Heavy EtOH use High purine diet	Gout is urate crystals in the joint causing fluctuant inflammation and pain; serum uric acid level is often elevated; CPDD, apatites, and Ca^{2+} oxalate can act similarly	First MTP, ankle, midfoot, or knee; exquisitely painful; rapid onset (within hours)	Joint aspiration and microscopy —negatively birefringent, needle-shaped uric acid crystals for gout	Colchicine or NSAIDs for acute attack; allopurinol for long-term control of recurrent gout; may use steroids if NSAIDs contraindicated
Seronegative spondyloarthropathies Psoriatic AS IBD-associated	HLA-B27 Psoriasis Male sex IBD Middle-age (20–40)	Autoimmune activation of synoviocytes, accumulation of inflammatory cells within the joint, and angiogenesis RF negative	Oligoarthritis with one large joint (knee); AS causes bilateral sacroiliitis; may also have dactylitis, enthesitis, and conjunctivitis	X-rays show erosion and bone production in characteristic distribution; MRI of pelvis/spine for AS	Physical therapy, NSAIDs, methotrexate, steroids, sulfasalazine, biologics
Hemarthrosis	Trauma Bleeding diathesis Anticoagulant use Scurvy	Bleeding into the joint; consider fracture of the joint if the synovial fluid is bloody and contains fat; repeated joint bleeding can cause synovial thickening, chronic inflammation, and joint deformity	Swelling, erythema, and pain on ROM of affected joint; may have soft tissue hematoma	Synovial fluid appears pink, red, or brown; it may include fat globules	Immobilization, ice, and compression; NSAIDs should be avoided for bleeding risk; can replace deficient clotting factors or intervene surgically

Table **17.13** Chronic Monoarthritis

Mechanism	Pathophysiology	Signs and Symptoms	Diagnostics	Treatment
Osteoarthritis	Slowly progressive and insidious degeneration of cartilage; development of bony spurs or osteophytes; can occur 2° to trauma (ACL injury)	Joint pain and brief stiffness after sleep or inactivity; pain occurs during activity and subsides with rest; erythema and warmth are minimal or absent; may have limited ROM, crepitus, and pain on weight-bearing	ESR is normal and synovial analysis reveals normal WBC count Radiographs show osteophytes at joint margins and narrowing of joint spaces	Initially treated with lifestyle changes (exercise and weight control), analgesia, NSAIDs, and corticosteroid injections; may proceed to surgical interventions such as arthroscopy and debridement or arthroplasty (joint replacement)
Internal derangement	Fragment of soft tissue or bone becomes interposed between the articular surfaces of the joint after trauma	Mild to moderate pain, swelling, and limited ROM of affected joint after trauma; locking of the joint and inability to weight bear	Derangement is detected by imaging (x-ray, CT, MRI)	Often requires surgical intervention (i.e., arthroscopy)
Infection	Mycobacterial and fungal, that is, joint involvement in Lyme disease (*B. burgdorferi*) can cause chronic monoarthritis—most often in the knee	Joint pain, swelling, erythema, and restricted ROM; may progress to involve several joints	Synovial fluid analysis: 10,000–30,000 = mycobacteria or fungus	Appropriate antibiotics, antifungal, or antiviral depending on etiology; may require surgical debridement
Tumor	Often juxta-articular benign or malignant neoplasms (osteoma or sarcoma); may be metastasis from prostate, breast, etc.	Localized pain and/or swelling with insidious onset; limited ROM may or may not be present; may have fatigue, weight loss, night sweats	X-ray may reveal areas of bone erosion; MRI will define tumor size and ext; CT is generally less useful than MRI	Surgical resection or radiation; may undertake a search for 1° neoplasm: CT chest/abdo, bone scan, etc.

APPROACH

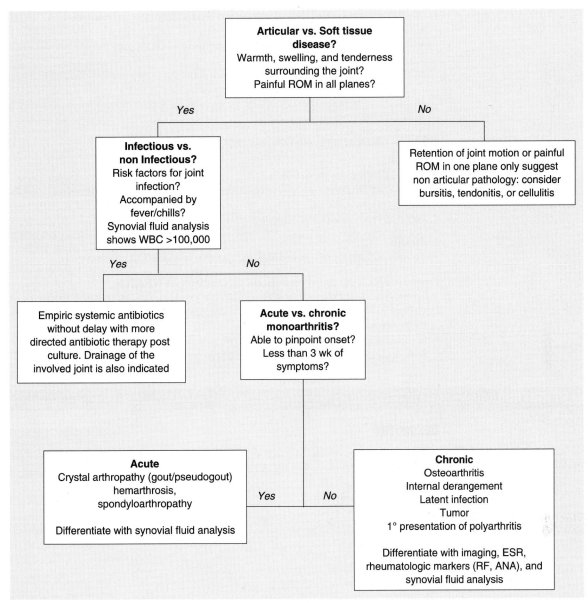

Figure 17.14 Approach to monoarticular joint pain.

APPLIED SCIENTIFIC CONCEPTS

GOUT VERSUS PSEUDOGOUT

Gout
- Acute inflammatory response to uric acid crystals in the joint accompanied by an elevated serum uric acid level.
- Episodic and mainly affects men, average attack lasts 7–9 d, and 90% of first gout attacks occur in the big toe (first MTP joint).
- Negatively bifringent, needle-like crystals on synovial fluid analysis.

CPDD (Pseudogout)
- Can be clinically indistinguishable from gout.
- Attacks are most often seen in the knee or wrist and are only rarely associated with hypercalcemia.
- Positively bifringent, rhomboid crystals on synovial fluid analysis.

SEPTIC ARTHRITIS

- *N. gonorrhoeae* is the most common cause of septic arthritis.
- Most of nongonococcal infections are caused by gram-positive aerobes
  - *S. aureus* (60%)
  - Anaerobic infection in immunocompromised patients and those with GI cancers and extremity wounds.
  - Mycobacterium, fungi (blastomycosis or *Candida*), and viruses (HSV, HIV, parvovirus) are more likely to induce chronic infections.
  - Infectious monoarthritis can also be caused by Lyme disease or spirochetes such as *T. pallidum* (syphilis).

NSAIDs—INDICATIONS AND CONTRAINDICATIONS

Function

- Inhibit prostaglandin synthesis
- Traditional NSAIDs (ASA, ibuprofen) block both cyclooxygenase pathways (COX-1 and COX-2)
- Newer NSAIDs selectively block the COX-2 pathway

Indication

- To treat inflammatory arthritides such as rheumatoid arthritis and gout

Contraindications and Precautions to Traditional NSAIDs

- GI toxicity (dyspepsia, PUD, bleeding), renal insufficiency, advanced hepatic impairment, CHF or HTN, known hypersensitivity, anticoagulants, chronic EtOH abuse, and platelet dysfunction.
- Should be avoided, or used with caution, in patients at high risk for CV disease and those with angina, HTN, fluid retention, or CHF.

POLYARTHRITIS

DEFINITION

- Pattern/evolution of joint involvement provide clues toward etiology
- Joint pain can be the first marker of a systemic illness

CAUSAL CONDITIONS

- Inflammatory
  - Infectious
  - Postinfectious (reactive)
  - Systemic rheumatic condition
- Noninflammatory

  See Figure 17.15.

APPROACH

INFLAMMATORY

Infectious

- Sequela of Group A *Strep* infection or transient viral infection involving large joints
- Several joints are affected in migratory pattern beginning in the legs and moving to the arms

Postinfectious (Reactive)

- 2–3 wk following infection of the GI or GU tract
- *Shigella, Salmonella, Campylobacter,* and *Chlamydia*
- Signs and symptoms:
  - **Reactive arthritis (Reiter's)**
  - Aseptic arthritides, both symmetric and additive
  - Involving mostly the joints of the lower extremity
  - Dactylitis and enthesitis are common

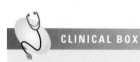

CLINICAL BOX

Reactive Arthritis (Reiter's)

Triad of:

- Nongonococcal urethritis
- Conjunctivitis
- Aseptic arthritis

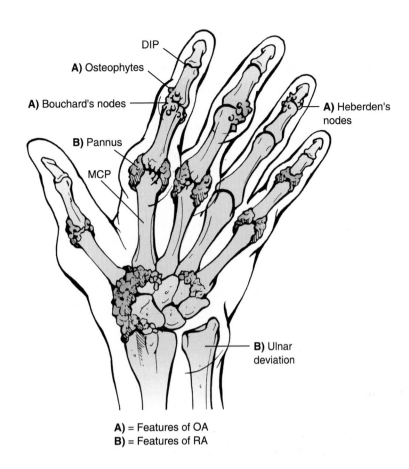

DIP

A) Osteophytes

A) Bouchard's nodes

B) Pannus

MCP

A) Heberden's
nodes

B) Ulnar
deviation

Figure 17.15 Rheumatoid arthritis
versus osteoarthritis.

A) = Features of OA
B) = Features of RA

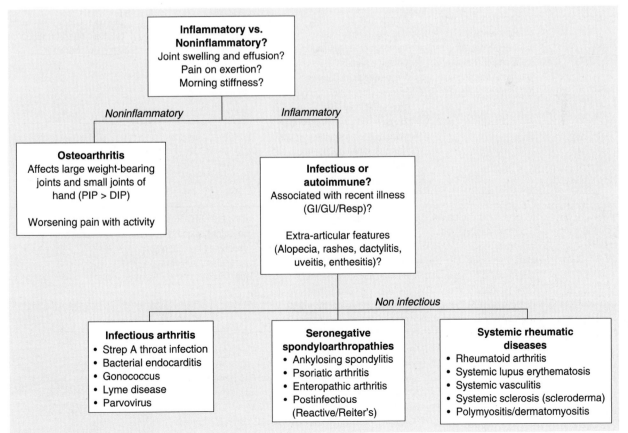

**Inflammatory vs.
Noninflammatory?**
Joint swelling and effusion?
Pain on exertion?
Morning stiffness?

Noninflammatory   *Inflammatory*

Osteoarthritis
Affects large weight-bearing
joints and small joints of
hand (PIP > DIP)

Worsening pain with activity

**Infectious or
autoimmune?**
Associated with recent illness
(GI/GU/Resp)?

Extra-articular features
(Alopecia, rashes, dactylitis,
uveitis, enthesitis)?

Non infectious

Infectious arthritis
• Strep A throat infection
• Bacterial endocarditis
• Gonococcus
• Lyme disease
• Parvovirus

**Seronegative
spondyloarthropathies**
• Ankylosing spondylitis
• Psoriatic arthritis
• Enteropathic arthritis
• Postinfectious
  (Reactive/Reiter's)

**Systemic rheumatic
diseases**
• Rheumatoid arthritis
• Systemic lupus erythematosis
• Systemic vasculitis
• Systemic sclerosis (scleroderma)
• Polymyositis/dermatomyositis

Figure 17.16 Approach to polyarthritis.

Systemic Rheumatic Conditions

Table **17.14**	**Approach to Systemic Autoimmune Rheumatic Diseases**			
	Etiology	**Clinical Signs**	**Investigations**	**Treatment**
Rheumatoid arthritis	Proliferation of synovial tissue forms a pannus which invades and destroys cartilage and bone M:F = 1:2.5	Morning stiffness (2+ h), warm and swollen joints, joint immobility, structural damage; rheumatoid nodules, 2° Sjögren's, interstitial fibrosis, pericardial abnormalities	Elevated ESR, RF, and CRP; joint destruction and deformity on x-ray	NSAIDs, corticosteroids, DMARDs (antimalarials, methotrexate, sulfasalazine, leflunomide, gold), biologics (e.g., TNF-α inhibitors)
SLE	Autoantibodies bind to proteins to form immune complexes which deposit in tissues and trigger inflammatory cascade M:F = 1:9	Nonerosive arthritis, photosensitive (butterfly) rash, discoid rash, hematologic disorders (anemia, leuco/lymphopenia, thrombocytopenia), oral ulcers, serositis, renal dysfunction, neurologic disorders, Raynaud phenomenon	CBC, serum Cr, urinalysis, ANA, anti-dsDNA, anti-Sm, antiphospholipid, no erosions on x-ray	NSAIDs, corticosteroids, antimalarials, azathioprine, cyclophosphamide, methotrexate Note: antimalarials may cause retinal toxicity and patients must have yearly eye exams; methotrexate can cause liver toxicity and LFTs need to be monitored
Systemic sclerosis (scleroderma)	Two types: diffuse (associated with malignant HTN) and limited; fibrosis of the skin with possible visceral organ involvement M:F = 1:3	Raynaud phenomenon, skin changes starting at fingers and toes and extending proximally; tightness, pruritus, pain, flexion contractures, friction rubs; can have interstitial lung disease, heart failure, or arrhythmias, or renal crises	ANA, anticentromere, antitopoisomerase, skin biopsy, Cr, GFR, PFTs, echocardiogram; Scl-70 is associated with ↑ interstitial lung disease	No drugs have been shown to change the course of the disease; Ca^{2+} channel blockers have been used for Raynaud's; physiotherapy and pain management for symptomatic relief
Vasculitis	Inflammatory destruction of blood vessels; Neutrophils invade vessel walls and degranulate leading to scarring and impediment of blood flow	Nonspecific arthralgias, myalgias, neuralgias, small vessel hemorrhage (lungs, kidneys), or palpable purpura **Wegener's:** medium-vessel, lung involvement, rapidly progressive glomerulonephritis). *Henoch–Schönlein purpura:* small-vessel, palpable purpura, arthritis, glomerulonephritis, and abdominal pain **Giant cell arteritis:** see Generalized Pain Disorders	Assess systemic involvement (lung, GI, kidney), biopsy of most accessible organ, ESR, CRP, ANCA (for Wegener's), serum cryoglobulins	Glucocorticoids (prednisone), cytotoxic drugs (azathioprine, cyclophosphamide)
Poly/ dermatomyositis	Muscle inflammation leading to damage and weakness; 15% association with underlying malignancy in older patients; bimodal distribution (10–15 and 45–60); M:F = 1:2	Myalgias, arthralgias, symmetrical muscle weakness with fatigue, morning stiffness, and anorexia; skin manifestations in dermatomyositis: Gottron's papules, heliotrope rash (eyelids), shawl sign, V-sign, dystrophic cuticles	Elevated ESR and CK; consider possibility of underlying malignancy, particularly in older individuals	Physical therapy, corticosteroids

NONINFLAMMATORY

Osteoarthritis

- Most common disease of the joints, one-third of 65+ patients have knee OA
- Cartilage degeneration over time progresses to defects in subchondral bone and bony spurs (osteophytes) then synovial inflammation
- Worsening pain with activity
- Common sites: weight-bearing joints—cervical and lumbar spines, small joints of the hand (DIPs, first CMC), hips, and knees

Investigations

Radiographs show osteophytes, asymmetric narrowing of joint spaces, subchondral sclerosis and cysts.

CLINICAL BOX

Limited Scleroderma (CREST)

- **C**alcinosis
- **R**aynaud phenomenon
- **E**sophageal dysmotility
- **S**clerodactyly
- **T**elangiectasias

CLINICAL BOX

Laboratory Investigations

RF

- AutoAb to IgG
- Positive in 70%–85% of RA patients
- Also positive in Sjögren's, SLE, cryoglobulinemia, and some nonrheumatologic conditions
- Can also be positive in healthy patients
- Not pathognomonic for disease!

ANA

- Positive in 95% of lupus
- 1 of 11 diagnostic criteria for SLE
- Nonspecific
- Also positive in RA, Sjögren's, hepatitis, TB, lymphoma

Anti-dsDNA

- Present in 60%–80% of SLE patients
- Highly specific
- Correlates with active kidney disease

ESR and C-reactive protein

- Nonspecific markers of inflammation

Management

- Weight loss and muscle strengthening
- Topical steroids for small joints
- Acetaminophen, NSAIDs, narcotics, intra-articular steroid injections
- Surgical intervention (arthroscopy, osteotomy, or arthroplasty)

PERIARTICULAR PAIN

DEFINITION

Pain originating from the soft tissue structures surrounding a joint but not from within the joint itself.

CAUSAL CONDITIONS

See Table 17.15 and 17.16.

APPROACH

WORK-RELATED INJURIES

History

What do you do?

How do you do it?

Are you worried? (your occupation has led to your injury)

Coworkers injured?

Satisfied with job?

Table **17.15**	Classification of Periarticular Pain	
Cause	**Characteristic**	**Causal Conditions**
Neuropathic Damage to nerves, spinal cord, or brain	Burning, tingling, numbness, hypersensitivity to temperature, constant, worse at night, unrelated to motion	Compartment syndrome Radiculopathy Neuropathy Postherpetic neuralgia Complex pain syndrome
Myopathic Damage to muscles, tendons, ligaments, or associated soft tissues	Tenderness, stiffness, weakness, muscle spasm, specific trigger points, worse with motion	Infectious • Fasciitis • Abscess • Osteomyelitis • Sepsis • Viral myalgias Degeneration/injury • Tendonitis • Bursitis • Epicondylitis • Muscle strain Idiopathic • Fibromyalgia • PMR • Dermato/polymyositis • Somatoform disorder • Hypermobility syndrome • Myofascial pain syndrome
Nociceptive Injury to body tissues such as incisions, fractures, and neoplasms	Aching, sharp, throbbing, may be constant or intermittent, worse with coughing and deep breathing	Neoplasm Leukemia Osteoporosis Multiple myeloma Osteomalacia

Table **17.16**	Causal Conditions of Periarticular Pain
Neuropathic Pain	
Radiculopathy	Impingement/damage to nerve roots; causes include disk herniation, spondylosis, spondylolisthesis, spinal neoplasm
Neuropathy	Damage to peripheral nerves; causes include infection, diabetes, B12 deficiency, neoplasm
Postherpetic neuralgia	Result of infection with herpes zoster—may be debilitating
Complex pain syndrome (aka reflex sympathetic dystrophy)	Persistent burning pain following injury accompanied by swelling, damage to skin and soft tissues, muscle wasting, bone loss, and sweating; Type I (peripheral injury) and Type II (proximal)
Degeneration/Injury	
Tendinosis	Pain associated with muscle contraction, swelling along the tendon sheath, point tenderness along the tendon
Bursitis	Inflammation in the sac of fluid between tendons, skin, and bone; result from trauma or repetitive motion; common in greater trochanteric bursa, knees, heels, elbows, and shoulders
Epicondylitis	Medial (golfer's elbow) or lateral (tennis elbow); Tendonitis of common wrist flexor (medial) or common wrist extensor (lateral)
Repetitive strain	May be a combination of myopathic and neuropathic pain; muscle imbalances and tightness, pain on soft tissue palpation

Management
- Improve work-station positioning (ergonomics)
- Avoid repetitive tasks
- Evaluate psychosocial factors (worker–employer/worker interactions)

MSK INJURIES

> **CLINICAL BOX**
>
> ### The "4 T"s of Tendon Injuries
>
> - **Tendonitis**—inflammation of tendon
> - **Tendinosis**—degeneration of tendon
> - **Tenosynovitis**—inflammation of tendon sheath
> - **Tendon rupture**—loss of functional integrity of tendon

HYPERMOBILITY SYNDROME/JOINT LAXITY

- Hyperextension of knees, elbows, or MCP joints
- Thought to be a disorder of collagen with ↓ joint capsule stability
- Idiopathic or associated with connective tissue disease (Marfan, Ehlers-Danlos)
- May be asymptomatic or present with soft tissue pain related to affected joints

GENERALIZED PAIN DISORDERS

FIBROMYALGIA

DEFINITION

- Characterized by chronic, diffuse pain, and sleep disturbance
- Etiology/pathophysiology unknown—hypotheses include inability to obtain restful sleep and genetic abnormalities in epi/norepinephrine or substance P
- Affects women between the ages of 30 and 50 disproportionately (F:M = 10:1)
- Patients report overwhelming fatigue and cognitive dysfunction—"fibromyalgia fog"
- Paresthesias, fine motor weakness, chest pain, Raynaud phenomena, and GI complaints can accompany fibromyalgia

CAUSAL CONDITIONS

Other conditions which mimic fibromyalgia include: drug-induced myopathy, thyroid disorders, PMR, RA, SLE, and PTSD.

Table **17.17** Differential Diagnosis of Fibromyalgia				
Depression	**Temperomandibular Syndrome (Clencher Syndrome)**	**Somatoform/Somatization Disorder**	**Regional Myofascial Pain Syndrome**	**Chronic Widespread Pain**
Major depression is a comorbidity in 30% of fibromyalgia patients; some patients may benefit from a referral to a psychiatrist or psychologist	TMJ complaints are common among fibromyalgia patients; may be due to muscle tightness, arthritis, ankylosis, or hypermobility of the TMJ	Psychologic disorder where mental health complaints (depression, anxiety, etc.) manifest themselves as physical symptoms; **see Chapter 19**	↓ ROM and regional, unilateral pain due to taut muscle bands; affected regions tender to palpation; treated with physiotherapy and targeted steroid injections	Idiopathic, widespread tenderness for >3 mo, not limited to tender points; may benefit from psychotherapeutic counseling

APPROACH

Diagnosis

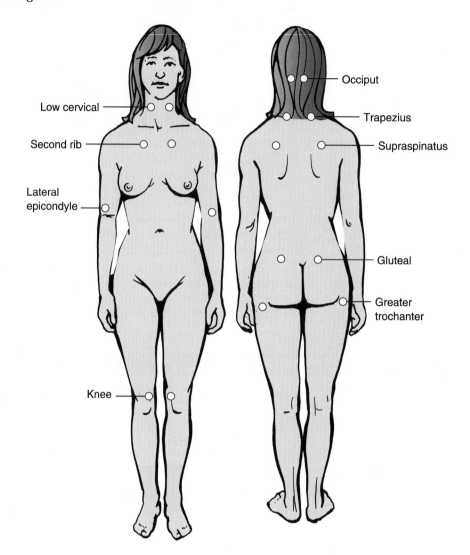

Figure 17.17 The patient must have widespread pain (left and right, above and below the waist, and axial skeleton pain) plus pain in 11/18 tender points upon digital palpation. Digital palpation should use ~4 kg of force—enough to blanch a fingernail. Examiners should examine the patient's face to evaluate pain instead of asking "is this tender?" There are no abnormal laboratory tests or imaging studies and the diagnosis is one of exclusion.

Management
- Patient education
- Sleep hygiene (regular hours, temperature regulation, limited noise, no stimulants)
- Exercise (walking, yoga, swimming) has been shown to reduce pain and fatigue
- Pharmacologic: TCAs (amitriptyline), gabapentin/pregabalin (Note: NSAIDs and corticosteroids are not efficacious and opioids should be avoided because of dependency risk)
- CBT, biofeedback therapy

PMR

DEFINITION

- Systemic inflammation (elevated ESR and anemia of chronic disease): constitutional symptoms (fever, malaise, anorexia), aches and pains in neck, shoulders, and pelvic girdle
- Presents in patients over the age of 50, more common in women
- Pathophysiology: nonerosive articular and periarticular synovitis
- Associated, in some cases, with temporal arteritis and anemia
- Rapid response to low-dose corticosteroids

CLINICAL BOX

Diagnosis of PMR requires ESR >50 mm/h and exclusion of:

- Connective tissue disease
- Rheumatoid arthritis
- Malignancy
- Infection

APPROACH

Management
- 10–15 mg/d of prednisone slowly tapered over 1–2 yr (if no response within 72 h, consider alternate diagnosis)
- Physiotherapy to maintain and restore ROM
- Temporal artery biopsy if vasculitis suspected (headaches, visual changes, scalp tenderness)

CLINICAL BOX

Adverse Effects of Corticosteroids

- Infection (check TB status)
- Osteoporosis
- Anxiety
- Hyperglycemia in diabetic patients
- Hypoadrenalism if withdrawn inappropriately

GIANT CELL ARTERITIS

DEFINITION
- Most common form of systemic vasculitis in elderly adults, common with PMR
- Affects extracranial branches of carotid artery (temporal artery)
- Causes headache, jaw claudication, fever, and visual symptoms such as amaurosis fugax—may lead to blindness if not promptly treated with glucocorticoids

APPROACH

Diagnosis
- Gold standard for diagnosis is temporal artery biopsy, but if suspected, treat first and biopsy later (bilateral biopsies within a week).

Management
- Requires higher doses of prednisone (40–60 mg/d initially then slow taper)
- May also require low-dose ASA (81 mg/d) initially

Giant cell arteritis can lead to blindness—treat promptly with glucocorticoids if suspected—diagnostic biopsy can be conducted later.

CHAPTER 18

Pediatrics

Naminder K. Sandhu, Dr. Tehseen Ladha, and Dr. Valerie G. Kirk

ABDOMINAL PAIN

CAUSAL CONDITIONS

CAUSES CATEGORIZED BY ACUTE VERSUS CHRONIC

Acute

Upper/Epigastric

- Liver: acute hepatitis
- Gallbladder: cholecystitis
- Pancreas: pancreatitis
- Lungs: pneumonia
- Stomach: foreign body ingestion, pyloric stenosis
- Functional

Lower

- Bowel: gastroenteritis, constipation, Meckel diverticulum, IBD, imperforate anus, HUS, HSP, foreign body ingestion
- Appendicitis*
- Mesenteric lymphadenitis

Table **18.1**	**Organic vs. Functional Pain**	
	Organic	**Functional**
Hx	Progressive	Poor Miss school Maladaptive coping
Pain	Away from midline +/− At night	Close to midline Not localized Not at night
Systemic or extraintestinal symptoms	Yes FTT possible	No
Bloody stools Emesis Diarrhea	Yes	No
Exam	+/− Abnormal	Normal
Labs	+/− Abnormal	Normal

---

* Emergencies!

- Urinary tract: UTI/pyelonephritis, urolithiasis
- Male GU: incarcerated inguinal hernia*, testicular torsion*
- Gynecologic: ectopic pregnancy, endometriosis, ovarian torsion*, pelvic inflammatory disease

Generalized

Peritoneal*: trauma, ruptured viscus, bacterial peritonitis

- Infantile colic
- Obstruction: Hirschsprung*, intussusception*, malrotation with volvulus*, constipation, Meckel diverticulum, adhesions, duodenal atresia Lungs: bacterial pneumonia
- Malabsorption: lactose intolerance, milk proteins, CF
- Infectious/inflammatory: gastroenteritis, HSP, HUS
- Metabolic: DKA
- Functional

Chronic

Upper/Epigastric

- Esophagus/stomach: GERD, water brash, infantile colic
- Functional

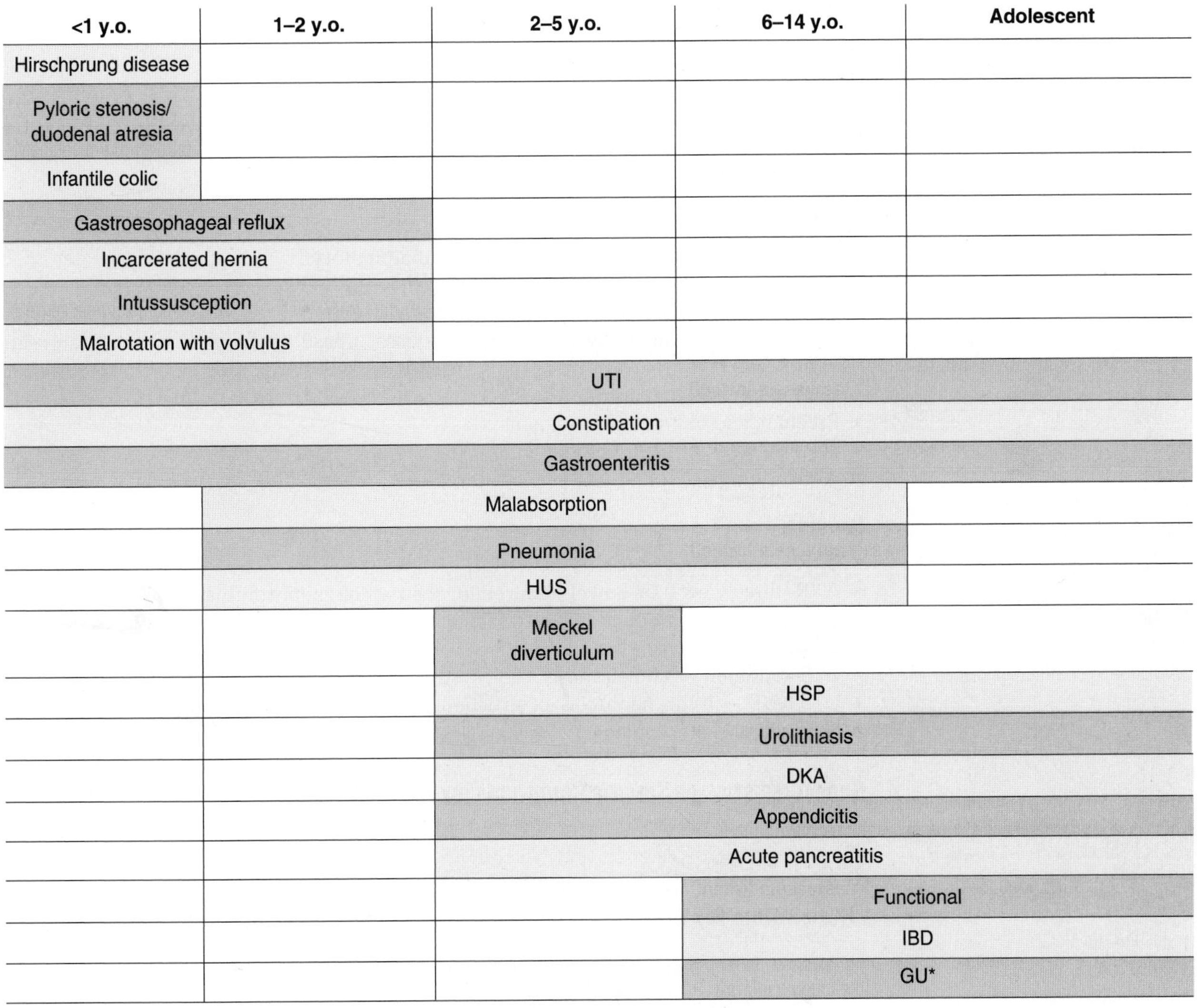

<1 y.o.	1–2 y.o.	2–5 y.o.	6–14 y.o.	Adolescent
Hirschsprung disease				
Pyloric stenosis/ duodenal atresia				
Infantile colic				
Gastroesophageal reflux				
Incarcerated hernia				
Intussusception				
Malrotation with volvulus				
UTI				
Constipation				
Gastroenteritis				
	Malabsorption			
	Pneumonia			
	HUS			
		Meckel diverticulum		
		HSP		
		Urolithiasis		
		DKA		
		Appendicitis		
		Acute pancreatitis		
			Functional	
			IBD	
			GU*	

* Includes testicular/ovarian torsion, endometriosis, ectopic pregnancy

Figure 18.1 Causes of abdominal pain by age.

Lower

- Bowel: IBD, malabsorption, bacterial overgrowth
- Functional

Generalized

- Infantile colic
- Obstruction: constipation
- Malabsorption: celiac, lactose intolerance
- Infectious/inflammatory: IBD, HSP, HUS
- Functional

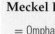

CLINICAL BOX

Meckel Diverticulum

= Omphalomesenteric duct remnant
- Symptoms rare
- Painless lower GI bleeding (40% to 60%)
- Intestinal obstruction (25%)
- Less common: diverticulitis, perforation + peritonitis

Diagnosis: 99mTc-pertechnetate scan

Treatment: surgical

Rule of 2s:
- Most common ~2 yr of age
- Affects 2% of population
- ~2 in. in length
- 2 ft proximal to ileocecal valve

CLINICAL BOX

Infants

Determine whether an acute organic cause for the pain exists and differentiate from infantile colic or constipation

Suspect GERD if have reflux + aspiration, esophagitis, or FTT

CLINICAL BOX

HUS Triad

1. Uremia
2. Thrombocytopenia
3. Microangiopathic hemolytic anemia

MANAGEMENT

LAB TESTS

- CBC and WBC differential → infectious/inflammatory
- Blood/urine cultures → sepsis
- Serum Lytes, glucose, Cr, BUN → metabolic
- Total/direct bilirubin, liver enzymes, amylase, lipase → hepatic, biliary, pancreatic pathology
- U/A → pyuria, hematuria
- Pregnancy test → ectopic pregnancy
- Stool → fecal fat, occult blood
- Antiendomysial antibodies → celiac disease

IMAGING

- CXR → pulmonary process
- AXR (three views) → bowel perforation, obstruction, nephrolithiasis, volvulus
- CT abdomen → appendicitis, pancreatitis, intra-abdominal abscess, mesenteric ischemia
- U/S abdomen → cholelithiasis, cholecystitis, intussusception, appendicitis
- U/S KUB → hydronephrosis, obstruction *(kidney/ureter/bladder)*
- U/S pelvis → gynecologic pathology

CHARACTERISTICS OF SPECIFIC CONDITIONS (BY AGE)

CLINICAL BOX

Indications for Emergency Surgery versus Medical Care

- Vascular compromise: strangulated hernia/torsion/necrotic bowel
- Obstruction (fixed): atresia/stenosis of GI tract
- Perforation (or risk/impending i.e., appendicitis)

DKA Precipitants

- Insulin deficiency
- Infection
- Ischemia
- Intoxication

Table **18.2**	Characteristics of Specific Conditions of Abdominal Pain (by Age)		
Condition	**Hx**	**Physical Exam**	**Investigations**
Hirschsprung disease	• Delayed meconium • FTT • Chronic constipation since birth	Abdominal distension Tight anal sphincter	Barium enema: narrow distal colon Definitive diagnosis by rectal biopsy: absence of ganglion cells
Pyloric stenosis	• Symptoms ~2–4 wk old • Poor feeding • Projectile nonbilious vomiting	FTT Possible palpable epigastric mass ("olive sign")	U/S: hypertrophied pylorus
Duodenal atresia	• Colicky abdominal pain + bilious vomiting within hours of birth (longer if stenosis vs. atresia)	Epigastric distension	AXR: "double bubble" sign
Infantile colic	• Rule of 3s: healthy infant who cries for >3 h/d, >3 d/wk, for >3 wk • See Crying/fussing child	Healthy appearing infant	No investigations Results normal
Gastroesophageal reflux/GERD	• Regurgitation/emesis, feeding aversion • "Colicky baby" • Apnea, stridor, aspiration • Sandifer syndrome: neck contortions with discomfort	+/− FTT (in GERD) +/− Hoarseness/stridor	Empiric antireflux therapy Upper GI series: anatomic abnormality Endoscopy: esophagitis pH probe
Incarcerated inguinal hernia	• Irritable and crying • Vomiting, abdominal distension • Groin pain • Classic Hx = swelling in inguinal area during periods of crying/straining	Abdominal distension/tenderness	Clinical U/S
Intussusception	• 3 mo–3 y.o. (up to 6 y.o.) • Paroxysmal, severe, crampy abdominal pain, inconsolable crying, drawing up legs • Episodes progressively more frequent +/− vomiting • Watery ("current jelly") stools • May behave normally between episodes; progressive lethargy	Abdomen benign/soft (+/− palpable sausage shaped RUQ mass)	Air contrast enema: obstruction, air fluid levels, absence of gas in RLQ Occult blood positive
Malrotation with volvulus	• Sudden onset bilious emesis, abdominal distension, melena	Abdominal distension/tenderness	AXR (barium enema): • Sigmoid: "coffee bean sign" • Cecal: small bowel dilation • Small bowel: "corkscrew" sign— best seen on CT Upper GI series: failure of duodenum to cross midline
UTI	• Irritability, fever, poor feeding • Vomiting or diarrhea • Flank or abdominal pain • Dysuria, urgency, frequency	Tender abdomen/flanks Fever	Urine R&M (WBC, nitrites, leukocyte esterase), C&S − culture/sensitivity Voiding cystogram, renal U/S after treatment
Constipation	• Rectal impaction • Lower, colicky, abdominal pain • Associated encopresis	Fecal mass on abdominal/rectal exam	AXR: fecal impaction
Gastroenteritis (70%–80% viral, 10%–20% bacterial, 5% parasitic)	• Fever, severe abdominal cramping pain, subsequent diarrhea	Soft, tender abdomen Fever possible	Stool C&S, stool O&P (ova & parasites)
Pneumonia	• Respiratory tract symptoms • N/V • Upper abdominal pain	Tachypnea, hypoxia, abnormal lung sounds	Possible ↑ WBC CXR: consolidation

(Continued)

Table **18.2** *(continued)*

Condition	Hx	Physical Exam	Investigations
HUS (*E. coli* 0157:H7 verotoxin—"Hamburger disease")	• Prodromal gastroenteritis, fever, bloody diarrhea • Irritability, lethargy, edema, pallor	Toxic, +/− uremic Tender abdomen Hypertension	CBC + blood smear: hemolytic anemia, ↓ plts Cr ↑ (ARF) U/A: proteinuria, hematuria
HSP	• Colicky abdominal pain associated with vomiting • Pain within week(s) of rash • Melena/hematochezia • Arthralgias • Rare complications: intussusception, pancreatitis, protein-losing enteropathy	Purpura rash on lower extremities, arthralgias	Leukocytosis, maybe thrombocytosis Occult blood positive ESR variably ↑ Hematuria Cr ↑
Urolithiasis	• Colicky flank pain, radiating to testes or labia • N/V, chills, ileus	Fever Tender abdomen +/− costovertebral angle	Radiopaque stones on AXR; CT gold standard U/S: obstruction of GU system, hydronephrosis
DKA	• Abdominal pain, N/V, anorexia • Dehydration • Altered LOC • Polyuria, polydipsia	Dehydration Diffuse abdominal tenderness Kussmaul breaths	↑ Glucose AG metabolic acidosis Positive urine/serum ketones +/− ↑ WBC, Cr, and BUN
Appendicitis	• Abdominal wall rigidity • Periumbilical pain, migrating to RLQ	Fever RLQ tenderness McBurney point +/− Peritonitis	U/S: thick-walled/dilated appendix, appendicolith CT: enlarged appendix, appendicolith, stranding
Pancreatitis	• Severe persistent pain radiating to back + vomiting (+/− bilious) • Fever, anorexia	Fever Tender, distended abdomen Periumbilical or flank bruising (hemorrhage)	↑ Lipase, ↑ WBC U/S: hypoechoic enlarged pancreas CT: edema, fat stranding, pseudocyst, necrosis, hemorrhage
Cholecystitis	• Pain steady, severe +/− radiate to shoulder/back • N/V, fever, anorexia • Fatty meal ingestion before onset of pain	Fever, tachycardia Tender abdomen +/− Murphy sign	U/S: thick wall, gallstones, dilated gallbladder
IBD	• FTT, anemia • Abdominal pain • Perianal disease • Bloody diarrhea • Arthritis	Tender abdomen; RLQ mass (Crohns); oral ulcers; perianal fistulae, anal tags, fissure; rash; arthritis	↑ WBC and plts, Anemia ↑ ESR, Depressed albumin Stool positive for blood, WBC
GU Testicular torsion	• Severe sudden onset testicular or scrotal pain, +/− inguinal/lower abdominal pain • Nausea, vomiting, fever • Pain awakens at night	Tender testicle, elevated +/− horizontally displaced	Scrotal doppler U/S: compromised flow
Ectopic pregnancy	• Sexual Hx • Missed periods	Painful internal pelvic exam +/− Peritonitis	Pregnancy test positive Pelvic U/S: ectopic pregnancy
Endometriosis	• Dysmenorrhea • Abnormal bleeding	General tenderness on internal exam	Pregnancy test negative Pelvic U/S: uterine tissue outside of uterus
Ovarian torsion	• Sudden unilateral abdominal/pelvic pain +/− N/V	Painful unilateral adnexa +/− Peritonitis	Pregnancy test negative Pelvic U/S: ovarian torsion

Table **18.3**	Management of Specific Conditions	
Condition	**Medical/Conservative Management**	**Surgical Management**
Constipation	• Diet modification, bowel routine	
Gastroenteritis	• Oral rehydration; treat etiology	
UTI	• Antibiotics	
Functional/infantile colic	• Patient/parent education, reassurance • Address psychosocial issues	
Pancreatitis	• Aggressive fluid resuscitation • Monitor/correct Lytes • NPO and NG decompression • Pain management • Broad-spectrum antibiotics if necrosis • Treat etiology	
HSP	• Bedrest, hydration, pain control • **Systemic corticosteroids** for severe **abdominal** pain	
HUS	• Monitor/correct fluids and Lytes • Red cell and Plt transfusions • Strict control of hypertension and nutrition; possible dialysis	
Acute intestinal obstruction	• Stabilize ABCs • IV fluid resuscitation • Broad-spectrum antibiotics if suspecting necrosis/perforation • NG tube decompression • Treat etiology	• If necrosis/perforation
Appendicitis	• IV antibiotics if perforated	• Appendectomy
Intussusception	• IV resuscitation, NG decompression • Reduction with air contrast enema	• If symptoms >24 h or signs of peritonitis
Incarcerated hernia	• If nonstrangulating: nonoperative reduction with sedation	• Surgical reduction if unable to reduce or frank peritonitis
IBD	• Immunosuppressive therapy (Azathioprine)	• Bowel resection if refractory to medical management
Pyloric stenosis		• Pyloromyotomy
Malrotation with midgut volvulus		• Ladd procedure
Duodenal atresia/stenosis		• Duodenoduodenostomy or duodenojejunostomy
Testicular torsion		• Removal or orchiopexy

DEPRESSED NEWBORN (CYANOSIS/HYPOXEMIA/HYPOXIA IN CHILDREN)

See also Chapter 20 (Respirology).

RATIONALE

- Physician must be prepared to manage "routine" delivery as well as newborn requiring resuscitation.
- Cyanosis is an ominous finding; the differentiation between peripheral and central is essential to mount appropriate management.

CAUSAL CONDITIONS

- Respiratory problems
- RDS (in premature infants)
- Birth asphyxia or CNS depression (maternal drugs)
- Meconium aspiration
- Sepsis
- Pneumothorax
- Severe anemia (erythroblastosis fetalis and secondary hydrops fetalis)
- Maternal causes
- Drugs (e.g., opiates)
- Diabetes mellitus
- Pregnancy-induced hypertension
- Congenital malformations/birth injury
- Shock/cyanosis/congenital heart disease
- Other (hypothermia, hypoglycemia, etc.)

APPROACH

Hx

- **Maternal:** illnesses, drug use, previous high-risk pregnancies, blood type and Rh status
- **Pregnancy:** infections, poly- or oligohydramnios, gestational age
- **Labor/delivery:** duration of rupture of membranes, hemorrhage, meconium, Apgar score, morphine administration, maternal fever

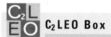 **C₂LEO Box**

Truth Telling

Recognize the duty to provide necessary emergency care where consent is unavailable.

- On occasion, the depressed newborn may be very premature, and resuscitation may be considered.
- On other occasions, continuing or discontinuing resuscitation may become an issue; may become necessary to seek guidance, due to a conflict between initiation and continuation of resuscitation and the duty to do no harm.

INVESTIGATIONS

- CBC, blood gas, Lytes, random glucose, blood/urine cultures, consider LP
- CXR
- Echocardiogram

MANAGEMENT

- Identify need of prompt respiratory support, and circulatory support (consider umbilical vein for quick venous access)
- Avoid hypothermia and hypoglycemia
- In the presence of thick meconium, clear from airway before ventilation
- Initiate investigations

Table **18.4**	APGAR Scoring System		
Sign	**0 Point**	**1 Point**	**2 Points**
Appearance (color)	Blue, pale	Body pink, extremities blue	All pink
Pulse	Absent	<100	>100
Grimace (reflex irritability)	No response	Grimace	Vigorous cry
Activity (muscle tone)	Flaccid	Some flexion of extremities	Active motion
Respiratory effort	Absent	Slow, irregular	Good, crying

CYANOSIS/HYPOXEMIA/HYPOXIA IN CHILDREN

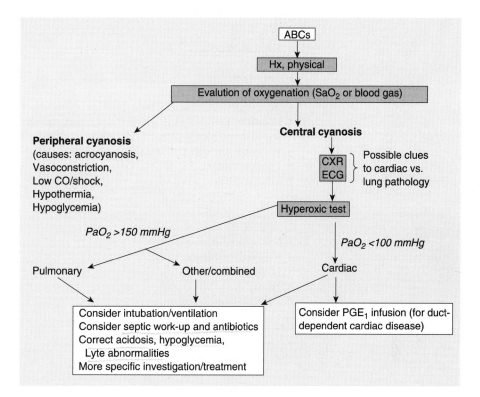

Figure 18.2 Approach to the cyanotic infant.

CLINICAL BOX

Peripheral versus Central Cyanosis

Central cyanosis = bluish discoloration visible in lips and mucous membranes signifying reduced SaO_2 of arterial blood.

- Caused by various mechanisms: hypoventilation, significant right-to-left intracardiac or intrapulmonary shunting, ventilation–perfusion mismatch, diffusion impairment (rare), inadequate transport of O_2 by the hemoglobin

Peripheral cyanosis = dusky or bluish tinge to extremities caused by impaired tissue delivery of adequately saturated blood in low-output states, polycythemia, or peripheral vasoconstriction.

- Process may be due to hypoxemia if central cyanosis also present

CAUSAL CONDITIONS

NEONATAL CYANOSIS

Pulmonary

Upper

- Choanal atresia
- TEF
- Laryngeal web

Lower

Congenital

- CDH — *congenital diaphragm hernie*
- Pulmonary hypoplasia
- CCAM — *congenital cystic adenomatos malformatio*

- Pulmonary sequestration
- Teratoma

Acquired

- RDS
- Aspiration
- TTN
- Pneumonia
- Pulmonary hemorrhage
- Pulmonary lymphangiectasia
- Location: elevated neck veins, third heart sound, laterally displaced point of maximal impulse, with or without pulmonary crackles/wheezes with or without pedal edema, with or without hepatomegaly, with or without cool extremities, ↓ pulse pressure
- Pneumothorax
- Pleural effusion

PPHN — Persistent pulmonary HTN

Miscellaneous

- Methemoglobinemia
- Metabolic acidosis
- Hypoglycemia
- Sepsis
- Polycythemia

Cardiac

- The five **T**s:
  - **T**ransposition of great arteries (TGA)
  - **T**etralogy of Fallot (TOF)
  - **T**otal anomalous pulmonary venous drainage (TAPVD)
  - **T**runcus arteriosus
  - **T**ricuspid atresia
- Pulmonary stenosis/atresia
- Ebstein anomaly (displacement of tricuspid valve toward apex of right ventricle)
- Left-to-right shunt with pulmonary edema
- Single ventricle states
- Low CO states

CNS

- Cerebral edema or hemorrhage
- Infection
- Hypoventilation
- Asphyxia
- Vocal cord paralysis or paresis

Peripheral cyanosis

- Vascular ("physiologic acrocyanosis")
- Sepsis
- Cardiogenic/septic shock
- Thrombosis
- Vasomotor instability
- Coarctation
- Aortic stenosis

INFANT/CHILD CYANOSIS

Pulmonary

Upper

Congenital

- Laryngotracheomalacia
- Subglottic stenosis
- Vocal cord paralysis

- Glossoptosis with micrognathia
- Choanal atresia

Acquired
- Croup
- Tracheitis

Lower
- Bronchiolitis
- Asthma
- CF
- Foreign body
- Aspiration
- Pneumonia
- Pneumothorax
- Pleural effusion
- Embolus

Cardiac
- Congenital heart disease
- Myocarditis
- Cardiomyopathy
- Dysrhythmia

CNS Depression
- Encephalitis
- Toxins
- Metabolic
- Neuromuscular

Peripheral Cyanosis
- Vascular (Raynaud, sepsis, thrombosis)
- Obstruction (superior vena cava syndrome, venous thrombosis, compartment syndrome)
- Hyperviscosity (polycythemia)

APPROACH

Hx

CLINICAL BOX

Risk Factors: Neonatal Disease

	Maternal Hx	
Risk factor	**Condition**
Diabetes	TTN, RDS, hypoglycemia
Drugs	Narcotic withdrawal
Pregnancy-induced hypertension	IUGR, polycythemia, hypoglycemia
Polyhydramnios	TEF — *Tracheoesophageal fistule*
Oligohydramnios	Pulmonary hypoplasia

	Labor and delivery	
Risk factor	**Condition**
Prolonged rupture of membranes	Sepsis, pneumonia
Anesthesia/analgesia	Depression, apnea, cyanosis
Asphyxia	Cerebral edema, metabolic acidosis
Chorioamnionitis	Sepsis
C/S without labor	TTN, RDS, PPHN
Breech	Trauma, Erb palsy with phrenic nerve palsy

If respiratory distress is not present at birth but develops over the first few hours, consider cardiac etiologies.

Newborn

Maternal Hx of illness in pregnancy, gestational age, delivery complications, presence of meconium, suction of infant, Apgar score, family Hx of congenital heart disease

Older Child
Acute versus chronic or recurrent cyanosis, lung or heart disease, foreign body or aspiration, fever, upper respiratory symptoms, exposure to medications/dyes/chemicals

PHYSICAL EXAM
Newborn
- Age of infant (ductus arteriosus closes by third day)
- Vital signs: peripheral pulses, BP, fever, tachypnea, tachycardia, beat-to-beat variability in HR
- Respiratory status: distress (tachypnea, grunting, flaring, retracting), air entry, stridor or wheeze, level of obstruction
- Perfusion: pallor, cyanosis, peripheral pulses, BP in all limbs, shock
- Ability to feed
- Cardiac: S2 may be loud and narrowly split in pulmonary hypertension; single S2 indicative of severe pulmonic stenosis or atresia, abnormal single-valve position (TGA), or presence of one large semilunar valve (i.e., truncus arteriosus)
- Evidence of CHF
- Abdomen: scaphoid (CDH), distension (bowel obstruction or ascites), hepatosplenomegaly (hemolytic disease), absence of bowel sounds (ileus)
- CNS: mental status, hypotonia (early sign of sepsis, asphyxia, or metabolic disorders), hypertonia (narcotic withdrawal)

Older Child
- Vital signs: hypotension or bradycardia (ominous signs), tachypnea
- Respiratory distress
- Obtundation of neurologic disease
- Perfusion: cyanosis, clubbing
- Cardiac: murmurs or extra heart sounds

INVESTIGATIONS
- Pulse oximetry: to detect the gradient across the ductus arteriosus: pulse oximeter probe over right hand and a lower extremity
- Arterial blood gases to determine oxygenation, ventilation, and acid–base status of infant
- CBC: rule out polycythemia, anemia, neutropenia, leukopenia, abnormal immature-to-total-neutrophil ratio, and thrombocytopenia as signs of sepsis
- Blood culture +/− LP if sepsis suspected
- Lytes: metabolic acidosis (e.g., closure of ductus in ductal-dependent cardiac disease)
- Urine metabolic and/or drug screen
- CXR (see below)
- ECG: arrhythmias
- Echocardiogram = gold standard in congenital cardiac lesions and pulmonary hypertension
- U/S: detect pleural effusion, eventration of diaphragm, and the size and location of liver and spleen

CXR
See Table 18.5.

Hyperoxia Test: Distinguishing Cardiac versus Respiratory Causes
- Indication: central cyanosis; infant's pulse oximeter reading is <85% in both room air and 100% O_2
- Method: arterial blood gas from a site distal to the ductus on room air and after 10 min of 100% O_2

    Note: Some cardiac defects such as TAPVD and hypoplastic left heart syndrome may respond. Severe pulmonary disease with a massive intrapulmonary shunt may not respond.

MANAGEMENT
- ABCs (and consider NICU/ICU admission if unstable/risk of deterioration)
- O_2 administration: air/O_2 blender + nasal cannula or O_2 hood—adjust flow and concentration of O_2 delivered based on Sao_2—aim for 90% to 95%, higher if PPHN suspected

CLINICAL BOX

Upper versus Lower Airway Obstruction

Upper
- Stridor
- Supraclavicular, submandibular, suprasternal retractions

Lower
- Intercostal, subcostal retractions
- Wheeze

CLINICAL BOX

Hyperoxia Test

- If there is right-to-left shunting in cyanotic heart disease, no amount of oxygenation in pulmonary circulation will alter desaturating effect of the shunt.
- A pulmonary defect causing cyanosis can be corrected by increasing inspired O_2.

CLINICAL BOX

Limitations of the Hyperoxia Test

- Not as reliable as echocardiogram and not as important as resuscitation and attendance to cardiorespiratory support, especially if in acidosis or respiratory distress
- Only saturations measured and not arterial Pao_2—use in conjunction with clinical assessment

Table **18.5**	CXR Signs and Diagnosis	
Sign	**Finding**	**Diagnosis**
Size and shape of heart	Egg shaped	Transposition of the great vessels
	Snowman sign	Total anomalous pulmonary venous return
	Boot shaped	Tetralogy of Fallot
	Cardiomegaly	Ebstein anomaly, cardiomyopathy, congestive cardiac failure
Pulmonary vascular markings	↑	Left-to-right shunt
	↓	Pulmonary stenosis, pulmonary atresia
Lung volume	Hyperinflated	Diaphragmatic paralysis, cystic lesions of lungs
	↓	Pneumothorax, atelectasis, pulmonary hypoplasia
Lung fields	Hazy with normal lung volume, ↑ parahilar markings, fluid in the horizontal fissure	TTN — Transient Tachipnea of NB
	Reticular granular pattern, air bronchograms	RDS (hyaline membrane disease)
	Fluffy infiltrates, patchy areas of atelectasis, areas of hyperinflation caused by air trapping	Meconium aspiration syndrome
Costophrenic angle	Air fluid level	Pleural effusion
Bony structures	Fractures of the ribs, humerus, or clavicles	

- Needle aspiration of the chest followed by chest-tube insertion in tension pneumothorax
- NPO + IV fluids (10% dextrose solution during first day of life)—maximize tissue perfusion
- If poor perfusion: administer 20 mL/kg normal saline bolus initially
- Monitor: vital signs (including Sao2), cardiorespiratory monitor, blood glucose
- Neutral thermal environment under a radiant warmer or incubator
- Orogastric or NG tube to: rule out TEF with esophageal atresia, empty the stomach, and prevent gastric distention
- If ductal-dependent congenital heart disease suspected and echocardiogram is not available, consider starting PGE1 infusion—intubation set up at bedside due to risk of apnea
- Risk of withholding infusion usually greater than associated risks
- No true contraindications except infants with TAPVD may worsen
- Treat metabolic acidosis
- Antibiotics in sepsis: ampicillin and cefotaxime or gentamicin, pending culture results
- Referral for specialized care

PDA
- Premature infants with hemodynamically significant PDA may require NSAID.
- Treatment surgical when PDA large except in patients with pulmonary vascular obstructive disease.
- Patients with large left-to-right shunts and pulmonary hypertension should be operated on early in life to prevent development of progressive pulmonary vascular obstructive disease.

Table **18.6**	Hyperoxia Test	
Response	**Interpretation**
Pao2 >150 mm Hg or Sao2 ↑ by 15%	Pulmonary disease likely also: polycythemia, sepsis, shock
Pao2 <100 mm Hg, rise by <30 mm Hg or Sao2 unchanged	Cardiac cause or PPHN likely

- Symptomatic PDA common problem in preterm infants → indomethacin (prostaglandin synthesis inhibitor) routinely used to close the PDA (and therefore left-to-right shunt)
- Note: Indomethacin does not close the PDA of full-term infants or children.
- "Tet spells" in patient with TOF — *Tetrology of Elob*

Hypoxemic/cyanotic spells characterized by: (a) sudden onset of cyanosis or deepening of cyanosis; (b) sudden dyspnea; (c) alterations in consciousness, from irritability to syncope; and (d) ↓ or disappearance of the systolic murmur

Treatment = O_2 and placing the patient in the knee-chest position → ↓ systemic venous return, may ↑ SVR, raising arterial SaO_2

DEVELOPMENT DISORDER/DELAY

DEFINITION

Developmental delay = child not reaching milestones at expected age (a symptom, not a diagnosis)

APPLIED SCIENTIFIC CONCEPTS

Table 18.7   Developmental Milestones

Age	Gross Motor	Fine Motor	Language	Social
Newborn	Raises head slightly, hands fisted	Tight grasp, follows to midline	Alerts to sound	Regards face
2–3 mo	Holds head in midline, lifts chest, supports on forearms	Follows past midline, holds hands open	Smiles to stroking or being spoken to, coos	Recognizes parent, moves arms actively to stimulus, anticipates feeds
4–5 mo	Rolls front-back/back-front, sits when propped, supports on wrists	Moves arms in unison to grasp, touches toy	Orients to voice, razzes	Enjoys looking at environment, reaches out for toys, laughs
6–8 mo	Sits unsupported, feet to mouth while supine	Reaches with one hand, transfers, raking grasp	Babbles, responds to name, indiscriminant dada/momma	Recognizes stranger
8–12 mo	Creeps, crawls, cruises, pulls to stand	Pincer grasp, probes with forefinger, holds bottle	Understands "no", waves	Explores environment, object permanence
12–18 mo	Walks alone, creeps upstairs	Throws objects, scribbles in imitation, builds two-block tower	Uses two words, runs unintelligible words together	Imitates, comes when called, cooperates with dressing, indicates wants
18–24 mo	Runs, throws toys, kicks balls, walks upstairs	Turns two pages at a time, spoon feeds self	Knows eight body parts, uses intelligible words in jargoning, >20 words	Copies tasks, plays alongside other children, seeks approval
2–3 yr	Walks up + down stairs, overhand throw	Turns pages one at a time, removes clothes, holds pencil	>50 words and 2-word sentences, 25% intelligible	Parallel play, imaginary play, gender aware
3 yr	Pedals tricycle, alternates feet up stairs	Dresses and undresses partially, copies circle	3-word sentences, minimum 250 words, knows own name, 75% intelligible	Group play, shares toys
4 yr	Hops, skips	Buttons, catches ball, copies square	Colors, asks questions	Tells tales, plays cooperatively
5 yr	Skips alternating feet, jumps over obstacles	Ties shoes, copies triangle	Prints first name	Plays competitive games, follows rules

CAUSAL CONDITIONS AND APPROACH

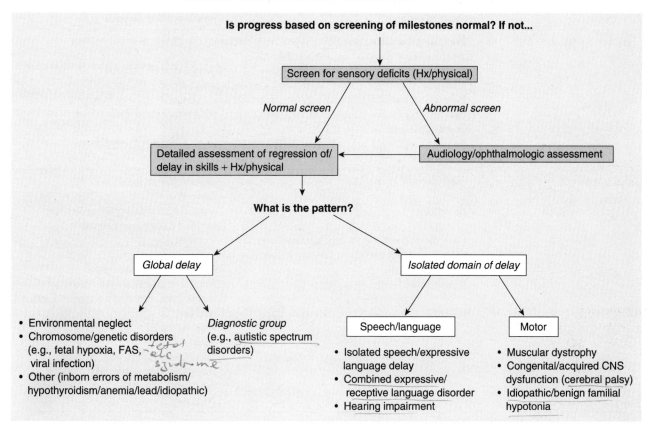

Figure 18.3 Causes and approach to developmental delay.

Hearing Impairment: Risk Factors

- NICU admission >48 h
- Recurrent/chronic otitis media
- Associated syndromic features
- Family Hx
- Bacterial meningitis
- TORCH infection
- Head trauma
- Birthweight <1,500 g
- Low Apgar score
- Ototoxic drugs
- Hyperbilirubinemia requiring exchange transfusion

Referral to audiologist or speech/language pathologist if:

- Does not react to sound in first 3 mo
- Does not respond to smiles and interactions at 4 to 6 mo
- Does not babble or try to talk or stops babbling by 12 mo
- No single words by 16 mo
- Uses more gestures than words or does not talk or understand simple words at 18 mo to 2 yr
- No two-word phrases by 24 mo
- Speech hard for strangers to understand or difficulty playing imaginary games at 3 to 4 yr
- Stutters or does not follow directions at 4 to 5 yr

Speech/Language Delay: Risk Factors

1. **Family/environmental:** family Hx of hearing or speech/language problems or cognitive limitation, children in foster care, family Hx of child maltreatment
2. **Genetic/congenital:** prenatal complications, prematurity, microcephaly, teratogen exposure, FAS, genetic disorders, dysmorphic features, positive toxicology screen at birth
3. **Medical conditions:** ear/hearing problems, oral motor/feeding problems, cleft lip/palate, tracheotomy, autism, FTT, ototoxic drugs, recurrent otitis/mastoiditis

Table **18.8**	Critical Clinical and Lab Findings in Developmental Delay	
	Assessment/Variable	**Relevance/Significance**
Historical risk factors	**Prenatal maternal factors:** alcohol or other drug/medication use, chronic or acute infectious exposure/illness, previous miscarriage or stillbirth **Perinatal:** obstetrical complications, prematurity, low birth weight, multiple gestation **Neonatal:** neurologic events, sepsis/meningitis, severe hyperbilirubinemia, hypoxia **Postnatal:** recurrent otitis media, poor feeding/growth, toxic exposure, head injury, meningitis **Family:** consanguinity, mental functioning, developmental delay, chromosomal abnormalities, deafness/blindness **Social:** family composition (teenage or single parent), stresses (e.g., alcohol), family violence, limited financial support, Hx of neglect of sexual abuse[a]	
Physical exam	Short stature Obesity Head size Facial dysmorphism: low set ears, epicanthal folds, thin upper lip, wide set eyes FTT, hepatomegaly Genitalia size Skin lesions MSK: muscle hypertrophy/wasting, contractures Neurologic: tone, ataxia	Williams, Turner, malnutrition Prader-Willi Some metabolic syndromes; small = any condition causing brain retardation Trisomies, FAS Metabolic/storage disorders Hypogonadism: Prader-Willi, Klinefelter, Charge association; macro-orchidism: fragile X syndrome Neurofibromatosis, Sturge-Weber syndrome, tuberous sclerosis Muscular dystrophies, cerebral palsy Hypertonic: neurodegenerative Hypotonic: Prader-Willi, Down, Angelman syndromes
Specific assessments after screening Visual assessment	Audiology assessment Visual impairment (e.g., ROP, septo-optic dysplasia, rubella, intracranial bleed) Cognitive assessment e.g., Wechsler intelligence scales, IQ Specific screening tools: e.g., M-CHAT (autistic spectrum disorders), DPN (FAS Diagnosis and Prevention Network) Educational assessment	Hearing impairment Mental retardation, learning disabilities Pervasive development disorders, FAS Learning disabilities
Lab/molecular testing	Newborn screening Plasma/urine a.a., homocysteine, etc.	Congenital hypothyroidism, PKU, biotinidase deficiency, CF, and others specific to provincial screening program Specific metabolic disorders
Neuromuscular	EMG, muscle biopsy EEG	Muscular dystrophies, familial hypotonia Epileptic disorder (e.g., infantile spasms)
Genetics	Genetic studies	E.g., trisomies, CF, 22q11 deletion, fragile X syndrome

[a]See Clinical Box Concerning Hx: Sexual Abuse/Neglect.

Refer for chromosomal/genetic, metabolic, or neurologic evaluation if:

- Delay in meeting developmental milestones
- Family Hx and concern
- Positive newborn screen
- Suspicious Hx (with risk factors) or physical exam

CONTROVERSIAL AND EVOLVING ETHICAL ISSUES IN PRACTICE: GENETIC TESTING

- Some children with developmental disorders caused by chromosome disorders or genetic syndromes and the issue of future genetic testing may arise

Concerning Hx: Sexual Abuse/Neglect

Extensive physical injury with Hx of minor trauma, recurrent/ multiple injuries, self-inflicted incompatible with child's development, delays in seeking treatment, dysfunctional behavior (overly compliant, pseudomature, acting out), substance abuse, poor school performance, regressive, emotional troubles, inappropriate sexual behavior

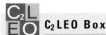 **C₂LEO Box**

Community Support Services and Resource Allocation
- Management of patients with developmental disorder resource intensive, some will have extremely high needs
- Resources may be limited, but need to be made available to them in a manner that is fair and equitable, without bias or discrimination
- Would benefit from improved government funding; advocacy for improvement in funding needs can be initiated at many levels by different advocates

- Manner in which discussed is nonjudgmental, with fair access to relevant and necessary information from appropriate sources provided
- Referral can be offered, considering one's moral boundaries, as well as consultation with ethics committees or boards

MANAGEMENT: DEVELOPMENTAL DELAY
Family Counseling
- Facilitate clarification, provide reassurance
- Support patient problem solving
- Education + specific parenting advice
- Suggest environmental intervention
- Provide links to resources
- Facilitate/interpret referrals

Academic Support
- Individualized educational plan

Speech/Language
- Speech therapy
- Amplification devices
- Family support
- Educational modification

Medical
- Motor: referrals, PT/OT, seizure control
- Diet
- Sensory: audiologist, ophthalmologist
- Behavior: check on sleep, aggression, psychotropic drug levels
- Infectious diseases (e.g., aspiration pneumonia) or immunizations
- Sexuality (education)
- Dermatology (examine all areas for decubitus ulcers and infection)

PEDIATRIC EMERGENCIES: ACUTELY ILL INFANT/CHILD

APPLIED SCIENTIFIC CONCEPTS
See Table 18.9.

OBJECTIVES
DIFFERENCE BETWEEN ADULT AND PEDIATRIC ORTHOPEDIC INJURIES
- Growing bones more ductile/stretchable
- Salter classification
- Unique fractures:
  - Plastic deformation: difficult to bend back
  - Greenstick injury
  - Buckle fracture
- Quicker healing

Table **18.9**	Special Considerations: Pediatrics vs. Adult Emergency Management
General anatomy	• Larger head → prone to injury, major source of heat loss; ↑ proportion of white matter (better brain plasticity) • Infants obligate nose breathers → secretions/blood in nasopharynx can cause significant distress • Neck: weaker muscles + supports greater mass • Thorax: more pliable, less overlying muscle and fat → contusions common, fractures rare • Rounded chest wall with flatter diaphragm → reduces excursion → minute ventilation ↑ by ↑ respiratory rate • Abdomen: less protected by muscle/fat → small forces may cause significant injury with minimal external evidence • Diaphragmatic breathers: gastric distension → may be difficult to ventilate if impaired diaphragmatic excursion/fatigued diaphragm • Surface area larger: heat loss significant • Smaller mass → greater force applied per unit body area in trauma
Airways and airway management	• Large occiput: passive flexion of C-spine → must maintain sniffing position • Larynx: more cephalad and anterior → cords difficult to visualize, position important! • Narrowest part of airway = cricoid cartilage → cuffed endotracheal tube not needed until 6–10 y.o. • Relative macroglossia
Response to hypovolemia	• Compensatory mechanism for hypovolemic shock: ↑ sympathoadrenal activity → tachycardia (and ↑ CO) + vasoconstriction • Early/compensated shock = still perfusing kidneys, brain, heart; BP last to be affected (amount of blood loss can be underestimated) • Eventually, ↑ HR + SVR → may impair coronary blood flow and ventricular filling, ↑ myocardial O_2 consumption → poorer myocardial function + tissue ischemia → sudden hypotension (uncompensated shock)

CLINICAL BOX

Signs Warranting Investigation of Abuse

General

- Evidence of trauma of different ages and specific shapes
- Delay in seeking medical help
- Any trauma without plausible or reproducible Hx: for example, subdural hematoma, cranial trauma, trauma to the eye, retinal hemorrhage, hyphema, internal organ trauma

Bruises

- Multiple, of different ages
- Before 9 mo of age
- Specific locations (face, buttocks, genitalia chest, back, etc.)
- Specific shape (linear, whorls, circular, etc.)
- Burns—immersion, perianal, cigarette

Fractures

- Neglected
- Of different ages
- With no plausible Hx
- Repeated in same location
- Unusual (e.g., posterior ribs, sternum, shoulder blades)
- Spiral or fragmentation
- Subperiosteal hemorrhage + callus formation
- Separation of growth plates

Sexual abuse

- Vaginitis, vaginal bleeding, genital injury
- Anal bleeding, chronic fissure
- Sexually transmitted disease (e.g., gonorrhea, human papilloma virus)
- Abnormal lesions in the genitor anal area
- Pregnancy

- Unique complications: growth arrest (physeal injury), progressive deformity (asymmetric physeal injury), overgrowth (2- to 10-y.o. group; physeal stimulation after diaphyseal fracture)

APPROACH

PHYSICAL EXAM

CLINICAL BOX

Pediatric Assessment Triangle

A = Appearance
  Tone, **I**nteractiveness, **C**onsolability, **L**ook/Gaze, **S**peech/Cry = "**TICLS**"

- Normal = alert, makes eye contact, interacts with environment, responsive, consolable, strong cry
- Abnormal = lethargic, "blank stare", "rag doll", does not interact, inconsolable, weak or muffled cry

B = work of Breathing
  Respiratory rate; position/posture (e.g., tripod or sniffing; retractions; nasal flaring; head bobbing); noises: snoring, grunting, wheezing, or stridor

- Normal = no abnormal rate, sounds, positioning or retractions
- ↑ = trouble oxygenating, ventilating or both
- ↓ = impending respiratory/cardiac arrest

C = Circulation
  Skin color: pink, pale, or cyanotic

- Normal = pink, capillary refill <3 s
- Abnormal = pale; mottled or cyanotic/ashen, capillary refill >3 s

Respiratory Failure
Respiratory

- Tachypnea, bradypnea, apnea
- Wheezing
- Grunting
- ↓/absent breath sounds
- Nasal flaring
- Retractions/indrawing
- Cyanosis

Neurologic

- Restlessness
- Irritability
- Headache
- Confusion
- Convulsions
- Coma

Cardiovascular

- Bradycardia or tachycardia
- Hypo/hypertension
- ↓ Capillary refill

General

- Fatigue
- Diaphoresis

Shock
Cardiovascular

- Tachycardia
- Hypotension (late in pediatric shock)

- Palpate distal and proximal pulses
- Decompensated shock: hypotension + diminished proximal pulses

CNS

- Reduced GCS
- Poor thalamic perfusion: loss of sympathetic tone
- Poor medullary flow: irregular respirations → gasping → apnea → respiratory arrest

Skin

- Gray/ashen/pale/cold/mottled
- Delayed capillary refill (>3 s)

Urinary Output

- ↓ (Normal urine output >1 mL/kg/h)

MSK System

- ↓ Spontaneous motor activity
- Flaccidity
- Prostration

INITIAL INVESTIGATIONS

- Hematology: CBC, type and cross-match
- U/A: gross and microscopic
- Chemistry: glucose, Lytes
- Microbiology: blood, urine, CSF cultures
- Pulse oximetry, blood gas
- Toxicology screen
- Radiology: C-spine films, CXR, CT head, chest, abdomen when indicated for trauma

MANAGEMENT

Airway

- Jaw thrust/chin lift (consider C-spine protection requirement)
- Suction nostrils, mouth, pharynx
- Oropharyngeal (or nasopharyngeal) airway if + upper airway noises or obstruction from prolapsed tongue
- Intubation (indications in side bar)

Breathing

- Assess: rate, chest rise, work of breathing, color, tracheal deviation, crepitus, flail segments
- 2 to 3 L nasal prongs **or** mask **or** nonrebreather mask (100% high-flow O_2)
- Bag mask ventilation if not breathing on own; decompress stomach through NG tube
- Positive pressure: CPAP or BIPAP
- Tension pneumothorax: decompress with large-bore needle through second intercostal space (midclavicular line) into pleural cavity
- Pneumo/hemothorax: chest tube in fourth intercostal space (anterior axillary line) → water seal

Circulation

- IV access: peripheral line first, if not central; alternative = intraosseous (see side bar)
- Cardiorespiratory monitor + oximeter
- sBP lower limits of normal: neonate <60, infant <70, otherwise (70 + 2 × age)
- Determine hematocrit, blood type, and cross-match
- Control external hemorrhage with direct pressure
- Fluid resuscitation for poor perfusion (hypotension[†] = late finding!): initial saline 20 mL/kg bolus → 3 mL crystalloid per milliliter external blood loss
- If not improved after three 20 mL/kg boluses: may need transfusion, inotropes (ICU); +/− possible surgical exploration
- Note: Do **not** restrict fluids for children with head injuries.

[†] Emergencies!

CLINICAL BOX

Indications for Airway Management/Intubation

1. Acute respiratory failure: PO_2 <60 mm Hg, Pco_2 >60 mm Hg, apnea, hypoventilation
2. Shock/severe metabolic acidosis
3. GCS <8
4. Airway protection
5. Other: burns, inability to control secretions, loss of gag reflex, SE/status asthmaticus, ingestions

status epilepticus

CLINICAL BOX

IV Access: Pediatrics

- External jugular
- Internal jugular
- Subclavian
- Antecubital
- Femoral
- Intraosseous

Disability
- AVPU scale: alert, verbal, painful, unresponsive
- Pediatric GCS
- Pupil size and reactivity

Exposure
- Remove all clothes
- Maintain warm ambient temperature and minimize heat loss

SPECIFIC PEDIATRIC EMERGENCIES

FEBRILE SEIZURES >5-MIN DURATION

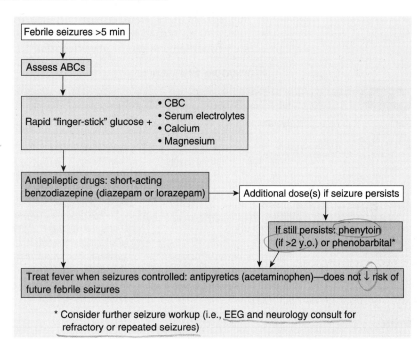

Figure 18.4 Pediatric febrile seizures >5-min duration.

SE

CLINICAL BOX

Status Epilepticus

30 min of continuous seizure activity or series of seizures without return to full consciousness between seizures

Stabilization

- Maintain adequate airway + normal gas exchange
- Treat hypoglycemia with glucose

Investigations

- Serum glucose, Lytes, calcium, magnesium
- Capillary/arterial blood gas
- A CBC and general chemical screen
- Urine and blood toxicology
- Serum AED levels
- Blood cultures and LP if evidence of systemic or CNS infection
- Urgent EEG: when uncertainty regarding presence of SE
- Neuroimaging when stable: CT to exclude mass lesion, MRI if the etiology of SE unknown
- Metabolic studies (i.e., rule out inborn errors of metabolism, when stabilized)

AEDs

- Are they currently on AEDs?
- Have they had SE in past? What medication worked?

Oral loading

1. Lorazepam 0.05 to 0.1 mg/kg IV (or midazolam 0.1 to 0.3 mg/kg IV)—if continue
2. Additional doses of lorazepam (up to a cumulative dose of 10 mg over 20 min)—if continue for 10 min after >2 × lorazepam
3. Fosphenytoin (maximum rate 150 mg/min) or phenobarbital
4. Valproic acid = second or third line

SHOCK

Resuscitation
- Assess and support the airway, respiration, and perfusion
- Supplemental O_2 (consider intubation) + continuous pulse oximetry

Monitoring Tissue Perfusion
- Arterial catheter may be inserted if BP is labile or restoration of arterial perfusion pressures is expected to be a protracted process.
- Central venous access for infusion of vasoactive medicines + monitoring CVP

Restoration of Tissue Perfusion
- IV fluids, packed red blood cells, and vasoactive agents
- IV fluids—40 to 60 mL/kg crystalloid solution push + repeat 20 mL/kg fluid boluses until signs of shock abate (urinary output; 1 to 2 mL/kg/h adequate)
- Vasopressors (second line)—augment peripheral vascular resistance: dopamine, norepinephrine, epinephrine, or phenylephrine

RESPIRATORY EMERGENCIES

Table 18.10   Upper Airway Disorders

Disease	Symptoms	Diagnosis	Treatment
Croup	URI Hoarse voice + barking cough Fever Stridor	Lateral neck x-ray: subglottic narrowing Frontal (AP) neck film findings: classic "steeple sign" in subglottic region	Supportive Nebulized racemic epinephrine for stridor Single-dose systemic steroid
Bacterial tracheitis	Preceding URI High fever Stridor, retractions Dysphagia Muffled, suppressed cough Toxic child	Clinical suspicion CXR: subglottic narrowing similar to croup Positive tracheal aspirate	Emergent intubation Empiric treatment IV antibiotics: nafcillin + ceftriaxone
Epiglottitis	Rapid evolution symptoms: fever, sore throat irritability, lethargy, drooling Dysphagia Severe stridor, airway obstruction Toxic child	Clinical suspicion Direct visualization in OR	Keep in position of comfort Intubate IV antibiotics—third/fourth generation cephalosporin Steroids not indicated
Retropharyngeal abscess	Prodromal nasopharyngitis + abrupt onset high fever, dysphagia, respiratory distress Drooling Meningismus	Lateral neck x-ray: widening of retropharyngeal space	IV antibiotics: nafcillin +/− cephalosporin (clindamycin for anaerobes) Emergent surgical drainage
Peritonsillar abscess	Sore throat Ipsilateral ear pain Trismus "Hot potato voice" Fever	Mass effect: deviated uvula Cervical adenopathy Fluctuance WBC elevated Throat culture positive	Surgical drainage or tonsillar aspiration IV antibiotics

CLINICAL BOX

Status Asthmaticus: Definition

Acute exacerbation of asthma that remains unresponsive to initial treatment with bronchodilators

Table **18.11**	**Lower Airway Disorders**		
Disease	**Symptoms**	**Diagnosis**	**Treatment**
Bronchiolitis	URTI symptoms, fever Irritability, poor feeding Tachypnea Tachycardia Cough, retractions, wheezing	CXR: variable findings	Humidified O$_2$ β-Agonists + nebulized racemic epinephrine may be helpful IV hydration
Asthma	Tachypnea or hypopnea if fatigued Wheezing, retractions Pulsus paradoxus Irritability/lethargy Tachycardia Hypoxia	Capillary/arterial blood gas: hypercapnea = ominous sign	O$_2$ β-Agonists Corticosteroids Anticholinergics Terbutaline Magnesium sulfate Intubation
Foreign body	Cough, wheeze, ↓ breath sounds	Hx choking episode (50%) CXR: persistent hyperinflation Mediastinal shift toward unaffected side Pulmonary infiltrates Air trapping	Basic life support Laryngoscopy + forceps removal Bronchoscopy Intubation with dislodgment of the object into bronchus

CLINICAL BOX

DDx of Wheeze

- Asthma
- Foreign body
- CF
- Bronchiolitis
- TEF
- Pneumonia

- Bronchopulmonary dysplasia
- CHF
- Mediastinal masses
- Pulmonary embolism
- Vascular anomalies
- Anaphylaxis/allergic reaction

PEDIATRIC EMERGENCIES: CRYING/FUSSING CHILD

DEFINITION

A young infant whose only symptom is crying/fussing challenges the primary care physician to distinguish between benign and organic causes.

CAUSAL CONDITIONS

- Functional/hunger/discomfort/irritability/colic
- Trauma (neglect/child abuse/fracture)
- Infections
- GI conditions (see **Abdominal Pain**)
  - Infection
  - Inflammation
  - Obstruction
  - Diarrhea
- Cardiac/respiratory
  - Congenital
  - Infective
  - Obstructive
  - Intracranial process

APPROACH

Hx

- Previous behavior, sleeping pattern
- Oral intake of food/drink
- Presence of fever, vomiting, diarrhea or constipation, urine output, shortness of breath → complete review of systems
- Medications received

PHYSICAL EXAM

Full physical exam with focus:

- Infection sites
- Intra-abdominal conditions
- ↑ Intracranial pressure
- Cardiac and respiratory disorders
- Sources of pain

INVESTIGATIONS: DIFFERENTIATE ACUTE VERSUS BENIGN

- CBC—leukocytosis
- Lytes, glucose—metabolic disturbance
- U/A—urologic problem
- CXR—pulmonary pathology
- Cultures, abdominal plain films or U/S, skeletal x-rays—if clinically indicated

MANAGEMENT

- Counsel caregivers of fussy/crying children without organic disease
- Select children who require follow-up for additional investigation, specific management, referral

SPECIFIC CONDITIONS

Infantile Colic

- Nonpathologic behavioral sign/symptom that begins in first weeks of life, peak age 2 to 3 mo

CLINICAL BOX

Infantile Colic: Rule of 3s

Healthy infant who cries for more than 3 h/d, >3 d/wk, for >3 wk

Characteristics

1. Severe, paroxysmal crying occurring mainly in late afternoon
2. Knees drawn up, fists clenched, +/− flatus expelled, facies pained, hypertonic posturing
3. Crying louder, higher, more variable in pitch and turbulent than noncolicky crying
4. Inconsolable

CLINICAL BOX

Crying: Hx

When does the crying occur?	How does it make you feel when your baby cries?
How long does it last?	How has the colic affected your family?
Directly after feeding: aerophagia or reflux	Valuate diet, stooling, urination, sleep pattern
What do you do when the baby cries?	Growth parameters
Is it a cry of pain or hunger?	Social situation and parent–infant interactions
How and what do you feed the baby?	

Management

- Typically self-limited; symptoms resolve within 4 to 5 mo of age
- Parental support, education, rest and relief
- Formulas:
  - Likely to be beneficial—whey hydrolysate milk
  - Unknown effectiveness—soy milk, casein hydrolysate milk, low lactose milk, low allergen diet by breastfeeding mothers, sucrose, herbal tea, reduced stimulation, ovol drops/gripe water

- Feeding techniques: frequent burping may reduce swallowed air
- Alternate sensory stimulation—pacifier, a ride in the car, a change of scenery, a swing, a warm bath, or a belly massage

5 S's: swaddling, **s**hushing, **s**ide or **s**tomach, **s**winging, **s**ucking (pacifier)

PEDIATRIC EMERGENCIES: HYPOTONIA/FLOPPY INFANT/CHILD

CAUSAL CONDITIONS

AMENABLE TO RAPID TREATMENT

- Lyte/metabolic (e.g., hypokalemia, hypermagnesemia, acidemia, hypoglycemia)
- Toxins/drugs

CENTRAL NEURAL DISEASE

- Cerebral malformations; neurodegenerative (leukodystrophy)
- Seizures, trauma (subarachnoid or subdural hemorrhage)
- Hydrocephalus/↑ intracranial pressure
- Infectious (encephalitis, abscess, meningitis)
- Neoplasms
- Hypoxic/ischemic encephalopathy
- "Benign congenital hypotonia"

PERIPHERAL NEURAL DISEASE

- Anterior horn cell (e.g., progressive spinal muscular atrophy, infarction, infection)
- Peripheral nerves/polyneuropathies (Guillain-Barré, Charcot-Marie-Tooth, trauma)
- Myoneural junction (myasthenia gravis, botulism)

CLINICAL BOX

UMN versus LMN Lesion

Central (UMN)	Peripheral (LMN)
↑ Tone	↓ Tone
Hyper-reflexia, clonus	Hypo/areflexia
↓ Muscle bulk	Fasciculations
Upwards plantar response	Downwards plantar response
No sensory loss	+/− Sensory loss

MUSCULAR DISEASE

- Muscular/myotonic dystrophy
- Congenital myopathies

Other genetic (trisomy 21, glycogen storage, Niemann-Pick, Tay-Sachs, Prader-Willi)

Table **18.12**	Selected Primitive Reflexes	
Reflex	**Fully Developed**	**Duration**
Palmar grasp	32 wk	2–3 mo
Rooting	36 wk	Less prominent after 1 mo
Moro	37 wk	5–6 mo
Tonic neck	1 mo	6–7 mo
Parachute	10–11 mo	Throughout life

APPROACH

1. ABCs (in acute situation)
2. Differentiate between generalized hypotonia and weakness/hyporeflexia
3. Rule out presence of acute/chronic conditions amenable to rapid treatment

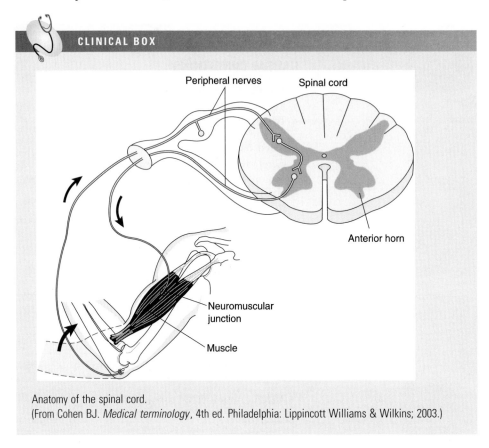

CLINICAL BOX

Anatomy of the spinal cord.
(From Cohen BJ. *Medical terminology*, 4th ed. Philadelphia: Lippincott Williams & Wilkins; 2003.)

Hx

- Antenatal: polyhydramnios (suggesting poor fetal swallowing), fetal akinesia (paucity of movement), malpresentation (breech)
- Perinatal: prematurity or birth asphyxia
- Postnatal and temporal profile/development: age and rapidity of onset, progression of symptoms, and distribution of involvement
- Family Hx: neuromuscular abnormalities, for example, congenital myotonic dystrophy, spinal muscular atrophy, metabolic disorders, familial dysautonomia

PHYSICAL EXAM

- Dysmorphic features, congenital defects
- Weight, length, head circumference
- Skin pallor, bruising, petechiae, evidence of trauma (e.g., traumatic myelopathy)
- Abnormalities of respiratory rate, pattern, diaphragmatic movement (e.g., congenital myopathies)
- Cardiomyopathy (e.g., carnitine deficiency)
- Organomegaly (e.g., acid maltase deficiency)
- Defects of genitalia, including hypogonadism (e.g., Smith-Lemli-Opitz syndrome)
- Contractures or laxity of joints (e.g., Ehlers-Danlos syndrome)

General: posture and level of alertness, spontaneous activity

Motor
- Facial weakness (e.g., congenital myotonic dystrophy)
- Ability to suck and swallow, character of cry, tongue fasciculations (spinal muscular atrophy)
- Respiratory difficulty

Tone
- Nature of hypotonia: posture of trunk, whether "frog-leg" position is present, muscle bulk, presence of fasciculation, head lag, examine flexion and extension of the joints
- Sphincter disturbance (spinal cord lesion)

Reflexes
- Primitive (Moro reflex, tonic neck response, palmar grasp, placing and stepping reactions) and deep—UMN or LMN lesion?

Sensation
- Abnormal sensation (neuropathy, spinal cord lesion)

Table **18.13**	**Further Investigation**	
Cause	**Clinical Exam**	**Investigations**
Central neural		Brain or spinal MRI EEG Chromosomal analysis Metabolic screen Molecular genetic testing LP, blood and urine cultures
Cerebral palsy (brain injury causing impaired motor function)	• Developmental delay, feeding problems, early hand preference, fisting, ↑ extensor tone in neck and back, asymmetrical crawl, wide-based gait, standing on toes	• MRI: periventricular leukomalacia
Down syndrome	• Central hypotonia	• Prenatal diagnosis, karyotype
Spinal muscular atrophy (degenerative disorder of anterior horn cells)	Three types based on degree of severity • Progressive neurologic deficit at any age • Varying inability to sit/walk, tongue fasciculations, strong alert face, weak limbs, areflexia	• Muscle biopsy: fiber type grouping, group atrophy • NCS: normal • EMG: giant action potentials • Diagnosis now made with molecular genetics
Spina bifida	• Weakness, spasticity, awkward gait, incontinence • Sacral dimple or hairy patch	• Spinal x-ray and MRI
Peripheral neural		CK Molecular genetic testing NCS EMG Muscle/nerve biopsy
Hereditary motor sensory neuropathy (Charcot-Marie-Tooth disease)	• Pes cavus, pes planus, toe walking, dropped foot • Examine parents as well	• NCS: slowed • EMG: signs of denervation • Molecular genetic testing
Acute inflammatory demyelinating polyneuropathy (Guillain-Barré syndrome)	• Acute ascending/proximal weakness in previously well child • Areflexia	• NCS: slowing and amplitude loss • LP: elevated protein and no cells in CSF
Myasthenia gravis (neuromuscular junction)	• Ocular involvement or generalized weakness • Preserved DTR	• Tensilon test (edrophonium) • Acetylcholine receptor antibodies
Muscular Myopathy (Duchenne, milder form Becker)	Muscular dystrophy • Proximal weakness, Gower sign (climbing up the legs using hands) • Pseudohypertrophied calves Myotonic dystrophy • Myopathic face also	• Elevated CK • EMG: myopathic findings • Muscle biopsy: degenerating and regenerating fibers with fibrosis • Genetics: mutation in dystrophin gene Xp21 (muscular dystrophy), trinucleotide repeats on Ch19 (myotonic)

INVESTIGATIONS

Conditions Amenable to Rapid Treatment

Lyte/metabolic imbalance—blood chemistry, glucose, TSH

Seizures—EEG, MRI

Infection—blood culture, LP

Intracranial bleeding—CT head

Hydrocephalus—CT head

MANAGEMENT

- Determine whether respiratory status is adequate or intubation required
- Treat cause if possible
- Possible referral to genetics or neurology
- Counsel families with afflicted children about management, prognosis, genetic implications
- Involve family and community resources

GENETIC CONCERNS

DEFINITION

Primary care physicians must provide counseling about risk factors (e.g., maternal age, illness, drug use) and refer for further evaluation if necessary.

CAUSAL CONDITIONS

CHROMOSOME DEFECTS

- Numerical: for example, Down syndrome
- Structural translocations, deletions and inversions: for example, Cri du Chat

MENDELIAN

- Dominant: for example, Huntington chorea, familial hypercholesterolemia, polycystic kidney disease
- Recessive: for example, CF (see below pedigree)
- X-linked: for example, hemophilia, Duchenne muscular dystrophy

Multifactorial conditions: for example, neural tube defects

APPLIED SCIENTIFIC CONCEPTS

DEFINITIONS FOR PATIENTS/PARENTS

- Mitosis—type of cell division where DNA is replicated and two daughter cells, genetically identical to original parent cells, are formed
  - Typical for all somatic cells (those other than the sperm or egg, which are germ-line cells)
- Meiosis—type of cell division where eggs and sperm are formed (limited to gametes)
  - Maternally and paternally derived chromosomes distributed independently in each cell
  - Two cell divisions occur versus mitosis; first a reduction division and second is like mitosis

ERRORS LEADING TO ANEUPLOIDY

- Human cell with 23 chromosomes (e.g., human ova or sperm) is in haploid state (n)
- In cells other than reproductive cells, 46 chromosomes are present in diploid state (2n)
- Polyploid = any number other than diploid number of chromosomes; usually not viable
- Aneuploid = cells deviating from multiple of the haploid number. For example, trisomy = presence of three of a particular chromosome rather than two, resulting from unequal division (nondisjunction) of chromosomes into daughter cells
- Most common numerical chromosomal anomalies in humans

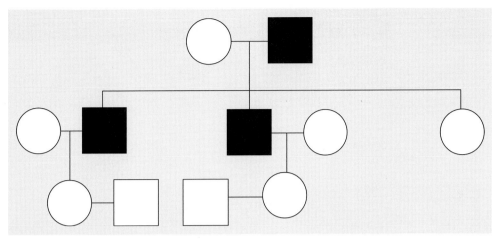

Figure 18.5 Three generation pedigree.

APPROACH

Hx

- Hx on proband/index case (clinically affected person) + each of first-degree relatives (parents, siblings, and offspring of proband)
- Prior obstetrical, medical, family Hx; exposure during current pregnancy; maternal age at delivery date
- Relatives with identical, similar, or associated features, or a genetically determined problem
- Consanguinity, ethnic origin of family (e.g., ↑ risk of Tay-Sachs in Ashkenazi Jews)
- Develop/interpret three generation pedigree

Investigations

Indications for Prenatal Diagnosis

- Positive screening tests: late maternal age (>35 y.o.), FTS, MSS, U/S evidence of prenatally diagnosable malformation
- Previous stillbirth, miscarriage, live birth with chromosomal disorder
- Family Hx of genetic disorder

Management

Option to refer to genetics

- Diagnostic confirmation
- Advice on further investigation if required
- Counseling regarding future risks and prenatal strategies for prevention of dysmorphic disorders

Referral to community resources, social support groups, etc.

CLINICAL BOX

Screening versus Diagnosis

Metal detector analogy: beep of detector does not mean you have a gun but that you need to search further.

Table **18.14**	**Screening for Chromosome Disorders**
Screening Test	**Indications**
Nuchal translucency (11–14-wk scan)	Screen for viability, age, location, risk of trisomies, neural tube defects
MSS (AFP + β-HCG + UE3)	Risk of trisomy 21, other trisomies, neural tube defects, prenatal U/S evidence of malformation
FTS (PAPP-A + β-HCG)	Replacing MSS—greatest sensitivity for trisomy 21
18–20-wk U/S scan	Detailed anatomic survey, biometry, extrafetal structures

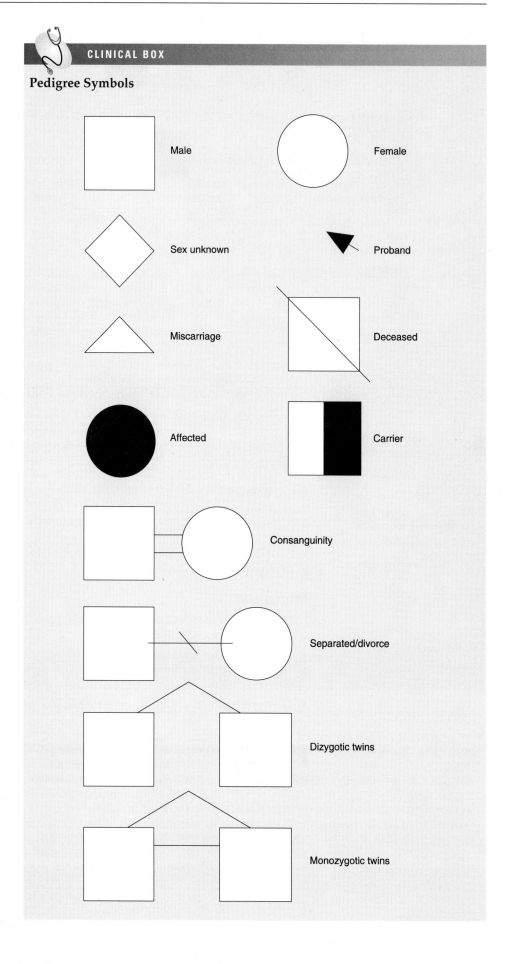

CLINICAL BOX

Pedigree Symbols

Male

Female

Sex unknown

Proband

Miscarriage

Deceased

Affected

Carrier

Consanguinity

Separated/divorce

Dizygotic twins

Monozygotic twins

Table **18.15** Prenatal Diagnostic Tests			
Available Prenatal Diagnostic Tests	**Investigations**	**Sensitivity**	**Risks**
Chorionic villus sampling (11 – 13 wk)	Karyotyping Fetal cells (for molecular/metabolic studies)	97.5%	Spontaneous abortion (1%) Lab failure (2%) Fetal limb injury
Amniocentesis (15–17 wk)	Karyotyping Fluid/fetal cells (for molecular/metabolic studies) AFP for neural tube defects	99.8%	Spontaneous abortion (0.5%) Amniotic fluid leak (1%) Lab failure (0.1%) Fetal limb injury
Cordocentesis (20 wk onwards)	Rapid karyotyping Fetal anemia	~100%	Spontaneous abortion (1%–2%) Preterm labor (5%–9%)
Fetal U/S	Structural defects Hydrops	17%–74%	—

Counsel patients regarding alternative reproductive options:

- For example, contraception, therapeutic donor insemination, donor ova, adoption, prenatal diagnosis with/without therapeutic termination of affected fetus

FAILURE TO THRIVE

DEFINITION

- FTT is a phrase that describes the occurrence of growth failure in either height or weight in childhood. Because FTT is attributed to children <2 yr whose weight is below the fifth percentile for age on more than one occasion, it is essential to differentiate normal from the abnormal growth patterns.
- FTT = inadequate physical growth involving a ↓ in height or weight in childhood or head circumference in <2 y.o.

CAUSAL CONDITIONS/APPROACH

PRENATAL

- Maternal: pre-existing conditions (diabetes, renal disease, etc.); use of drugs, tobacco, alcohol
- Pregnancy: placental insufficiency, intrauterine infections
- Genetic: chromosomal abnormalities and syndromes

POSTNATAL

See Figure 18.6.

APPROACH

Hx

- Determine onset of FTT and association with other factors
- Prenatal: maternal hypertension, drugs, smoking, infections
- Birth: lack of appropriate weight gain, IUGR, positive newborn screen
- Diet: low volume of feeds, food/formula intolerance, poor accessibility to nutrition, dyspnea/tachypnea on feeds
- Development: social interactions, developmental delay in any domain
- Behavior: irritability, easily fatigued
- Family: chronic conditions, height/weight of family members
- GI problems: diarrhea, vomiting, colic, jaundice, dysphagia
- Chronic conditions: for example, cerebral palsy, any affecting major organs, chronic infections, allergies, chronic lung disease, obstructive sleep apnea
- Psychosocial: living environment, family structure, Hx of abuse/neglect, family substance abuse, violence, beliefs about child rearing, level of education

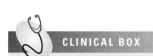

CLINICAL BOX

Social Risk Factors for Poor Growth

- Emotional deprivation due to parental withdrawal, rejection, or hostility
- Economic problems affecting nutrition, living conditions, and parental attitudes
- Exposure to infections or toxins
- Maladaptive behaviors: problems establishing regular feeding times
- Caregiver mood disorders
- Chaotic home environment due to alcohol/drug abuse, violence, sexual abuse

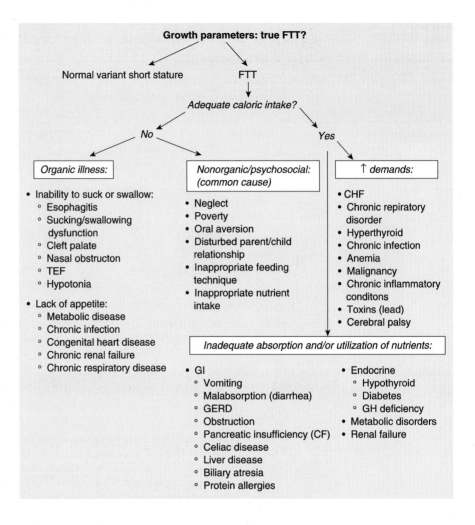

Figure 18.6 Approach to FTT.

PHYSICAL EXAM

Plot growth parameters, observe infant's behavior and parental interaction. Full physical exam with attention to:

- General: edema, wasting, hypotonia, skin/hair color/texture changes, signs of Vit deficiency, dysmorphic features, mental status changes
- Respiratory distress, cough, tonsillar hypertrophy
- Heart murmurs
- Hepatomegaly, abdominal distension

INVESTIGATIONS

Psychosocial versus Organic?
- 3-d dietary record, dietician consult

Suck/Swallow/Feeding Issues?
- PT/OT observed feed

Pre/Perinatal Causes?
- TORCH screen, HIV if appropriate
- Chromosomal tests
- Molecular genetic testing
- Cranial U/S Genetics consult

Malabsorption/Utilization?
- GI
  - CBC and differential
  - Protein and albumin
  - INR (low Vit K)

- Fe, ferritin
- Antiendomysial antibodies, IgA
- Stool for lipid globules, reducing substances
- 72-h fecal fat
- ESR +/− CRP
- LFTs
- Sweat chloride, Sao$_2$, sleep study
- Metabolic
  - Metabolic screen
  - Serum/urine a.a.
  - Molecular genetic testing

↑ Demands/Lack of Appetite Due to Chronic Illness?

- Renal failure: U/A, Cr, Lytes
- Infections: HIV/other viral serology, stool cultures, IgGs
- Congenital heart disease: associated clinical findings + cardiac imaging
- Respiratory: sweat chloride
- Endocrine: TSH low, FT4 high

Endocrine

- TSH high, FT4 low
- Glucose
- Insulin tolerance test: GH deficiency
- Bone age

Renal

- U/A
- Cr
- Lytes

MANAGEMENT

- Hospitalization and interdisciplinary approach
- Consultation of subspecialists for example, metabolics, neurology
- Continue management of comorbidities, if any
- Counseling and education for example, dietician, PT
- Connect with community resources

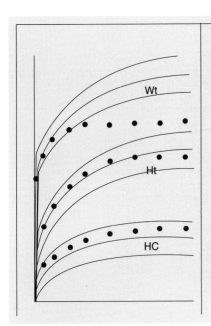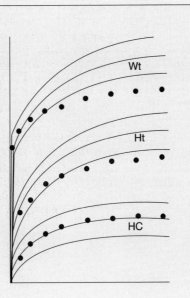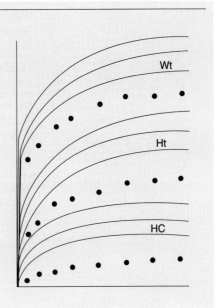

Figure 18.7 Interpreting growth parameters.

Table 18.16	Interpreting Growth Parameters		
Patterns	**I**	**II**	**III**
Head circumference	Normal	Normal	↓
Height	Normal or ↓	↓	↓
Weight	↓, low for height	↓, proportional to height	↓, proportional to height
Appearance	Malnourished	Healthy	Stunted
Growth chart	See Figure 18-9		
Etiologies	See all of the above	Endocrinopathy Dwarfism —constitutional or deprivation Normal variant short stature—not true FTT	Early onset FTT: • IUGR • Chromosomal/genetic abnormality • Perinatal insults

DYSMORPHIC FEATURES

DEFINITION

3/100 infants born with genetic disorder or congenital defect

CAUSAL CONDITIONS

CLINICAL BOX

Teratogens
Drugs and chemicals

Alcohol	Lead
Aminoglycosides	Methylmercury
Aminopterin	Penicillamine
Antithyroid agents	Tetracycline
Bromine	Thalidomide
Cortisone	Valproic acid
Warfarin	Heroin
Retinoic acid (Accutane)	
DES	

Physical agents
Ionizing radiation (x-rays)

Maternal conditions
Autoimmune disease
Diabetes
Malnutrition
PKU

Infectious organisms
Coxsackie virus
Cytomegalovirus
HSV
Parvovirus
Rubella
T. gondii
T. pallidum (syphilis)

TERATOGENIC DISORDERS (SEE CLINICAL BOX TERATOGENS)

Chromosomal Disorders

1. Down syndrome
2. Turner syndrome
3. Fragile X chromosome
4. Klinefelter syndrome
5. Idiopathic/sporadic

APPROACH

Hx

- Prenatal maternal factors: alcohol/drug/medication use, teratogen exposure, chronic or acute infection, previous miscarriage or stillbirth
- Perinatal: obstetrical complications, prematurity, low birth weight, multiple gestation
- Neonatal: neurologic events, sepsis/meningitis, severe hyperbilirubinemia, hypoxia
- Postnatal: recurrent otitis media, poor feeding/growth, toxic exposure, head injury
- Family: consanguinity, mental functioning, developmental delay, chromosomal abnormalities, deafness/blindness

Indications for Antenatal Screening

- Maternal age >35 y.o.
- Family Hx diagnosed chromosomal/genetic disorder, developmental delay
- Antenatal teratogen use
- Informed choice of patients

MANAGEMENT

- Explain alternatives for dealing with the risk of recurrence
- Counsel families or assist with literature search
- Discuss with parents long-term care: depends on diagnosis/prognosis

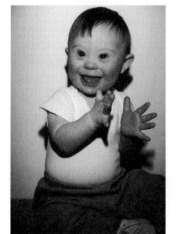

Figure 18.8 Down syndrome.
(From Nettina SM. *The Lippincott manual of nursing practice*, 7th ed. Lippincott Williams & Wilkins; 2003.)

Table **18.17**	Down Syndrome		
General Information	**Hx**		**Investigations**

• Various chromosomal abnormalities possible: nondisjunction (94%), translocation (4%), and mosaicism (2%)
• Shortened life expectancy
• Congenital heart disease, the major cause of morbidity and early mortality
• ↑ Risk of recurrent respiratory infections, epilepsy, intestinal obstruction, and leukemia
	• Parental age, previous eyeglass prescriptions, occlusion therapy, onset of strabismus and/or nystagmus, previous external infections and treatment modalities, tearing, and photophobia
	• Review pulmonary, GI, cardiovascular, and neurologic systems
			• Prenatal U/S, amniocentesis, karyotype
			• Fetal U/S
			  • Cystic hygroma colli
			  • Cardiac defects
			  • Duodenal obstruction
			  • Hydrops fetalis
			  • Prune belly anomaly
			• Detection of carriers: when translocation detected in the parents, risk of recurrence depends on type of translocation and carrier parent's gender
			• Anticipatory care (side bar)

Physical exam			
• Flat occiput, short broad neck • Ears: dysplastic ears • Eyes: epicanthal folds, upward slanting of palpebral fissures • Ocular findings: amblyopia, high refractive errors, strabismus, nystagmus, Brushfield spots, cataracts, glaucoma • Nose: small nose, depressed nasal bridge • Mouth: protruding tongue, high-arched palate, dental abnormalities • Extremities: short fifth middle phalanx, single palmar creases, sandal foot • MSK: joint hyperextensibility, neuromuscular hypotonia, dry skin • CNS: wide range of IQs • Cardiac: congenital heart defects			See Figure 18.8

CLINICAL BOX

Down Syndrome Anticipatory Care

TSH	Hypothyroid
Testicular exam	Tumors
Eye exam	Strabismus, amblyopia, cataracts
Echocardiogram	Septal defects
Flexion-extension cervical spine x-ray	Atlanto-occipital instability
Clinical +/− polysomnogram	Sleep apnea
Otolaryngology	Recurrent ear infections

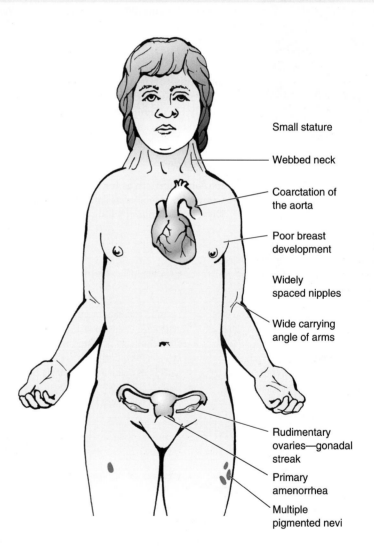

Small stature

Webbed neck

Coarctation of the aorta

Poor breast development

Widely spaced nipples

Wide carrying angle of arms

Rudimentary ovaries—gonadal streak

Primary amenorrhea

Multiple pigmented nevi

Figure 18.9 Turner syndrome.

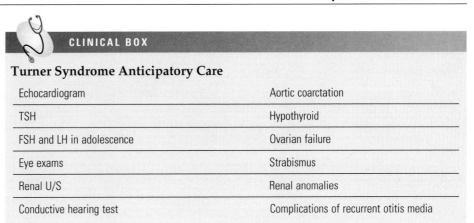

CLINICAL BOX

Turner Syndrome Anticipatory Care

Echocardiogram	Aortic coarctation
TSH	Hypothyroid
FSH and LH in adolescence	Ovarian failure
Eye exams	Strabismus
Renal U/S	Renal anomalies
Conductive hearing test	Complications of recurrent otitis media

Table 18.18 Turner Syndrome

General Information	Hx	Investigations
• Most with pure 45X spontaneously abort; those who survive to birth may have mosaicism • **Not** associated with advanced maternal age • Mortality ↑ due to aortic coarctation and other CVS disease • Life expectancy reduced • Renal anomalies may predispose to UTIs or hypertension	• Unexplained short stature • Adrenarche at normal age but breast development absent • Primary or secondary amenorrhea with unexplained infertility	• Fetal U/S: nuchal cystic hygroma, horseshoe kidney, left-sided cardiac anomalies, posterior hairline, nonimmune fetal hydrops • Prenatal or postnatal karyotype • Anticipatory care (side bar) • [O]

Physical exam

• Short stature, webbed neck • Eyes: ptosis, strabismus, amblyopia, cataracts • Ears: dysplastic external ears, serous otitis media is more common • Thyroid: goiter (hypothyroidism) • Dermatology: hypoplastic or hyperconvex nails, excessive nevi, loose skin folds • MSK: shield chest, cubitus valgus (↑ carrying angle), wide-spaced nipples, congenital hip dysplasia, scoliosis • GI bleeding: intestinal vascular malformations, ↑ incidence of Crohns and ulcerative colitis • Ovarian failure: no breast development by age 12; pubic hair development normal • Hypertension: coarctation of aorta, renal anomalies • Cardiac: coarctation of aorta, bicuspid aortic valve, aortic dissection	See Figure 18.9

CLINICAL BOX

Fragile X Syndrome Anticipatory Care

Speech/language, PT/OT, psychologic evaluation	Low IQ + learning disabilities
Eye assessment	Strabismus, nystagmus
Hearing and otolaryngology	Recurrent otitis media
Regular cardiac auscultation	Mitral valve prolapse
BP monitoring	Hypertension
Testicular exam	Macro-orchidism
MSK exam	Joint laxity and scoliosis
Full mutation females	Precocious puberty, emotional status, genetic counseling + discussion of reproductive alternatives

Table 18.19 Fragile X Syndrome

General Information	Hx	Investigations

• Trinucleotide expansion (CGG repeated sequence) within *FMR1* gene
• Very common cause of developmental delay
• Diagnosis often made/considered in early school years
	• Family Hx: multiple male relatives with mental retardation or ataxia/tremors
	• Cognitive: typically mild-to-severe mental retardation (20–70), less severe in females; IQ ↓ with age
	• Neuropsychologic:
	  • Developmental delays after reaching early milestones
	  • Autistic-like behavior (hand flapping, perseveration, echolalia, and avoidance of eye contact)
	  • Features of ADHD, obsessive-compulsive disorder, and/or sensory integration disorder
	  • Seizure disorder (20%)
	• Recurrent nonspecific issues e.g., otitis media, apnea, sinusitis
		• Definitive diagnosis = molecular investigation
		• Cytogenetics: Xq27.3 fragile site → confirm with DNA testing
		• Molecular genetics: determine exact number of CGG triplet repeats (southern blot or PCR)
		• Anticipatory care (side bar)

Physical Exam

Most findings notable only after onset of puberty
- Growth: early growth spurt but adult height average or slightly below
- Craniofacial: long thin face, facial asymmetry, large head circumference, prominent forehead and jaw
- Mouth: dental overcrowding and high-arched palate
- Ears: large and prominent
- Eyes: strabismus
- Extremities: hyperextensible finger joints, hand calluses, double-jointed thumbs, a single palmar crease, and pes planus
- Back and chest: pectus excavatum and scoliosis
- Genitals: macro-orchidism universal in adult males
- Cardiac: heart murmur/click consistent with mitral valve prolapse

Table 18.20 Klinefelter Syndrome

General Information	Hx	Investigations

• 47,XXY 80%–90% cases, mosaicism (46,XY/47,XXY) in 10%
• Variants (rare): 48XXYY, 48XXXY, 49XXXYY, 49XXXXY
• May have ↑ frequency of extragonadal germ cell tumors
	• Infertility and gynecomastia most common complaints leading to diagnosis
	• Other: fatigue, weakness, erectile dysfunction, osteoporosis, language impairment, academic difficulty, subnormal libido, poor self-esteem, and behavior problems
		• Cytogenetics
		  • 80%–90% 47,XXY
		  • 10% mosaics
		• Hormone testing
		  • High plasma FSH, LH, and estradiol levels
		  • Low plasma testosterone; ↑ in response to administration of β-HCG subnormal
		• Anticipatory care (side bar)

Physical Exam

- Growth: infants/children have normal heights, weights, and head circumferences; height velocity ↑ by age 5, and adult height usually taller than average
- Extremities: disproportionately long arms and legs
- CNS: normal intelligence → low (IQ ↓ by 15 per extra X), minor developmental and learning disabilities (70%)
- Psychiatric: anxiety, depression, neurosis, psychosis
- Dental: taurodontism (enlargement of molar teeth by extension of the pulp) in 40%
- Hypogonadism: sparse facial/body/sexual hair, high-pitched voice, female type fat distribution, testicular dysgenesis
- Gynecomastia; risk of breast carcinoma 20× normal
- Infertility/azoospermia
- Osteoporosis
- Cardiac and circulatory: mitral valve prolapse (55%), varicose veins (40%), venous ulcers, hypercoagulability

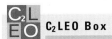
CLINICAL BOX

Klinefelter Syndrome Anticipatory Care

Testosterone, FSH, LH in adolescence	Infertility
Developmental/behavioral assessment	Possible cognitive delay
Breast exam + teach self-exam	Gynecomastia, ↑ risk breast cancer

- Multidisciplinary services, family support, possible academic support and child placement
- Anticipatory guidance
- Option of genetics referral:
  - Diagnostic confirmation
  - Advice on further investigation, if required
  - Counseling regarding future risks and prenatal strategies for prevention of dysmorphic disorders

AMBIGUOUS GENITALIA

DEFINITION

Genetic males with 46, XY genotype but having impaired androgen sensitivity of varying severity may present with features that range from phenotypic females to "normal" males with only minor defects in masculinization or infertility. Primary care physicians may be called upon to determine the nature of the problem.

APPLIED SCIENTIFIC CONCEPTS

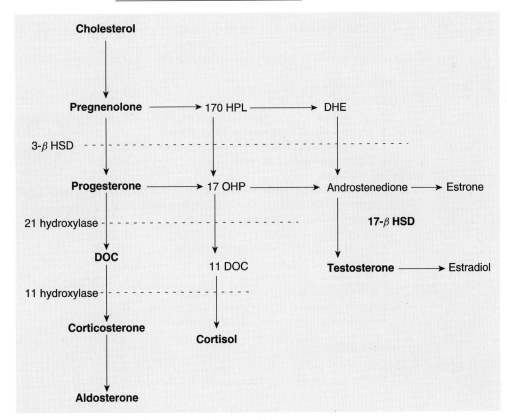

Figure 18.10 Applied scientific concepts: ambiguous genitalia.

APPROACH

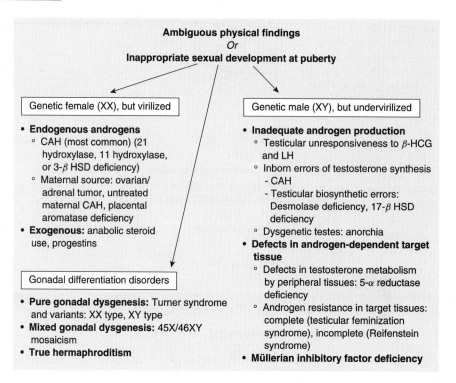

Figure 18.11 Approach to ambiguous genitalia.

Hx

- Family Hx of genital ambiguity, females with infertility or amenorrhea, early death of infants
- Prenatal exposure to androgens (progesterone, danazol, testosterone), maternal virilization in pregnancy (placental aromatase deficiency)
- Consanguinity (↑ recessive disorders like CAH, 5-α reductase deficiency)

Physical Exam

- External genitalia
  - Size and degree of differentiation of the phallus: clitoromegaly or hypospadias, hooded
  - Urethral meatus: perineal urogenital sinus
  - Labioscrotal folds separated or fused at the midline
  - Pigmented labioscrotal folds
- Gonads
  - Palpable? Impalpable raises suspicion of virilized female with CAH or anorchia or persistent müllerian duct syndrome in genetic male
  - Location: inguinal gonads
- Rectum
  - Rectal exam may allow palpation of the cervix and uterus, confirming internal müllerian structures
  - The uterus is relatively enlarged in a newborn because of the effects of maternal estrogen, permitting easy identification.
- Secondary sexual characteristics in adolescents
  - Gynecomastia in males, virilization (hirsutism, acne) in females

Investigations

- Lab
  - DHEA, androstenedione, testosterone: elevated in CAH
  - 5-α reductase levels: undervirilized genetic male
  - ACTH stimulation test: negative in CAH
  - Lytes: hyponatremia or hypokalemia of CAH
  - Karyotype: establish patient's chromosomal sex

- Imaging
  - U/S pelvis/kidneys:uterus? Müllerian structures? adrenals enlarged in CAH
  - Genitogram or exploratory laparotomy/gonadal biopsy (rare): internal ductal anatomy

MANAGEMENT

- Counsel parents on the importance of early gender assignment in order to prevent potential harm in psychosocial development.
- Consult pediatric urologists for advice on gender assignment: genital reconstruction
- Hormone replacement therapy (corticosteroids in CAH)
- Prenatal diagnosis with future pregnancy
- Community resources, social support groups, and so on.

NEONATAL JAUNDICE

See also Chapter 9.

DEFINITION

Jaundice, usually mild unconjugated bilirubinemia, affects nearly all newborns. Up to 65% of full-term neonates have jaundice at 72 to 96 h of age. Although some causes are ominous, the majority are transient and without consequences.

APPROACH

Hx

- Presentation: onset and duration
- Pregnancy, labor and delivery—maternal illness or drug intake, trauma, delayed cord clamping, Apgar
- Family Hx: jaundice, hematologic or metabolic disorders, anemia, liver disease
- Postnatal: breastfeeding, sepsis, loss of stool color, medications, signs/symptoms of hypothyroidism/metabolic disease

PHYSICAL EXAM

- Jaundice: cephalocaudal progression
- Vital signs
- Hydration status
- Neurologic deficits: lethargy, hypotonia, seizures, altered cry
- Hepatosplenomegaly, ascites, shock, dark urine, pale stools, petechiae (See Figure 18.13)

MANAGEMENT

See Table 18.21.

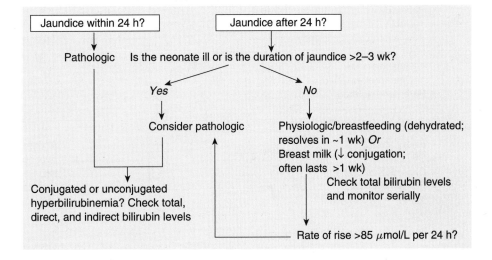

Figure 18.12 Approach to neonatal jaundice.

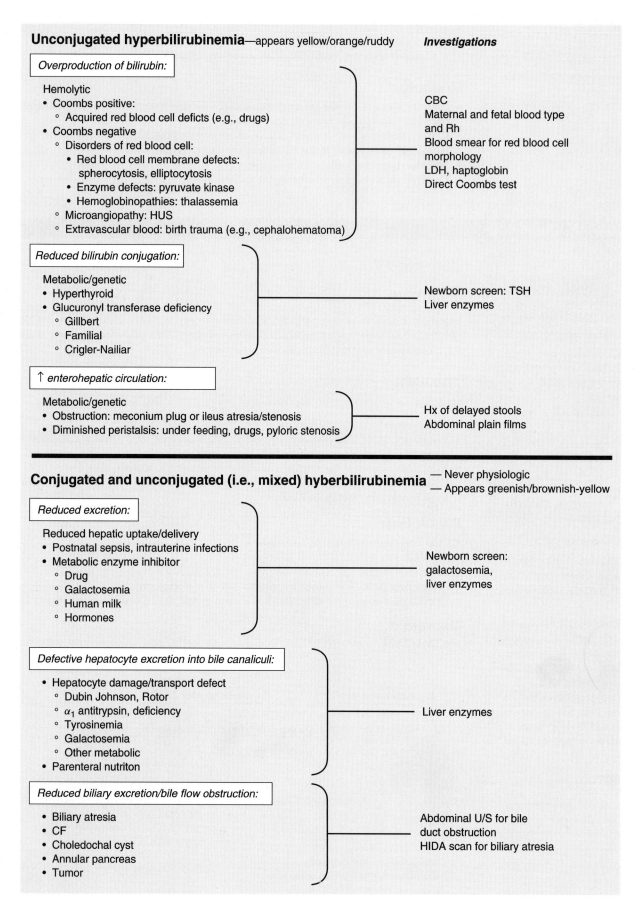

Unconjugated hyperbilirubinemia—appears yellow/orange/ruddy

Investigations

Overproduction of bilirubin:

Hemolytic
- Coombs positive:
  - Acquired red blood cell defects (e.g., drugs)
- Coombs negative
  - Disorders of red blood cell:
    - Red blood cell membrane defects: spherocytosis, elliptocytosis
    - Enzyme defects: pyruvate kinase
    - Hemoglobinopathies: thalassemia
  - Microangiopathy: HUS
  - Extravascular blood: birth trauma (e.g., cephalohematoma)

CBC
Maternal and fetal blood type and Rh
Blood smear for red blood cell morphology
LDH, haptoglobin
Direct Coombs test

Reduced bilirubin conjugation:

Metabolic/genetic
- Hyperthyroid
- Glucuronyl transferase deficiency
  - Gillbert
  - Familial
  - Crigler-Nailiar

Newborn screen: TSH
Liver enzymes

↑ enterohepatic circulation:

Metabolic/genetic
- Obstruction: meconium plug or ileus atresia/stenosis
- Diminished peristalsis: under feeding, drugs, pyloric stenosis

Hx of delayed stools
Abdominal plain films

Conjugated and unconjugated (i.e., mixed) hyberbilirubinemia
— Never physiologic
— Appears greenish/brownish-yellow

Reduced excretion:

Reduced hepatic uptake/delivery
- Postnatal sepsis, intrauterine infections
- Metabolic enzyme inhibitor
  - Drug
  - Galactosemia
  - Human milk
  - Hormones

Newborn screen:
galactosemia,
liver enzymes

Defective hepatocyte excretion into bile canaliculi:

- Hepatocyte damage/transport defect
  - Dubin Johnson, Rotor
  - α_1 antitrypsin, deficiency
  - Tyrosinemia
  - Galactosemia
  - Other metabolic
- Parenteral nutriton

Liver enzymes

Reduced biliary excretion/bile flow obstruction:

- Biliary atresia
- CF
- Choledochal cyst
- Annular pancreas
- Tumor

Abdominal U/S for bile duct obstruction
HIDA scan for biliary atresia

Figure 18.13 DDx for pathologic jaundice.

Table 18.21   Management of Neonatal Jaundice

Treatment	Principle	Advantages	Disadvantages
Phototherapy	Photoisomerization to water soluble isomers	• Relatively safe for mild-to-moderate hyperbilirubinemia • Readily accessible	• Contraindicated in conjugated hyper-bilirubinemia ("bronze baby") • Potential for burns, retinal damage • Loose stools • Dehydration • Skin rash and tanning • Significant separation of the infant and parents
Exchange blood transfusion	Reserved for dangerously high levels Removes and replaces partially hemolyzed and antibody-coated erythrocytes	• Most rapid method of treatment	• NEC • Thrombocytopenia • Coagulopathy • Arrhythmias • Infection • Death
Pharmacological	Heme oxygenase inhibitors (metalloporphyrins) Hepatic enzyme inducers: phenobarbital, IVIg (isoimmune hemolytic disease)	• May reduce need for exchange blood transfusion	• Experimental at present • Takes a few days for effect • Sedative

Neonatal Serum Bilirubin Nomogram

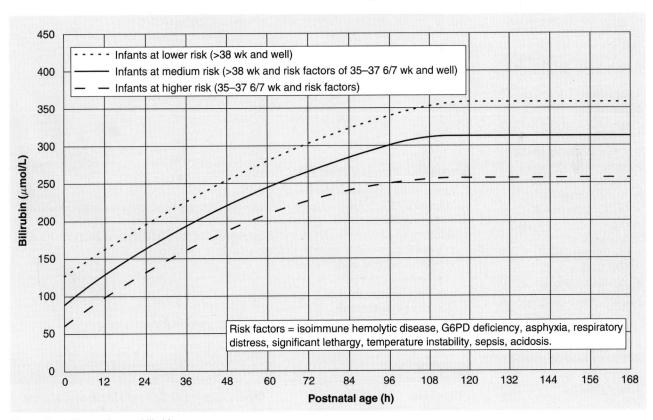

Figure 18.14 Neonatal serum bilirubin nomogram.

NONREASSURING FETAL STATUS (FETAL DISTRESS)

RATIONALE

Nonreassuring fetal status (FHR pattern) occurs in 5% to 10% of pregnancies; early detection/management can reduce serious consequences.

CAUSAL CONDITIONS

CLINICAL BOX

NST

- Fetal movements associated with accelerations of FHR
- Reactive/reassuring NST = two or more FHR accelerations, >/=15 bpm above the baseline and lasting >/=15 s within 20-min period

CLINICAL BOX

Causes of IUGR

Maternal factors
- Severe maternal starvation during pregnancy
- Chronic hypoxemia
- Prothrombotic hematologic/immune disorders
- Medical conditions and obstetrical complications associated with vasculopathy
- Infections (e.g., TORCH)
- Substance abuse
- Toxins

Fetal factors
- Chromosomal abnormalities or genetic syndromes
- Major congenital anomalies
- Multiple gestation

Placental insufficiency
- Abnormal uteroplacental vasculature
- Chronic inflammatory lesions
- Abruptio placenta
- Thrombophilia-related pathology
- Placental structural anomalies

CLINICAL BOX

Indications for Fetal Monitoring

Maternal conditions
- Antiphospholipid syndrome
- Poorly controlled hyperthyroidism
- Hemoglobinopathies,
- Cyanotic heart disease
- SLE
- Seizure disorder
- Chronic renal disease
- Type 1 diabetes
- Hypertensive disorders

Pregnancy-related conditions
- Pregnancy-induced hypertension
- Gestational diabetes
- ↓ Fetal movement
- Oligohydramnios
- Polyhydramnios
- IUGR
- Post-term pregnancy
- Moderate to severe isoimmunization
- Previous fetal demise
- Multiple gestation
- Placenta previa

DETERMINING NONREASSURING FETAL STATUS

1. Antepartum risk factors (as above)
2. Prenatal U/S(s): growth, placental condition, amniotic fluid volume, anatomic defects
3. NST—see side box
4. Fetal biophysical profile: 30-min U/S assessment of fetal activity and amniotic fluid
   - Valid from viability to term; predicts perinatal mortality
   - Indications/test of choice for:
     - Nonreactive NST
     - Post-term pregnancy
     - ↓ Fetal movement
   - Any other suggestion of fetal distress or uteroplacental insufficiency

Table **18.22**	**Fetal Biophysical Profile**
Component	**Criteria Required for Score of 2 (If Not Met, Score 0)**
1. Fetal breathing movements	One episode of rhythmic breathing lasting 30 s
2. Fetal tone	One episode of extension of extremity with return to flexion
3. Gross body movement	Three discrete movements
4. Amniotic fluid pocket	Single vertical pocket >2 cm in two axes
5. NST (not required if above components are normal)	Reactive

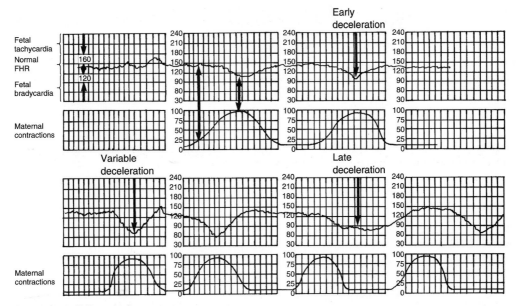

Figure 18.15 FHR monitoring.

(From Beckmann CRB, Ling FW, Laube DW et al. *Obstetrics and gynecology*, 4th ed. Baltimore: Lippincott Williams & Wilkins; 2002.)

5. FHR monitoring during labor
   - Baseline FHR: tachycardia (>160 bpm for >10 min) or bradycardia (<120 bpm for >10 min)
   - Variability
   - Accelerations
   - Decelerations
   - Fetal scalp blood sampling (for pH):
     - If nonreassuring FHR pattern, specificity to rule out asphyxia high
     - Sensitivity and positive predictive value of identifying hypoxic–ischemic encephalopathy low

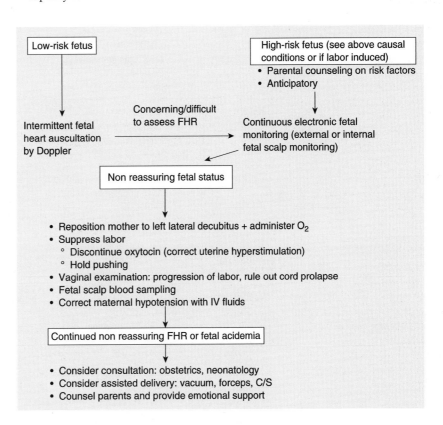

Figure 18.16 Approach to fetus with nonreassuring signs.

Significance of Decelerations

- **Early:** benign, for example head compressions
- **Variable:** cord compression
- **Late:** hypoxia

Consequences of Fetal Nonreassuring Status

- **Short term:** fetal acidosis and hypoxia
- **Long term:** hypoxic–ischemic encephalopathy, cerebral palsy

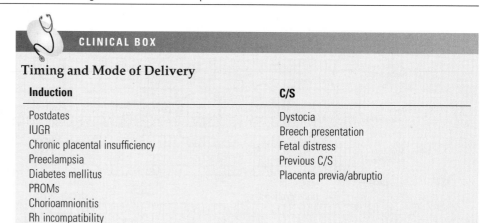

Timing and Mode of Delivery

Induction	C/S
Postdates	Dystocia
IUGR	Breech presentation
Chronic placental insufficiency	Fetal distress
Preeclampsia	Previous C/S
Diabetes mellitus	Placenta previa/abruptio
PROMs	
Chorioamnionitis	
Rh incompatibility	

- Suggested guidelines: pH >7.25, observe labor; pH 7.20 to 7.25, repeat within 30 min; pH <7.20, prepare for C/S

APPROACH

MANAGEMENT OF POST-TERM PREGNANCY (>42 WK)

- Labor induction: sweeping/stripping of membranes (does not modify risk for cesarean delivery and maternal and neonatal infections were not ↑)

Table **18.23**	Management of Infectious Diseases during Pregnancy that May Impair Fetal Development	
Infection	**Possible Fetal Consequences**	**Management during Pregnancy**
Toxoplasmosis	Chorioretinitis Mental retardation Hydrocephalus Stillbirth	Antibiotic therapy involving spiramycin
Other: syphilis	Hydrops Bone lesions Hepatosplenomegaly Keratitis Rash	Penicillin G (for any stage of syphilis) Monitor VDRL monthly
Rubella	Cataracts "Blueberry muffin" rash Congenital heart disease	Prevention—early prenatal testing Counsel about congenital anomalies Treatment of newborn supportive Vaccination of mother
Cytomegalovirus	90% newborns asymptomatic Periventricular calcification Hearing loss IUGR	Good hygiene (e.g., hand washing) Otherwise expectant Does not warrant C/S
Herpes simplex virus (HSV)	Skin, eye, mouth involvement Encephalopathy Severe coagulopathies	Acyclovir C/S if active lesions in third trimester
Varicella zoster	Limb hypoplasia Chorioretinitis Growth retardation Cataracts	Varicella zoster Igs within 72 h of infection Acyclovir also an option
Parvovirus B19	Hydrops	Expectant; fetal transfusion if hydrops
Hepatitis B	Prematurity Low birth weight	HBIG to neonate at birth + vaccine at 1, 6 mo

- Prostaglandin: cervical ripening and labor induction
- NST and amnionic fluid volume assessment
- Delivery if: evidence of fetal compromise or oligohydramnios

PREMATURITY

RATIONALE

<10% of babies born prematurely in North America account for >50% of all perinatal morbidity and mortality.

CAUSAL CONDITIONS/RISK FACTORS

MATERNAL

- **Past** pregnancies
  - **Prior preterm birth** = most significant
  - Spontaneous abortion in second trimester
- **This** pregnancy
  - Infections (bacterial vaginosis, GBS, TORCH, etc.), preeclampsia, PROM
  - Drugs: smoking, substance abuse
  - Disease: chronic medical illnesses
  - Diet: inadequate weight gain during pregnancy
  - Demographics: low socioeconomic status; non-Caucasian race

IATROGENIC (INDICATED INDUCTION OF LABOR)

- Uterine
  - Incompetent cervix
  - Excessive enlargement (hydramnios)
  - Malformations (leiomyomas, septate)
- Placental
  - Bleeding (previa, abruption)
  - Insufficiency

FETAL

- Multiple gestation
- Congenital/genetic anomalies
- Chorioamnionitis
- Threatened abortion/vaginal bleeding in early pregnancy

APPROACH

See Table 18.24.

LONG-TERM RISKS

- Cognitive and behavioral problems at school age (lower IQ, ADHD)
- Very/extreme prematurity: cerebral palsy; < normal visual acuity, and/or hearing loss

  Investigations for precipitants + prediction of premature birth:

1. Routine prenatal screening: for example, preeclampsia (BP, U/A), fetal U/S
2. Cervical U/S: length inversely proportional to risk of preterm delivery,
3. length >30 cm of high negative predictive value for preterm labor <34 wk
4. Fetal fibronectin: positive value in cervicovaginal fluid (as early as 8 to 22 wk) = powerful predictor of subsequent preterm birth

FURTHER MANAGEMENT OF PREMATURE INFANTS

- Nutrition
  - Human milk → ↓ risk of late-onset sepsis, NEC, bacteremia, other infections
  - 2,000 IU oral Vit D daily until transitioned to Vit D-fortified milk/formula
  - Comorbidities may require ↑ calories to maintain growth
- Counsel parents about immediate and long-term health problems
- Coordinate health care facilities for short- and long-term care

CLINICAL BOX

Low Birth Weight versus Prematurity

- **Low birth weight** = neonates born too small (<2,500 g)
- **Preterm** or **premature** = neonates born too early (<37 wk)

CLINICAL BOX

PDA

Shunts blood flow left to right → ↑ flow through pulmonary circulation and ↓ perfusion of systemic circulation

CLINICAL BOX

NEC

Specific findings
- Feeding intolerance, vomiting
- Bloody stools
- Abdominal distention, tenderness
- Pneumatosis intestinalis on AXR

Management
- NPO and NG decompression
- Oxygenation +/− mechanical ventilation
- IV fluids to replace third-space GI losses
- Broad-spectrum antibiotics
- Indications for surgery = evidence of necrosis: perforation, fixed dilated loop of bowel on serial radiographs, progressive deterioration

Table **18.24** Immediate Neonatal Health Problems	
Problems[a]	**Management**
Respiratory abnormalities • RDS • Apnea or prematurity • Chronic lung disease	Continuous cardiopulmonary monitoring Oxygenation Assist ventilation with PEEP, CPAP May require endotracheal surfactant May require caffeine stimulation if apneic
PDA	Volume expansion (possible inotropes) Systemic steroids
IVH Fragile germinal matrix; grades of severity	Screening + diagnosis by U/S on first day Supportive—avoid hemodynamic instability + conditions impairing cerebral autoregulation Follow-up serial imaging
ROP Developmental vascular proliferative disorder	Spontaneous regression common Avoidance of high PaO$_2$ Laser photocoagulation or cryotherapy if severe Follow-up eye exams
NEC	See clinical box NEC
Jaundice	Phototherapy (see Neonatal Jaundice)
Hypothermia	Plastic bags/wrap within minutes after birth
Hypoglycemia	Blood glucose monitoring routinely until feedings established and glucose values normalized
Hypocalcemia	Calcium supplementation
Infection (e.g., GBS)	Full septic workup Empiric antibiotic therapy

[a]Risks ↓ with ↑ gestational age.

CHILDHOOD COMMUNICABLE DISEASES

DEFINITION

Communicable diseases common in childhood; vary from mild inconveniences to life-threatening disorders; physicians need to differentiate between these common conditions and initiate management.

CAUSAL CONDITIONS

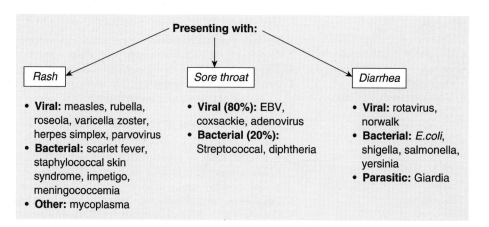

Figure 18.17 Causal conditions: communicable diseases.

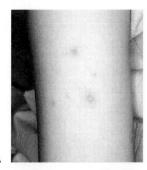

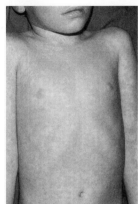

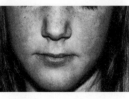

A

B

C

Figure 18.18 Examples of rash: communicable Disease. **A:** Chicken pox. **B:** Measles. **C:** Erythema infectiosum. (A. From Fleisher GR, Ludwig W, Baskin MN. *Atlas of pediatric emergency medicine.* Philadelphia: Lippincott Williams & Wilkins 2004; B. Copyright NMSB/Custom Medical Stock Photography; and C. From Goodheart HP. *Goodheart's photoguide of common skin disorders*, 2nd ed. Philadelphia: Lippincott Williams & Wilkins; 2003.)

COMMUNICABLE DISEASES

RASH

Chicken Pox: VZV

- Prodrome of mild fever and other systemic symptoms
- Generalized, polymorphous, pruritic, vesicular rash ("dew drop on a rose petal")
- Latency in dorsal root ganglia during primary infection → reactivation = "shingles"
- Primary infection usually results in life-long immunity
- Transmission: direct contact
- Incubation period: 10 to 21 d
- Contagious 1 to 2 d before onset of rash, until crusting of lesions

Measles: Morbillivirus

- Fever, cough, coryza, conjunctivitis (3Cs), diffuse maculopapular rash, transient enanthemas (Koplik spots)
- Rash starting on face and spreading caudally
- Risk of death from respiratory and neurologic complications
- Transmission: respiratory droplet
- Incubation period: 8 to 12 d

Erythema Infectiosum (Fifth Disease): Parvovirus B19

- Prodrome of fever, malaise, myalgias ~7 d prior
- Red "slapped cheek" rash with circumoral pallor
- Maculopapular, lace-like, pruritic rash on trunk, moving peripherally
- Other manifestations: polyarthropathies, anemia (immunocompromised), transient aplastic crisis (if have hemolytic anemia), hydrops fetalis (in first trimester of pregnancy)
- Transmission: respiratory droplets, blood (products), vertical transmission
- Incubation period: 4 to 14+ d

Herpes Simplex: HSV 1 or 2 (beyond Neonatal Period)

- Primary infection usually asymptomatic
- Gingivostomatitis most common: fever, irritability, tender lymphadenopathy, ulcerative enanthem
- Genital herpes in adolescents
- Recurrence: grouped vesicles periorally or genital, conjunctivitis, herpetic whitlow
- Transmission: direct contact with secretions from lesions, sexual intercourse
- Incubation period: 2 d to 2 wk

Impetigo: GABHS, *S. aureus*

- Pruritic/tender vesicular/pustular lesions rupturing into honey-colored crust
- Often secondary infection
- Bullous impetigo due to *S. aureus*
- Complications: glomerulonephritis
- Transmission: direct contact
- Incubation period: as rapid as 12 h

Roseola Infantum (Baby Measles): Human Herpes Virus 6

- High fever: 3 to 5 d → generalized maculopapular rash spreading from trunk to extremities, sparing face
- Transmission: likely droplet
- Peak incidence: 6 to 24 mo old
- Incubation period: 9 to 10 d

SORE THROAT

GABHS: S. pyogenes

- Acute onset sore throat, fever, headache, odynophagia, abdominal pain, N/V, anterior cervical lymphadenopathy
- Transmission: droplet
- Incubation period: 2 to 5 d
- No longer contagious within 24 h of antimicrobial therapy initiation

Important Nonsuppurative Sequelae of Streptococcal Infections

Acute rheumatic fever

Jones criteria for diagnosis: two major **or** one major + two minor

Major criteria
- Carditis
- Polyarthritis
- Chorea
- Subcutaneous nodules
- Erythema marginatum

Minor criteria
- Fever
- Arthralgia
- Prolonged PR interval on ECG
- ↑ Acute-phase reactants (ESR and CRP)

Scarlet fever
- Acute onset fever, sore throat, strawberry tongue
- 24 to 48 h after pharyngitis, rash in groin, axillae, neck → nonpruritic, nonpainful, confluent erythematous sandpaper-like; rarely systemic effects
- Fades after 3 to 4 d
- Treat as for pharyngitis × 10 d

Postinfectious glomerulonephritis

Infectious Mononucleosis: EBV
- Fever, exudative pharyngitis, lymphadenopathy, hepatosplenomegaly, atypical lymphocytosis
- Transmission: close personal contact
- Incubation period: 30 to 50 d

Diphtheria (*C. diphtheriae*)
- Extremely rare since development of childhood immunization
- Nasopharyngitis or laryngotracheitis; cutaneous form rare
- Low-grade fever and gradual onset over 1 to 2 d
- Complications: upper airway obstruction, toxic myocarditis, peripheral neuropathies
- Transmission: droplet
- Incubation period: 2 to 7+ d

APPROACH

Hx
- Presenting features of infection: rash, sore throat, or diarrhea
- Immunization status
- Hx of contacts, travel, farm visits, ingestion of unpasteurized milk or uncooked meat, source of water supply

INVESTIGATIONS
- Viral serology: detection of viral antigens and/or antibodies to virus
  - Can be assessed through blood sample, skin lesion scraping, nasopharyngeal secretions, throat swab, and so on.
  - For example, measles or parvovirus IgM
- Rapid diagnostic test: for example, rapid streptococcal test (based on group A carbohydrate antigen)
- Use of enzyme immunoassay, PCR, and/or direct fluorescent antibody staining techniques
- Bacterial, viral, fungal cultures
- Stool analysis: bacterial culture/sensitivity, O&P, fecal occult blood

Sexually Transmitted Diseases

Evaluate fully individuals and contacts with:

- Gonorrhea
- Syphilis
- HIV
- Chlamydia trachomatis (reportable)

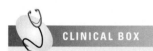

If Considering Congenital Infection

Ask about pregnancy and delivery, maternal Hx of fever, rash, flu-like illness, genital herpes, cleaning cat litter, and so on.

Key Objective

Determine incubation period and possible route of communication

- Trichomonas vaginalis
- Condylomata acuminata
- Herpes

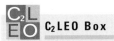 **C₂LEO Box**

Statutory Requirements of Physicians

Certain communicable diseases/infectious diseases require statutory reporting to the Public Officer of Health.

MANAGEMENT

Table **18.25**	Management of Specific Communicable Diseases	
Disease	**Diagnostic Techniques (In Addition to Clinical Assessment)**	**Management**
Chicken pox (VZV)	• Vesicle scraping for direct fluorescent antibody test • Serum IgG (retrospective diagnosis)	• Supportive; avoid salicylates (risk of Reye syndrome) • Acyclovir for immunocompromised • Consider postexposure immunization/VZIG in high-risk patient within 72 h **Control measures:** airborne + contact precautions until vesicles resolve/crust over
Measles (morbillivirus)	• IgM serology	• No antiviral therapy available • Standard + airborne precautions for 4 d after rash onset **Control measures:** • Universal immunization • Ig can be used in susceptible person within 6 d of exposure
Herpes simplex (human HSV 1 and 2)	• Viral culture—secretions, blood, or CSF • Rapid viral test • HSV 1, 2 serology • PCR of CSF	• Opthalmic drug for eyes; consult opthalmology • Genital herpes: oral antiviral therapy • IV acyclovir for immunosuppressed or 21 d if CNS involvement **Control measures:** • Contact precautions if severe mucocutaneous disease • If recurrent HSV infection, cover active lesions
Impetigo (*S. aureus*, GABHS)	• Culture of lesion scrapings	• Topical mupirocin; systemic antibiotics if extensive • Keep wound clean, avoid direct contact of lesions **Control measures:** avoid direct contact of lesions
Erythema infectiosum (parvovirus B19)	• Parvovirus B19 serology	• Supportive **Control measures:** • No longer infectious when clinical manifestations present • Standard + droplet precautions
Roseola (human herpes virus 6)	• No reliable technique	• Supportive (treat fever)
Strep pharyngitis (GABHS)	• Throat swab culture	• Treat primarily to prevent sequelae! • Penicillin drug of choice; ampicillin or amoxicillin • Erythromycin or first-generation cephalosporin if penicillin allergy **Control measures:** home from school until 24 h after starting antibiotics + droplet precautions
Infectious mono (Ebstein-Barr virus)	• Rapid monospot (heterophil antibodies) • Serology	• Avoid contact sports until spleen no longer palpable • Acyclovir not useful **Control measures:** standard precautions if hospitalized

CLINICAL BOX

Incompletely Immunized Child

- Lapse in schedule: does not require reinstitution of entire series; continue at next visit as if usual interval has lapsed
- If status unknown, consider disease susceptible and initiate appropriate immunizations without delay in schedule corresponding to person's current age

Immunization

CLINICAL BOX

Principles of Immunization

Active immunization
- Administration of all/part of microorganism or modified product of organism (e.g., toxoid, purified antigen) to evoke immunologic response mimicking that of natural infection
- Vaccines incorporating intact infectious agent may be live (attenuated) or killed (inactivated)

Passive immunization
- Administration of preformed antibody to recipient (e.g., Ig)
- Indications: immunosuppressed, antibody deficiency disorders, therapeutically when disease already present, postexposure situations

---

Table **18.26**	Recommended Canadian Infant/Child Immunization Schedule (*National Advisory Committee on Immunization, 2005*)									
Age	**DTaP-IPV**	**HiB**	**Pneu-C**	**Men-C**	**MMR**	**Var**	**HepB**	**DTap**	**Flu**
2 mo	▫	▫	▫	▫			Infancy: three doses or Preteen/teen: two to three doses if not yet given		
4 mo	▫	▫	▫	▫					6–23 mo
6 mo	▫	▫	▫	▫					▫
12 mo			▫	▫ if not yet given	▫	▫			One to two doses
18 mo	▫	▫			▫				
4–6 yr	▫				▫ or				
14–16 yr								▫	

HiB conjugate; Pneu-C (7-valent);
MMR (live, attenuated)—contraindications: immunocompromised, pregnancy, allergy;
Var (live, attenuated)—contraindications: immunocompromised, pregnancy, allergy;
DTap (adult formulation);
Flu = influenza.

ABNORMAL STATURE

DEFINITION

To define any growth point, children should be measured accurately and each point (height, weight, and head circumference) plotted.

SHORT STATURE (NORMAL VARIANT)

Familial
- Height <3 percentile
- Family Hx of short stature
- Normal Hx and physical exam
- Growth velocity >5 cm/yr
- Puberty at normal age
- Bone age[§] = chronologic age

Constitutional
- Height <3 percentile
- Family Hx of late puberty
- Normal Hx and physical

[§] Emergencies!

CLINICAL BOX

Normal Variant Short Stature

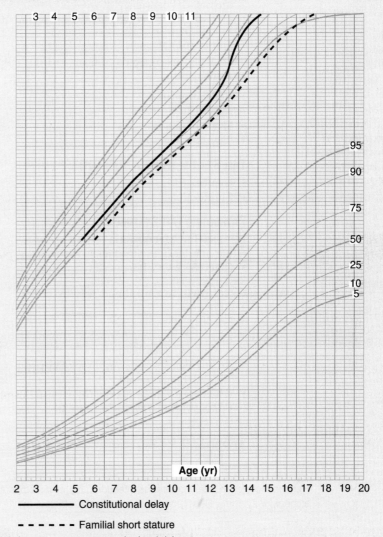

Familial short stature versus constitutional delay.

- Growth velocity >5 cm/yr
- Puberty late
- Bone age < chronologic age

PATHOLOGIC SHORT STATURE

Proportionate

IUGR

- Genetic syndromes (e.g., Turner syndrome)
- Congenital infection (e.g., TORCH)
- Placental insufficiency
- Drugs (e.g., nicotine, alcohol)

Postnatal

- Chronic malnutrition
- Psychosocial deprivation
- Drugs (corticosteroids, amphetamine)
- Radiation

Hx Suggesting IGF-1 Excess (Gigantism)

- Obesity
- Macrognathia/prognathism
- Swollen hands and feet, nose, coarse facial features
- Frontal bossing
- Hyperhidrosis
- Joint symptoms (hypertrophic arthropathy)
- Peripheral neuropathies (e.g., carpel tunnel syndrome)
- Headaches, visual problems
- Hypertension
- Left ventricular hypertrophy, cardiomyopathy
- Benign tumors including uterine myomas, prostatic hypertrophy, colon polyps
- Frequently associated endocrinopathies (e.g., hypogonadism, impaired glucose tolerance, hyperprolactinemia)

- Chronic illness: GI (celiac, Crohns), cardiopulmonary (CHF, CF), renal, hematology (severe anemia), infectious (recurrent, immunodeficiency syndrome)
- Endocrine: hypothyroid (most common endocrine cause), GC excess (Cushing syndrome), GH deficiency
- Precocious puberty (accelerated early growth and epiphyseal closure)

Disproportionate

Short limbs, exaggerated lumbar lordosis, epiphyseal growth plates do not respond to growth factors

- Achondroplasia
- Scoliosis
- Spinal radiation
- Rickets

TALL STATURE (NORMAL VARIANT)

- Familial
- Constitutional: precocious puberty (tall as child, short as adult)

PATHOLOGIC TALL STATURE

Intrauterine Macrosomia
- Intrauterine hyperinsulinism: for example, poorly controlled maternal diabetes mellitus
- Other: Beckwith-Wiedemann syndrome

Overgrowth in Childhood/Adolescence
- GH excess
- Pituitary adenoma (98%)
- Excess GH releasing hormone secretion/growth factor activity
  - Excess of other hormones
- Sex steroids deficiency or insensitivity (e.g., CAH)
- Thyroid: hyperthyroid
- Primary exogenous obesity (hyperinsulinism)
  - Other: MEN I, McCune-Albright

APPROACH

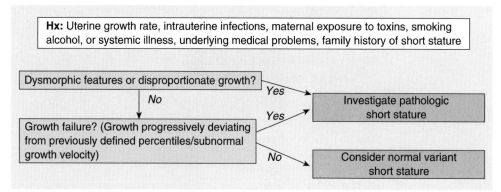

Figure 18.19 Approach to abnormal stature.

PHYSICAL EXAM
- Standing height, arm span, lower versus upper segment (difference is standing height minus distance from top of pubic symphysis to floor)
- Disproportionate or proportionate abnormal growth?
- Calculate growth velocity, and relationship between chronologic age and height age
- Dysmorphic features

INVESTIGATIONS
- CBC and ESR, U/A, Lytes and Cr, TSH and FT4, prolactin
- Skeletal radiographs—bone age (x-ray of left hand)

- Cytogenetic studies (karyotype, especially in girls)
- Chronic systemic illness labs (based on organ system, when indicated)
- Endocrine testing
  - Serum IGF-1 (low in GH deficiency)
  - Provocative GH testing: insulin tolerance or arginine test (subnormal serum GH response indicates GH deficiency)
  - 24-h urine-free cortisol or dexamethasone suppression test (subnormal values in GC deficiency)

MANAGEMENT

- Patients in need of specialized care—counsel families/children
- Specific to etiology: for example, hormone replacement in GH or GC deficiency, manage chronic illness
  - Use of exogenous sex steroids to promote epiphyseal fusion in children with tall stature very controversial; treatment otherwise conservative

SUDDEN INFANT DEATH SYNDROME

DEFINITION

- Sudden death of an infant younger than 1 yr that remains unexplained after thorough investigation, including Hx, autopsy, exam of the death scene.
- Devastating event for parents, caregivers and health care workers. It is imperative that the precursors, probable cause, and parental concerns are extensively evaluated to prevent recurrence.

CAUSAL CONDITIONS

TRUE SIDS

- Nonmodifiable possible risk factors: abnormal arousal/sleep pattern, long QT, ethnicity (higher incidence in minorities), siblings of infants who have died of SIDS, prematurity
- Modifiable risk factors: **maternal smoking**, prone sleep position

MIMICKING SIDS

- CNS (infection, seizure disorder, trauma, AV malformation, tumor)
- O_2 delivery
- Cardiac: cardiomyopathy, myocarditis, congenital malformation
- Pulmonary: pneumonia/bronchiolitis/bronchitis, airway abnormality
- Sickle cell anemia
- Nonaccidental trauma: battering, poisoning, Münchhausen by proxy
- Other: sepsis, hyperthermia, metabolic decompensation (underlying metabolic disease), hepatitis, adrenal disease, GI disease

SIDS is a diagnosis of exclusion: rule out nonaccidental trauma as a part of DDx.

MANAGEMENT

- Immediate resuscitative measures
- Important observations at the scene: as the position of the infant, marks on the body, body temperature and rigor, type of bed or crib and any defects, amount and position of clothing and bedding, room temperature, type of ventilation and heating, and reactions of the caretakers
- Short-/long-term bereavement management for parents/family
- Evaluate fully, but with compassion and empathy, possible causes (careful Hx and physical exam)
  - Rule out underlying illness of all systems
  - Rule out child abuse
  - Postmortem exam
- Referral and/or consultation for infants and families at risk that is bereavement issues, genetic counseling
- Child protection, if appropriate

PREVENTION

- "Back-to-Sleep" (supine sleeping position)
- Remove soft objects/loose bedding from crib; provide firm sleep surface
- Do not smoke during pregnancy
- Separate but proximate sleeping environment
- Avoid overheating
- Avoidance of home monitor use (no evidence suggesting reduction in risk)

ABNORMAL TEMPERATURE

DEFINITION

- Fever in children is the most common symptom for which parents seek medical advice. While most causes are self-limited viral infections it is important to identify serious underlying disease and/or those other infections amenable to treatment.
- Acute fever usually either viral (low grade, moderate fever) or bacterial (high grade, chills, rigors)

CAUSAL CONDITIONS

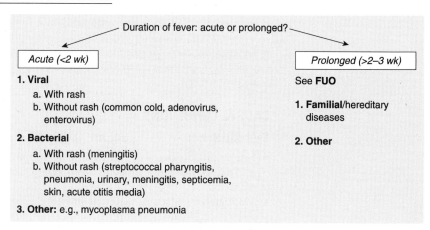

Figure 18.20 Abnormal temperature: causal conditions.

APPROACH

Hx

- Symptoms of sepsis (nonspecific): fever, chills, and constitutional symptoms of fatigue, malaise, anxiety, altered mental status (most consistent clinical feature)
- Localizing symptoms:
  - Head and neck—earache, sore throat, sinus pain/congestion, nasal congestion/exudate, lymphadenopathy
  - Chest—cough, pleuritic chest pain, dyspnea
  - Abdominal/GI—abdominal pain, nausea, vomiting, diarrhea
  - Pelvic/GU—pelvic/flank pain, discharge, dysuria, frequency, urgency
  - Bone/soft-tissue—focal pain or tenderness, focal erythema, edema, fluctuance

PHYSICAL EXAM

- ABCs, vital signs
- Findings suggestive of focal infection

INVESTIGATIONS

- Throat swab for culture: bacterial pharyngitis
- Blood culture: bacteremia
- CXR: consolidation = pneumonia
- U/A: leukocytes, nitrites
- Urine culture: UTI

- Stool culture, O&P: bacterial, parasitic, protozoan gastroenteritis
- Joint aspiration: septic joint
- Joint x-ray: osteomyelitis
- LP: meningitis, encephalitis

CLINICAL BOX

LP

Indications of LP	Contraindications to LP
1. Suspected CNS infection	1. ↑ Intracranial pressure
2. Suspected subarachnoid hemorrhage	2. Skin infections over puncture site
3. Therapeutic ↓ of CSF	3. Suspected intracranial mass lesion
4. Sampling of CSF for any other reason	4. Uncontrolled bleeding diathesis

SEPSIS/SEPTIC SHOCK

- SIRS present if abnormalities in two of the following: temperature, HR, respiratory rate, peripheral leukocyte count
- Sepsis = presence of SIRS in the setting of infection
- Severe sepsis = sepsis with evidence of end-organ dysfunction due to hypoperfusion
- Septic shock = sepsis with persistent hypotension despite fluid resuscitation → tissue hypoperfusion

CLINICAL BOX

Physical Signs of Sepsis

Early sepsis: peripheral vasodilation (tachycardia, bounding pulses, warm extremities, adequate capillary refill)

Later sepsis: stroke volume and CO ↓ → poor distal perfusion (cool extremities, delayed capillary refill, altered mental status, ↓ urine output)

Septic shock (inadequate organ function/perfusion):
- Alteration in mental state
- Hypoxemia (PaO_2 <72 mm Hg at FiO_2 0.21)
- Elevated plasma lactate
- Oliguria (<0.5 mL/kg/h)

DIAGNOSIS OF SEPSIS

>/= two of the following **in setting of infection:**

- Temperature >38°C (100.4°F) or <36°C (96.8°F)
- Tachycardia (>2 SD above the mean for age)
- Tachypnea (>2 SD above the mean for age)
- WBC >12,000 cells/mm^3 or <4000 cells/mm^3 or >10% band forms

MANAGEMENT

1. Resuscitate
   - Assess and support the airway, respiration, and perfusion
   - Supplemental O_2 (consider intubation) + continuous pulse oximetry
2. Monitor/restore tissue perfusion
   - Arterial catheter if BP labile or if restoration of arterial perfusion pressures expected to be protracted process
   - IV fluids: 40 to 60 mL/kg crystalloid solution push + repeat 20 mL/kg fluid boluses (adequate urinary output: 1 to 2 mL/kg/h)

Antibiotics Contraindicated in Children

- **Floroquinolones:** impair bone/cartilage growth
- **Tetracyclines:** staining of teeth, damage growing cartilage
- **Sulfonamides** (in neonates): kernicterus

CLINICAL BOX

Streptococcal Infection

Must be treated due to important sequelae! See **Childhood Communicable Diseases** topic.

- Vasopressors (second line)—dopamine, norepinephrine, epinephrine, or phenylephrine
- Consider central venous access
3. Eradicate infection
   - Collect appropriate cultures
   - Initiate empiric regimen of broad-spectrum antimicrobial agents

MANAGEMENT

- Key: treat fever based on presumed diagnosis/pathogen for several days/weeks
- ASA not recommended due to risk of Reye syndrome.*

CLINICAL BOX

Endemic, Epidemic, Pandemic

- **Endemic** = disease constantly present to a degree in people of certain class or living in a particular location
- **Epidemic** = affecting many individuals in a community or a population simultaneously
- **Pandemic** = epidemic occurring over very wide area, crossing international boundaries, affecting large numbers

CLINICAL BOX

Highest Risk Populations

- Children 6 mo to 5 y.o.
- Pregnant women
- Adults >/= 50 y.o.
- Adults with chronic conditions, immunosuppressed
- Persons who live with or care for persons at high risk

CLINICAL BOX

Reye Syndrome

- Acute hepatic encephalopathy + fatty infiltration of liver and kidneys
- Associated with ASA ingestion by children with varicella or influenza

Table **18.27**	**Management of Febrile Illness**	
Infection	**Common Bacterial Pathogen(s)**	**Empiric Antibiotic Treatment**
Meningitis	*N. meningitides, S. pneumoniae*, HiB (now rare)	Third-generation cephalosporin
URTI	Pharyngitis: GABHS Acute otitis media: *S. pneumoniae*, NTHI, *M. cattarhalis*	Penicillin Amoxicillin
Pneumonia	*S. pneumoniae*, GABHS; atypicals	Cefuroxime or amoxicillin; macrolides
UTI	*E. coli*	TMP-SMX; cephalexin or cefixime
Septic arthritis	*S. aureus*	Cloxacillin
Endocarditis	*S. viridans* (native valve)	IV oxacillin or nafcillin

---

* Emergencies!

Table **18.28**	**Special Topic: Influenza**
Characteristics of influenza epidemics	• Winter months • Begins abruptly, peaks over 2–3 wk, lasts for 2–3 mo • Influenza A more extensive and severe • Vaccination ↓ hospitalizations for cardiac and cerebrovascular disease • Complications: bacterial pneumonia, ear infections, sinus infections, dehydration, and worsening of chronic medical conditions
Prophylaxis	• **Annual immunization** = key in high-risk populations[a] • Antiviral drugs in patients not immunized or who may have suboptimal response to vaccine (chemoprophylaxis, see below)

Chemoprophylaxis	• May be useful for prevention in unimmunized children
	• **Not** to substitute for vaccination in high-risk individuals
	• Target groups when influenza active in community:
	  • High-risk children who have been vaccinated with no time to mount immune response
	  • High-risk children in whom vaccine contraindicated
	  • Immunocompromised children who may not respond to inactivated influenza vaccine
	  • Control of influenza outbreaks in a closed setting e.g., institution

Treatment	• Antivirals do not ↓ duration of illness but may ↓ risk of complications or need for hospitalization
	• Indications:
	  • ↑ Risk of severe or complicated influenza (+/− vaccination)
	  • Healthy children with severe illness

Antiviral drugs	• Neuraminidase inhibitors (oseltamivir [Tamiflu]) • M2 inhibitors (amantadine and rimantadine)

[a]See clinical box Highest risk populations.

FEVER OF UNKNOWN ORIGIN

See also Chapter 11.

DEFINITION

Unlike acute fever (<2 wk), which is usually either viral (low grade, moderate fever) or bacterial (high grade, chills, rigors) in origin, FUO = illness of 3 wk or more without an established diagnosis despite appropriate investigation.

CAUSAL CONDITIONS

INFECTIONS (~1/3 OF CASES)

- Systemic
  - Endocarditis
  - TB
  - Bacteremia
  - Miscellaneous rare infections (patients with HIV, travel abroad)
- Localized
  - Abscess
  - Contiguous spread (e.g., liver, subphrenic from hepatobiliary, bowel, retroperitoneal abscess)
  - Hematogenous spread (e.g., splenic)
  - Perinephric/renal
  - Osteomyelitis
  - CNS infections (meningitis, cerebritis)

NEOPLASMS (~1/3 OF CASES)

- Lymphoma/leukemia
- Solid (renal cell, hepatoma/metastases)

Multisystem (Connective Tissue Disease)

- Collagen disease (SLE, rheumatoid arthritis, vasculitis)
- Granulomatous (sarcoidosis, giant cell arteritis, Kawasaki)
- Miscellaneous (drug, factitious)

APPROACH

Hx

- Fever
  - Duration, height, pattern of fever, response to antipyretics
  - Localizing and associated symptoms/signs
- Past medical Hx + immunization record
- Travel Hx
- Animal exposure, insect bites
- Past exposure (e.g., TB), ill contacts
- Immunosuppression
- Medications (e.g., antimicrobial drugs)
- Contact with toxins or high-risk patients/contact or high-risk behaviors

Physical Exam

- Skin lesions and rashes: petechiae (infectious endocarditis, other bacteremias, and viral and rickettsial infections)
- Conjunctivitis (infectious mononucleosis, lupus erythematosus, TB)
- Oropharynx: pharyngeal hyperemia without exudate → infectious mononucleosis; gingival hypertrophy → leukemia or Langerhans cell histiocytosis
- Bone tenderness (e.g., osteomyelitis or malignancy)
- Rectal, external genitalia, and pelvic exam (pelvic abscess or tumor)

Investigation

Rule out common causes of fever first!

Blood
- CBC + peripheral smear: high or low counts are abnormal
- Lytes, urea, Cr, and hepatic enzymes: hydration status, metabolic/renal/liver pathology
- ESR, CRP: inflammatory process
- ANA/rheumatoid factor: connective tissue disease
- Bone marrow biopsy: if abnormal CBC/smear → possible malignancy

Urine
- U/A: UTI, nephritic/nephrotic syndrome
- CSF

LP
- Suspected meningitis or encephalitis

Microbiology
- Selective viral serology (e.g., HIV, HSV, EBV, CMV, hepatitis) +/− molecular testing
- Tuberculin skin test
- Blood culture: aerobic and anaerobic bacteria
- Urine culture

Imaging
- CXR: infiltrate, lymphadenopathy
- CT head, spine: mass lesion, ↑ intracranial pressure
- CT abdomen: abscess, tumor

Management

- Consistent with underlying cause—therapeutic trial without firm diagnosis is counter-productive!

- Select patients in need of specialized care
- Treatment of sepsis: see **Fever in a child**

APPLIED SCIENTIFIC CONCEPTS

Table **18.29**	Fever, Hyperpyrexia, and Hyperthermia
Concept	**Definition**
Fever	↑ Body temperature that exceeds the normal daily variation and occurs **in conjunction with** ↑ **in hypothalamic set point**
Hyperpyrexia	Fever >41.5° C (>106.7 °F) • Occurs in patients with severe infections, CNS hemorrhages
Hyperthermia	**Unchanged (normothermic) setting of the thermoregulatory center** in conjunction with uncontrolled ↑ in body temperature exceeding body's ability to lose heat • Mechanisms: exogenous heat exposure and endogenous heat production

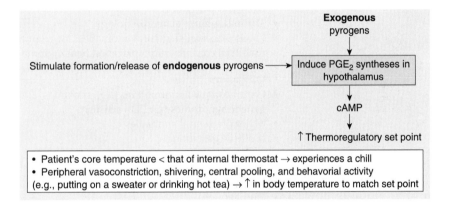

Figure 18.21 Pathophysiology of fever.

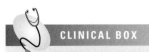

CLINICAL BOX

Exogenous versus Endogenous Pyrogens

Exogenous pyrogens
- Fever-producing substances from outside the body
- Examples = bacteria, bacterial endotoxin, antigen–antibody complexes, yeast, viruses

Endogenous pyrogens
- Produced by body (neutrophils, monocytes, hepatic Kupffer cells, splenic sinusoidal cells, alveolar macrophages, and peritoneal lining cells)
- Examples = pyrogenic cytokines interleukin 1, interleukin 6, tumor necrosis factor, interferon α

MECHANISM OF ANTIPYRETIC AGENTS

Synthesis of PGE_2 depends on COX via substrate arachidonic acid → antipyretics = COX inhibitors

1. Nonsteroidal anti-inflammatory agents (indomethacin, ibuprofen): excellent antipyretics
2. Acetaminophen: poor COX inhibitor in peripheral tissue but oxidized in brain → new form inhibits COX
3. GCs:
   - Reduce PGE_2 synthesis by inhibiting the activity of phospholipase A_2 (preventing release of arachidonic acid)
   - Block transcription of mRNA for pyrogenic cytokines

ABNORMAL WEIGHT

DEFINITION

- May be long-term sequelae for both IUGR and the infant large for the gestational age
- Low birth weight the most important risk factor for infant mortality, and significant determinant of infant and childhood morbidity
- LGA = infant with birthweight >90% for gestational age
- SGA = infant with birthweight <10% for gestational age
- Macrosomia = excessive growth regardless of gestational age, usually defined as birth weight >4,000 or 4,500 g
- IUGR = fetus that has not reached its growth potential because of genetic or environmental factors; results in birth of SGA infant

CAUSAL CONDITIONS

SGA (INCLUDES IUGR)

Maternal Factors

- Severe maternal starvation during pregnancy
- Chronic hypoxemia (pulmonary disease, cyanotic heart disease, severe anemia)
- Prothrombotic hematologic/immune disorders (e.g., antiphospholipid syndrome)
- Medical conditions (e.g., nephropathy, collagen vascular disease) and obstetrical complications (e.g., preeclampsia) associated with vasculopathy
- Viruses and parasites (e.g., TORCH)
- Substance abuse
- Toxins (e.g., medications such as warfarin, anticonvulsants, antineoplastic agents, folic acid antagonists)
- Demographic variables: race, pregnancy at the extremes of reproductive life, maternal age at first childbirth, nulliparity or grand multiparity, and previous delivery of SGA newborn

Placental Insufficiency

- Abnormal uteroplacental vasculature
- Chronic inflammatory lesions
- Abruptio placenta
- Thrombophilia-related pathology
- Gross placental structural anomalies: for example, single umbilical artery, velamentous umbilical cord insertion, placental hemangioma

Fetal Factors

- Chromosomal abnormalities (e.g., trisomies, autosomal deletions, ring chromosomes) or genetic syndromes (e.g., Dwarfism)
- Major congenital anomalies
- Multiple gestation

LPA

Maternal

- Familial
- Poorly controlled diabetes: excessive delivery of nutrients to the fetus, resulting in fetal hyperglycemia, hyperinsulinemia, and ↑ growth, particularly of insulin-sensitive tissues
- Maternal obesity
- Excessive maternal weight gain during pregnancy (normal is 25 to 35 lb)
- Multiparity: occurs more often as parity ↑
- Previous delivery of LGA infant
- Race and ethnicity: Hispanic and white newborns larger than black infants

Fetal

- Fetal disorders (e.g., Beckwith-Wiedemann syndrome, Sotos syndrome)
- Prolonged gestation
- Male fetus
- Rare: twin-twin transfusion syndrome

APPROACH

Hx

Prenatal

- Maternal: demographics, drug/teratogen use/exposure, chronic illnesses, obstetrical Hx (previous and current: gestational hypertension/HELLP, diabetes, etc.), family Hx genetic abnormalities
- Fetal: multiple gestation, fundal height measurements, intrauterine infections, results of prenatal screening

Delivery/Postnatal

Method of delivery, complications during delivery (e.g., hypoxia, birth trauma), Apgar

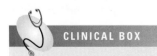

CLINICAL BOX

Normal fundal height = age of gestation (in cm) +/− 2 cm (at 12-wk gestation and beyond)

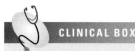

CLINICAL BOX

Classification of IUGR

Symmetric: early in gestation and usually caused by intrinsic factors (e.g., congenital infections or chromosomal abnormalities)

Asymmetric: reduced body weight and relatively normal length and head growth; abnormal growth typically begins in late second/third trimesters

CLINICAL BOX

Gestational Age Assessment—Ballard Score

- Extent of creases on the sole of the foot
- Presence and size of a breast nodule
- Features of scalp hair
- Characteristics of ear cartilage
- Appearance of genitalia
- Neurologic assessment of posture, active and passive tone, and reflexes

Physical exam alone is not sufficient to make or exclude the diagnosis of IUGR.

PHYSICAL EXAM

- Weight, length, head circumference in relation to gestational age on growth chart
- Gestational age assessment
- Vital signs, respiratory stability, level of alertness
- General inspection for abnormal movement of limbs, dysmorphic features and/or structural defects
- SGA infants with IUGR: symmetric or asymmetric IUGR
- LGA infants: assess for brachial plexus injury, clavicular fracture, other birth-related injuries

INVESTIGATIONS

Prenatal

- Prenatal U/S estimation of fetal weight = single best test to screen for and diagnose SGA/IUGR
- Also assesses abdominal circumference, body proportions, amniotic fluid volume
- Fetal karyotyping: if IUGR early (<32 wk), severe (<third percentile), or accompanied by polyhydramnios or structural anomalies
- Assessment for thrombophilic disorders may be considered if IUGR recurrent, early, severe, or with positive maternal/family Hx
- Doppler studies (umbilical artery) not useful for screening and diagnosis
- Use to identify small fetus at risk for adverse perinatal outcome (preterm birth, neonatal intensive care admission, asphyxia, etc.)
- To distinguish constitutionally small fetus from fetus with IUGR at risk for perinatal compromise

Postnatal

- CBC and hematocrit
- Blood gases
- Blood glucose (hypoglycemia)
- Chemistry
- Blood/urine/CSF cultures as indicated
- Drug screen
- Genetics: karyotype, metabolic testing if suspicious

MANAGEMENT

SGA/IUGR

- Anticipate complications: delivery should be planned at a perinatal center
- Prompt resuscitation, including clearing the airway of meconium if needed

Table **18.30** Complications of Abnormal Weight	
SGA	**LGA**
1. Difficult cardiopulmonary transition: beware perinatal asphyxia, meconium aspiration, or PPHN	1. ↑ Risk of cesarean delivery, severe postpartum hemorrhage, and vaginal lacerations
2. Complications of prematurity: e.g., NEC, RDS	2. Birth injury: brachial plexus injury +/− shoulder dystocia, clavicular fracture
3. Impaired thermoregulation	3. Perinatal asphyxia
4. Hypoglycemia: risk correlates with severity of growth restriction	4. Hypoglycemia (due to hyperinsulinemia)
5. Polycythemia: risk ↑ with severity of growth restriction (hypoxia → ↑ erythropoietin)	5. Polycythemia: hyperinsulinemia → oxidative demands → fetal hypoxia → ↑ erythropoietin
6. Impaired immune function	6. ↑ Perinatal mortality
7. Perinatal mortality: ↑ as growth restriction becomes more severe; congenital malformations, perinatal asphyxia, and transitional cardiorespiratory disorders	7. Minor congenital anomalies: talipes calcaneovalgus, hip subluxation
8. Long-term risk of impaired growth (e.g., short stature) and neurodevelopment (e.g., lower IQ) • More common if neonatal complications (e.g., asphyxia) and infant premature	8. May have propensity for adult obesity

- Avoid heat loss by immediate drying and placement under a radiant warmer
- Appropriate therapy for disorders of transition, including meconium aspiration pneumonia, myocardial dysfunction, or PPHN
- Enteral feeding early in healthy infants; in those with severe perinatal asphyxia, are ill, or do not tolerate enteral feeds, provide parenteral feeds
- Monitor for hypoglycemia serially
- Monitor ionized calcium levels (SGA infants who are premature or have birth asphyxia at risk for hypocalcemia) and supplement appropriately
- Specific attention to congenital malformations, chromosomal abnormalities, congenital infection

LGA
- If no contraindications, such as perinatal depression or other illness, feed early to avoid hypoglycemia and monitor glucose levels; measure hematocrit to detect polycythemia
- Preventive strategies: reduce risk factors (see above **Causal conditions**)

CHAPTER 19

Psychiatry

Dr. Gwyneth Zai, Dr. Clement Zai, Dr. John Teshima,
Dr. James L. Kennedy, and Dr. W.L. Alan Fung

ATTENTION DEFICIT HYPERACTIVITY DISORDER/LEARNING DISORDER

RATIONALE

- 5% to 10% of school-age population has developmental and behavioral problems.
- Long waiting lists for child psychiatrists often result in family physicians providing medical care for these children.

CAUSAL CONDITIONS AND APPROACH

See Figure 19.1.

INVESTIGATIONS

- Blood: CBC—electrolytes, anemia/infection, renal function, thyroid function, lead
- Urinalysis—toxin/drug: alcohol, marijuana
- Child abuse
- Neurologic consult—hearing, vision
- Mental status
- History from family, teacher with consent
- Family history

MANAGEMENT

Table **19.1** Treatment Options for ADHD		
Biologic	**Psychological**	**Social**

- Medications:
  - Atomoxetine
  - Mixed amphetamine salts
  - Methylphenidate
  - Dextroamphetamine
  - Pemoline[a]
  - Clonidine (α-adrenergic agonist)
  - TCAs
  - Bupropion
- Sleep
- Nutrition support
	- Counseling (individual, group and family)	- Structured activities
		- Behavioral management
		- Parent, child, and teacher education
		- Academic support

[a]Not available in Canada.

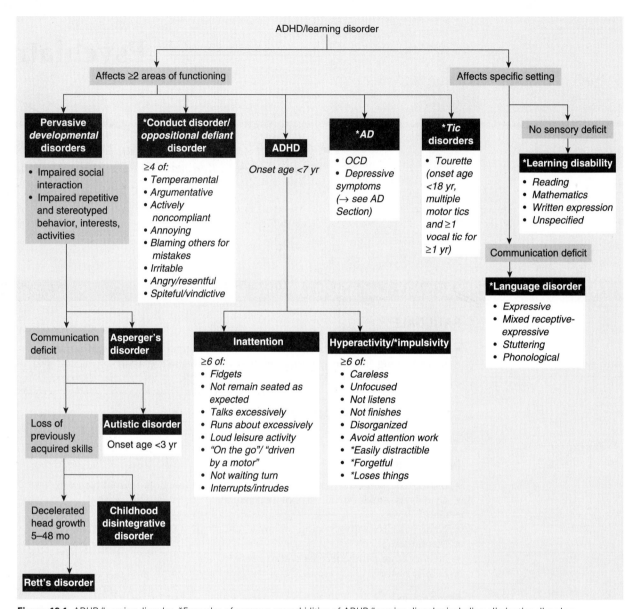

Figure 19.1 ADHD/learning disorder. *Examples of common comorbidities of ADHD/learning disorder including elimination disorders.

ANXIETY DISORDERS

ASC Box

Etiology of AD

- An exaggerated fear response has been postulated in the etiology of AD.
- Research studies have focused on the specific regions of the brain that coordinate fear and store memory for future exposure to the same stimuli, namely, the amygdala and hippocampus.
- Neurotransmitters that connect these brain regions have also been studied extensively including the dopaminergic, serotonergic, glutaminergic, and GABAergic systems.

RATIONALE

- Anxiety is part of the human adaptive reactions to external threats by activating the sympathetic nervous system—fight or flight.

- Anxiety becomes pathological if:
  - Fear is out of proportion to severity of threat.
  - When social and/or occupational functioning is/are impaired.

CAUSAL CONDITIONS

See Figure 19.2.

APPROACH

GENERAL OBSERVATIONS AND PHYSICAL EXAMINATIONS

- Mental status examination: body language, psychomotor retardation/agitation (fidgeting, moving about, hand-wringing, nail biting, hair pulling, lip biting, tremor), decreased eye contact, flat/restricted affect, suicidal/homicidal ideation/plan/intent
- Examine vital signs, pupils, and skin for diaphoresis, stigmata of drug and/or alcohol use, thyroid gland, and weight loss

INVESTIGATIONS

Table **19.2** Investigations for AD	
Test	**Finding/Interpretation**
CBC	• To rule out anemia and/or infection
Electrolytes	• To rule out electrolyte imbalance
BUN, creatinine	• To rule out renal failure
Fasting blood glucose	• To rule out hyper or hypoglycemia
Cortisol level	• To rule out adrenal abnormalities
Thyroid (TSH)	• To rule out hyper or hypothyroidism
Toxicology/drug screen	• Alcohol • Cannabis • Opioid • Amphetamine • Cocaine • Other stimulants
Urinalysis	• Drugs (see above)
Neurologic consult	• Headache to rule out brain lesions, masses, or hemorrhage
CXR	• Shortness of breath to rule out lung diseases
ECG	• Chest pain to rule out acute coronary syndrome
CT head	• Headache to rule out brain lesions, masses, or hemorrhage

CLINICAL BOX

AD Treatment

- SSRIs/SNRIs = Start with low dose slowly and aim for higher doses and longer duration to treat anxiety than depression.
- Exposure therapy is highly effective for phobia and OCD if the patient has insight.
- Avoid bupropion to treat anxiety.

MANAGEMENT

Table **19.3** Treatment Options for AD		
Biological (meds)	**Psychological**	**Social**
• Benzodiazepines • SSRIs/SNRIs (venlafaxine) • SSRIs • TCAs • MAOIs • Buspirone • Mirtazapine 30–45 mg	Requires insight into disorders: • Exposure therapy • CBT • Psychotherapy • Group therapy • Family therapy	• Support group • Community resources • Family involvement

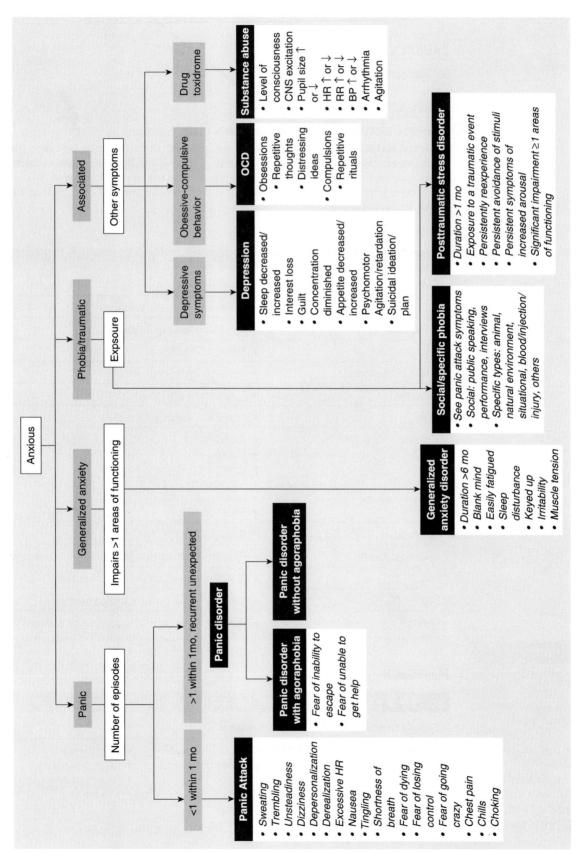

Figure 19.2

PERSONALITY DISORDERS

DEFINITION

- An enduring pattern of inner experience and behavior that deviates markedly from the expectations of the individual's culture; manifested in two or more of cognition, affect, interpersonal functioning, and impulse control
- Inflexible and pervasive across a range of situations
- Causes distress or impaired functioning not necessarily for the person with PD, but for those around him/her
- Usually at least age 18 yr for diagnosis, but pattern well established by adolescence or early adulthood
- Associated with many complications, such as depression, suicide, violence, brief psychotic episodes, multiple drug use, and treatment resistance

DSM-IV CRITERIA

CLINICAL BOX

General Diagnostic Criteria

1. Behavior deviates markedly from individual's cultural expectations. Inflexible and pervasive across a broad range of personal and social situations, manifesting in ≥ 2 of:
   - Cognition (perception and interpretation of self, others, and events)
   - Affect (range, intensity, lability, and appropriateness of emotional response)
   - Interpersonal functioning
   - Impulse control
2. Often leading to clinically significant distress or impairment in social, occupational, or other important areas of functioning
3. Stable and of long duration with onset tracing back to at least adolescence or early adulthood
4. Not better accounted for by other psychiatric disorders
5. Not due to direct physiologic effects of a substance or a GMC such as head injury

CLUSTER A: ECCENTRIC (ODD) AND "MAD"

Paranoid PD (0.5%–3%) = ≥ 4 Diagnostic Criteria from "SUSPECT"
- **S**: Spouse fidelity suspected
- **U**: Unforgiving and bearing grudges
- **S**: Suspicious of others
- **P**: Perceives attack on his/her character not apparent to others and reacts quickly
- **E**: Enemy or friend (suspects associates and friends)
- **C**: Confides in others feared
- **T**: Threats perceived in benign events

Schizoid PD (2%7%) = ≥ 4 diagnostic criteria from "SOLITARY"
- **S**: Shows emotional coldness to others
- **O**: Omits from social events
- **L**: Lacks friends
- **I**: Involved in solitary activities
- **T**: Takes pleasure in few activities
- **A**: Appears indifferent from praises and criticisms
- **R**: Restricts from close relationship
- **Y**: Yanks himself/herself from social interactions

Schizotypal PD (3%–5.6%) = ≥ 5 diagnostic criteria from "ME PECULIAR"
- **M**: Magical thinking or odd beliefs
- **E**: Experiences unusual perceptions
- **P**: Paranoid ideation
- **E**: Eccentric behavior or appearance
- **C**: Constricted (or inappropriate) affect
- **U**: Unusual (odd) thinking and speech

- **L**: Lacks close friends
- **I**: Ideas of reference
- **A**: Anxiety in social situations
- **R**: Rule out psychotic disorders and pervasive developmental disorder

CLUSTER B: DRAMATIC (IMPULSIVE/EMOTIONAL) AND "BAD"

Antisocial PD (3% in males; 1% in females) = ≥3 diagnostic criteria from "CORRUPT"
- **C**: Conformity to law lacking
- **O**: Obligations ignored
- **R**: Reckless disregard for safety of self or others
- **R**: Remorse lacking
- **U**: Underhandedness (deceitful, lies, cons, others)
- **P**: Planning deficit (impulsive)
- **T**: Temper (irritable and aggressive)

Borderline PD (2%–4%) = ≥5 diagnostic criteria from "PRAISE"
- **P**: Paranoid ideas
- **R**: Relationship instability
- **A**: Abandonment fear, anger outbursts, affective instability
- **I**: Impulsiveness, identity disturbance
- **S**: Suicidal behavior
- **E**: Emptiness

Histrionic PD (1.3%–3%) = ≥5 diagnostic criteria from "PRAISE ME"
- **P**: Provocative or sexually seductive behavior
- **R**: Relationships considered more intimate than they are
- **A**: Attention (uncomfortable when not the center of attention)
- **I**: Influenced easily
- **S**: Style of speech (impressionistic, lacks details)
- **E**: Emotional liability and shallowness
- **M**: Make up (physical appearance used to draw attention to self)
- **E**: Exaggerated emotions (theatrical)

Narcissistic PD (2%) = ≥5 diagnostic criteria from "SPECIAL"
- **S**: Special (believes he or she is special and unique)
- **P**: Preoccupied with fantasies of unlimited success, power, brilliance, beauty, or ideal love
- **E**: Entitlement (strong sense)
- **C**: Conceited (grandiose sense of self-importance)
- **I**: Interpersonal exploitation
- **A**: Arrogant (haughty)
- **L**: Lacks empathy

CLUSTER C: ANXIOUS AND "SAD"

Avoidant PD (0.5% −1.6%) = ≥4 diagnostic criteria from "AVOIDER"
- **A**: Avoid occupational activities
- **V**: View self as inept, unappealing, or inferior
- **O**: Occupies with fear of rejection or criticism in social situations
- **I**: Inhibits from new interpersonal relationships
- **D**: Difficulty initiating new projects due to lack of self-confidence
- **E**: Embarrassment prevents new activity or taking personal risks
- **R**: Restraints in intimate relationships due to fear of being shamed

Dependent PD (1.6% −6.7%) = ≥5 diagnostic criteria from "DEPENDENT"
- **D**: Difficulty in making everyday decisions without advice and reassurance from others
- **E**: Excessive length to obtain nurturance and support
- **P**: Preoccupies with thoughts of taking care of self
- **E**: Exaggerated fears of being left to care for self
- **N**: Needs others to assume responsibility for most major areas of his/her life
- **D**: Difficulty in expressing disagreement
- **E**: Ending one relationship immediately seeks urgently for another
- **N**: Not able to initiate projects due to lack of self-confidence
- **T**: Take care of me is his/her motto

Obsessive-compulsive PD (3%–10%) = ≥4 diagnostic criteria from "LAW FIRMS"

- **L**: Loses point of activity due to preoccupation with details
- **A**: Ability to complete tasks compromised by perfectionism
- **W**: Worthless objects unable to discard
- **F**: Friendships and leisure activities excluded due to a preoccupation with work
- **I**: Inflexible, scrupulous, overconscientious on ethics, values, or morality, not accounted for by religion or culture
- **R**: Reluctant to delegate unless others submit to exact guidelines
- **M**: Miserly toward self and others
- **S**: Stubbornness and rigidity

CAUSAL CONDITIONS

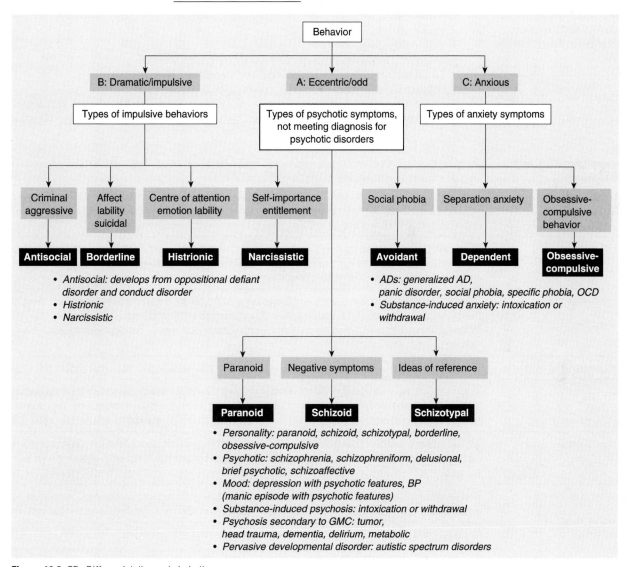

Figure 19.3 PD. *Differential diagnosis in italics.*

APPROACH

INVESTIGATIONS

- Routine blood work: CBC + differentials, thyroid function test (TSH, T3/T4), electrolytes, magnesium, calcium, phosphates, renal function test (creatinine, BUN), fasting glucose, hemoglobin A1C, liver function test (AST, ALT, ALP, albumin, INR, bilirubin), lipid profiles (LDL, HDL, TG), ESR, folate, vitamin B_{12}
- Urine drug screen
- Additional screening: neurologic consultation, CXR, ECG, EEG, CT/MRI of head

CLINICAL BOX

Differentiating from Other Psychiatric Disorders

- Onset: early onset (late adolescent to early adulthood)
- Duration: chronic for life, long enduring patterns of behavior
- Natural history: nonepisodic, nonfluctuating
- Functioning: pervasive across all functioning in life, affecting social, occupational, and interpersonal functioning
- Insight: egosyntonic

Avoid medications that can be abused (benzodiazepines, opioids) or can be fatal in overdose (TCA).

MANAGEMENT

- Psychoeducation
- Psychotherapies
- Dialectical behavioral therapy (especially for borderline PD)
- Social skills training (for schizotypal and dependent PD)
- Substances and alcohol abuse counseling (for antisocial PD)
- Pharmacotherapy: low-dose antipsychotics (for schizotypal and borderline PD), low-dose antidepressants, low-dose anxiolytics

Table **19.4** Psychotherapies	
Psychodynamic Psychotherapy	Interpersonal and relational intervention used to help patients in problems of living, increasing individual sense of well-being and reducing subjective discomforting experience; based on experiential relationship building, dialog, communication, and behavior change that are designed to improve the patient's mental health
Family/couple therapy	Works with families and couples in intimate relationships to nurture change and development with structural focus of here-and-now by reestablishing parental authority, strengthening normal boundaries, rearranging alliances, and emphasizing family relationships as an important factor in psychological health
Supportive therapy	Relies on the empathetic and supportive relationship between the patient and the therapist: to reduce anxiety, to strengthen defense mechanisms to assist day-to-day functioning, to enhance self-esteem, clarification, confrontation, rationalization, reframing, encouragement, rehearsal/anticipation, decatastrophizing, and allowing "ventilation" of frustrations
Group therapy	Develops goals of self-understanding, self-acceptance, increasing social skills, and creating a microcosm of society
CBT	Modifies cognitions, assumptions, beliefs, and behaviors, with the aim of influencing disturbed emotions; with behavioral component including systemic desensitization, flooding, positive reinforcement, negative reinforcement, extinction, and punishment; and with cognitive component including theory, goal setting, and thought record
Insight-oriented therapy	Involves intensive analysis of the unconscious aspects of psychology, emotions, and behaviors, exploring the inner conflicts caused by childhood loss or trauma, providing understanding and insight into ways of dealing with loss and conflict, and to develop more appropriate coping mechanisms
Interpersonal therapy	Brief psychological treatment for depression to improve the quality of the patient's relationships, focusing on unresolved grief and conflicts in his/her life that differ from his/her expectations, and overcoming social isolation
Brief therapy	Emphasizes on a specific problem with direct intervention

MOOD DISORDERS

RATIONALE

- Depression is one of the top five diagnoses in primary care.
- Depressed mood occurs in some individuals as a normal reaction to grief, but in others it is considered abnormal because it interferes with the person's daily function.
- It is necessary to detect depression, initiate treatment, and refer to specialists for assistance when required.

DEFINITION

- Mood disorders are defined by the presence of episodes, which represent a combination of symptoms comprising a predominant mood state such as major depressive, manic, mixed, and/or hypomanic
- Age of onset: 20s to 30s
- Prevalence 5% to 15% with female-to-male ratio of 2:1
- 50% recurrence after first episode, 70% to 75% after the second episode, and 90% after the third episode without treatment; 20% recurrence with antidepressant treatment
- Fourth leading cause of global disability (WHO) and estimated as second by 2020
- Second reason for prescription (with hyperlipidemics being the first)
- Depression worsened many GMC in morbidity and mortality
- Higher in urban than in rural (lower income and lower support)
- Only 40% consults with family physicians of which only 25% receive treatment

CAUSAL CONDITIONS

- Adjustment disorder with depressed mood
- Dementia (associated with aphasia, apraxia, agnosia, and/or disturbance in executive functioning with planning, organizing, sequencing, and abstracting)
- Posttraumatic stress disorder (reexperiencing traumatic event with anxiety symptoms and can be complicated with depressive symptoms)

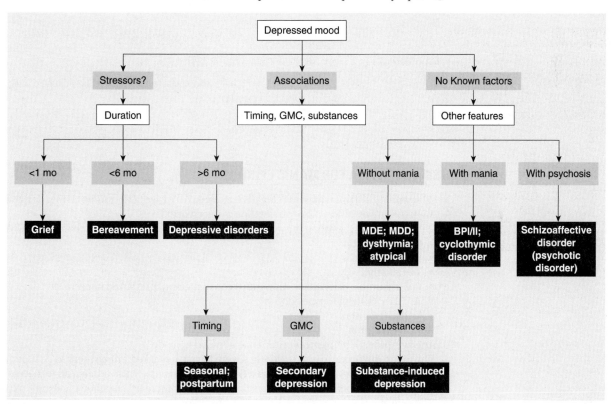

Figure 19.4 Differential diagnosis of mood disorders.

DSM-IV CRITERIA FOR MDE

1. At least five of the following symptoms (**MSIGECAPS**) with at least one of depressed mood or anhedonia presented within the same 2-wk period with a change from previous functioning:
   - **M**: mood depressed
   - **S**: Sleep decreased or increased
   - **I**: Interest decreased (anhedonia)
   - **G**: Guilt
   - **E**: Energy decreased
   - **C**: Concentration decreased

- **A**: Appetite decreased or increased
- **P**: Psychomotor agitation or retardation
- **S**: Suicidal ideation
2. The symptoms do not meet criteria for a mixed episode.
3. The symptoms cause clinically significant distress or impairment in social, occupational, or other important areas of functioning.
4. The symptoms are not due to the direct physiological effects of a substance or GMC.
5. The symptoms are not better accounted for by bereavement and other psychiatric disorders.

Table **19.5**	**Causes of Secondary Mood Disorders (VITAMINN CDE)**
Vitamin disorders	Wernicke, beriberi, pellagra, pernicious anemia
Infectious	Encephalitis/meningitis, hepatitis, pneumonia, tuberculosis, syphilis
Trauma	Brain injuries
Autoimmune	SLE, polyarteritis nodosa
Metabolic	Porphyria, Wilson, diabetes
Intoxication/withdrawal	Opioids, benzodiazepines
Neoplastic	Pancreatic cancer, carcinoid, pheochromacytoma
Neurological	Huntington, multiple sclerosis, tuberous sclerosis, degenerative (vascular, Alzheimer's, Parkinson's), epilepsy, stroke, CVA
Cardiovascular	Cardiomyopathy, CHF, MI, CAD
Drugs	Antihypertensives, antiparkinsonian, hormones, steroids, antituberculous, interferon, antineoplastic
Endocrine	Hypothyroidism, hyperthyroidism, hypopituitarism, SIADH

DSM-IV CRITERIA FOR MANIC EPISODE

1. Abnormally and persistently elevated, expansive, or irritable mood lasting for at least 1 wk (or any duration if hospitalization is necessary)
2. At least three of the following symptoms or four if the mood is only irritable (**GSTPAID**)
   - **G**: Grandiosity
   - **S**: Sleep decreased
   - **T**: Talkative
   - **P**: Pleasurable activities with painful consequences, pressured speech
   - **A**: Activity level increased
   - **I**: Ideas (flight of)
   - **D**: Distractible
3. The symptoms do not meet criteria for a mixed episode.
4. The mood disturbance is sufficiently severe to cause marked impairment in occupational functioning or in usual social activities or relationships with others, or to necessitate hospitalization to prevent harm to self or others, or there are psychotic features.
5. The symptoms are not due to the direct physiologic effects of a substance (such as drug abuse, medications, and/or other treatment), or a GMC.

MIXED EPISODE

- Criteria met for both manic episode and MDE nearly every day for 1 wk.
- Criteria 4 and 5 of manic episodes are met.

HYPOMANIC EPISODE

- Criterion 1 of a manic episode is met but duration is at least 4 d.
- Criteria 2 and 5 of manic episodes are met.
- Episodes associated with an uncharacteristic decline in functioning that is observable by others.

- Change in function is **not** severe enough to cause marked impairment in social or occupational functioning or to necessitate hospitalization.
- Absence of psychotic features

MDD

1. Presence of a single MDE (vs. recurrent with the presence of two or more separate MDE as considered by an interval of at least two consecutive months in which criteria are not met for a MDE)
2. MDE is not better accounted for by schizoaffective disorder and is not superimposed on schizophrenia, schizophreniform disorder, delusional disorder, or psychotic disorder not otherwise specified.
3. There has never been a manic episode, a mixed episode, or a hypomanic episode.

Table **19.6**	**Features/Specifiers of MDD**
Psychotic	With the presence of hallucinations or delusions
Chronic	Lasting for 2 or more yr
Catatonic	With at least two of motoric immobility, excessive motor activity, extreme negativism, or mutism, peculiarities of voluntary movement, echolalia, or echopraxia
Melancholic	With quality of mood depressed distinctly that is worse in the morning with early morning awakening, nonreactive mood, marked weight loss, excessive guilt, psychomotor retardation
Atypical	With reactive mood, increased sleep, overeating/weight gain, leaden paralysis, rejection hypersensitivity
Postpartum	Occurs in 10% of mothers, typically from 4 wk lasting for 2–6 mo with residual symptoms lasting up to 1 yr, and may present with psychosis, mania, and MDE
Seasonal	With pattern of onset at the same time each year, usually recurrent onset in autumn/winter with remission in spring/summer

DYSTHYMIA (6%)

1. Depressed mood for most of the day, depressed for more days than not, as indicated either by subjective account or observation by others, for at least 2 yr
2. At least two of the following while depressed:
   - Poor appetite or overeating
   - Insomnia or hypersomnia
   - Low energy or fatigue
   - Low self-esteem
   - Poor concentration or difficulty in making decisions
   - Feelings of hopelessness
3. During the 2-yr period of the disturbance, the person has never been without the symptoms in criteria 1 and 2 for more than 2 mo at a time.
4. No MDE has been present during the first 2 yr of the disturbance.
5. There has never been a manic episode, a mixed episode, or a hypomanic episode, and criteria have never been met for cyclothymic disorder.
6. The disturbance does not occur exclusively during the course of a chronic psychotic disorder, such as schizophrenia or delusional disorder.
7. The symptoms are not due to the direct physiologic effects of a substance or a GMC.
8. The symptoms cause clinically significant distress or impairment in social, occupational, or other important areas of functioning.

BIPOLAR DISORDERS (BPs)

- **BP I**—disorder in which at least one manic or mixed episode has occurred commonly accompanied by at least one MDE but not required for diagnosis
- **BP II**—disorder in which there is at least one MDE and at least one hypomanic episode without past manic or mixed episode

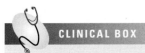

CLINICAL BOX

Risk Factors for MDD

Sex (F > M), age (onset in 25–50 yr age group), family history (depression, alcohol abuse, sociopathy), childhood experiences (loss of parent before age 11, negative home environment with abuse or neglect), personality (insecure, dependent, obsessive), recent stressors (illness, financial, legal), postpartum (<6 mo), lack of intimate/confiding relationships, or social isolation

CYCLOTHYMIA

- Presence of numerous periods of hypomanic and depressive symptoms while not meeting criteria for MDE for at least 2 yr and never without symptoms for more than 2 mo
- No MDE, manic, or mixed episodes and no evidence of psychosis
- Not due to a GMC or substance use
- Symptoms cause clinically significant distress or impairment in social, occupational, or other important areas of functioning.

APPROACH

GENERAL OBSERVATIONS AND PHYSICAL EXAMINATIONS

- Mental status examination: psychomotor retardation/agitation (fidgeting, moving about, hand-wringing, nail biting, hair pulling, lip biting), decreased eye contact, depressed mood and flat/restricted affect, slowness of speech/thought, suicidal/homicidal ideation/plan/intent
- Examine vital signs, pupils, and skin for previous suicide attempts, stigmata of drug and/or alcohol use, thyroid gland, and weight loss.

INVESTIGATIONS

- Blood works = CBC, electrolytes, BUN, creatinine, fasting blood glucose, liver profiles, thyroid profiles (TSH), toxicology/drug screen (alcohol, cannabis, opioid, amphetamine/stimulant or cocaine withdrawal or intoxication)
- Urinalysis, urine drug screen
- Additional screening: neurologic consultation, CXR, ECG, CT scan as indicated

TREATMENT

Table **19.7**	Treatment Options for Mood Disorders		
Biologic (meds)	**Med Dosage**	**Psychological**	**Social**

SSRIs	• 20–60 mg of fluoxetine, paroxetine, and citalopram
	• 50–200 mg of sertraline and fluvoxamine
	• 10–20 mg of escitalopram
		Requires insight into disorders
		• CBT
		• Psychotherapy
		  • Interpersonal psychotherapy
		  • Psychodynamic psychotherapy
		  • Group therapy
		  • Family therapy
			• Support group
			• Community resources
			• Family involvement

TCAs	• 50–150 mg of nortriptyline • 150–300 mg of amitriptyline, imipramine, and desipramine		
MAOIs	• 45–90 mg of phenelzine • 20–60 mg of tranylcypromine • 450–900 mg of moclobemide		
Venlafaxine	• 75–375 mg		
Bupropion	• 150–300 mg		
Mirtazapine	• 30–45 mg		
Also consider ECT.			

PSYCHOTIC PATIENT/THOUGHT DISORDERS

RATIONALE

Psychosis refers to a mental disorder that is marked by deranged personality and loss of contact with reality, often with delusions, hallucinations, or illusions, with schizophrenia being the most severe (1% of the general population).

CAUSAL CONDITIONS

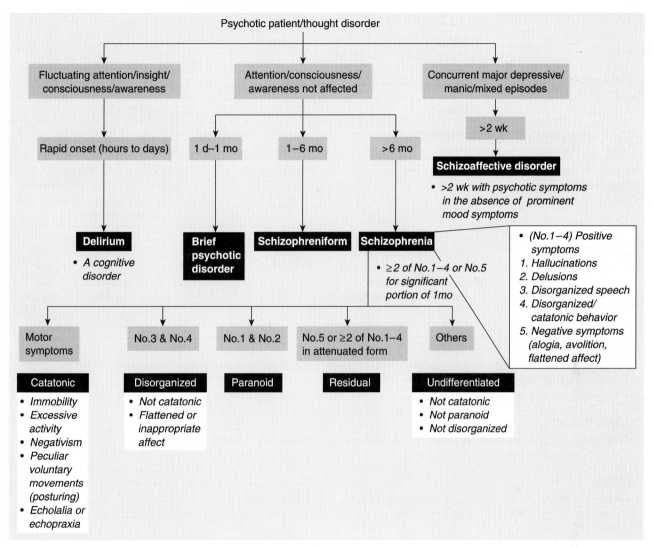

Figure 19.5 Psychotic patient/thought disorder.

DIFFERENTIAL DIAGNOSES

- Substance-induced (intoxication or withdrawal): alcohol, steroids, hallucinogens, lead
- History of pervasive developmental disorders: autistic spectrum disorder
- Concurrent major depressive, manic, or mixed episodes: schizoaffective disorder and mood disorder with psychotic features
- GMC: tumor, head trauma, dementia, metabolic

APPROACH

INVESTIGATIONS

- Routine blood work: CBC + differentials, thyroid function test (TSH, T3/T4), electrolytes, magnesium, calcium, phosphates, renal function tests (creatinine, BUN), fasting glucose, hemoglobin A1C, liver function test (AST, ALT, ALP, albumin, INR, bilirubin), lipid profiles (LDL, HDL, TG), ESR, folate, vitamin B12
- Urine drug screen, urinalysis
- Additional screening: neurologic consultation, CXR, ECG, EEG, CT/MRI of head

MANAGEMENT

Continuous monitoring (See Table 19.8)

Table **19.8**	Management of Psychotic Patient/Thought Disorders

PHARMACOLOGIC

Important notes

- Titrations
- Oral (peak plasma levels after 1–4 h) or intramuscular (peak plasma levels after 30 min with clinical effects starting after 15–30 min)
- Poor subjective response predicts poor compliance—may need long-acting forms

Antipsychotics	Indications	Contraindications	Adverse Effects
Typical—high potency (haloperidol, fluphenazine)	Positive symptoms; pregnancy (haloperidol)	Preexisting movement disorder/TD	Higher risk of EPS/TD; hyperprolactinemia
Typical—low potency (chlorpromazine, thioridazine)	Positive symptoms	Preexisting movement disorder/TD	Lower risk of EPS/TD; postural hypotension, sedation, anticholinergic (blind as a bat, mad as a batter, dry as a bone, red as a beet, hot as a hare)
Atypical (olanzapine, risperidone, ziprasidone[a], clozapine, quetiapine, amisulpride[a], aripiprazole[a])	Positive or negative or cognitive symptoms; preexisting movement disorders sensitivity (quetiapine or clozapine); treatment refractory (clozapine); suicidality (clozapine)	Diabetes (relative not absolute)	Low risk of EPS/TD; Weight gain/hyperglycemia/hyperlipidemia/diabetes/sedation; agranulocytosis (clozapine—need weekly CBC for 6 mo then $\geq$ biweekly CBC); prolonged QT interval (especially quetiapine—need ECG monitoring)

PSYCHOSOCIAL

- Psychodynamic psychotherapy—explore conflicts, resistance, defenses, sense of self, relationships
- Supportive psychotherapy—reassure, explain, clarify, guide, and suggest
- CBT—same as supportive except also to gradually help patient challenge their delusional beliefs by examining evidence for them

HOSPITALIZATION

- For suicidal or aggressive patients and patients who cannot care for themselves outside hospital
- For stabilization of acute episodes

OTHERS

- Psychoeducation for patient, caregiver, and family about nature and natural history of psychosis
- Rehab and day programs, case management, supportive housing, ACT teams, community support groups for patients and family members, sheltered work programs
- Emotional support
- Select patients who need specialized care

[a]Not available in Canada.

 C₂LEO Box

Ethics

- Psychotic patients will require treatment with psychotropic medications and the patient's beliefs on this issue must be evaluated first.
- State and provide support with disclosure of difficult news: interpret side effects and health risks with the use of recommended medications.
- Psychotic conditions are usually chronic, difficult to manage, and require extensive resources. However, select patients for referral, hospitalization, and emergency care in a manner that is fair and equitable, without bias or discrimination. Also, describe to the patient the impact of cost restraint in a supportive way.

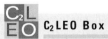 **C₂LEO Box**

Law

- The same fundamental legal rights that are binding on the physician will apply to a patient who is psychotic.
- Consent is mandatory with patient who is psychotic. Consent should be obtained after discussion with the patient concerning anticipated effects, risks, alternatives available, and information about delegation of care.
- Necessary treatment without consent is to be provided to a psychotic patient only in a medical emergency.
- For a patient who is psychotic, information disclosure may be permitted by law (e.g., ability to drive).
- Duty of care for a psychotic patient is expected until the doctor/patient relationship is ended through an appropriate process. The physician may be held vicariously liable for others (nurses, etc.) who are under the physician's delegation.
- Mental Health Act may need to be implemented to enforce observation or treatment.

SEXUALLY CONCERNED PATIENT/GENDER IDENTITY DISORDER

RATIONALE

The social appropriateness of sexuality is culturally determined. The physician's own sexual attitude needs to be recognized and taken into account to deal with the patient's concern in a relevant manner. The patient must be set at ease to make possible discussion of private and sensitive sexual issues.

CAUSAL CONDITIONS

Sexual Dysfunctions (Male and Female)
- See Chapters 14 and 21 for details.
- Arousal/desire problems (inhibition of sexual desire): medication-induced (antidepressants), medical diseases, psychiatric disorders
- Coital pain problems (dyspareunia): vaginal atrophy, imperforate hymen, trauma
- Orgasm related (premature ejaculation/ejaculation failure/anorgasmia)
- Erectile dysfunction (impotence)
- Vaginismus and/or sexual phobias

Sexual Paraphilias
Sexual arousal, fantasies, sexual urges or behavior involving nonhuman objects, suffering or humiliation of oneself or one's partner, children, or others

- Rarely self-referred, and often come to medical attention through interpersonal or legal conflict
- Person usually has more than one paraphilia with only 5% of paraphilia diagnoses attributed to women.
- Typical presentation begins in childhood or early adolescent, increasing in complexity and stability with age but decreasing with advancing age although with chronic presentation, and may increase with psychosocial stressors.

Gender Identity Disorder
Typical Presentation
- Gender identity is set in most people by age 2 or 3 yr of age
- Strong and persistent cross-gender identification
- Repeated stated desire or insistence that one is of the opposite sex
- Preference for cross-dressing, cross-gender roles in make-believe plays
- Intense desire to participate in the stereotypical games and pastimes of the opposite sex
- Strong preference for playmates of the opposite sex
- Significant distress or impairment in functioning and persistent discomfort with his or her sex or gender role
- Prevalence: 1 in 11,000 men; 1 in 30,000 women
- Sex ratio: M:F = 3–5:1

- Prognosis depends on age of onset and intensity of symptoms
- Boys: develop the disorder before age 4 yr
- Cross-dressing may be present
- Girls: most give up masculine behavior by adolescence
- One third to two thirds would develop homosexuality (fewer females than males)

Table **19.9** Subtypes of Paraphilia	
Subtype	**Definition**
Exhibitionism	Recurrent urge of behavior to exposure one's genitals to an unsuspecting person
Fetishism	Use of nonsexual or nonliving objects or part of a person's body to gain sexual excitement
Frotteurism	Recurrent urge or behavior of touching or rubbing against a nonconsenting person
Voyeurism	Recurrent urge or behavior to observe an unsuspecting person who is naked, disrobing, or engaging in sexual activities, or may not be sexual in nature at all
Pedophilia	Sexual attraction to prepubescent or peripubescent children
Sexual masochism	Recurrent urge or behavior of wanting to be humiliated, beaten, bound, or otherwise made to suffer for sexual pleasure
Sexual sadism	Recurrent urge or behavior involving acts in which the pain or humiliation of the victim is sexually exciting
Transvestite fetishism	Sexual attraction toward the clothing of the opposite gender
Paraphilia not otherwise specified	• Necrophilia: sexual attraction to corpses • Zoophilia: sexual attraction to animals • Coprophilia: sexual pleasure from feces • Urophilia: sexual pleasure from urine and urination

DSM-IV Criteria for Gender Identity Disorder
1. Strong and persistent cross-gender identification (not merely a desire for any perceived cultural advantages of being the other sex)
   - In children, the disturbance is manifested by four or more of:
     - Repeated stated desire or insistence that one is of the opposite sex
     - In boys, preference for cross-dressing or stimulating female attire; in girls, insistence on wearing only stereotypical masculine clothing
     - Strong and persistent preferences for cross-sex roles in make-believe plays or persistent fantasies of being the other sex
     - Intense desire to participate in the stereotypical games and pastimes of the opposite sex
     - Strong preference for playmates of the opposite sex
     - In adolescents and adults, the disturbance is manifested by symptoms such as a stated desire to be the other sex, frequent passing as the other sex, desire to live or be treated as the other sex, or the conviction that one has the typical feelings and reactions of the other sex
2. Persistent discomfort with his or her sex or sense of inappropriateness in the gender role of that sex.
   - In children, the disturbance is manifested by any of the following:
     - In boys, assertion that his penis or testes are disgusting or will disappear, or assertion that it would be better not to have a penis, or aversion toward rough-and-tumble play, and rejection of male stereotypical toys, games, and activities
     - In girls, rejection of urinating in a sitting position, assertion that she has or will grow a penis, or assertion that she does not want to grow breasts or menstruate, or marked aversion toward normative feminine clothing

- In adolescents and adults, the disturbance is manifested by symptoms such as preoccupation with getting rid of primary and secondary sexual characteristics (e.g., request for hormones, surgery, or other procedures to physically alter sexual characteristics to simulate the other sex) or belief that one was born the wrong sex

3. The disturbance is not concurrent with a physical intersex condition.
4. The disturbance causes clinically significant distress or impairment in social, occupational, or other important areas of functioning.
5. Gender identity disorder not otherwise specified.
   - Intersex conditions (e.g., Turner, Klinefelter, partial androgen insensitivity syndrome, congenital adrenal hyperplasia)
   - Cross-dressing behavior that is transient and stress-related
   - Persistent preoccupation with castration or penectomy without a desire to acquire the sex characteristics of the other sex

LESBIAN AND GAY PATIENTS

- Sexual orientation describes the degree of a person's erotic attraction to people of the same sex (homosexual), opposite sex (heterosexual), or both sex (bisexual).
- Individuals may fall anywhere along a continuum between exclusive homosexuality and exclusion heterosexuality.
- Homosexuals and bisexuals undergo a developmental process of identity formation.
  - Sensitization—sensation of being different from one's peers
  - Identity confusion—after puberty, awareness of same-sex attraction may conflict with social expectations
  - Identity assumption—self-definition as homosexual or bisexual, but not yet fully accepted
  - Commitment—self-acceptance and comfort with identity, disclosure to family, social, and occupational settings

DISABILITY AND SEXUALITY (SEXUAL ATTRACTION TO DISABILITY)

- Rarely of public concern
- Psychotherapy for distressed individuals presenting for treatment by advocating the preplanned thought stopping, substitution of appropriate behaviors, and introspection methods
- Testosterone-lowering medications might be of small benefits, if in acute distress

SEXUAL ADDICTION (SEXUAL COMPULSION)

- Criteria = loss of control, continue despite adverse consequences, compulsive and obsessive behaviors, craving for more, preoccupation, sacrifice obligations and activities for behavior, develop tolerance, distress/anxiety/restlessness/irritability if unable to engage in behavior
- Cycle of preoccupation, ritualization, compulsive sexual behavior, and despair
- Consequences = social, emotional, physical, legal, financial/occupational
- Risk factors = trauma, neurochemistry (relationship of depression, anxiety, and OCD), social conditioning and imprinting, developmental impairments, interaction of loneliness, anger, boredom, and spiritual rebellion, psychodynamic perspective

CHILD/ADOLESCENT SEXUALITY

- Refers to sexual feelings, behavior, and development in children/adolescents

AGING AND SEXUALITY

- Sexuality changes with increasing age
- Females sexuality decreases while males' sexuality tends to be unchanged throughout life

APPROACH

GENERAL OBSERVATIONS AND PHYSICAL EXAMINATIONS

- Observe for general appearance, appropriateness of behavior, body language, distress, agitation, masculine/feminine features

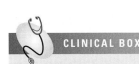

CLINICAL BOX

Physical, Psychological, and Sexual Developmental Processes

There is great fluidity and variability in the outcome with only a small proportion becoming transsexuals or transvestites, and with the majority of affected children eventually developing a homosexual orientation or heterosexual orientation without transvestism or transsexualism.

- Examine vital signs, puberty staging, thyroid gland, weight changes, drug and/or alcohol use (needle injection, alcohol breath), concentrate on neurologic examinations (especially peripheral neuropathy), and genital examinations

INVESTIGATIONS

- Blood works = CBC, electrolytes, BUN, creatinine, fasting blood glucose, liver profiles, thyroid profiles (TSH), toxicology/drug screen (alcohol, opioid, amphetamine/stimulant or cocaine withdrawal or intoxication), FSH/LH, GH
- See Chapters 6, 14, and 21 for details.
- Additional screening: neurologic/endocrinology/gynecology/urology consultations, CXR, ECG, CT scan as indicated

MANAGEMENT

- A full assessment including family evaluation to identify emotional, behavioral, and separation problems is essential, and unresolved issues in the child's environment are often present such as loss.
- Direct assessment and treatment of other underlying disorders including GMC and psychiatric disorders should be promptly initiated.
- Testosterone = control of sexuality, fantasies, and behavior; also increases the frequency, duration, and magnitude of spontaneous and nocturnal erections
- Antiandrogenic drugs such as medroxyprogesterone (long-acting contraceptive Depo Provera) have been used to reduce sex drive in men but they have many unpleasant side effects including breast growth, headaches, weight gain, and reduction in bone density.
- SSRIs, lithium have been used to reduce impulse control problems and/or sexual obsessions, and psychostimulants have been used to augment the effects of SSRIs in paraphiliacs.
- Psychotherapy including individual or group therapy and behavioral modification should aim to assist development, particularly that of gender identity, by exploring the nature and characteristics of the atypical organization of the child's or adolescent's gender identity, and focusing on ameliorating the comorbid problems and difficulties in the child's life while reducing the distress being experienced by the child.
- Recognition of the person's inability to control the compulsion, acceptance of the disease and its consequences, and willingness to learn from others in recovery with commitment to change should be discussed.
- Therapist should also provide recognition and acceptance of the gender identity problem and remove its secrecy, while providing guidance for the child's sense of gender identity and support for the family in tolerating uncertainty and anxiety in relation to the gender identity development and how best to manage it.
- Referral for assessment and/or treatment in a multidisciplinary gender identity specialist service should be made if the criteria of gender identity disorder are met.
- Referral to a pediatric endocrinologist for the purpose of physical assessment, education about growth and endocrinologic problems, and involvement in any decision about physical interventions should be considered.

SUICIDAL BEHAVIOR

RATIONALE

- Psychiatric emergencies are common and serious problems. Suicidal behavior is one of several psychiatric emergencies, which physicians must know how to assess and manage.
- **Suicide:** The act of intentionally terminating one's own life for numerous reasons such as psychiatric disorders, boredom, substance abuse, shame, avoiding pain or other undesirable fates, and financial difficulties
- Suicidal ideation → plan → intent (final common pathway)

CAUSAL CONDITIONS

Prevalence

1. Psychiatric disorder (>90%)
   - Depression = 15% lifetime risk in depression and higher in BP
   - Substance abuse = 15% lifetime risk, especially with alcohol

- Psychotic disorders = schizophrenia (10% to 15% risk), delusions, paranoia, command hallucinations, loss of rational thinking
- PD = borderline and antisocial
- Panic/AD = especially in panic disorder
- Delirium = altered level of consciousness
2. Psychosis (delusions, paranoia, command hallucinations)
3. Previous suicide attempts
4. Sociocultural factors
   - Marital status (never married, widow, separated, divorced)
   - Other (older, women/abused women, previously abused children, unemployed/unskilled, physical illness, family history of suicide, Native Canadians, live alone, lost loved one, anniversary of loss, lacking social support)

Table **19.10** Acute and Chronic Risk Factors

Acute Risk		Chronic Risk	
Precipitants	**Current Mental Status**	**Demographics**	**Psychiatric History**
• Recent loss/separation	• Active suicidal ideation	• Age >65 yr old with highest risk and late adolescent 16–19 yr of age with second highest risk	• Mood disorder
• Poor health	• Suicide intent		• Schizophrenia
• Unwilling to accept help	• Suicide plan		• Substance abuse (alcohol)
• Feeling hopeless	• Preparations for death	• Sex = M > F (3:1) in completed suicide and F > M (4:1) in attempted suicide	• Impulsivity
• Lack of coping strategies	• Psychosis		• Irritability/violence
• Suicide of another person	• Depression	• Single, widowed, or divorced	• Past suicide attempts (strongest predictor)
		• Unemployed or retired	• Prior admissions
		• Lack of social support	• Family history of suicide

APPROACH

GENERAL OBSERVATIONS AND PHYSICAL EXAMINATIONS

- Mental status examination: eye contact, psychomotor retardation/agitation (fidgeting, moving about, hand-wringing, nail biting, hair pulling, lip biting), distress, restlessness, depressed mood and flat/restricted effect, suicidal/homicidal ideation/plan/intent
- Examine vital signs, pupils, and skin for previous suicide attempts, stigmata of drug and/or alcohol use, thyroid gland, and weight loss.

INVESTIGATIONS

- Blood works = CBC, electrolytes, BUN, creatinine, fasting blood glucose, liver profiles, thyroid profiles (TSH), toxicology/drug screen (alcohol, cannabis, opioid, amphetamine/stimulant or cocaine withdrawal or intoxication)
- Urinalysis, urine drug screen
- Additional screening: neurologic consultation, CXR, ECG, CT scan as indicated

MANAGEMENT

Treatment

- Treat the underlying disorders including GMC or other psychiatric disorders with depression being the most common.
- Biological = medications
  - Antidepressants (SSRIs, TCAs, MAOIs, venlafaxine, bupropion, mirtazapine)
  - Antipsychotics (typical, atypical)
- Psychological (requiring insight to disorders) = CBT, psychotherapy
- Social = support group, community resources, family involvement

MANAGEMENT OF RISK

See Table 19.11.

Table **19.11**	Management Based on Suicidal Risk		
Low Risk	**Intermediate Risk**	**High Risk**
• Reinforce importance of talking • Going to ER when needed • Calling crisis line • Staying with a supportive person • Availability and back up • Instil **hope**!	• Low-risk interventions • Increase frequency of contact • Involve social supports/family • Avoid alcohol or other triggers • Consider voluntary hospitaliza- tion	• Intermediate risk interventions • Mental Health Act forms— Form 1 or 2 in Ontario • Police involvement

 C₂LEO Box

Euthanasia

- Active euthanasia and physician-assisted suicide are both illegal in Canada.
- When faced with these issues, physicians should reassure the patients that they will not be abandoned and that continuous care will be provided indefinitely.
- Psychiatric referral should be considered as these patients are more likely to be depressed than having unbearable pain.
- A clear distinction must be made between terminating life-sustaining treatment(s), which is legal in Canada under special circumstances.

FAMILY VIOLENCE

See also Chapter 8.

RATIONALE

- **Domestic violence** = intentional controlling or violent behavior (physical, sexual, or emotional abuse, economic control, or social isolation of the victim) by a person who is/was in an intimate relationship with the victim
- The victim lives in a state of constant fear and is terrified about when the next episode of abuse will occur.
- Despite this, abuse frequently remains hidden and undiagnosed because patients often conceal that they are in abusive relationships.

CAUSAL CONDITIONS/RISK FACTORS

Preexisting Vulnerabilities

- Women/pregnant (trauma victims, chronic abdominal pain/headaches)
- Elders with injuries
- Children with injuries
- Head injuries
- Others (past violence, former victim of abuse, intellectual functioning, family and cultural influences, impulsivity)

Psychiatric/Medical Disorders

- Psychosis (e.g., delusions of persecutory or jealous types, command hallucinations)
- Substance-related (e.g., abuse/dependence, intoxication, withdrawal, substance-induced–psychotic/mood/anxiety/cognitive disorders)
- PD (e.g., antisocial, borderline, narcissistic, paranoid)
- Mood disorders (e.g., manic phase of BP, agitated depression)
- Cognitive disorders (e.g., delirium, dementia)
- ADs (e.g., OCD, generalized AD, social phobia)
- Attention deficit and disruptive behavior disorders (e.g., ADHD, oppositional defiant disorder, conduct disorder)

- Pervasive developmental disorders/autistic spectrum disorders
- Developmental disability/mental retardation
- Impulse control disorders (e.g., intermittent explosive disorder)
- Medication-induced (e.g., akathisia)
- Other GMC related (e.g., Huntington, neuropsychiatric SLE)
- Socioeconomic cultural factors
- Chronic medical conditions/disability

APPROACH

GENERAL OBSERVATIONS AND PHYSICAL EXAMINATIONS

- Partner refuses to leave examination room and answers questions for the patients
- Signs of imminent violence in partner: threats, paranoid ideas, yelling, pacing, agitated behavior
- Mental status examination: avoidance of eye contact, fearfulness, evasive behavior, psychomotor retardation/agitation (fidgeting, moving about, hand-wringing, nail biting, hair pulling, lip biting), hostility, distress, restlessness, depressed mood and flat/restricted effect, suicidal/homicidal ideation/plan/intent
- Examine vital signs (tachycardia), pupils (drug-related), and skin for scars/wounds/bruises, stigmata of drug and/or alcohol use, and weight loss (chronic suffering)
- Examine location of injuries (usually central, breasts, abdomen, genitals), forearm defensive wounds, bruises of different ages

INVESTIGATIONS

Table **19.12**	**Investigation in Violence**
Test	**Finding/Interpretation**
CBC	• To rule out anemia and/or infection
Electrolytes	• To rule out electrolyte imbalance, dehydration, starvation
Thyroid (TSH)	• To rule out hyper or hypothyroidism
INR, PTT, coagulation status	• To rule out coagulopathy
Toxicology/drug screen	• Alcohol • Cannabis • Opioid • Amphetamine • Cocaine • Other stimulants
Urinalysis	• Drugs (see above)
CXR	• To rule out fractures
Other x-ray	• To rule out limb fractures
CT	• Headache to rule out brain lesions, masses, or hemorrhage

MANAGEMENT

- Determine immediate and short-term risk to victim.
- Provide validation, support, and counseling.
- Offer referral (e.g., hospital social worker, local domestic hotline, domestic violence advocates, institutional and community resources, specialists such as psychiatrists) to discuss options and safety issues and plans.
- Educate patient about what to do in case of emergency and range of support services available.
- Leave the room and obtain assistance from security or police if partner is violent.
- Physician's legal responsibility to report potential victims of violent patients only with patient's consent because of patient–physician confidentiality.

Physician must report to CAS or other related society if family violence involves children.

- Carefully document details of abuse.
- Select patients in need of referral to a specialist, prepare safety plans, and offer referral to community services.

ADULT ABUSE/SPOUSE ABUSE

See also Chapter 8.

RATIONALE

- Abuse of power in a relationship involving domination, coercion, intimidation, and the victimization of one person by another
- Most spouse abuse: wife abuse (some abuse of husbands has been reported)
- 10% of women in a relationship with a man have experienced abuse
- Of women presenting to a primary care clinic, almost one third reported physical and verbal abuse

CATEGORIES

PHYSICAL

Pushing, hitting, biting, burning, locking out, abandoning in an unsafe place; resulting in pain, injury, sleep deprivation, disablement, and murder

SEXUAL

Forced unwanted sexual activity: rape, sex with objects, friends, animals, mimic pornography, wear more provocative clothes, and so on

- Rape of wives
- Rape of women (may be associated with other crimes or nonsexual abuse)
  - Sexual sadists
  - Exploitive predators
  - Inadequate men
  - Men with displaced expression of anger and rage

EMOTIONAL OR PSYCHOLOGICAL

Constant criticism; threats to hurt, kill; extreme jealousy, denying friendships, outside interests, or activities; time accounting; and so on

ECONOMIC

Not allowing money, denying improvement in earning capacity, detailed accounting of spending, etc.

CAUSAL CONDITIONS/RISK FACTORS

- See Family Violence section in Chapter 8.
- History of hyperalertness, sleeping or eating disturbances, fatigue, mood swings, phobias, somatization, startle response
- Past experiences of sexual assault, family violence, or child sexual abuse

APPROACH

GENERAL OBSERVATIONS AND PHYSICAL EXAMINATIONS

(see Family Violence section in Chapter 8)

INVESTIGATIONS

(see Family Violence section in Chapter 8)

- Diagnose wife/husband abuse and assess the role in etiology of other health concerns; assess immediate and short-term risk to victim.
- Determine whether the husband/wife comes from a violent home or was abused himself, feels threatened at home, work, or with peers.

MANAGEMENT

See Family Violence section in Chapter 8.

CHILD ABUSE, PHYSICAL/EMOTIONAL/SEXUAL/NEGLECT/SELF-INDUCED

See also Chapter 8.

DEFINITION/RATIONALE

- Intentional harm to a child by the caregiver
- Part of the spectrum of family dysfunction, leading to significant morbidity and mortality
- Abuse causes physical and emotional trauma, and may present as neglect
- Increased index of suspicion in children suffering from traumatic injury or have psychological or social disturbances (e.g., aggressive behavior, stress disorder, depressive disorder, substance abuse, etc.)

CATEGORIES

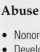

CLINICAL BOX

Mental Health Act Forms (Form 1 in Ontario)

- When in doubt, fill in Form 1 for further reassessment.
- There is an increased risk of suicidality with the initiation of antidepressant treatment; therefore, close monitoring or follow-up is required.

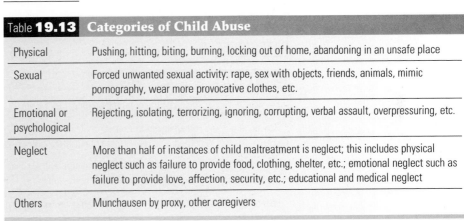

Table **19.13**	**Categories of Child Abuse**
Physical	Pushing, hitting, biting, burning, locking out of home, abandoning in an unsafe place
Sexual	Forced unwanted sexual activity: rape, sex with objects, friends, animals, mimic pornography, wear more provocative clothes, etc.
Emotional or psychological	Rejecting, isolating, terrorizing, ignoring, corrupting, verbal assault, overpressuring, etc.
Neglect	More than half of instances of child maltreatment is neglect; this includes physical neglect such as failure to provide food, clothing, shelter, etc.; emotional neglect such as failure to provide love, affection, security, etc.; educational and medical neglect
Others	Munchausen by proxy, other caregivers

CLINICAL BOX

Manifestations of Abuse

- Nonorganic failure to thrive
- Developmental delay
- Starvation/dehydration
- Poor hygiene
- Dental caries
- School truancy
- Dysfunctional social relationships
- Speech and language difficulties
- Emotional and behavioral problems

CAUSAL CONDITIONS/RISK FACTORS

- See Family Violence section in Chapter 8.
- Family dynamics: nonloving, tension, stressful
- Parental characteristics: emotional, explosive, angry, irritable, aggressive
- Refusal by parent to have child interviewed alone
- Inconsistent or implausible history, vague or lacking in detail history, changing history, no history at all offered, attribution of injuries to siblings

APPROACH

GENERAL OBSERVATIONS AND PHYSICAL EXAMINATIONS

- See Family Violence section in Chapter 8.
- Signs of physical, sexual, or other abuse (e.g., cutaneous markings, burns, bruises, etc.) or emotional and behavioral signs of abuse
- Manifestations of abuse

INVESTIGATIONS

See Family Violence section in Chapter 8.

MANAGEMENT

- Assess and secure the child's safety.
- If warranted (even based on suspicion alone), report to appropriate social service department or refer to child welfare (e.g., CAS).
- Document events carefully.

Must differentiate child abuse from cultural therapy such as "cupping," "coining," "spooning," etc.

- Recognize potential physical and psychological sequelae of physical and sexual abuse including child's growth and health, psychiatric issues, peer acceptance, dysfunctional family.
- Treatment options and outcomes for victims and perpetrators including the involvement of police, CAS, etc.
- Work with interdisciplinary team (involving mental health worker, social worker, nutritionist, behavioral/developmental specialist, education specialist, visiting nurse, etc.) and access community services.
- Strategies for prevention of child abuse including family counseling, parental counseling and education, social support, community support, etc.
- See Family Violence section in Chapter 8 for further details.

Physician must report to CAS or other related society if family violence involves children.

ELDERLY ABUSE

See also Chapter 8.

RATIONALE

- An act or omission that results in harm to the elderly person's health or welfare
- Three types of abuse: domestic, institutional, and self-neglect

CATEGORIES

Table **19.14**	**Categories of Elderly Abuse**
Physical	Pushing, hitting, biting, burning, locking out of home, abandoning in an unsafe place
Sexual	Forced unwanted sexual activity: rape, sex with objects, friends, animals, mimic pornography, wear more provocative clothes, etc.
Emotional or psychological	Constant criticism, threats to hurt, kill, extreme jealousy; denying friendships, outside interests or activities, time accounting, etc.
Economic	Not allowing money, denying improvement in earning capacity, taking money out of account, etc.
Abandonment, neglect, and self-neglect	

CAUSAL CONDITIONS/RISK FACTORS

- See Family Violence section in Chapter 8.
- Must rule out GMC

APPROACH

GENERAL OBSERVATIONS AND PHYSICAL EXAMINATIONS
- Observe for distress, agitation, restlessness, and affect.
- Examine for bruises, bites, burns, lacerations, and other injuries.

INVESTIGATIONS
- See Family Violence section in Chapter 8.
- Dementia workup (see Dementia section in Chapter 12).

MANAGEMENT
- Decide whether hospitalization is necessary or alternative accommodation (if there is concern for patient safety)
- Legal implications of elderly abuse might include police involvement and law.
- Counsel and assist caregiver; provide information and education in accessing community services.
- Multidisciplinary approach to intervention
- See Family Violence section in Chapter 8 for further details.

Pulmonary Medicine

*Erika Dianne Penz, Brandie Laurel Walker, Farah Ramji,
and Martha Ainslie*

DYSPNEA

RATIONALE

Table **20.1**	**Resp States**
Dyspnea	• Subjective experience of shortness of breath • Common with both pulmonary and cardiac dz
Tachypnea	↑ Rate of breathing (>12–20 breaths/min)
Hyperpnea	Deep and rapid breathing
Hyperventilation	An ↑ in alveolar ventilation leading to an alveolar CO_2 level below normal

APPLIED SCIENTIFIC CONCEPTS

- Respiration is controlled in the medulla with inputs from
  - Cortical (voluntary) control
  - Mechanical/stretch receptors in chest wall and diaphragm
  - P_{CO_2}/pH chemoreceptors in the medulla
  - P_{CO_2}, P_{O_2}, pH receptors in the carotid body and aortic arch

ASC Box

O_2 Transport

O_2 is primarily transported by hemoglobin, only a small portion is transported by solution.

ASC Box

Physiology of Dyspnea

Multiple mechanisms lead to the sensation of dyspnea:

- Mechanical receptors in chest wall that feedback to Resp motor neurons
- Lung stretch receptors
- Irritant receptors in bronchial mucosa activated by stimulation of bronchial mucosa and ↑ muscle tone and flow
- Central and peripheral chemoreceptors (even in the absence of activation of Resp muscles)

CAUSAL CONDITIONS

Table 20.2	Anatomic Differential Dx of Dyspnea	
System	**Mechanism**	**Differential Dx**
Cardiac	Myocardial dysfunction	• Ischemic or hypertensive cardiomyopathy • Dilated cardiomyopathy • Infiltrative • Restrictive • Congenital • Diastolic dysfunction
	Arrhythmia	• Atrial fibrillation
	Pericardial dz	• Tamponade • Constrictive pericarditis
	↑ cardiac output	• Pregnancy • Hyperthyroid • Anemia
	Valvular heart dz Deconditioning	
Pulmonary	Airways	• Asthma • Anaphylaxis • Obstructive lung dz (COPD)
	Parenchyma	• Alveoli (infectious, RDS, vasculitis) • Diffusing membrane (interstitial pulmonary dz—sarcoid, scleroderma, fibrosis, inhalational, radiation or drug related) • Pneumonia • Aspiration
	Vasculature	• Pulmonary capillaries (PE)
	Pleura	• Pl Eff • Pneumothorax, hemothorax
	Neuromuscular	• Guillain-Barré, myasthenia gravis, hypokalemia • Spinal cord injury • ASA toxicity • Metabolic acidosis • Hypokalemia
	Chest wall	• Kyphos-scoliosis • Obesity • Ankylosing spondylitis
Other		• Anemia • Anxiety • Carbon monoxide

APPROACH

- Differentiate cardiac versus pulmonary versus other causes of dyspnea
- See Acute and Chronic Dyspnea for specific etiologies

CLINICAL BOX

Important History Points

- Smoking history
- Past medical history (heart dz, pulmonary dz)
- Exposures (sick contacts, immunocompromised, occupational, infections, irritants, allergies)
- Time course of Sx (acute versus chronic)
- Exacerbating and alleviating factors

Table **20.3**	History Clues to Differentiate Dyspnea
Breathing Description	**Associated Condition**
Heavy breathing	Deconditioning
Chest tightness	Obstructive (asthma), MI
↑ effort of breathing	COPD, asthma, myopathy
Air hunger, need to breath	CHF, PE, moderate to severe asthma
Suffocating	Pulmonary edema
Paroxysmal nocturnal dyspnea	CHF, asthma
Rapid, shallow breaths	Interstitial dz

CLINICAL BOX

Brain Natriuretic Peptide

- Used to help differentiate heart failure from pulmonary dyspnea
- BNP is released by myocytes being stretched
- No level that fully differentiates CHF and other causes, but levels >500 pg/mL considered positive for CHF, and levels <100 likely not CHF (gray area in between)

Table **20.4**	Clinical Findings of Dyspnea		
Resp exam			
Auscultation		Stridor	Aspiration, anaphylaxis
		Crackles	Pulmonary edema
		Wheeze	Asthma, COPD
		Bronchial breath sounds	Consolidation
		Whispered pectoriloquy, egophony	Consolidation
Percussion		Dullness	Pneumonia, Pl Eff
		Hyper-resonant	Pneumothorax, COPD
Palpation		Fremitus	↑ Consolidation
			↓ Consolidation with blocked airway, COPD, pneumothorax, and Pl Eff
Cardiovascular exam			
↑ JVP		CHF, PE	
Extra heart sounds (S3, S4, murmurs)		CHF, valvular heart dz, pulmonary hypertension	
Displaced PMI			
Tachypnea		PE, CHF	
Pulus paradoxus		Tamponade, COPD, asthma	
Others			
Homan sign		Pain with foot dorsiflexion (DVT)	
Clubbing		ILD, lung cancer, cyanotic heart dz	

CLINICAL BOX

Hct

Hct to exclude anemia as cause for dyspnea

Table **20.5**	Systematic Approach to CXR to Avoid Subtle Abnormalities
View	Demographics (age, sex, history)
	Identify projection (PA, AP, Lat, portable, insp/exp, Lat decubitus)
	Heart magnified more on AP
	Patient position (upright vs. supine)
Technique	Insp effort (six ribs anteriorly, ten ribs posteriorly)
	Rotation (compare heads of clavicles)
	Penetration (should see the vertebral bodies through the cardiac silhouette)
Survey	Soft tissues
	Bony tissues
	Heart and vasculature
	Lung fields and pleura
	Beneath diaphragms

ACUTE DYSPNEA

CLINICAL BOX

Normal ABGs

pH	7.4 (7.36–7.44)
PCO₂	40 (37–42) mm Hg
HCO₃	24 (22–26) mmol/L
PO₂	80–100 mm Hg

CLINICAL BOX

Helpful Tests

- D-dimer—if negative, less likely to be PE
- BNP—positive in CHF
- ABG
- CBC
- CXR
- CT—PE
- V̇Q̇ scan
- ECG
- Echocardiography
- PFTs/spirometry
- C-ANCA suggests Wegener granulomatosis
- P-ANCA
- Troponin

CLINICAL BOX

Aspiration

- Need insp and exp x-ray views to look for evidence of gas trapping suggestive of foreign body
- Supportive therapy
- May require intervention (i.e., foreign body removal)

RATIONALE

- A limited number of conditions cause shortness of breath that occurs over minutes to hours
- Accurate, timely Dx is important as it permits swift treatment that can limit morbidity and mortality

CAUSAL CONDITIONS

see Dyspnea

APPROACH

SIMPLIFIED APPROACH TO ABGs

1. pH acidemic or alkalemic?
2. Resp or metabolic?
   In Resp cause, P_{aCO_2} and pH change in opposite directions.
3. Appropriate compensation?
   - Acute Resp acidosis: P_{CO_2} ↑ by 10, H_{CO_3} ↑ by 1
   - Chronic Resp acidosis: P_{CO_2} ↑ by 10, H_{CO_3} ↑ by 3
   - Acute Resp alkalosis: P_{CO_2} ↓ by 10, H_{CO_3} ↓ by 2
   - Chronic Resp alkalosis: P_{CO_2} ↓ by 10, HCO_3 ↓ by 4
   - If compensation is over- or under-expected result, consider mixed etiology
4. If metabolic acidosis, what is anion gap $[Na] - ([Cl] + [HCO_3])$, normal is 14 ± 2
5. What is the delta gap—change in anion gap minus change in HCO_3

   If a positive gap exists (>+6), suggests another metabolic process such as metabolic acidosis. If negative gap exists (<−6), then nonanion gap acidosis exists.

Table **20.6**	**Compensation in Resp Acid–Base Imbalance**	
	HCO₃ (mmol/L)	**Pco₂ (mm Hg)**
Acute resp acidosis	↑ by 10	↑ by 1
Chronic resp acidosis	↑ by 10	↑ by 3
Acute resp alkalosis	↓ by 10	↓ by 2
Chronic resp alkalosis	↓ by 10	↓ by 4

ᵃIf compensation is over-or under-expected result, consider mixed etiology

Table **20.7**	**Causes of Resp Acid–Base Imbalance**
Causes of Resp acidosis	**Resp Alkalosis**
<ul><li>CNS depression</li><li>Neuromuscular disorders</li><li>Upper and lower airway abnormalities</li><li>Lung parenchyma abnormalities</li><li>Thoracic cage abnormalities</li></ul>	<ul><li>Hypoxia: pneumonia, pulmonary edema, restrictive lung dz</li><li>Primary hyperventilation: CNS disorders, drugs (salicylates) sepsis, hepatic failure</li></ul>

STATUS ASTHMATICUS

- Markers of severity—inability to speak full sentence, use of accessory muscles, pulsus paradoxus, inability to lie flat, normal to elevated CO_2
- ABG for severe cases
- Supportive therapy—O_2

- Continuous short-acting β_2-agonist (salbutamol) until significant clinical response plus anticholinergic such as ipratropium bromide initially (1st 72 h)
- Steroids recommended for all exacerbations for 7–10 d
- If not responding to inhaled therapy, can try epinephrine SC 0.3–0.4 mL (1:1000) q30 min × 3 times
- May require ICU

PULMONARY EMBOLISM

See Unilateral Edema.

ACUTE EXACERBATION OF COPD

- Defined as sustained worsening of dyspnea, cough, or sputum production leading to ↑ use of maintenance medications
- Treat with oral or IV steroids for 14 d
- Abx if ↑ sputum, purulence, or volume.
- If uncomplicated, likely pathogens are *H. flu*, *M. catarrhalis*, *Strep pneumo*
- First line Abx are **amoxicillin**, **doxycycline**, **septra** or second or third cephalosporins
- Second line β lactam, Resp fluoroquinolone

Complicated COPD

- FEV1 <50% predicted
- >4 exacerbations/yr
- Ischemic heart dz
- Home O_2
- Chronic oral steroids
- Abx within 3 mo
- 1st choice β lactam/β lactamase, fluoroquinolone
- May require consultation with a respirologist.

PNEUMONIA

- Determine Abx treatment based on most likely pathogen
- Assess for immunosuppression (i.e., HIV, solid organ transplant, chronic steroids, immune suppressive drugs)
- CAP: if no comorbidities, likely organisms *Strep pneumo*, *H. flu*, and atypicals including *C. pneumoniae*, *M. pneumoniae*, and *L. pneumophila*.
- In uncomplicated outpatients (i.e., those without chronic pulmonary dz) first line treatment is extended spectrum macrolide or *doxycycline*
- In complicated outpatients (i.e., those with COPD and recent Abx use) treat with Resp fluoroquinolone such as *levofloxacin*, (second line is *amoxicillin-clavulanate* or second generation cephalosporin and macrolide)
- Hospitalization based on pneumonia severity index score
- Hospital acquired pneumonia (>48 hr) are more likely to be caused by resistant organisms or gram negative bacteria—need broad-spectrum Abx

ARDS

- Manifestation of various acute lung injuries
- 4 criteria are as follows:
  1. Acute onset
  2. Bilateral patchy airspace dz
  3. PCWP <18 mm Hg, or no clinical evidence of ↑ LVEDP
  4. Pao_2/Fio_2 <200
- Characterized by pulmonary edema, Resp distress, and hypoxemia.
- Etiologies include aspiration/toxic inhalations, sepsis, shock, trauma, DIC, embolism, drugs, and head trauma.
- Treat underlying disorder, immediate intensive care, aggressive supportive therapy

ASA TOXICITY

- Suspect if combination of metabolic acidosis and concurrent Resp alkalosis
- Mild toxicity characterized by nausea and vomiting, abdominal pain, and tinnitus
- More serious toxicity results in hyperthermia, tachypnea, Resp alkalosis and metabolic acidosis, hypoglycemia, hyperkalemia, seizure, coma, and death

- Cardiopulmonary arrest due to pulmonary edema is the most common cause of death in ASA overdose
- Decontamination of gut with charcoal
- Alkalinize the urine, dialysis indicated for severe toxicity

VASCULITIS

- Wegener granulomatosis and microscopic polyangiitis are characterized by pauci-immune necrotizing and crescentic glomerulonephritis and pulmonary capillaritis
- Need specialist referral and hospitalization for high-dose steroids and pulsed cyclophosphamide to induce remission, followed by slow taper

CHRONIC DYSPNEA

RATIONALE

- May be more difficult to determine etiology than with acute dyspnea
- Often patients have cardiopulmonary dz

CAUSAL CONDITIONS

see Dyspnea

CLINICAL BOX

Indications for Cardiopulmonary Exercise Testing

- Used to evaluate and differentiate cardiac and pulmonary pathology
- Cardiac exercise test including measurements of Resp O_2 uptake, CO_2 production, and ventilation (respiration rate, tidal volume, and minute ventilation)
- Considered medically necessary in evaluation of CHF patients being considered for heart transplant, differentiation of cardiac and pulmonary causes of ↓ exercise tolerance, or exercise induced dyspnea

---

APPROACH

Characteristics	0: At risk	I: Mild	II: Moderate	III: Severe	IV: Very severe
	FEV 100% FEV$_1$ 100%	FEV$_1$ ≥80% predicted	FEV$_1$ 50–80% predicted	FEV$_1$ 49–30% FEV$_1$ 30–50% predicted	FEV$_1$ <30% predicted

Education, self-management, avoidance of risk factors, vaccines, stop smoking

Add SABA when needed

Add LABA
Rehabilitation

Add inhaled steroids

- Long-term supplemental Oxygen
- Surgery
- End-of-life care

Figure 20.1 Steps in management of COPD.

COPD

- Affects 4% of Canadian adults
- Caused by smoking
- In nonsmokers, or patients with early presentation, consider α-1 antitrypsin deficiency
- Progressive, partially reversible airway obstruction with systemic effects and characterized by ↑ exacerbations

Drug Treatment for COPD

Mild:

1. SABA
2. Tiotropium or LABA and SABD

Moderate: tiotropium and LABA and SABA prn Severe: tiotropium and LABA with inhaled corticosteroid, ± theophylline and SABA prn

Criteria for Home O_2 Therapy

- Evaluate for hypoxemia if FEV1 <40%
- Use long-term O_2 therapy
- (>15 h/d) if:
- PaO_2 ≤55, or <60 with cor pulmonale

Drug Therapy for Smoking Cessation

- Nicotine replacement
- Bupropion
- Varenicline

- Diagnose early through spirometry on patients who:
  - Are smokers or exsmokers >40
  - Have persistent cough/sputum
  - Have frequent Resp infections
  - Have progressive shortness of breath with exertion

Smoking Cessation

Stages of change:

1. Precontemplation: not interested in quitting, explore disadvantages of smoking, give personalized counseling
2. Contemplative: plan on quitting in next 6 mo
3. Preparation: quit date <1 mo, prescribe pharmacologic agents, create a plan of action, and review high-risk situations
4. Action: within 6 mo of quitting, encourage and review plan of action
5. Maintenance

ILD

Classified by its pathology

X-ray approach of ILD takes into consideration:

1. Distribution of dz
2. Nodular versus reticular
3. Lymph node involvement
4. Presence of effs

Dx of IPF suggested by:

- Restrictive pattern on PFT testing, and impaired gas exchange
- Bibasilar reticular abnormalities with minimal ground glass on HRCT
- BAL or transbronchial biopsy that does not support alternate Dx
- Exclusion of other causes (i.e., drug toxicities, exposures)

Requires referral to respirologist for definitive Dx.

Table 20.8 X-ray Patterns of ILD

Peripheral Bibasilar Reticular Patterns	Nodular Pattern
• IPF (UIP) • Asbestosis • Pulmonary fibrosis associated with connective tissue dz • Chronic hypersensitivity	• Fungal dz • Metastatic dz/lymphangitic carcinomatosis • Silicosis • Sarciodosis • Histiocytosis X

BRONCHIECTASIS

- Permanent dilatation of the airways caused by inflammation and destruction of airway walls)
- Results in persistent infection
- Etiology includes obstruction, postinfection, and conditions that result in chronic infection and poor drainage (i.e., cystic fibrosis)
- Should be followed by a specialist

PEDIATRIC DYSPNEA/RESPIRATORY DISTRESS

Ensure patent airway and check for signs of cyanosis.

RATIONALE

- Resp distress is a very common pediatric emergency
- Important to recognize and intervene early, as young children and infants can quickly become fatigued and fail to compensate
- Resp distress is characterized by ↑ work of breathing or hypoventilation

CAUSAL CONDITIONS

See Figure 20.2.

Table **20.9**	**Causal Conditions of Pediatric Dyspnea**
Upper airways	• Croup • Foreign body aspiration • Laryngeal edema/spasm/epiglottitis • Retropharyngeal abscess • Choanal atresia
Lower airways/pulmonary problems	• Ttracheitis/bronchiolitis • Pneumonia atelectasis • Asthma/bronchospasm • RDS of the neonate • Tracheoesophageal fistula
Pulmonary vasculature	• PE
Pl problems	• Pl Eff/empyema • Pneumothorax
Neurologic/Chest wall	• Opiates • ↑ ICP • Neuromyopathy • Diaphragmatic hernia • Massive ascites • Severe scoliosis

APPROACH

Key is to understand likely etiologies in each age group.

APPROACH TO RESP DISTRESS IN THE DELIVERY ROOM

Transient Tachypnea of the Newborn
- Due to inadequate clearance of fluid from the lung
- Fluid in the airspaces and extra-alveolar interstitium results in a ↓ in pulmonary compliance and ↑ airway resistance
- Usually happens within 2 h of delivery
- Supportive management as this is self-resolving and benign

RDS
- Caused by a ↓ amount of surfactant (premature)
- Progressive atelectasis occurs because the infant cannot generate the ↑ insp pressure required to cause inflation of the alveoli
- Can test amniotic fluid before delivery to assess risk of RDS
- Needs specialist care, can give surfactant, or use nasal CPAP

Persistent Pulmonary Hypertension
- Due to elevated pulmonary vascular resistance that leads to a right-to-left shunt (through foramen ovale and the ductus arteriosus)
- Results in hypoxemia

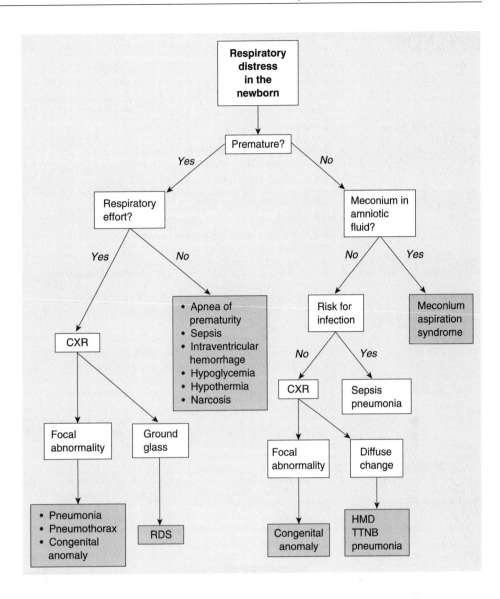

Figure 20.2 Approach to Resp distress in the newborn.

Breathing of meconium can result in severe aspiration pneumonia; therefore, eliminate meconium before stimulating breathing.

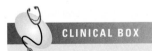

Warning Signs of Resp Failure

- Cyanosis
- Obtundation
- ↓ Chest wall motion
- Tachypnea, bradypnea, or apnea

- Manifested as severe cyanosis and tachypnea
- Infant needs urgent cardiac evaluation

Meconium Aspiration
- If meconium is present in the amniotic fluid, need to suction the oropharynx when the head is delivered.

APPROACH TO STRIDOR
See Table 20.10.

APPROACH TO WHEEZE
See Table 20.11.

Asthma
See Table 20.12 and Figure 20.3.

Diagnostic tests
- AP/Lat CXR—should be ordered in every person presenting with wheeze
- PFTs
  - Detect flow limitation
  - Quantify response to bronchodilators
  - Flow volume loop (insp + exp) in older children to determine presence, degree, and location of airway obstruction

Table 20.10	Approach to Stridor
Croup	• Most common cause of barking cough for children aged 6 to 36 mo • Caused by inflammation of upper airway and larynx • Usually viral (parainfluenza) but may be allergic, or super infection with bacteria, often has low-grade fever • Treatment for severe cases with stridor is racemic epinephrine, hospitalization • "Spasmodic croup" is due to laryngeal spasms
Foreign body aspiration[a]	• Common 1–2 yr of age; coughing and choking often precede Sx • May cause stridor in upper airway, but could manifest as wheeze or infection if lodged in lower airway • Bronchoscopy required to remove object
Epiglottitis	• 2–7 y.o., high grade fever, dysphagia, drooling, sore short • Usual etiology is bacterial (often H. influenzae) • Neck x-ray to examine soft tissue may be helpful • Needs admission for careful observation, Abx
Retropharyngeal abscess	• Complication of bacterial pharyngitis; high fevers, swallowing difficulty, refusal to feed, sore throat, Resp distress
Choanal atresia	• Congenital deformity of the posterior portion of the nasal passage • If bilateral, can cause Resp distress in the newborn, as infants are obligate nose breathers • Requires surgery
Laryngomalacia	• Common cause of stridor soon after birth, due to collapse of epiglottis or arytenoid cartilages during inspiration • Benign and self-limiting condition, supine position worsens Sx
Peritonsillar abscess	• Infection between tonsils and superior constrictor muscles; adolescents/preadolescents, severe throat pain, trismus, dysphagia, trouble speaking
VCD	• Can be congenital or secondary to trauma at birth; can have unilateral or bilateral dysfunction; unilateral associated with weak cry; associated with CNS abnormalities
Subglottic stenosis	Can be congenital or acquired; difficult to distinguish between asthma if Sx not present initially in neonatal period
Others[a]	Laryngeal cysts, webs, hemangiomas, papillomas, tracheal stenosis

[a]Can present as stridor or wheeze

CLINICAL BOX

Signs Suggesting Exclusion of Asthma

- Wheezing associated with feed
- Neonatal Resp distress ± ventilatory support
- Neonatal neurodysfunction
- Intractable wheezing not responding to bronchodilator
- Difficulty swallowing ± recurrent vomiting
- Onset early in infancy

Table 20.11	Approach to Wheeze
Tracheomalacia	• Congenital insufficiency of tracheal rings resulting in collapse of intrathoracic part of the lumen during expiration • Presents as wheeze or exp stridor
Tracheitis	• May occur due to bacterial super infection (S. aureus) after a viral infection
Bronchiolitis	• Usually caused by Resp syncytial virus • Affects children <2 y.o. • Child gets cough, wheezing, and shortness of breath over ~2 d • Treatment is supportive
Pneumonia	• In bacterial pneumonia the process is more likely focal, whereas in viral or atypical the presentation may be more diffuse and peribronchial • Common bacteria include S. aureus, H. influenzae, and S. pneumoniae. • Common viral causes include CMV, herpesvirus, and enterovirus in newborns; CMV, RSV, influenza, and parainfluenza; and adenovirus in children

Table **20.12**	**Causal Conditions of Wheeze in Pediatrics**	
	Acute	**Chronic**
Functional	Infection (bronchiolitis, laryngotracheobronchitis, bacterial tracheitis)[a] Foreign body aspiration[a] Asthma	Aspiration syndromes (foreign body, GERD, swallowing disorders, fistula) Bronchopulmonary dysphagia VCD
Structural		Tracheobronchomalacia Vascular compression Vascular ring Tracheal stenosis/web

[a]Most common in children

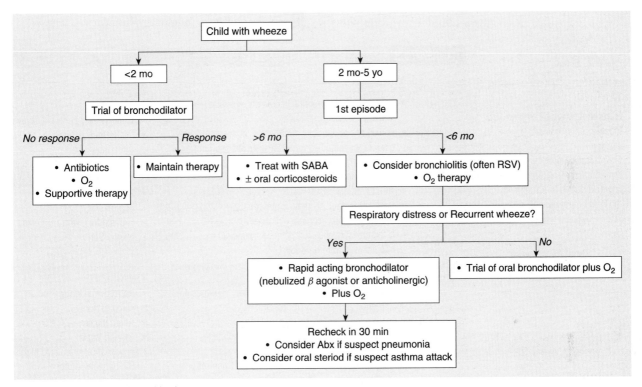

Figure 20.3 Approach to child with wheeze.

UPPER RESPIRATORY TRACT DISORDERS: WHEEZE

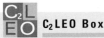

C₂LEO Box

Physicians' Legal Liability for Negligence

A physician may fail to recognize that wheezing does not equate to asthma. In an acute situation, life-threatening illnesses should be considered (epiglottitis, mechanical airway obstruction).

RATIONALE

- Wheezing is a sign of obstructing airway and indicates a pathological process. Requires sufficient airflow to produce sound. Absence of wheeze in acute asthma can be ominous sign.
- Stridor is a high pitched sound caused by oscillation of narrowed airway, signifying significant obstruction of large airways, and always should prompt urgent airway evaluation

APPROACH

HISTORY

- Associated with cough, dyspnea, ± chest tightness ↑ probability of asthma
- Postnasal drip or reflux Sx

- History of cardiac dz or signs of CHF
- History of cancer or Sx suggestive of malignancy

  Interpreting PFTs:

- PFTs routinely look at three main variables
- Flow—FVC, FEV1, FEV1/FVC ratio (used in evaluating whether there is obstructive etiology)
- Volume—TLC, RV, FRC (used in evaluating restrictive or obstructive lung dz)
- Diffusion—DLCO
  1. FVC is normal at 80–100 (excludes restrictive lung dz) If the FVC is reduced, could be due to restriction or gas trapping
  2. FEV1: 80–100 normal (not obstructive)
  3. FEV1/FVC ratio is normal if >0.80 (ratio declines with age) (if normal, then not an obstructive pattern)
  4. An adequate bronchodilator response is 12%–15% improvement in FEV1 and 200 mL
  5. ↑ RV suggests gas trapping
  6. DLCO is ↓ in pulmonary fibrosis, emphysema, pulmonary vascular dz, anemia

ASC Box

Three potential anatomic areas for obstruction:

1. Extrathoracic upper airways (nose to extrathoracic trachea)
2. Intrathoracic upper airways (intrathoracic trachea)
3. Lower airways (intrathoracic airways below carina)

Table 20.13 Wheeze versus Stridor

	Wheeze		Stridor
Character	• Monophonic—constant acoustical character—signifies large airway obstruction • Polyphonic—variable quality and acoustical character—signifies small airway obstruction • Inspiration or expiration • High pitched or low pitched • Airway of any size • Large: Constant acoustic character • Small: Variable acoustic character • If localized in one part of chest, consider neoplasm or foreign body		• Monophonic • Loudest over central airways • Inspiration, expiration, or throughout • Large airway—intrathoracic or extrathoracic • Insp stridor—extrathoracic obstruction • Exp stridor—intrathoracic obstruction

Causes	Acute
	• Asthma
	• Infection
	  • Bronchitis
	  • Viral infection
	  • Pneumonia
	• Foreign body
	  • Aspiration
	  • Esophageal
	• CHF
		Chronic
		• Asthma—postnasal drip
		• COPD
		• Gastroesophageal reflux
		• Recurrent aspiration
		• Pulmonary edema
		• Cystic fibrosis
		• VCD
		• ILD
		• Retained foreign body
			• VCD[a]
			• Retrosternal goiter/tumor compression
			• Angioedema
			• Foreign body[a]
			• Croup[a] (brassy cough, night Sx, previous upper Resp tract infection
			• Epiglottitis[a]
			• Hypertrophied tonsils[a]

[a]Most common in children

Table 20.14 Lung Volumes

	Normal	Obstruction–Hyperinflation	Restriction
VC (L)	6.0	4.0	4.0
TLC (L)	8.0	10/0	5.0
FRC (L)	4.0	7.0	3.0
RV (L)	2.0	6.0	1.0

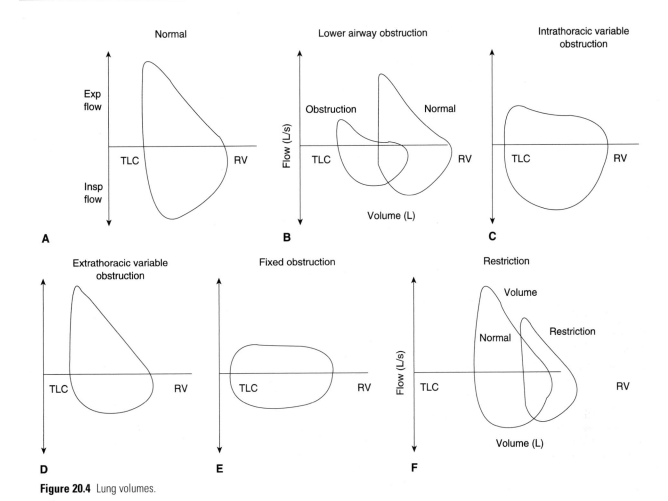

Figure 20.4 Lung volumes.

Always consider potential complete airway obstruction possible in stridor.

MANAGEMENT

STRIDOR

- Emergent airway evaluation—direct laryngoscopy/bronchoscopy
- Prepare for establishing an emergency airway
- Patients must remain under direct observation

WHEEZE

- Patient unstable? (RR >30, accessory muscles, becoming fatigued, CO_2 retention)
- Consider emergent airway with intubation
- Stable—use history to determine cause

MANAGEMENT OF ACUTE WHEEZE/ASTHMA

- O_2 (titrate to achieve Sao_2 >90%
- Short-acting β-agonist (4–8 puffs q20 min or nebulizer 2.5—5 mg q20 min, continuous if severe)
- Prednisone 60 mg PO for suspected asthma exacerbation
- Ipratropium (MDI 4—8 puffs q30 min or nebulizer 0.5 mg q30 min × 3, combined with β- agonist)
- Magnesium 2 g IV over 20 min (in very severe asthma exacerbations)

CYANOSIS/HYPOXEMIA/HYPOXIA

See also Chapter 18.

RATIONALE

Table **20.15** Cyanosis Definitions	
Cyanosis	• Physical sign of bluish coloration of the skin due to the presence of >50 g/L of deoxygenated hemoglobin in blood vessels near the skin surface • O_2 saturation of arterial blood falls below 85%
Hypoxemia	• An abnormal deficiency in the concentration of O_2 in arterial blood • Can be reversed with supplemental O_2
Hypoxia	• Total body is deprived of O_2

CAUSAL CONDITIONS

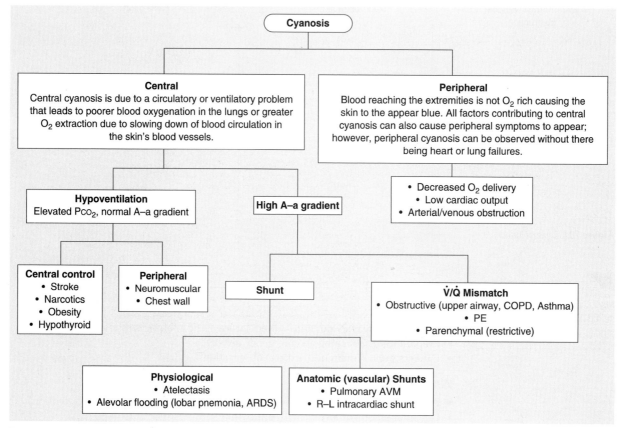

Figure 20.5 Classification of cyanosis.

APPROACH

- Patient will show signs of dyspnea, confusion, altered consciousness, cardiac arrhythmias, cyanosis, diaphoresis, and tachypnea.
- Dx requires ABGs and CXR.
- Patients who have these S should be treated with supplemental O_2.

CLINICAL BOX

Outcome criteria for a trial of long-term O_2 use in chronic hypoxia:

- $Po_2 < 54.7$ mm Hg
- $Pco_2 > 45.0$ mm Hg
- $FEV_1 < 1.51$
- $FVC < 20.1$

CLINICAL BOX

- Hazards of O_2 therapy: CO_2 retention and subsequent hypercapnia hazard.
- CO_2 retention in patients with COPD and O_2 toxicity can occur with high concentration of O_2 over long periods

CLINICAL BOX

Alveolar-Arterial Gradient

(A-a gradient)
   Used to compare the causes of hypoxemia.

- Normal <10 mmHg, but can range from 5–20 mm Hg in a normal individual.
- An ↑ A-a gradient suggests a diffusion defect, $\dot{V}/\dot{Q}$ (ventilation/perfusion) defect, or right-to-left shunt.

$$A - a \text{ gradient} = PA_{O_2} - Pa_{O_2}$$

$$PA_{O_2} = \text{alveolar } P_{O_2} \text{ (calculated from the alveolar gas equation)}$$

$$PA_{O_2} = (760 - 47) \times F_{I_{O_2}} - Pa_{CO_2}/0.8 \text{ (or 1)}$$

$$Pa_{O_2} = \text{arterial } P_{O_2} \text{ (from ABGs)}$$

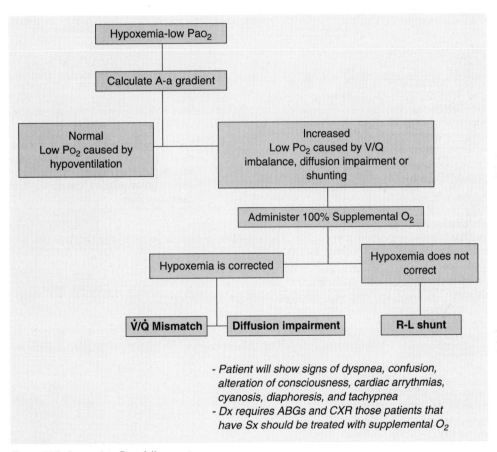

Figure 20.6 Approach to Resp failure.

COUGH

RATIONALE

- Chronic cough is a common problem causing patients to require medical attention.
- Most common causes are postnasal drip, asthma, and gastroesophageal reflux.

CAUSAL CONDITIONS

See Table 20.16.

APPROACH

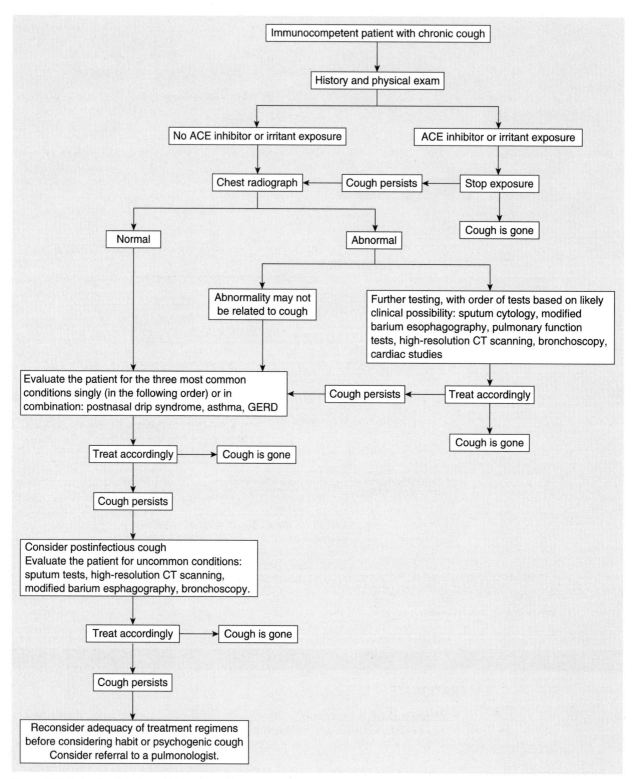

Figure 20.7 Evaluation of patient with chronic cough.

ASC Box

- Cough reflex
- Cough receptors (mechanical and chemical) from:
  - Resp epithelium
  - Pericardium
  - Esophagus
  - Diaphragm
  - Stomach
- Stimulate through afferent nerves the medullary cough center that activates exp muscles through efferent nerves.

Table **20.16** **Causal Conditions of Cough by Etiology**		
Chronic	**Acute**
Upper Resp	Infectious
• Postnasal drip	• URTI
• Gastroesophageal reflux	• Bronchitis
• Chronic sinusitis	• Pneumonia
• Drugs (ACE inhibitors)	
• Foreign body (more common in children)	
Pulmonary	Irritant
• Obstructive airway dz (asthma, chronic bronchitis, bronchiectasis, cystic fibrosis)	• Noxious fumes
• Lung neoplasm	• Smoke
• Chronic lung infections (lung abscess, TB, aspiration)	• Foreign body
• ILD	
Cardiac —CHF	

CXR

Smoker

- Abnormal CXR may suggest bronchiectasis and bronchogenic carcinoma and a CT scan should be performed for these Dx.
- Patients with a normal CXR with recurring Sx of chronic cough should consult a pulmonologist for PFT.

Nonsmoker

- Normal CXR of a nonsmoker often rules out the likelihood of pneumonia, infiltrative dz, or bronchiectasis.
- Consider postnasal drip syndrome with upper Resp tract and sinus Sx as a possible cause.
- Management of postnasal drip syndrome by combination of decongestants and antihistamine.
- If treatment is successful, patient should continue for 2 wk and then discontinue when Sx subside; if Sx continue asthma should then be considered as a potential cause.
- Cough may be the sole manifestation of asthma, for Dx and management, see "Lower Resp Tract Disorders."
- Heartburn, hoarseness of voice, or early morning cough could suggest GERD; 24-h esophageal pH monitoring may be conducted or medical management with proton-pump inhibitors should be considered.
- Other causes may include pneumonia or bronchitis when chronic cough is followed with purulent sputum.

BLOOD IN SPUTUM

RATIONALE

- Expectoration of blood or blood-streaked sputum.
- Massive hemoptysis occurs at expectoration >100—600 mL of blood over a 24-h period, when there are identifiable features of hemodynamic instability, altered gas exchange, or Resp difficulties.

APPLIED SCIENTIFIC CONCEPTS

- Although a disproportionate amount of blood flow in the pulmonary arteries, (almost the entire cardiac output but at low pressure), to the much smaller blood flow at high pressure through the bronchial arteries, >90% of the time, hemoptysis originates from the bronchial arteries.
- The pulmonary arteries supply nutritive blood supply for the airways, hilar lymph nodes, visceral pleura, and some of the mediastinum.

CAUSAL CONDITIONS

Table **20.17**	Causal Conditions of Hemoptysis
Airway dz	
Inflammatory	• Bronchitis (acute, chronic) • Bronchiectasis, lung abscess, cystic fibrosis
Neoplasms	• Bronchogenic carcinoma • Endobronchial metastatic carcinoma (melanoma, breast, renal, colon) • Bronchial carcinoid • Kaposi sarcoma (in patient with AIDS)
Other	• Foreign body • Trauma
Pulmonary parenchymal dz	
Infectious	• TB, necrotizing pneumonia, mycetoma, aspergilloma
Inflammatory/immune	• Goodpasture, pulmonary hemosiderosis, Wegener, lupus
Other	• Coagulopathy, iatrogenic, cocaine, endometriosis
Cardiovascular	
Elevated capillary pressure	• Mitral stenosis, tricuspid endocarditis, LV failure
Other	• Pulmonary embolus with infarction, AV malformation

CLINICAL BOX

Nosebleeds and Hoarseness of Voice

• Suggest bleeding from upper Resp tract

APPROACH

HISTORY

- Anticoagulation use
- Sx of CHF
- Infectious Sx
- Immunosuppression
- HIV risk factors
- Travel history
- Chronic cough and sputum suggestive of bronchiectasis
- Sx to suggest PE
- Wt loss, fever, night sweats suggestive of malignancy
- Smoking history
- GI and nasal Sx to suggest alternate source of blood

CLINICAL BOX

Coffee-Ground Emesis

Hematemesis is occasionally difficult to distinguish from hemoptysis as blood from a Resp source may be swallowed and present as coffee-ground emesis.

PHYSICAL

Table **20.18**	Points on Physical Exam
Lung cancer	Cachexia, clubbing, Horner syndrome, SVC syndrome, unilateral vocal cord paralysis
Bronchiectasis	Clubbing, primary lung cancer, lung abscess, chronic lung dz, lung metastases
Wegener	Nasal discharge, nasal septum perforation, saddle nose deformity, palpable purpura, polyarthralgias, joint tenderness, rash, mononeuropathy, active urine sediment, renal failure, hematuria
Infections	Fever, bronchial breath sounds, toxic changes
PE	Pl rub, right-sided heart failure

In massive hemoptysis (>200 mL/d), ensure adequacy of ventilation and hemodynamic stability first and consult a specialist.

GENERAL APPROACH

1. Determine if blood is coming from bronchial region, lungs, upper Resp tract, nasopharynx, or GI tract.
2. If bleeding not from lungs, examine upper Resp system.
3. Upper GI work-up needed when the bleeding source is unclear.

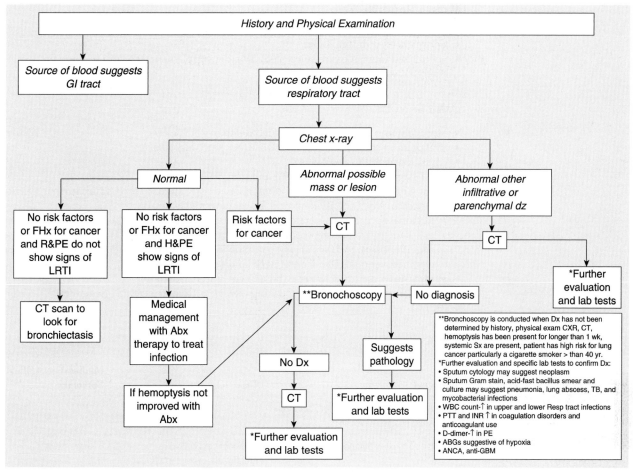

Figure 20.8 Approach to Dx of blood in sputum.

FURTHER EVALUATION AND SPECIFIC LAB TESTS

Table **20.19** Diagnostic Tests to Confirm Etiology of Hemoptysis	
Sputum Cytology	**Neoplasm**
Sputum Gram stain, acid-fast bacillus smear and culture	Pneumonia, lung abscess, TB, and mycobacterial infections
WBC	↑ in upper and lower RTI
PTT and INR	Coagulation disorders and anticoagulant use
D-dimer	PE
ABG	Hypoxia
ANCA, anti-GBM	Autoimmune

MANAGEMENT OF HEMOPTYSIS

NONSPECIFIC HEMOPTYSIS

- Evaluate ABCs and stop hemoptysis by treating underlying cause.
- If normal CXR, monitor on outpatient basis.
- If abnormal CXR, follow-up with CT and consider referral to specialist for bronchoscopy.

Massive Hemoptysis

- Maintain ABCs
- Consult with pulmonologist
- Specialized intensive care suggested, consider supplemental O_2 and prepare for possible emergent surgery

LUNG CANCER

- Most common cause of cancer-related death in both sexes
- 85% occur in smokers (asbestos exposure + smoking ↑ risk)
- Classified as SCLC and NSCLC
- TNM staging to classify treatment and prognosis
- Staging of SCLC by CT chest, abdomen, bone scan, and CT/MRI brain; further imaging indicated in NSCLC only if clinical Sxs suggest metastatic dz
  - Regional spread is associated with Pl Effs, tracheal obstruction, hoarseness, dysphagia, Pancoast syndrome(common in apical tumors, involves brachial plexus, causes shoulder pain), SVC syndrome(common in central tumors, leads to SVC compression, dyspnea, venous distension of neck, and swelling of face)
  - Metastases common to brain, bone, liver, adrenal, skin
- Paraneoplastic syndromes: Cushing (SCLC), hypercalcemia (squamous), SIADH (SCLC)

Table 20.20   **Classification of Lung Cancers**

Cancer and Staging	At Dx (%)	Definition	Treatment	Median Survival/5-yr Survival
Small cell	25%	Usually presents as disseminated, but often chemoradiation sensitive		
• Limited		One side of chest within one radiation port	Radiation and chemo ± prophylactic cranial irradiation	1–2 yr
• Extensive		Beyond one radiation port	Chemo	1 yr
Nonsmall cell	75%	Adenocarcinoma (35%) Squamous cell carcinoma (30%) Large cell carcinoma (10%)		
• I	10%	Isolated lesion and size	Surgery ± chemo	>60%
• II	20%	Hilar node involvement	Surgery ± radiation chemotherapy	40%–50%
• IIIA	15%	Mediastinal spread but resectable	Neoadjuvant chemo ± radiation, then surgical resection	10%–20%
• IIIB	15%	Unresectable		
• IV	40%	Metastatic	Chemo and/or supportive care Palliative radiation	1%

LOWER RESPIRATORY TRACT DISORDERS

RATIONALE

Sx of chest tightness, cough, wheeze, and dyspnea are often indicative of a lower Resp tract disorder.

CAUSAL CONDITIONS

See Table 20.21.

tomic Classification of LRT Disorders

	Differential Dx
dz)	• COPD (emphysema and chronic bronchitis) • Asthma • Bronchiectasis • Cystic fibrosis
	• Aspiration • Bronchiolitis • Cystic fibrosis
	• ILD
	• PE
	• Pulmonary edema

mmon Sx to Differentiate LRT Disorder on History

	PND, chest tightness, cough, waxing and waning Sx, seasonal variation, Sx exacerbated by cold, exercise, dust
	Dyspnea is hallmark Sx, particularly on exertion; chronic cough, sputum production, prior history of smoking, frequent Resp infections
sis	Chronic Resp infections, chronic cough, purulent sputum production, fever, weakness, Wt loss, dyspnea (less frequently), hemoptysis
CHF	Orthopnea, PND, leg swelling, dyspnea on exertion, fatigue
Interstitial lung	Progressive dyspnea on exertion then at rest, hypoxia (later stages), dry cough, wheeze uncommon, occupational/drug exposure, autoimmune history
Aspiration	History of stroke/seizure, neuromuscular dz, ETOH or drug abuse affecting level of consciousness, use of sedating medications, elderly, GERD
PE	Sudden dyspnea on exertion or rest, leg swelling, risk factors for DVT

See Table 20.23.

ASTHMA

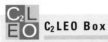

C₂LEO Box

Physicians' Legal Liability for Negligence
Failure to properly assess and ascertain the severity of a patient's asthma and to pursue the appropriately aggressive treatment for this potentially lethal illness is not initiated in a timely manner.

• Paroxysmal or persistent Sx including dyspnea, wheeze, chest tightness, cough, and sputum production
• Variable airflow limitation
• Presence of hyper-responsive airways

CLINICAL BOX

Properly Controlled Asthma

• Daytime Sx <4/wk
• Nighttime Sx <1/wk
• Capable of normal physical activity, no work absence
• Mild/few exacerbations
• Rescue puffer <4 dose/wk
• FEV1 <90% of patient's best

Table **20.23**	**Findings on Physical Exam and CXR to Differentiate LRT Disorders**	
	Physical Exam	**CXR Findings**
Asthma	Can be associated with nasal polyps Often normal Wheeze or quiet chest (in severe cases)	Often normal
COPD	• Normal—mild dz. • Prolonged expiration on forced exhalation (>6 s)—moderate–severe • ↑ AP diameter—moderate–severe • Paradoxical breathing—severe • Pulmonary HTN with right-sided failure (RV heave, loud S2, fixed split S2, JVP distension, leg swelling)—severe	• ↑ AP diameter (bronchitis) • Hyperinflation (flat diaphragm) • Evidence of bullae
Bronchiectasis	• Nasal polyps and evidence of sinusitis may be present • Rales at lung bases	• Sometimes normal • Dilated bronchi • Tram tracks (thin parallel lines coming from hilum)
CHF	Bibasilar crackles, elevated JVP, S3 gallop, evidence of valvular dz?, leg swelling	Vascular redistribution to apical area, fluid in the fissures, fluffy opacities,(unilateral or bilateral), pl Eff, curly B lines
Interstitial lung	Clubbing (IPF), fine crackles, evidence of rheumatological dz, RV failure in severe dz	• Variable findings
Aspiration	Crackles (often right sided but can be bilateral), wheeze, fever	• Can range from minimal findings to pneumonia and/or ARDS
PE	Fever, tachypnea, tachycardia, (hypotension, elevated JVP, pulsus in large PE)	Often normal; may have evidence of Hampton's hump if infarction of lung

Table **20.24**	**Diagnostic Testing for Asthma**
Spirometry	To diagnose asthma, reversible airway obstruction should be present, with FEV1 being the gold standard for measuring reversibility. Bronchodilator response is measured by repeating spirometry 15–30 min after inhalation of bronchodilator; 12%–15% or 200 mL ↑ in FEV1 is positive response.
PF measurements	Can be done at home; >10% variability in PF during day is usually diagnostic of asthma
Methacholine challenge	Used if history suspicious for asthma but normal spirometry; positive test exists when a ↓ in FEV1 of 20% or more occurs after low dose inhaled methacholine
Allergy testing	Indicated when any concern re induction of Sx due to exposure to indoor allergens.

Table **20.25**	**Treatment of Asthma**
Step	**Treatment**
1. Mild intermittent	• Sx <=2 times/wk, <=2 times/mo nighttime, normal lung function • No long-term control, short-acting β-agonist for Sx relief
2. Mild persistent	• Sx >2 times/wk, >2 times/mo nighttime, activity may be affected, normal PF/FEV1 but PF variability 20%–30% • Low dose inhaled corticosteroid plus short-acting β-agonist for Sx relief
3. Moderate persistent	• Daily Sx, daily use of β-agonist, activity affected, exacerbations >2 times/wk, nighttime >1 time/wk, FEV1 60%–80% predicted or PF variability >30% • Medium dose inhaled corticosteroid or low–medium dose inhaled corticosteroid with long-acting β-agonist plus short-acting β-agonist for Sx relief
4. Severe persistent	• Continual Sx, limited physical activity, frequent exacerbations, nighttime Sx frequent, FEV1 <60% predicted or PF variability >30% • High–dose-inhaled corticosteroid and long-acting bronchodilator ± anti-IgE treatment such as omalizumab ± leukotriene recepter antagonist ± oral corticosteroids

Reasons for Poor Asthma Control

- Lack of education about asthma and medication
- Not using objective measures to assess control (PF or FEV1)
- Poor adherence

ASTHMA MANAGEMENT

All patients:

- Education on trigger avoidance
- Action plan
- Proper use of inhalers (see Table 20.25)

APPLIED SCIENTIFIC CONCEPTS

Table 20.26   Cellular Mechanisms of Asthma and Treatment

	Role	Pharmacologic Interventions
Mast cells	• Early phase allergen response by crosslinked IgE activation • Release of histamine, tryptase, leukotriene, and cytokines • Smooth muscle contraction	• β_2 agonists/anticholinergics for smooth muscle relaxation • Anti-IgE ab to prevent activation
Eosinophils	• Late phase allergen response • Release of MBP, ECP, leukotrienes • Airway narrowing and hyperactivity, mucous secretion	• Leukotriene receptor antagonists (mast cells and eosinophil action)
T-cells	• Initiation and sustaining airway inflammation • Th2 immune deviation (IL-4,13)	• Corticosteroids to inhibit proinflammatory cytokines

PLEURAL EFFUSION/PLEURAL ABNORMALITIES

PL EFF

- A Pl Eff signifies an imbalance between the formation and removal of Pl fluid.
- This can result from pulmonary, Pl, or extrapulmonary dz.
- Most common Sx is dyspnea; less commonly is cough or chest pain.

ASC Box

- Pl fluid
  - Pl fluid has low protein concentration (<2 g/dL); pH and glucose similar to that of blood.
  - Is formed primarily from the parietal pleura. Turnover of fluid depends on vascular and interstitial fluid exchange.
  - Hydrostatic pressure of the parietal pleura is 30 cm H_2O (similar to systemic circulation) whereas hydrostatic pressure of the visceral pleura is similar to that of the pulmonary circulation (10 cm H_2O). The fluid therefore moves from parietal toward visceral pleura.
  - Oncotic pressure is similar in both (25 cm H_2O).

CAUSAL CONDITIONS

Light's Criteria for Exudates

- Pl fluid protein divided by serum protein >0.5
- Pl fluid LDH divided by serum LDH >0.6
- Pl fluid LDH > two thirds the upper limits of normal serum LDH

Table **20.27** Exudative versus Transudative Pl Eff	
Exudative (DELII MICE)	**Transudative**
• Results primarily from inflammation in lung/pleura or impaired lymphatic drainage, including movement of fluid from extrathoracic spaces • Local factors	• Imbalance of hydrostatic and oncotic pressures in the chest, including movement of fluid from extrathoracic spaces (peritoneal/retroperitoneal) • Systemic factors

• **D**rugs (amiodarone, nitrofurantoin, cytotoxic)
• **E**xtrapulmonary
• **I**nfectious[a]
  • Empyema
  • Parapneumonic
  • Abscess
  • TB
• **L**ymphatic abnormalities
• **M**alignancy[a]
  • Carcinoma,
  • Lymphoma
  • Mesothelioma
  • Chylothorax
• **I**nflammatory
  • Pancreatitis
  • PE
  • Sarcoidosis
  • Radiation
  • ARDS
  • Asbestos
  • Uremic pleurisy
• **I**atrogenic
• **C**onnective tissue dz
• **E**ndocrine
	• CHF[a]
	• Cirrhosis
	• Nephrotic syndrome
	• Peritoneal dialysis
	• Hypoalbuminemia
	• Constrictive pericarditis
	• Atelectasis
	• SVC obstruction

[a]Most common in children

APPROACH

See Figure 20.9.

THORACENTESIS

> **CLINICAL BOX**
>
> **Common Tests for Pl Fluid Analysis**
>
> **Pl**
> • LDH
> • Total protein
> • Glucose
> • pH
> • Cell count
> • Differential
> • Cytology (Gram stain)
>
> **Serum**
> • LDH
> • Total protein
> • Glucose
>
> **Rare**
> • Amylase
> • Chylomicrons
> • Triglycerides
> • AFB smear and culture (yields Dx ~40% of cases)

> **CLINICAL BOX**
>
> **Thoracentesis Relative Contraindications and Complications**
>
> **Contraindications**
> • Bleeding diathesis
> • Anticoagulation
> • Small volume Pl fluid
> • Mechanical ventilation
> • Active skin infection
>
> **Complications**
> • Pneumothorax (10%)
> • Re-expansion pulmonary edema
> • Hemothorax

> **CLINICAL BOX**
>
> **Indications for CT scan**
>
> • Parapneumonic Eff not responding to Abx
> • Suspicion of lung malignancy

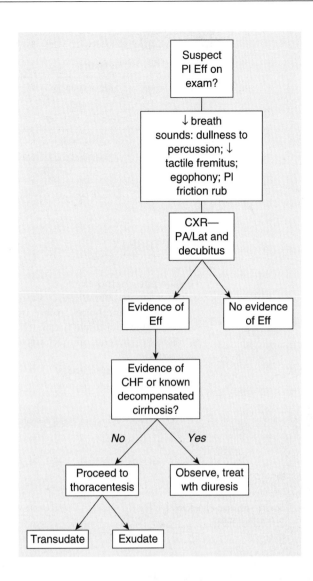

Figure 20.9 Approach to Pl Eff.

Table **20.28**	**Analysis of Pl Fluid**		
pH <7.3	**Glucose Level <1.66 mmol/L**	**Glucose between 1.66 and 2.77 mmol/L**	**Bloody Pl Effs**
Malignancy	Empyema	Malignant Eff	1. Hemothorax
TB	Rheumatoid pleurisy	TB pleuritis	Defn: Hct Pl Eff $\geq$0.5 Hct serum
Empyema		Esophageal rupture	• Iatrogenic
Complicated		Lupus pleuritis	• Trauma
parapneumonic			• Rib fracture
Eff			• Ruptured AVM
Esophageal			• Dissecting AA
rupture			• Requires drainage urgently
Rheumatoid			2. Bloody Pl Eff
pleurisy			• Malignancy
			• Mesothelioma
			• PE
			• Benign asbestos
			• Post op cardiac Sx
			• Post cardiac injury

Table **20.29**	**Eff in Setting of Pneumonia**	
	Definition	**Treatment**
Uncomplicated	Culture negative Free flowing pH >7.2	Observe if <10 mm, clinically stable or improving, no loculation seen
Complicated	Does not resolve with Abx alone, pH <7.2 or loculated and culture negative	Chest tube
Empyema	pH <7.2 Culture positive or Gram stain ± pus	Chest tube

PNEUMOTHORAX

- Air in Pl space
- Tension pneumothorax
  - Rapid, labored breathing, cyanosis, tachycardia, hypotension, tracheal shift away from side of pneumothorax, absent breath sounds ipsilateral side, JVP distended, pulsus paradoxus, abdominal distention
  - Suspect in patients on mechanical ventilation or noninvasive ventilation with sudden deterioration
- Spontaneous pneumothorax
  - May have variable degree of Sx, depending on size

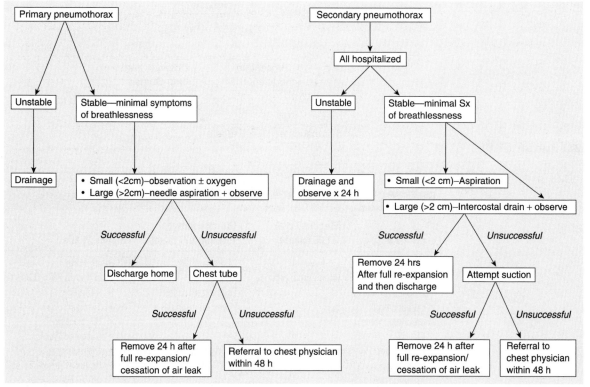

Figure 20.10 Approach to pneumothorax.

UNILATERAL/LOCAL EDEMA

RATIONALE

- Thrombosis is a common problem. Approximately 70% of patients with PE have asymptomatic DVT.
- Case fatality rates range from 1% to 5%.

- Post-thrombotic syndrome (chronic pain, swelling, ulceration of skin) can occur in up to one third of patients with DVT, with latency up to as late as 10 yr.
- Thrombi that result in clinically significant PE are almost always located in the proximal veins of the legs, but can also begin as calf vein thrombi that extend proximally.

CAUSAL CONDITIONS

Conditions that can mimic DVT:

- Lymphatic obstruction
- Ruptured popliteal cyst
- Cellulitis
- Postphlebitic syndrome
- Trauma
- Thyroid dz

APPROACH

HISTORY

- Triad of calf pain, edema, pain on dorsiflexion of foot (Homan sign)—1/3 of patients
- If suspicious for PE, (dyspnea, pleuritic chest pain, RR >20, cough, hemoptysis), consider more objective testing
- Often asymptomatic

WELL'S CRITERIA FOR DVT

Table **20.30** Well's Criteria for DVT	
Sx	Score
Active cancer (ongoing treatment, Dx within 6 mo, palliative care)	1
Paresis, paralysis, or recent plaster cast	1
Immobilization of lower extremity	1
Recently bedridden for >3 d and/or major surgery within 4 wk	1
Localized tenderness over distribution of deep veins	1
Entire leg swollen	1
Calf swelling >3 cm compared with asymptomatic side, measured at 10 cm below tibial tubercle	1
Pitting edema (greater in symptomatic leg)	1
Collateral superficial veins (nonvaricose)	1
Alternative Dx as likely or greater than that of DVT	− 2

Table **20.31** Well's Pretest Probability of DVT		
Score	Risk	Probablity
0	Low	3%
1–2	Moderate	17%
>3	High	75%

WELL'S CRITERIA FOR PE
See Tables 20.32 and 20.33.

DVT may be a presenting feature of malignancy.

Malignancy is found most often in patients without obvious cause for DVT, recurrent idiopathic thrombosis, and in patients older than 60.

CLINICAL BOX

Establish Risk factors for DVT

- Pregnancy
- Malignancy
- Hip surgery
- Major knee surgery
- Immobilization
- Oral contraceptives
- Nephrotic syndrome
- Sepsis
- Anticardiolipin ab
- Protein C, S, antithrombin deficiency
- Previous VTE

Table **20.32** Well's Criteria for PE	
• Clinical signs or Sx of DVT • PE as likely as alternative Dx	3 pts
• HR >100 bpm • Immobilization or surgery within 4 wk • Prior DVT or PE	1.5 pts
• Hemoptysis • Malignancy	1.0 pt

Table **20.33** Pretest Probability for PE		
Pts	**Risk**	**Probablity**
0–2 pts	Low	3%
2–6 pts	Intermediate	20%
>6 pts	High	60%

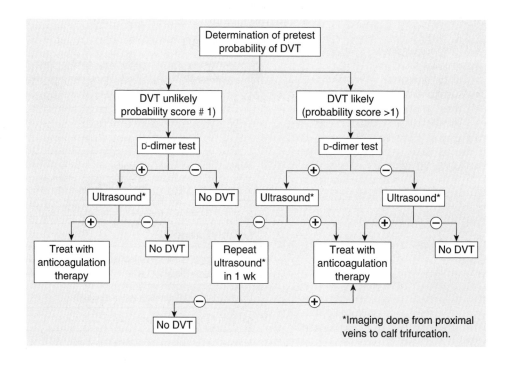

Figure 20.11 Approach to DVT.

LAB INVESTIGATIONS

- CBC, lytes, INR, PTT, ABG, CXR, ECG, D-DIMER
- Specialist should be consulted before a CT scan or bronchoscopy are performed, patient has massive hemoptysis or when hemoptysis is recurrent.

MANAGEMENT OF DVT/PE

- Heparin–works immediately by inhibiting activated coagulation factors
- Coumadin–works slowly by inhibiting synthesis of vitamin K dependent coagulation factors
- Need to follow INR with target of 2.0–3.0

Table **20.34** Heparin Unfractionated versus LMWH	
Unfractionated Heparin	**LMWH**
Inhibits both thrombin and factor Xa	Inhibits specifically factor Xa
Requires frequent monitoring of PTT	Does not require monitoring
Difficult to maintain therapeutic range	More reliable dose relation Lower incidence of thrombocytopenia Can be administered in community

INDICATIONS FOR ANTICOAGULATION

- If DVT or PE is suspected, anticoagulation with heparin or LMWH should be administered until diagnostic evaluation is complete.
- Warfarin (Coumadin) should be administered for long-term anticoagulation use but needs to be overlapped with heparin for 5–7 d, until INR therapeutic is 2.0–3.0.
- Length of treatment
  - VTE after time-limited factor (surgery, transient immobilization)—treat for 3 mo
  - Idiopathic DVT/PE—treat for 6 mo
  - If ongoing risk factors (immobility, cancer, multiple risk factors), second event—treat for life
- Complications: Bleeding, thrombocytopenia (HIT) with use of heparins, osteoporosis with long-term high-dose unfractionated heparin, drug interactions with warfarin, teratogenicity with warfarin

Table **20.35** Thromboprophylaxis		
Risk	**Situation**	**Prophylaxis**
Low 0.4% DVT 0.2% PE	• Minor surgery in patients <40 yr with no risk factors	• Early ambulation
Moderate 2%–4% DVT 1%–2% PE	• Minor surgery in patients with risk factors • Minor surgery in patients aged 40–60 with no risk factors	• Low dose unfractionated heparin 5,000 U q12 h • LMWH—dalteparin 2,500 U q.d. or enoxaparin 20 mg q.d. • Intermittent pneumatic compression stockings
High 4%–8% DVT 2%–4% PE	• Surgery in patients >60 yr with no risk factors • Surgery in patients aged 40–60 with risk factors	• Low dose unfractionated heparin 5,000 U q8 h • LMWH—dalteparin 5,000 U q.d. or enoxaparin 40 mg q.d. • Intermittent pneumatic compression stockings + elastic stockings
Very high 10%–20% DVT 4%–10% PE	• Surgery in patients >40 yr with multiple risk factors • Hip or knee arthroplasty • Major trauma • Acute spinal cord injury	• LMWH—dalteparin 5,000 U q.d. or enoxaparin 40 mg q.d. • Oral dose of Coumadin (INR 2-3) • Intermittent pneumatic compression stockings/elastic stockings + low dose heparin/LMWH

APPROACH TO CELLULITIS

See Table 20.36.

Table **20.36**	Classification of Cellulitis	
Class	Clinical findings—acute and progressive onset of painful, hot, swollen, red area of skin; rarely bilateral Leg is commonest site with an obvious portal of entry	Treatment 1st line/2nd line(penicillin allergy)
I	No systemic signs of illness	Cloxacillin 500 mg q.i.d. PO\clarithromycin 500 mg PO b.i.d.
II	Systemically ill OR systemically well with comorbidity	Cloxacillin 2 g q.i.d. IV\clarithromycin 500 mg IV b.i.d. or clindamycin 600 mg IV t.i.d.
III	Systemically unwell with comorbidities that may complicate course of therapy	Cloxacillin 2 g q.i.d. IV\clarithromycin 500 mg IV b.i.d. or clindamycin 900 mg IV t.i.d.
IV	Sepsis syndrome or life-threatening infection.	Penicillin 2–4 M units q4 hourly IV + ciprofloxacin 400 mg b.i.d. IV + clindamycin 900 mg t.i.d. IV

ALLERGIC REACTIONS

- Information on allergic reactions can be found under various topics in this book.
- This chapter considers the topics together, as people with allergic rhinitis or atopic dermatitis have an ↑ likelihood of developing asthma or Resp atopy.
- Atopy is a genetic condition resulting from hypersensitivity reactions to allergens.
- Also see Food Allergy in Chapter 9 and Anaphylaxis in Chapter 5.

APPLIED SCIENTIFIC CONCEPTS

MAST CELLS

- Have very high affinity receptor for IgE on surface (coated with IgE ab).
- When allergen binds to IgE on surface of mast cell, get crosslinking leading to activation of the mast cell.
- Activation leads to release of preformed mediators (stored in granules) such as histamine, proteoglycans (heparin), and serine proteases.
- Activated mast cells makes and releases prostaglandin D2, leukotriene C4, and cytokines

HISTAMINE CAUSES

- A dilatation of postcapillary venules
- Bronchial and smooth muscle contraction
- An ↑ in nasal mucus production
- ↑ in blood vessel permeability leading to edema

CAUSAL CONDITIONS

See Table 20.37.

APPROACH

The approach to atopy and allergy largely depends on the severity of the reaction. Common allergy associated conditions and management are outlined below. Education is the most important intervention.

- Reading food labels
- Avoiding high-risk situations such as buffets
- Wear medic-alert bracelet
- May need self-injectable adrenaline (especially if previous allergic reaction resulting in Resp or cardiovascular effects, but may want to have if peanut or tree nut allergy, if an allergic reaction has occurred to a small trace of allergen, or if individual is far from medical care)
- Know the early warning signs of allergic reaction

CLINICAL BOX

Common Food Allergies

- Peanuts
- Tree nuts
- Eggs
- Cows milk
- Wheat
- Fish
- Shellfish
- Sesame

CLINICAL BOX

Other Common Allergies

- Drugs (Abx)
- Insect venom
- Radiocontrast media
- Latex

Table **20.37**	Allergies
Generalized	See Anaphylaxis
Localized	
Skin (see Chapter 4)	• Dermatitis/atopy/pruritus • Urticaria • Angioedema
Resp	• Rhinorrhea • Wheezing • Angioedema
Gastrointestinal tract	• Food intolerance • Celiac dz

RHINORRHEA

See also Rhinorrhea in Chapter 7.

- Characterized by sneezing, itchy eyes, rhinorrhea
- Due to the inhalation of airborne antigens to which patient has been previously sensitized (and has made IgE ab)
- Very common cause of physician visits and lost days from school and work
- Up to 50% of patients with asthma and up to 30% of patients with eczema have allergic rhinitis
- Careful history to elicit likely allergen, seasonal, perennial, or occupational features
- Rhinitis can also be due to infectious causes, perennial nonallergic causes, and others such as hormonal (pregnancy, hypothyroid), drug induced, associated with food, or mechanical causes
- May treat with nasal steroids

ANGIOEDEMA

- Rapid swelling of skin, mucosa, and submucosal tissue
- Commonly associated with allergy (to foods or drugs such as ACE inhibitors) but exists in an hereditary form
- If rapidly progressing, requires emergency management (see Anaphylaxis)

WHEEZING

- Differential Dx of wheeze includes:
  - Asthma
  - Foreign body
  - Aspiration
  - GERD
  - Cystic fibrosis
  - Bronchitis
  - Tumor
  - COPD
- Atopy is a predictor of persistent asthma
- Take a history to elicit family history of atopy and physical exam to look for atopic dermatitis
- Can do skin-prick testing to identify allergens

ATOPIC DERMATITIS

Chronic inflammatory skin condition (see Allergy section in Chapter 4)

CHAPTER 21

Urology

*Al'a Abdo, Dr. Julien Letendre, Dr. Thierry Lebeau,
and Dr. François Bénard*

DYSURIA AND PYURIA

RATIONALE

- Frequency: micturition at short intervals; it may result from ↑ urine formation, ↓ bladder capacity (secondary to loss of elasticity, edema, or residual urine) or lower urinary tract irritation.
- Dysuria
  1. Difficulty with micturition (the true definition)
  2. Sometimes used to denote pain or discomfort on micturition
- Bacteriuria: presence of bacteria in urine; does not preclude invasion of urinary tissue.
- UTI: Microbial infection, usually bacterial, of any part of the urinary tract.
- Pyuria: Presence of at least 5 (for men) or 20 (for women) leukocytes/high-power field on the microscopic exam of a urine sample.

CLINICAL BOX

Significance of UTI in Different Groups

Gender	Females	• Often normal in healthy females (shorter urethra and its perineal positioning) • Often coincides with sexual activity
	Males	• Generally signal an underlying problem (stasis from obstruction, vesical urolithiasis, etc.)—the long male urethra and the bactericide properties of prostate secretions generally protect against bacterial invasion
Age	Children	• Prepuce ↑ chances of UTI 10-fold before age of 6 mo) • Vaginal voiding (urinating with legs adducted causing backflow of urine into vagina) causes a change in the local flora as well as perineal humidity which can predispose to UTIs. • Consider certain etiologies: *obstruction (PUV, UPJ obstruction) and VUR*
	Elderly	• Stasis from obstruction (BPH) • Menopause • Catheterization

---

CAUSAL CONDITIONS

1. Urinary tract involvement (UTI is the most common cause)
2. Prostatitis
3. Infections (or inflammation) outside the urinary tract

Table **21.1**	**Classification of UTI**	
Classification	**Categories**	**Explanation**
Anatomic	Upper Lower	Pyelonephritis • Cystitis • Urethritis (sometimes indistinguishable from cystitis) • "Bacterial prostatitis"
Clinical	Uncomplicated Complicated	Healthy, nonpregnant women **All other UTIs** • Male • Pregnant women • Children with underlying congenital anomaly • DB mellitus • Immunosuppressed • Renal insufficiency • Urolithiasis • Debilitated patient • Abnormal urinary apparatus or function • Recent instrumentation catheterization/surgery • Nosocomial/institution acquired (generally, bacteria are more virulent and more resistant to Abx) • Resistant bacterial strains
Clinical/chronologic classification	Isolated (sporadic)	• First infection or remotely occurring infection • Most common type
	Unresolved bacteriuria	Urine not sterilized after Abx Tx Causes Bacterial resistance/inadequate Abx Tx (multiple organisms) Azotemia (poor excretion of Abx into urine) Rapid reinfection (another organism) Patient noncompliance Papillary necrosis (unable to concentrate Abx in urine) Infected calculi, tumor, foreign object
	Recurrent	• Repeated infection (after treatment) interrupted by a period of sterile urine **Relapse** Within 2 wk of Tx Same bacteria • Usually signals the presence of a predisposing condition **Reinfection** >2 wk after Tx

CLINICAL BOX

Risk Factors for UTI

Age (years)	Sex	Major Risk Factor
<1	♂ Male and female	Uncircumcised Anatomic anomalies
<5	Male and female	Anatomic anomalies (VUR, obstruction)
6–15	Male and female	Functional anomalies (dysfunctional voiding)
16–35	Female	**Sexual intercourse**
36+ (especially elderly)	Female	Gynecologic surgery, genital prolapse
	Male Male and female	Obstruction (BPH) Catheterization, surgery

4. Overactive bladder
5. Other—less frequent causes
   - Radiation cystitis
   - Chemotherapy (iatrogenic)
   - Neoplasm
   - Foreign bodies

APPROACH

- When a patient presents with frequency, dysuria and/or pyuria, an investigation for UTIs must be performed.
- In the history, look for irritative symptoms, past UTIs, and risk factors according to sex and age.
- The definitive diagnosis relies on the **urinalysis** (+ nitrites, + esterase, + hematuria) **and urine culture**.
  - Urine culture should be performed in the following situations: complicated UTI, recurrent UTI, upper UTI, or febrile UTI.
- In children, an abdominal ultrasound can be performed to look for signs of obstruction (dilation of the collecting system—HN and hydroureter—and thickening of the vesical wall); a VCUG can be used to detect VUR; a *99mTc-DMSA scan can be used to identify acute pyelonephritis* or renal scarring, and to evaluate the function of each kidney separately.

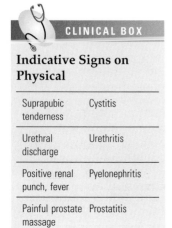

CLINICAL BOX

Indicative Signs on Physical

Suprapubic tenderness	Cystitis
Urethral discharge	Urethritis
Positive renal punch, fever	Pyelonephritis
Painful prostate massage	Prostatitis

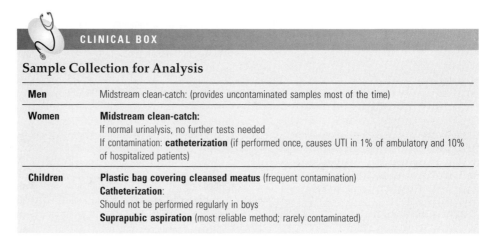

CLINICAL BOX

Sample Collection for Analysis

Men	Midstream clean-catch: (provides uncontaminated samples most of the time)
Women	**Midstream clean-catch:** If normal urinalysis, no further tests needed If contamination: **catheterization** (if performed once, causes UTI in 1% of ambulatory and 10% of hospitalized patients)
Children	**Plastic bag covering cleansed meatus** (frequent contamination) **Catheterization:** Should not be performed regularly in boys **Suprapubic aspiration** (most reliable method; rarely contaminated)

Table **21.2**	**Indications for Additional Investigation and/or Referral in UTI**
Male	All male patients (boys and men)
Female	• **Recurrent** or **persistent** UTI • Girls <5 yr
Male and female	• Persistent fever after adequate treatment • Evidence of obstruction • Gross hematuria • History of calculi

OVERACTIVE BLADDER

- When infections and cancer have been ruled out, overactive (unstable) bladder should be considered.
  - The patient will present with: frequency + urgency ± incontinence.
  - By definition, there is no evidence of an underlying pathological process.
  - The diagnosis is clinical. However, uninhibited bladder contractions may be demonstrated on urodynamic studies.

Table **21.3**	Cystitis versus Pyelonephritis	
Finding	**Cystitis**	**Pyelonephritis**
Dysuria (pain) irritative symptoms	+ (More abrupt onset)	±
Fever	(Or low grade)	+ (high)
Chills	−	+
Pyuria	+	+
Bacteruria	+	+
Hematuria (micro or macro)	+ In 50% of cases (generally micro)	±
Bacteremia	−	+
Renal punch	−	+
Complication	• Evolution to pyelonephritis • Relapse of infection • Bacterial persistence	• Bacteremia and septic shock • Renal parenchymal damage (pyonephrosis, renal abscess) • Papillary necrosis
Predisposing factors	• Female • Obstruction • Indwelling catheters • Sexual intercourse • Urolithiasis • Foreign objects	• Previous cystitis • VUR • Nephrolithiasis

+, finding present; −, not present; ±, may or may not be present.

Table **21.4**	Differentiation of Acute Pain at Micturition in Women		
	Bacterial Cystitis	**STD**	**Vaginitis**
Onset	Acute	Acute	Gradual
Associated symptoms	Suprapubic pain	Nonspecific	Pruritus
Exam	Nonspecific	Vaginal discharge (leucorrhea)	
Urinalysis	Pyuria >90% Hematuria in 50%	Pyuria (occasionally) No hematuria	No pyuria
Definitive diagnosis	Urine culture	Physical exam points to PID and Gram stain, culture or PCR of cervical and urethral samples (see Chapter 14).	Gram stain and culture of discharge (see Chapter 14).

(Adapted with permission from Siroky MB, Oates RD, Babayan RK. *Handbook of urology*, 3rd ed. Philadelphia: Lippincott Williams & Wilkins; 2004.)

Tx

UTIs

- Empiric antibiotherapy should be started (and adjusted for the culture if it is available).
- Although the same bacteria that cause uncomplicated cystitis also cause uncomplicated pyelonephritis, the consequences of inappropriate treatment in the latter are far more dangerous; therefore, TMP–SMX is not the first line of therapy (*see Table below*)

Asymptomatic Bacteriuria

- Absolute indications
  - **Pregnancy**
  - Immunocompromised patients
  - Renal transplant patients

- Relative indications
  - Urologic instrumentation, endoscopy, or surgery
  - Children, especially those with VUR
  - Patient with neurogenic bladder
  - Patient with indwelling catheter

Table **21.5**	Empiric Antibiotherapy for UTIs				
	Type of Infection		**Abx**	**PO versus IV**	**Length of Tx**
Uncomplicated	Acute cystitis	First line: If allergy or high incidence of resistance:	TMP–SMX Ciprofloxacin	PO	3 d
	Acute pyelonephritis	Mild: Severe:	Ciprofloxacin Ciprofloxacin + third generation cephalosporin	PO IV	7–14 d
	If gram-positive on Gram stain	Assume *Enterococci* If severe:	Amoxicillin ± clavulanate Amoxicillin + clavulanate + gentamicin	PO IV	
Complicated	Cystitis or pyelonephritis	Generally more resistant organisms:	Third generation cephalosporin or ciprofloxacin	IV	
	If gram-positive on Gram stain	Assume *Enterocci*	Ampicillin + gentamicin		

CLINICAL BOX

Pathogens Responsible for UTIs

UTI	Bacteria	Percentage
Uncomplicated	*E. coli*	53–79
	Proteus mirabilis	4–5
	Staphylococcus saprophyticus	3
	Klebsiella spp.	2–3
	Other Enterobacteriaceae	3
Complicated	*E. coli*	26–29
	Enterococci	13–17
	Pseudomonas aeruginosa	9–16
	Klebsiella spp.	8–10
	Other Enterobacteriaceae	9–11

INDICATIONS FOR HOSPITAL ADMISSION IN PYELONEPHRITIS

1. Infection + obstruction
2. Complicated UTIs (depending on the severity of the disease and the comorbidities)
3. Pregnancy
4. Inability to maintain hydration or to tolerate oral medication
5. Severe pain or debilitation
6. Failure of outpatient treatment
7. Lack of follow-up or compliance
8. Diagnostic uncertainty
9. Comorbid illness

Infection and obstruction in pyelonephritis is a medical emergency.

All patients presenting with anatomic abnormalities, urolithiasis, suspected cancer, urinary obstructions, and foreign objects that are not readily removable and overactive bladder should be referred to a urologist (see Table 21.2).

HEMATURIA

RATIONALE

- Three or more RBC per HPF is considered an abnormal presence of blood in urine and may arise from any site along the urinary tract.
- Must be investigated as it may be a sign of serious underlying disease.
- Classified as microscopic or gross.

APPLIED SCIENTIFIC CONCEPTS

- Normal glomerular capillaries filter blood molecules based on their size and electrical charge.
  - The basement membrane's negatively charged proteoglycans repel molecules with negative electrical charge-like albumin.
- Activation of the humoral and cellular immunity pathways, and complement system alters those properties allowing albumin and RBC to be filtered and reach Bowman's capsule, resulting in proteinuria and hematuria.

CAUSAL CONDITIONS

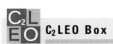

C₂LEO Box

Negligence
The DDx for persistent hematuria ranges from benign to malignant and therefore it cannot be ignored or assumed to be benign (e.g., UTI).

Table **21.6**	**DDx of Hematuria**		
	Extraglomerular		
	Collecting System	**Renal**	**Glomerular**
Transient	• UTI • Stones • Exercise induced • Trauma • Endometriosis • Appendicitis • Diverticulitis • Anticoagulants[a]	• UTI • Exercise induced • Trauma • Anticoagulants[a] • Thromboembolism (e.g., renal artery embolism, revel vein thrombosis)	**Isolated:** (e.g., Alport syndrome, IgA nephropathy) **Postinfections:** postinfectious gram-negative (e.g.,poststreptococcal) **Systemic involvement:**
Persistent	**Benign** • Benign bladder and ureteral polyps **Malignant** • Bladder cancer • Prostate cancer • Ureteral cancer	**Tumors** • RCC • TCC • Wilm's tumor **Tubulointerstitial** • Polycystic kidney disease • Infection (pyelonephritis) **Vascular** • Papillary necrosis • Sickle cell disease • Arteriovenous malformation	Systemic lupus erythematosus Vasculitis

[a]The incidence of hematuria in patients on anticoagulants is similar to that of patients not receiving anticoagulants. They still need to be investigated.

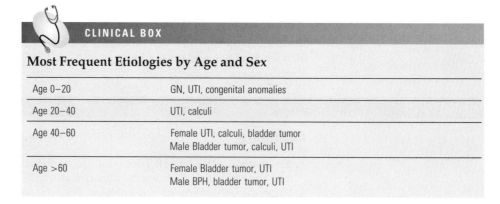

CLINICAL BOX

Most Frequent Etiologies by Age and Sex

Age 0–20	GN, UTI, congenital anomalies
Age 20–40	UTI, calculi
Age 40–60	Female UTI, calculi, bladder tumor Male Bladder tumor, calculi, UTI
Age >60	Female Bladder tumor, UTI Male BPH, bladder tumor, UTI

CLINICAL BOX

Causes of Non–RBC Red Urine

HEME +	HEME −
Hemoglo-binuria	**Drugs**
Dialysis	Sulfa drug
Hemolysis	Nitrofu-rantoin
Myoglo-binuria	Salicylates
Rhabdomyo-lysis	Phenytoin
Rifampin	**Foods**
Trauma	Beets
	Food coloring
	Metabolites
	Bilirubin
	Porphyrin

APPROACH

MICROSCOPIC HEMATURIA

- The first step is to confirm the presence of RBCs in the urine.
- Dipstick is highly sensitive (>90%), but less specific than microscopic evaluation.
- Distinguishing a renal from a urologic disease is an important step of the evaluation.

Silent hematuria originating from a urologic tumor is usually *intermittent*. Therefore the *spontaneous resolution should not be a reassuring sign.*

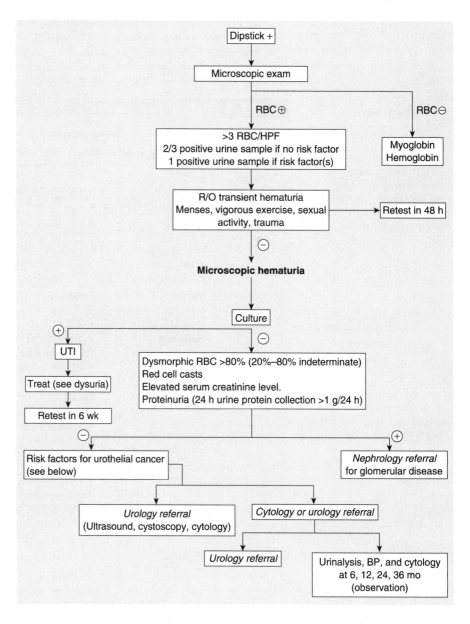

Figure 21.1 Evaluation of microscopic hematuria.

Establish hemodynamic stability first when evaluating gross hematuria.

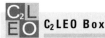 **C₂LEO Box**

Informed Consent

Patient should be informed that once exclusion of UTI has been established, it is critical to differentiate extra- and glomerular hematuria, which is best accomplished by an experienced physician to examining the urine sediment. This information must be discussed before more invasive and/or expensive investigations can be recommended.

 CLINICAL BOX

Urothelial Cancer Screening

- Routine urinalysis screening in asymptomatic individuals is not recommended by the Canadian Task Force on the periodic health exam.
- Urine cytology is recommended for all patients with risk factors presenting with hematuria. Not recommended for routine screening.

 CLINICAL BOX

Urothelial Cancer Investigation

If a bladder tumor is discovered, imaging the upper urinary tract is essential because there is 2%–5% chance of synchronous lesion.

GROSS HEMATURIA

- The timing of hematuria during micturition may indicate the site of the bleeding.
  - **Initial** suggests a urethral lesion
  - **Terminal** suggests bleeding from the bladder neck or trigone
  - **Total** suggests a source from the bladder or above
- If a history of trauma is present, CT scan of the kidneys must be part of the workup (see Urinary Tract Injuries in Chapter 5).
- Gross hematuria requires a urology referral (cystoscopy/IVP or CT scan)

SPECIAL CONSIDERATIONS

UROTHELIAL CARCINOMA

- Affects the bladder (>90%), the pelvis, and ureter (<10%)
- Bladder TCC is the fourth most common cancer in men in Canada
- Risk factors
  - **Cigarette smoking** is the major risk factor.
  - Occupational exposure to dyes (benzenes or aromatic amines)
  - History of gross hematuria
  - Age >40
  - Previous urologic disorder
  - History of irritative symptoms
  - History of recurrent UTI despite appropriate use of Abx

RENAL CELL CARCINOMA

- Accounts for 80% of renal tumors
- Paraneoplastic syndromes occur in 10%–40% of RCC
  - Erythrocytosis (EPO)
  - Hypercalcemia (PTH)
  - Hypertension (renin)
  - Stauffer syndrome (hepatic cell dysfunction)
  - Hormone production (cortisol, prolactin, insulin, gonadotropins)

 CLINICAL BOX

RCC Classic Triad

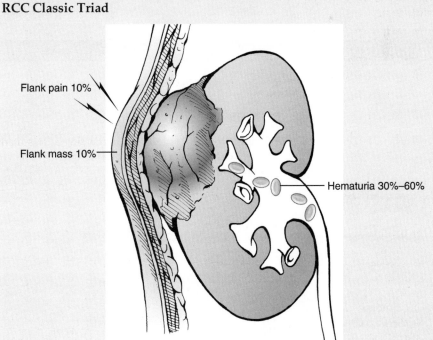

Flank pain 10%

Flank mass 10%

Hematuria 30%–60%

UROLITHIASIS

See also Renal colic.

- Factors influencing stone formation:
  - ↑ Ion concentration (hypercalcemia, hyperuricosuria, hyperoxaluria)
  - ↓ Urine volume (dehydration)
  - *Low pH* favors uric acid stones, *high pH* favors calcium phosphate and struvite stones
  - ↓ Inhibitory factors (hypocitraturia, hypoMg, others—Tomm–Horsfall)
- Recurrent stones:
  - History: number of previous episodes, onset of previous episodes, bowel disease, gout, DB, medications, and family history.
  - Investigation:
    - Serum: electrolytes, calcium, phosphate, uric acid, PTH
    - 24-h urine collection: urine volume, pH, calcium, creatinine, sodium, phosphate, oxalate, citrate, uric acid, ± cystine
  - General measures for prevention of recurrent urolithiasis
    - ↑ Fluid intake >2 L/d
    - ↓ Animal protein intake
    - Restrict sodium intake (2–3 g/d)
    - Do not restrict calcium intake (if <2 g/d)
    - ↓ Dietary oxalate (tea, coffee, chocolate, beer, spinach, nuts, cranberries)

CLINICAL BOX

Clinical Presentation of Urolithiasis

- Asymptomatic stone
- Acute episode/renal colic
- Microscopic hematuria (rare presentation form; consider other causes of hematuria even if an asymptomatic stone is present)
- Chronic urinary infection
- Acute urinary infection
- Bladder stone (irritative and obstructive symptoms, hematuria, suprapubic pain)

POLYURIA AND POLYDIPSIA

See also Polyuria in Chapter 6.

DEFINITIONS

- Urinary frequency: Urination occurring at less than 2-h intervals, associated with subjective complaint of urinating too frequently. The volume of urine excreted is normal or diminished.
- Polyuria: Excreting large volumes of urine (>2 mL/kg/h).

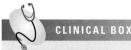

CLINICAL BOX

Causes of Polyuria

1. Water diuresis
   a. Excessive intake
   b. Excessive loss—DB insipidus
2. Osmotic diuresis
   a. Sugar—DB mellitus
   b. Urea—chronic renal disease
   c. Salts, organic anions

APPROACH

See Table 21.7.

CLINICAL BOX

Labs for Polyuria

Urinalysis: to differentiate between water and osmotic diuresis.

Dehydration test: to distinguish between nephrogenic and central DB insipidus (fasting glycemia).

Table **21.7**	Frequency versus Polyuria			
Problem		**Mechanism**	**Cause**	**Associated Symptoms**
Frequency	↓ Capacity of bladder	↑ Bladder sensitivity to stretch because of inflammation	Infection, stones, tumor, foreign body in bladder	Burning on urination, urinary urgency, sometimes gross hematuria
		↓ Elasticity of the bladder wall	Infiltration by scar tissue or tumor	
		↓ Cortical inhibition of bladder contractions	Motor disorders of the CNS, such as a stroke	Urgency; neurologic symptoms such as weakness or paralysis
	Impaired emptying of bladder, with residual urine in the bladder	Partial mechanical obstruction of the bladder neck or proximal urethra	Most commonly BPH; also urethral stricture and other obstructive lesions of the bladder or prostate	Prior obstructive symptoms: hesitancy in starting urinary stream, straining to void, reduced size and force of the stream, and dribbling during or at the end of urination
		Loss of peripheral nerve supply to the bladder	Neurologic disease affecting the sacral nerves or nerve roots, e.g, diabetic neuropathy	Weakness or sensory defects
Polyuria	Deficiency of ADH	Central DB insipidus	A disorder of the posterior hypothalamus	Thirst and polydipsia, often severe and persistent; nocturia
	Renal unresponsiveness to ADH	Nephrogenic DB insipidus	A number of kidney diseases, including hypercalcemic and hypokalemic nephropathy; drug toxicity, e.g., from lithium	
	Solute diuresis	Electrolytes, such as sodium salts	Large saline infusions, potent diuretics, certain kidney diseases	Variable
		Nonelectrolytes, such as glucose	Uncontrolled DB mellitus	Thirst, polydipsia, and nocturia
	Excessive water intake		Primary polydypsia	Polydipsia tends to be episodic Thirst may not be present Nocturia is usually absent

(Adapted with permission from Bickley LS, Szilagyi PG, Stackhouse JG, eds. *Bates' Guide to Physical Exam and History taking*, 8th ed. Philadelphia: Lippincott Williams & Wilkins; 2002.)

 CLINICAL BOX

Detrusor versus Outlet

Always consider UI as an imbalance between the relationship of the bladder and the outlet.

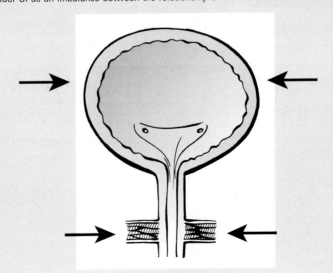

URINARY INCONTINENCE

See UI in Chapter 14.

RATIONALE

UI is the involuntary loss of urine. It may occasionally be related to serious disease, and often causes significant psychosocial impairment.

CAUSAL CONDITIONS

CLINICAL BOX

Neurogenic Bladder

Neurologic lesions to consider with neurogenic bladder

- MS
- Trauma (including iatrogenic)
- Stroke
- DB mellitus
- Other

CLINICAL BOX

Transient Causes of Incontinence: DIAPPERS

- **D**elirium
- **I**nfection
- **A**trophic urethritis or vaginitis
- **P**harmaceuticals (drugs)
- **P**sychogenic
- **E**xcessive urine output
- **R**estricted mobility
- **S**tool impaction

Table **21.8**	Classification, Pathophysiology, and Causal Conditions of UI			
Classification				
Wein	**Clinical**	**Mechanism**	**Pathophysiology and Associated Causes**	

Failure to store	**Urgency**	Bladder overactive (detrusor contracts without inhibition)	1. Irritation of bladder
			  a. Infection, stone, cancer, etc.
			2. Hyperreflexia (neurogenic bladder)
			  a. By definition, always related to neurologic defect
			    i. Trauma/surgery
			    ii. Congenital
			3. Other
			  a. Iatrogenic
			  b. Idiopathic (bladder instability): by definition, not related to neurologic defect	

	Stress	Insufficient outlet pressure	1. Lack of support from pelvic floor
			  a. **Multiple vaginal deliveries**
			  b. Iatrogenic
			    i. **Gynecologic surgery**
			    ii. Prostatectomy
			    iii. Pelvic irradiation
			2. Neurologic lesion
			  a. Thoracolumbar spine (Σ)
			    i. Affects inner sphincter (smooth muscle), therefore, UI mostly at night
			  b. Peripheral nerve (pudendal)
			    i. Radical prostatectomy	

Failure to empty	**Overflow**	Bladder underactive (detrusor atony)	1. Neurologic lesion (trauma or other)
			  a. Sacral region of spine (S2-5)
			  b. Peripheral nerves (pudendal or pelvic nerve)
			2. Congenital defect
			  a. Spina bifida	

		Outlet obstruction (mechanical hindrance of flow)	1. Extrinsic obstruction
			  a. **BPH**
			  b. Advance prostate cancer
			2. Intrinsic obstruction
			  a. **Urethral stenosis**
			    i. Transurethral surgery
			    ii. Postinfectious (STD)
			3. Congenital
			  a. PUV (boys)	

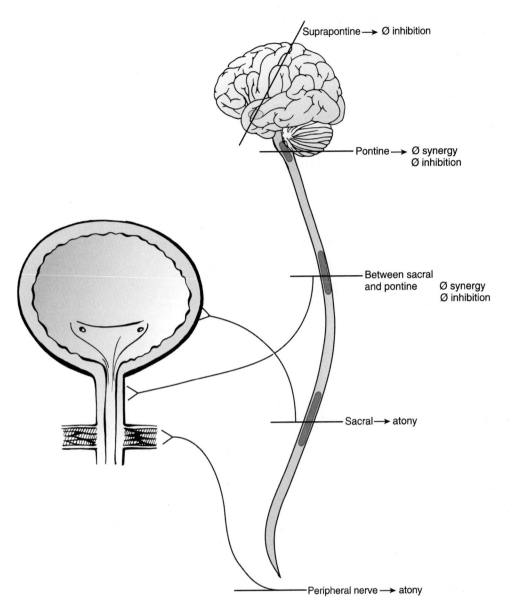

Suprapontine → Ø inhibition

Pontine → Ø synergy
Ø inhibition

Between sacral
and pontine   Ø synergy
Ø inhibition

Sacral → atony

Peripheral nerve → atony

Figure 21.2 Bladder/sphincter innervation and dysfunction.

Table **21.9**	**Stress versus Urgency UI**	
	Stress Incontinence	**Urgency Incontinence**
Definition	Involuntary urine leakage with efforts such as coughing, sneezing, laughing, lifting, etc.	Involuntary urine leakage accompanied by a pressing need to urinate (urgency)
Pathophysiology	An ↑ in abdominal pressure (effort) is transmitted more to the bladder, than it is to the urethra (because of anatomic abnormality of the pelvic floor, which has become unable to adequately support the urethra)	Uninhibited (involuntary) bladder contractions that cause a rise in intravesical pressure, which, when higher than urethral resistance, will cause leakage
Most common causes	• Multiple vaginal deliveries • Vaginal and paraurethral atrophy after menopause. • Postpartum pelvic floor repair	• Cystitis, urethritis • Vesical polyps, carcinoma, calculi • Psychogenic • Stroke, dementia, parkinsonism
Treatment	• Pelvic floor exercises • Pessaries and surgery	• Bladder retraining • Pelvic floor exercises • Anticholinergics

APPROACH

Tx

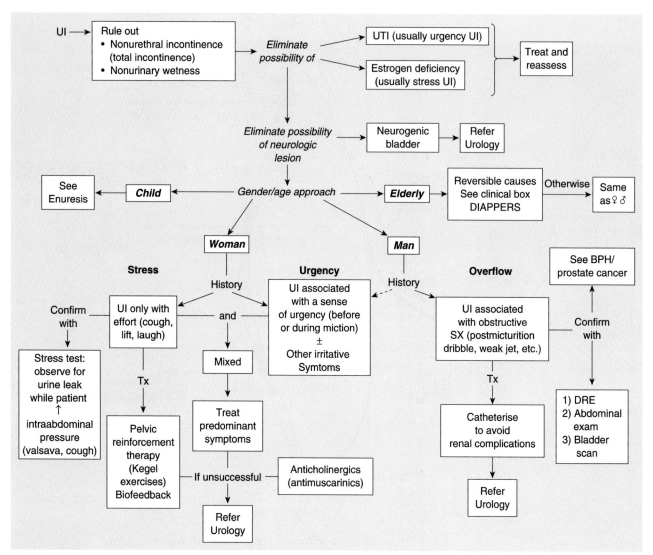

Figure 21.3 Approach to UI.

CLINICAL BOX

Important Aspects of the Physical Exam
- Abdominal
  - Sign of overdistended bladder; measure postvoid residual (use BladderScan)
- DRE
  - Anal sphincter tone
  - Size, consistency, and symmetry of prostate
- Pelvic
  - Speculum: look for fistulae, prolapse, vaginal mucosal atrophy
- Neurologic
  - R/O serious CNS disease (MS) or peripheral nerve disease (DB, trauma)
  - Bulbocavernous reflex (if absent, signals pathology between S2-4. Absent in 2% of men and 30% of women)

Table **21.10**	Tx of UI
Stress UI	1. Kegel exercises 2. Pessaires 3. Surgical correction
Urgency UI	1. Treat underlying cause (infection, cancer) 2. Bladder training 3. Anticholinergics (oxybutynin, tolterodine)
Overflow	1. Immediate catheterization to avoid complications 2. Treat underlying cause (obstructive/neurologic)

URINARY OBSTRUCTION

CLINICAL BOX

Renal Insufficiency

When patients present with renal insufficiency differentiate an obstructive from a nonobstructive acute renal insufficiency.

RATIONALE

- Classification of urinary obstruction
  - Acute or chronic
  - Complete or partial
  - Unilateral (usually upper tract) or bilateral (usually lower tract)
  - Site
- The presentation and the consequences of urinary obstruction depend on its nature and location.

CAUSAL CONDITIONS

CLINICAL BOX

Urinary Obstruction and Renal Function

Although unilateral urinary obstructions have repercussions on the same side collecting system and kidney, global renal function stays normal as long as the other kidney and urinary tract are normal.

Table **21.11**	Causes of Urinary Obstruction	
Child	Urethra	• Posterior urethral valve • Meatus stenosis • Stricture • Phimosis
	Junctions	• Megaureter • UPJ obstruction
Adult	Urethra Bladder Upper urinary tract	• Post-STD stenosis • Calculi • Calculi • Pregnancy
Elderly	Lower urinary tract	• Postinstrumentation scarring (stricture) • Prostatic (BPH/cancer) • Calculi • Vesical tumor involving the bladder neck or ureteral orifices • Local extension of prostate or cervix cancer occluding ureteral orifices
	Upper urinary tract	• Pelvic lymph nodes • Retroperitoneal fibrosis or tumor

ASC Box

Hypertension

- Hypertension due to unilateral obstruction is secondary to systemic vasoconstriction resulting from activation of renin-angiotensin.
- Hypertension due to bilateral obstruction is secondary to volume expansion.

APPROACH

Table **21.12**	**Signs and Symptoms of Urinary Obstruction**	
Urinary Tract	**Symptoms**	**Signs**

Lower tract	• Voiding LUTS
	  • Hesitancy
	  • ↓ Force and caliber of stream
	  • Terminal dribbling
	  • Suprapubic pain
	• Hematuria
	• Acute urinary retention
		• Hypertension
		• Palpable bladder
		• Palpable stricture of the urethra
		• DRE
		  • Atony of anal sphincter
		  • Benign or malignant enlargement of prostate

Upper tract	• Flank colicky pain and radiation • Gross total hematuria • GI symptoms (nausea/vomiting) • Fever/chills	• Hypertension • Palpable enlarged kidney (HN) • Pelvic mass • Renal tenderness

ASC Box

Acute versus Chronic Obstruction

- Acute obstruction of the urinary tract does not result in HN due to a relative noncompliance of the collecting system. Therefore, the obstruction causes an elevation of pressure within the collecting system resulting in pain.
- Owing to its gradual process, chronic obstruction presents with HN and relatively no pain.

INVESTIGATIONS

- Urinalysis, urine culture, CBC, serum creatinine, BUN, electrolytes, blood glucose, ±PSA

CLINICAL BOX

DDx of Elevated PSA
- BPH
- Prostate cancer
- Prostatitis
- Acute urinary retention
- DRE/prostate biopsy/TRUS
- Cystoscopy/catheterization
- Ejaculation

Table **21.13**	**Investigations for Urinary Obstruction Based on Signs and Symptoms**
Lower Urinary Tract Assessment (Patients with LUTS)	**Upper Urinary Tract Assessment (Patients without LUTS)**

• Bladder scan/urinary catheter
• Retrograde urethrogram
• Cystoscopy
• Urodynamics study
	• Ultrasound
	  • If patient presents with renal insufficiency, hematuria, recurrent UTI, prior urinary tract surgery, and history of urinary stones
	  • Assessment of HN, bladder residual, and prostate volume
	• CT scan
	• IVP

SPECIAL CONSIDERATIONS

RENAL COLIC

Also see Urolithiasis in Hematuria.

- Clinical presentation according to stone location in renal colic.
- Three typical locations:
  1. Infundibulum or ureteropyelic stone: flank pain
  2. Mid ureteral stone (at the crossing of the iliac vessels): groin pain and RLQ pain (DDx appendicitis, ectopic pregnancy)
  3. Low ureteral stone (at the ureterovesical junction): flank pain, scrotal pain (or at labia majora) and irritative urinary syndrome (urgency, burning, frequency)

Location of Renal Colic

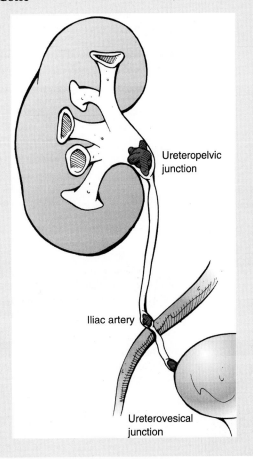

Ureteropelvic junction

Iliac artery

Ureterovesical junction

Fever and kidney stone

- Urinary obstruction with septic state (acute pyelonephritis) is a **urologic emergency.**
- Urine flow must be restored to prevent septicemia and pyonephrosis which may lead to chronic renal failure or death (percutaneous nephrostomy or ureteral catheter).

INVESTIGATION

- Mandatory lab tests
  - Urinalysis: hematuria almost always present, if absent (15%) reconsider diagnosis
  - WBC
  - Serum creatinine
- Imaging
  - IVP
  - Uroscan (no contrast and identifies other causes of abdominal pain)

Acute Tx

- Conservative
- Calculus <4 mm has a 90% chance of passing spontaneously versus <10% for a 1 cm stone
  - NSAID
  - Flomax (α_1-adrenergic blocker)—controversial
  - Analgesics
  - Hydration (>2 L/d)
- Surgical—Urology referral
  - Presence of infection or nonprogression (usually 2 wk depending on size, localization, symptoms, and social factors such as airplane pilots or travelers)
  - Extracorporeal lithotripsy, ureteroscopic stone extraction, and percutaneous nephrolithotomy

BPH AND PROSTATE CANCER

PSA versus DRE for Prostate Cancer

PSA testing is more sensitive than DRE for the detection of prostate cancer. PSA screening detects a large majority of prostate cancers; however, a significant percentage of early prostate cancers (10%–20%) will be missed by PSA testing alone.

Table **21.14**	**BPH versus Prostate Cancer**	
	BPH	**CaP**
Epidemiology	At autopsy 20% at age 45 50% at age 55 80% at age 80	Latent CaP 40% Clinical CaP 10% Death from CaP 3%
Risk factors	Family history	Old age/black men/cigarette smoking
Pathology	Hyperplasia of transition zone (100%)	Adenocarcinoma (95%): • Peripheral zone (60%–70%) • Transition zone (10%–20%) • Central zone (5%–10%) TCC (4%)

Clinical presentation	• Asymptomatic
	• LUTS (50% at 75):
	  • Obstructive (mechanical)
	  • Irritative (from detrusor hypertrophy and hyperplasia)
		• Asymptomatic
		• LUTS (locally advanced disease)
		• Bone pain (metastasis—osteoblastic lesions)

Physical Exam	DRE (see below)	DRE (induration)
Labs	• Urinalysis (R/O hematuria and infection) • Serum creatinine (10% of BPH present with renal failure) • PSA (controversial)	PSA
Investigation	• **None** needed • Cystoscopy if considering surgery • Upper tract imagining if complications present (hematuria, infection, stones, RI)	• TRUS • TRUS-guided needle biopsy • Bone scan (if PSA >10–20 ng/mL)
Treatment	**Medical** • α-Blockers • 5α-Reductase inhibitors **Surgical** • TURP • Other minimally invasive—open simple prostatectomy	According to staging **Local** • Radical prostatectomy • Radiation therapy **Metastasis** • Hormonal therapy
Prognosis	If moderately to severely symptomatic and no treatment initiated, risk of developing urinary retention ↑	Highly variable. Natural history is poorly understood Obviously some staging correlation exists

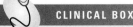

Coronal View of Normal Prostate and BPH

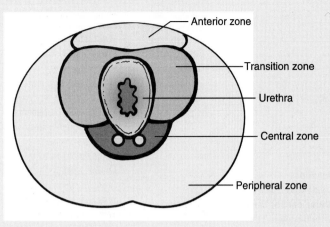

Gleason Score

Gleason score grades histological findings in prostate pathology. Most important assessment with staging for prognosis.

- 6 = Highly differentiated
- 7 = Moderately differentiated
- 8–10 = Poorly differentiated

Prostate Cancer Screening
- The USPSTF concludes that the evidence is insufficient to recommend for or against routine screening for prostate cancer using PSA testing or DRE. (I recommendation.)
- The USPSTF found good evidence that PSA screening can detect early-stage prostate cancer, but mixed and inconclusive evidence that early detection improves health outcomes.
- Screening must be discussed with patients individually. Physicians should explain the invasiveness of the investigations following an abnormal PSA and the possibility of complications, as well as the possibility of false-negative results. Furthermore, physicians should inform patients that a positive result may lead to treatment that may or may not improve their life expectancy.

SCROTAL MASS

Testicular Cancer Risk Factors
- Cryptorchidism (up to 14-fold)
- Testicular atrophy
- Testicular dysgenesis
- Caucasian (five whites for one black)

RATIONALE
- Although scrotal masses refer to various conditions, the words "scrotal mass" imply directly testicular cancer. Whereas it is relatively uncommon when all age groups are considered (only 1.1% of malignant tumors in Canadian men), it is the most common malignancy of the young men (age 24–34).
- Recent advances in management have resulted in dramatic improvement in survival rate (approximately 95% survival).

CAUSAL CONDITIONS
See Table 21.15.

APPROACH

History of a Scrotal Mass
- Past history
  - Undescended testicle/cryptorchidism
  - Infertility
  - Previous testicular tumor
- Present illness
  - Trauma
  - Change in scrotal size
  - Difficulty voiding
  - Breast tenderness

Scrotal Mass Differentiation
- Intratesticular and extratesticular
- Solid and cystic (transillumination)
- Painless and painful

Table **21.15**	DDx of Scrotal Mass		
System/Region	**Etiology**	**Pain**	**Transillumination**
Inguinal	Inguinoscrotal hernia	−(+ if strangulated)	−
Scrotum/testis **Cystic/soft solid**	Hydrocele	−	+
	Epididymal cyst (spermatocele)	−	+
	Varicocele	−	−
	Hematocele (trauma)	+	−
	Torsion	+++	−
	Idiopathic scrotal edema	−	+
	Testicular malignancy	−(+ if hemorrhage into the tumor)	−
	Acute epididymitis	++	−
	Chronic epididymitis	+	−
	Granulomatous orchitis/ testicular abscess	+	−
	Testicular rupture (trauma)	+++	−

+, present and −, not present.

R

Intratesticular Mass
An intratesticular mass is considered **testicular cancer** until proved otherwise (< 5% of testicular mass are benign).

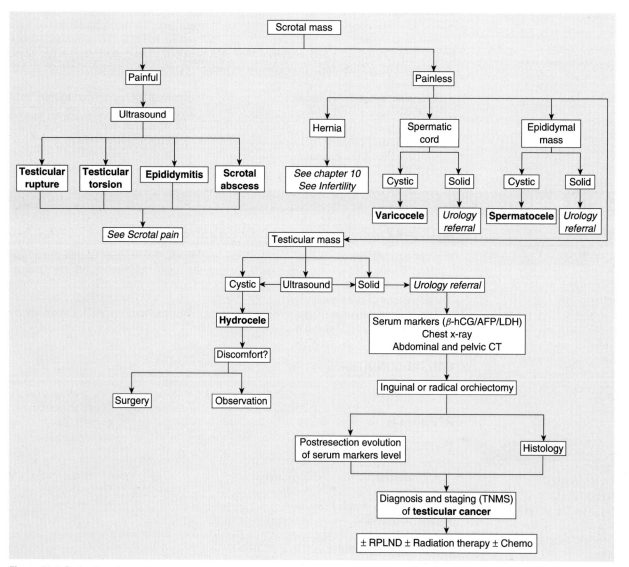

Figure 21.4 Evaluation of scrotal mass.

Invasive Procedures
Trans-scrotal biopsy and hydrocele needle aspiration should be avoided due to the risk of cancer seeding.

Testicular cancer is often misdiagnosed for other testicular pathologies (mainly epididymitis, hydrocele, and testicular trauma). Awareness of the physician is mandatory.

SCROTAL EXAM

- To examine a scrotum, palpating and identifying the intrascrotal contents is key.
  - Testicle and epididymis (located posteriorly and superiorly to the testicle)
  - Spermatic cord (standing position allows searching for a varicocele)
  - External inguinal ring (standing with a Valsalva)
  - Prostate (rectal exam)
- If testicular cancer is suspected
  - Abdomen including inguinal lymph nodes
  - Chest
    - Gynecomastia
    - Supraclavicular node (See Figure 21.4)

CLINICAL BOX

Testicular Cancer Screening

The Canadian Task Force on preventive health care considers the data insufficient to recommend for or against routine screening or self-examination (C recommendation).

USPSTF recommends against routine screening for testicular cancer in asymptomatic adolescent and adult males. (D recommendation)

Table 21.16 Painless Scrotal Mass other Than Testicular Cancer

Scrotal Mass	Definition	Etiologies	Clinical Presentation	Investigation	Treatment
Hydrocele	Collection of fluid between the layers of the tunica vaginalis	Idiopathic reactive • Tumor • Epididymitis/orchitis • Trauma	• Painless scrotal mass • Swelling may ↑ during the day • May present as a cord hydrocele • Testis not always palpable	**Ultrasound** if unsure diagnosis or risk factors for testicular cancer	Surgical repair if symptomatic or testicular atrophy
Communicating hydrocele	Incomplete obliteration of the processus vaginalis allowing peritoneal fluid to pass.	Congenital	• Usually self-resolves before the first year of life • May be associated to an indirect hernia	Not necessary	No therapy before 1 yr of age; surgical correction if inguinal hernia
Spermatocele/epididymal cyst	• Sperm filled collection of the epididymis • Spermatozoids may be present	Idiopathic Associated with von-Hippel–Lindau disease	Painless smooth and round scrotal mass located superior to the testis	Not necessary	Surgical excision if symptomatic
Chronic epididymitis	Persistent or recurrent infection of the epididymis	Recurrent UTI mostly associated with urethral stricture	Tender, indurated epididymis associated with an infected semen	• No puncture in men desiring fertility	Conservative (Abx, NSAID, sitz baths) versus total epididymectomy
Varicocele	Dilated and tortuous veins of the pampiniform plexus of the spermatic cord	Primary Secondary: • Renal tumor (left) • Vena cava obstruction (right) • Retroperitoneal fibrosis	• Painless "bag of worms" • 90% left-sided • Accidental discovery • Infertility investigation • *Assess testicular volume*	• Not necessary • Semen analyses if infertility	Surgical ligation if testicular atrophy or infertility

Varicocele

- A right-sided varicocele or a persistent varicocele after dorsal decubitus should prompt an evaluation of the retroperitoneum.
- R/O malignancy.

CLINICAL BOX

Ultrasound Imaging

When testis exam is impossible to due to a large hydrocele, an ultrasound should be done to R/O testicular cancer.

CLINICAL BOX

Torsion of the Testicular Appendix

Although the clinical presentation is similar to testicular torsion of the cord, it presents no danger to the testis. Classic sign is the "blue dot sign," which consists of the infracted appendix. Self-resolves.

CLINICAL BOX

Cremasteric Reflex

Cremasteric reflex consists of the rapid elevation of the ipsilateral testis created by gently scratching the inner superior thigh with a stick.

SPECIFIC CONSIDERATIONS

TESTICULAR CANCER

- Classification
  - Germ cell tumors: seminoma/embryonal cell carcinoma/teratoma/choriocarcinoma/mixed
  - Non–germ cell tumors: Leydig cell tumor/lymphoma
- Clinical presentation
  - Painless lump 50%
  - Diffuse pain with swelling and hardening of scrotum 30%
  - Acute pain 10%
  - Systemic involvement 10%
- Associated signs
  - Reactive hydrocele 10%
  - Gynecomastia 5%
- Lymphatic spread
  - If tumor confined to the testis = retroperitoneal nodes
  - If tumor locally spreads to epididymitis or cord = pelvic and inguinal nodes
- Most frequent metastasis occurs to the lung, liver, bones (blastic lesions), and kidneys

SCROTAL PAIN

RATIONALE

Only a few true urologic emergencies exist, of which testicular torsion present with scrotal pain. Consequences may be serious. Therefore, quickly identifying testicular torsion and distinguishing it from other conditions causing scrotal pain (e.g., acute epididymitis) is important.

CAUSAL CONDITIONS

Table **21.17**	**DDx of the Acute Scrotum**
Testis	Orchitis
	Hemorrhage into testicular tumor
	Testicular rupture (trauma)
Testicular appendix	Torsion of testicular appendix
Epididymis	Acute epididymitis
Spermatic cord	Testicular torsion
Tunica vaginalis	Hematocele (trauma)
Inguinal	Incarcerated/strangulated inguinal hernia

APPLIED SCIENTIFIC CONCEPTS

See Figure 21.5.

APPROACH

Tx

- Ultrasound versus radionuclide imaging
  - Color Doppler ultrasound exam is the imaging method of choice for the evaluation of the acute scrotum: it allows to assess anatomy as well as the blood flow to the testis.

- Natural history of testicular torsion
  - Irreversible ischemic injury to the testis may begin as soon as 4 h after occlusion of the cord. If vascular supply is reestablished within 4–8 h, slight changes will appear on sperm analyses. If it is reestablished after **8 h**, there is a significant risk of testicular atrophy.

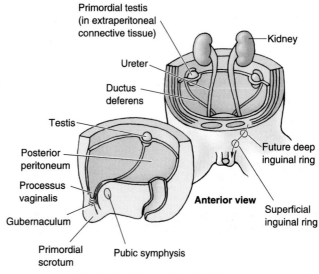

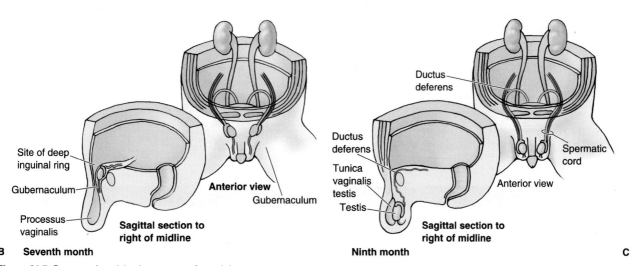

Figure 21.5 Descent of testicles into scrotum from abdomen.

CLINICAL BOX

Manual Detorsion

The examiner should try to twist or "unscrew" the testis (outward, toward the thigh). Manual detorsion may not totally correct the rotation that has occurred, and prompt exploration is still indicated.

Table **21.18**   **Testicular Torsion versus Acute Epididymitis**

	Testicular Torsion	Acute Epididymitis	
Epidemiology	1/4,000 Mostly preadolescent boys	Sexually active <35 yr	>35 yr Urinary catheter
Risk factors	Cryptorchidism Congenital anomaly	Behavioral risk for STD	Bacteriuria Urethra stricture
Etiology	Idiopathic	*Chlamydia* or *gonorrhea*	*E. coli* and other gram-negative
Clinical presentation	Acute onset of pain (minutes) Possible previous self-resolving episodes of scrotal pain	Gradual onset of scrotal pain and swelling (hours) Urethral discharge may be present History of sexual exposure	
Physical exam	• Absence of cremasteric reflex • Bell-clapper deformity (testis long axis is transverse from shortening of spermatic cord from torsion)	• Presence of cremasteric reflex • Prehn sign (pain relived with elevation of testicule) • Epididymis swelling	
Labs	Not useful	• Gram stained urethral smear • Gram stain of a midstream urine specimen	
Radiology	• Radionuclide scanning • Color duplex Doppler ultrasonography	Ultrasound (±Doppler to R/O testicular torsion)	

Treatment	• Manual detorsion
	• Surgical exploration is mandatory
	  • Restores vascular supply and
	  • Bilateral orchiopexy is performed to prevent further episodes
		For epididymitis secondary to STD
		• Ceftriaxone, 250 mg IM × 1
		• Tetracycline, 500 mg PO q.i.d. × 10 d
		• Doxycycline, 100 mg PO b.i.d. × 10 d
		• Evaluate partners
			For epididymitis secondary to bacteriuria
			• Promptly administer broad-spectrum antimicrobial agent
			• (e.g., TMP–SMX, quinolone)
			• Investigate causes of bacteriuria

Complication	• Testicular atrophy • Infertility	• Testicular atrophy • Infertility • Scrotal abscess • Chronic epididymitis	

MALE INFERTILITY

For female infertility see Chapter 14.

RATIONALE

- Infertility is defined as the inability to conceive after **1 yr** of intercourse without contraception. It affects approximately 15% of couples.
- Both partners must be investigated: a male factor is solely responsible for approximately 20% of infertility problems whereas male and female factors are involved in 30%–40%.

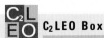 **C₂LEO Box**

Ethics

Infertility is a "couple" issue that demands nonjudgmental discussion by the physician on the evolving ethical issues surrounding advanced reproductive technologies. If certain issues are outside the physician's personal moral bounds, the infertile couple should be referred to another physician.

APPLIED SCIENTIFIC CONCEPTS

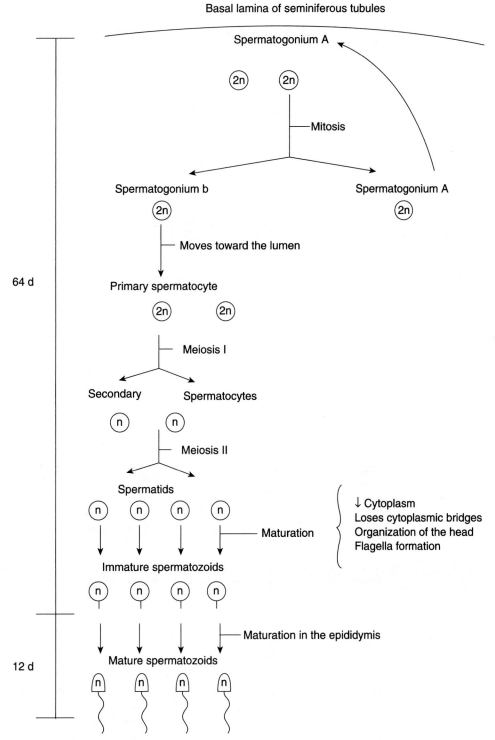

Figure 21.6 Spermatogenesis.

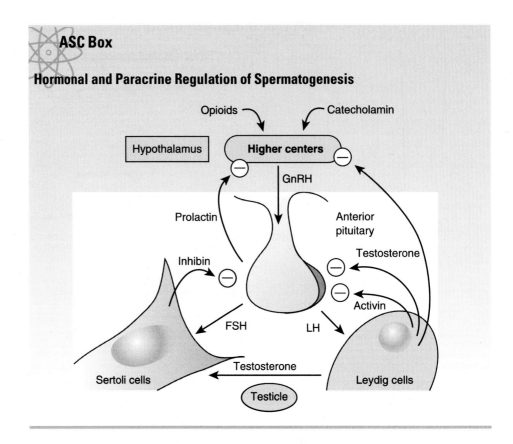

ASC Box

Hormonal and Paracrine Regulation of Spermatogenesis

CAUSAL CONDITIONS

Male infertility may occasionally be the presenting manifestation of an underlying life-threatening condition such as testicular cancer and pituitary tumors.

CLINICAL BOX

Correctable Causes of Male Infertility

Varicocele is the most common cause of male infertility. Approximately 40% of male seen for infertility have a varicocele.

More than 50% will have an improvement of their semen analysis after varicocelectomy.

Table **21.19**	**DDx of Male Infertility**	
Pretesticular	*Hypothalamic disease*	Gonadotropin deficiency (Kallmann syndrome)
		Congenital hypogonadotropic syndromes
	Pituitary disease	Pituitary insufficiency
		Hyperprolactinemia
		Endogenous/exogenous hormones
Testicular	Chromosomal (e.g., Klinefelter syndrome [XXY], microdeletion)	
	Cryptorchidism	
	Testicular injury	
	Viral orchitis	
	Varicocele	
	Radiation	
	Drugs (e.g., ROH/lithium/α blockers/tricyclic/CCB/steroid)	
Posttesticular	*Obstruction*	Congenital (e.g., CF)
		Acquired (e.g., vasectomy/groin surgery/infection)
		Functional (e.g., nerve injury/drugs)
	Sperm motility or function	Immotile cilia
		Maturation defects
		Immunologic infertility
		Infection
	Disorders of the coitus	Impotence
		Hypospadias
		Timing and frequency

APPROACH

Table **21.20** History and Physical Exam	
History	**Exam**
Medical history	***Genital***
Genetic disease	Testis <4 cm Testicular mass
Cryptorchidism	Varicocele
History of torsion	Absent *vas deferens*
Reproductive history	Hypospadias
Sexual history (STDs)	***Other***
Systemic diseases (eg., DB)	Prostate pain or mass (DRE)
Prior surgeries	Abnormal hair distribution
Habits	Gynecomastia
Drugs/cigarettes/toxic exposure	
Hot bath/truckers	
History	
Coital frequency and timing	
↓ Libido	
Difficult erection	
Blood or pain with ejaculation	
Absent ejaculation	
Use of lubricants	

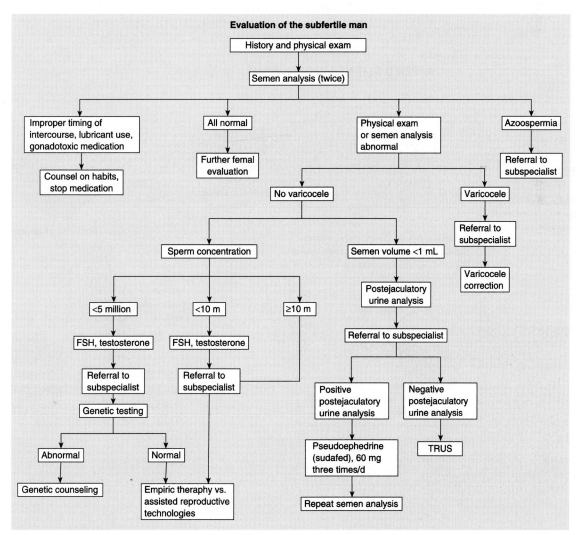

Figure 21.7 Evaluation of subfertile male. (Image reproduced with permission from Kolettis PN. Evaluation of the subfertile man. *Am Fam Physician.* 2003;67(10):2170.)

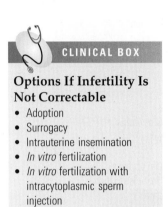

Options If Infertility Is Not Correctable
- Adoption
- Surrogacy
- Intrauterine insemination
- *In vitro* fertilization
- *In vitro* fertilization with intracytoplasmic sperm injection

Table **21.21**	Semen Analysis (WHO Strict Criteria)
Characteristics	**Reference Values**
Ejaculate volume	>1.5 mL
pH	>7.2
Sperm concentration	$>20 \times 10^6$/mL
Total sperm count	$>40 \times 10^6$/ejaculate
Motility	>50% grade A or B or >25% with progressive motility within 60 min of ejaculation
Morphology	>14% normal
White blood cells	$<1 \times 10^6$/mL

IMPOTENCE/ERECTILE DYSFUNCTION

RATIONALE

- ED is the inability of the male to achieve and/or maintain penile erection and thereby engage in copulation;
- Impotence: ED experienced 75% of the time.
- ED/impotence may be a manifestation of serious disease (vascular, neurologic, psychological).

APPLIED SCIENTIFIC CONCEPTS

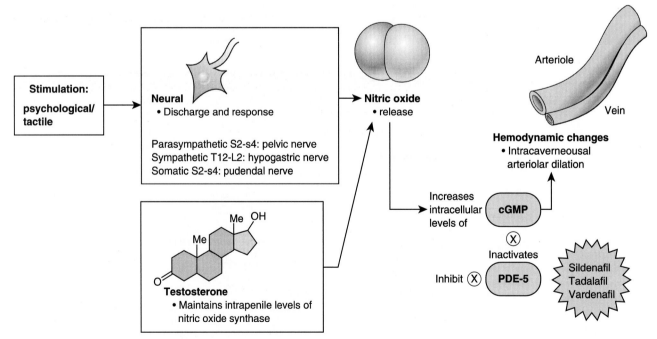

Figure 21.8 Physiology of erection and site of action of major drugs.

CLINICAL BOX

Mnemonic of Causal Condition of ED: IMPOTENCE

Inflammatory: prostatitis, urethritis, stricture
Mechanical: chordee, Peyronie disease, phimosis
Postoperative: iatrogenic (radical prostatectomy)
Occlusive: arteriogenic
Traumatic: pelvic fracture, urethral rupture
Endurance: cardiovascular diseases
Neurologic: neuropathy, temporal lobe epilepsy, MS
Chemical: ROH, marijuana, prescription drugs (e.g., SSRIs, β-blockers, thiazides, hormone modulators, 5α-reductase inhibitors)
Endocrine: Testicular failure, pituitary failure, hyperprolactinemia; **DB** (through vaso-occlusive, neurologic, and psychological factors—very common) (see Chapter 6)

APPROACH

- It is capital to consider the psychological component of ED, both in the assessment of the condition and in the management of the patient.
- History
  1. R/O psychogenic ED through the history (persistence of night erections, emotional stress, performance anxiety).
  2. Be alert to risk factors of cardiovascular disease and DB: Smoking, obesity, alcoholism, genetic predisposition, and so on.
  3. Rarer causes of ED should equally be considered:
     a. Testosterone deficiency (hypogonadism, testicular failure)
     b. Hyperprolactinemia
- The physical exam should include a thorough neurologic exam including the bulbocavernous reflex.
- Labs (according to the WHO) should include fasting glycemia, HbA1c, lipid profile, and total testosterone.

CLINICAL BOX

Specific PDE 5 Inhibitors

(Sildenafil, Tadalafil, Vardenafil)

Mechanism of action

PDE5 inhibitor → ↑ cGMP → ↑ smooth muscle relaxation → ↑ erection (see Figure)

Counter indications

- Absolute
  - Patients using nitrates (e.g., nitroglycerine for CAD)
- Relative
  - Very low blood pressure (borderline)
  - Liver or renal insufficiency
  - Patients using drugs that inhibit cytochrome P450

Adverse effects

Headache, facial flushing, nasal congestion, altered vision, and dyspepsia.

TX

1. Addressing the psychological component and patient counseling and education should be the first step of management in all patients.

2. Pharmacotherapy: drugs used to treat ED
   i. PDE5 inhibitors.
   ii. Intracavernous injections (smooth muscle relaxants and vasodilators) should only be used after evaluation by an urologist.
   iii. Androgen replacement is only appropriate for patients with documented androgen deficiency (e.g., hypogonadism).
3. Vacuum devices.

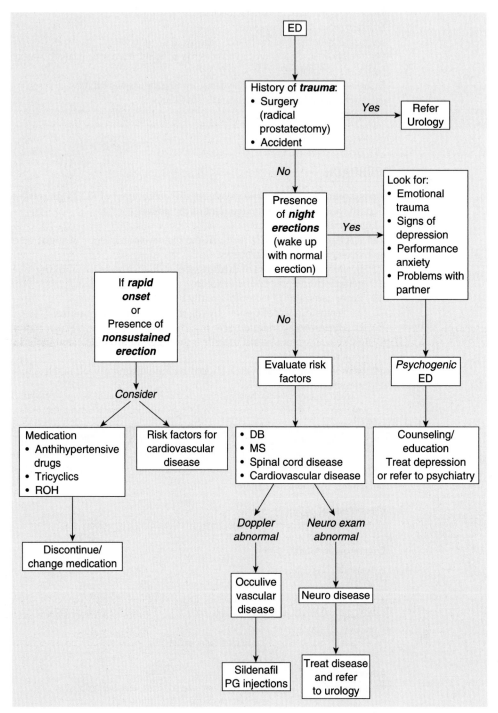

Figure 21.9 Tx of ED.

PRIAPISM

See Table 21.22.

Table **21.22**	Classification of Priapism	
Priapism	**Ischemic *Low-Flow***	**Nonischemic *High-Flow***
Pathophysiology	Venous congestion and enhanced blood viscosity	Excessive arterial inflow to the penis
Associated conditions	Sickle cell disease Vasoactive drugs Neoplasic disease Spinal cord injury	Trauma Vasoactive drugs Penile surgery Neurologic conditions
Features	Painful corpora Rigid erection Tender penis	Nonpainful corpora Tumescence Nontender penis
Diagnostic		
Blood from the Corpus Cavernosum	Dark blood (Po_2 <30, Pco_2 >60 and pH <7.25)	Red blood (Po_2 >90, Pco_2 <40 and pH <7.40)
Color Doppler	Minimal or absent blood flow	Normal or high blood flow

Treatment (>4 h)	1. Needle aspiration
	   Intracavernous injection of an
	   α-adrenergic agent
	2. If >48–72 h, surgical shunting
		Observation (62% of spontenous resolution)
		Selective arterial embolization
		Surgical

ED	Frequent	Less common

ENURESIS

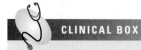

CLINICAL BOX

Classification of Enuresis

- Diurnal or nocturnal
- Primary (never been consistently dry at night) or secondary (resume wetting after 6 mo of continence/dryness)

RATIONALE

- Enuresis is the repeated voiding of urine into a child's clothes or bed after the developmental (not necessarily chronologic) age of **5 yr old**. It must either occur twice a week during a 3-mo period or it must cause significant distress and impairment (according to the DSM).
- Although most children with enuresis will have no apparent organic cause, a screening is necessary to R/O neurologic or anatomic disease, or developmental deficits.

APPLIED SCIENTIFIC CONCEPTS

See Figure 21.10.

CAUSAL CONDITIONS

Table **21.23**	Causal Conditions of Enuresis	
Classification		**Common Causes**
Primary	Nocturnal	• Idiopathic • Familial • Bladder dyssynergia
	Diurnal + nocturnal	• Anatomic abnormality • Neurologic disorder developmental conditions • Bladder dysfunction
Secondary	Nocturnal Diurnal + nocturnal	• Psychogenic/stress • UTIs • DB mellitus, DB insipidus

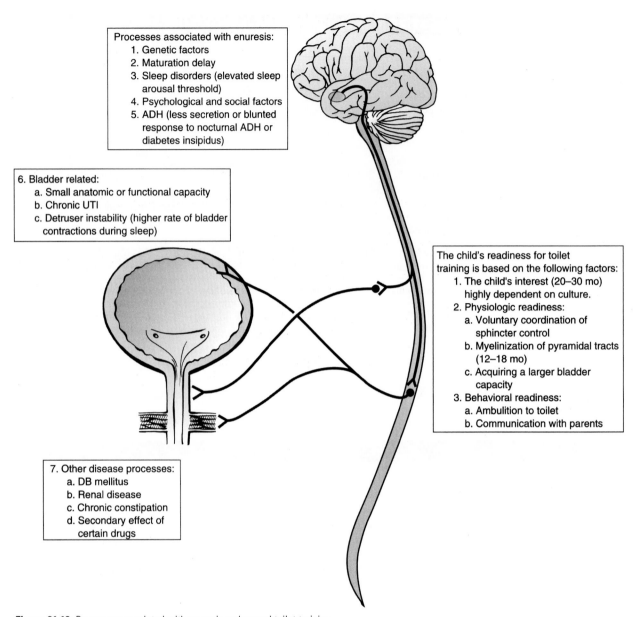

Processes associated with enuresis:
1. Genetic factors
2. Maturation delay
3. Sleep disorders (elevated sleep arousal threshold)
4. Psychological and social factors
5. ADH (less secretion or blunted response to nocturnal ADH or diabetes insipidus)

6. Bladder related:
   a. Small anatomic or functional capacity
   b. Chronic UTI
   c. Detruser instability (higher rate of bladder contractions during sleep)

The child's readiness for toilet training is based on the following factors:
1. The child's interest (20–30 mo) highly dependent on culture.
2. Physiologic readiness:
   a. Voluntary coordination of sphincter control
   b. Myelinization of pyramidal tracts (12–18 mo)
   c. Acquiring a larger bladder capacity
3. Behavioral readiness:
   a. Ambulition to toilet
   b. Communication with parents

7. Other disease processes:
   a. DB mellitus
   b. Renal disease
   c. Chronic constipation
   d. Secondary effect of certain drugs

Figure 21.10 Processes associated with enuresis and normal toilet training.

APPROACH

HISTORY

1. Family history of enuresis
2. Stressful conditions and contributory psychosocial factors (moving of the family, divorce/death in the family, birth of a sibling, etc.)
3. Known medical conditions
   a. Neurologic
   b. Urinary
   c. GI
4. Urinary signs or symptoms
   a. Hesitancy
   b. Dribbling
   c. Painful micturition

PHYSICAL EXAM

1. Regular abdominal and genital exam.
2. Rectal exam if the child has chronic constipation.

3. Spine (lumbosacral) to R/O spina bifida, tethered cord.
4. Observation of voiding for obstructive signs.

LABS

Urinalysis (see UTIs) to screen for:

1. UTIs
2. Renal disease
3. DB mellitus

TX

- Educate parents about the potential psychological side effects this condition may have on the child.
- Treat underlying conditions. Treatment of chronic constipation may be the only solution required.
- There are three basic treatment approaches:
  1. Conditioning therapy (good success rate, low relapse)
     a. Enuresis alarms (a device which senses urine in the child's underwear and alerts him when liquid is detected)
     b. Conditioned awakening and timed voiding at specific hours of the day.
  2. Reward system: Bladder stretching by having the child progressively refrain from urinating for longer periods of time coupled with a reward.
  3. Pharmacotherapy: (good short-term success rate, high relapse)
     a. DDAVP
     b. Oxybutynin (used with bladder stretching exercises)

Table of Normal Lab Values

Blood

Coagulation (Hemostasis)

Bleeding time (Ivy)	<9 min
INR	0.9–1.2
PTT	28–38 s
PT	10–13 s

Hemogram

Hct	
Female	0.370–0.460
Male	0.420–0.520 Hb
Hb	
Female	123–157 g/L
Male	140–174 g/L
MCV	80–100 fL
MCH	27–34 pg
Platelet count	130–400 × 109/L
RBCs	
Female	4.0–5.2 × 1,012/L
Male	4.4–5.7 × 1,012/L
RDW	11.5%–14.5%
Reticulocyte count	20–84 × 109/L
Erythrocyte sedimentation rate (Westergren)	
Female	1–20 mm/h
Male	1–13 mm/h
White blood cells and differential	
WBC	4–10 × 109/L
Segmented neutrophils	2–7 × 109/L
Band neutrophils	<0.7 × 109/L
Basophils	<0.10 × 109/L
Eosinophils	<0.45 ×109/L
Lymphocytes	1.5–3.4 ×109/L
Monocytes	0.14–0.86 ×109/L

Chemical Constituents

Albumin (serum)	35–50 g/L
Alkaline phosphatase (serum)	35–100 U/L
Aminotransferase (transaminase) (serum)	
Alanine (ALT; SGPT)	3–36 U/L
Aspartate (AST; SGOT)	0–35 U/L
γ-Glutamyl transferase	
Female	10–30 U/L
Male	10–35 U/L
Amylase (serum)	<160 U/L
HCO_3 (serum)	24–30 mmol/L

Bilirubin (serum)
   Direct (conjugated) $<7\ \mu mol/L$
   Total $<26\ \mu mol/L$
Calcium (serum)
   Total   2.18–2.58 mmol/L
   Ionized   1.05–1.30 mmol/L
Chloride (serum)   98–106 mmol/L
Cholesterol (serum) <5.2 mmol/L
LDL <3.37 mmol/L
HDL >0.9 mmol/L
Cortisol   160–810 mmol/L
CK (serum)   5–130 U/L
Cr (serum)
   Female $50–90\ \mu mol/L$
   Male $70–120\ \mu mol/L$
Ferritin $10–250\ \mu g/L$
Folic (Folate)   7–36 mmol/L
Glucose fasting (serum)   3.3–5.8 mmol/L
Hemoglobin A1C   4%–6%
Iron (serum) $11–32\ \mu mol/L$
LDH (serum)   95–195 U/L
Lipase (serum) <160 U/L
Magnesium (serum)   0.75–0.95 mmol/L
Osmolality (serum)   280–300 mmol/kg
Oxygen saturation (arterial blood) (Sao₂)   96%–100%
Paco₂ (arterial blood)   35–45 mm Hg
Pao₂ (arterial blood)   85–105 mm Hg
pH   7.35–7.45
Phosphorus (inorganic) (serum)   0.8–1.5 mmol/L
Potassium (serum)   3.5–5.0 mmol/L
PSA $0–4\ \mu g/L$
Protein (serum)
   Total   60–80 g/L
   Albumin   35–50 g/L
Sodium (serum)   135–145 mmol/L
Thyroid-stimulating hormone (sensitive)   0.4–5.0 mU/L
T3 (free)   3.5–6.5 pmol/L
T4 (free)   8.5–15.2 pmol/L
TIBC $45–82\ \mu mol/L$
Transaminase—see Aminotransferase
Triglycerides (serum) <2.20 mmol/L
TnT $<0.01\ \mu g/L$
Urea nitrogen (BUN) (serum)   2.5–8.0 mmol/L
Uric acid (serum) $180–420\ \mu mol/L$
Vitamin B₁₂   74–516 pmol/L

Cerebrospinal Fluid

Cell count $<4 \times 106/L$
Glucose   2–4 mmol/L
Proteins (total)   0.20–0.45 g/L

Urine

Calcium <7.3 mmol/d
Chloride   110–250 mmol/d
Creatinine   6.2–17.7 mmol/d
Osmolality   100–1200 mOsm/kg
Potassium   25–120 mmol/d
Protein <0.15 g/d
Sodium   25–260 mmol/d

List of Abbreviations

ABBREVIATION	EXPANSION
↑	Increase
SaO_2	Oxygen saturation
#	Fracture
#	Number of
$\Normal$	Normal
↓	Decrease
⁻Na	Sodium deficit
♀	Female
♂	Male
1°	Primary
17-OH-P	17 Hydroxy progesterone
2°	Secondary
2 h PPG	Two-hour postprandial glucose
5-HIAA	5-Hydroxyindoleacetic acid
5-HT	Serotonin
5-HT3	5-Hydroxytryptamine
99mTc	Technetium-99 m
AA	Afferent arteriole
AA	Aortic aneurysm
AAA	Abdominal aortic aneurysm
AACG	Acute angle closure glaucoma
AAT	Activity as tolerated
ab	Antibody/antibodies
ABC	Airway, breathing, circulation
Abdo	Abdomen, abdominal
ABG	Arterial blood gas
ABI	Ankle brachial index
AbN	Abnormal
ABO	Blood group system of groups A, AB, B and O
Abx	Antibiotic
Abx Tx	Antibiotherapy
AC	Alternating current
AC	Activated charcoal
AC	Air conduction
AC	Acromioclavicular
AC Fossa	Antecubital fossa
AC/A	Ratio of accommodative convergence/accommodation
AC/MDAC	Activated charcoal/multidose activated charcoal
ACA	Anterior cerebral artery
ACD	Acute adrenal insufficiency
ACE	Angiotensin converting enzyme
ACEI	Angiotensin converting enzyme inhibitor
AChR	Acetylcholine receptor
ACL	Anterior cruciate ligament
ACLS	Advanced cardiac life support

ACS	Acute coronary syndrome
ACT	Assertive community treatment
ACTH	Adrenocorticotropic hormone
AD	Advanced directive
AD	Anxiety disorder
ADH	Antidiuretic hormone, Vasopressin
ADHD	Attention deficit/hyperactivity disorder
ADL	Activity of daily living
ADLs	Activities of daily living
ADM	Abductor digiti minimi
AED	Antiepileptic drug
AF	Atrial fibrillation
AFB	Acid fast bacillus
AFFIRM	Atrial fibrillation follow-up investigation of rhythm management
AFI	Amniotic fluid index
AFib	Atrial fibrillation
AFL	Atrial flutter
AFP	Alpha fetoprotein
AFV	Amniotic fluid volume
Ag	Antigen
AG	Anion gap
AGUS	Atypical glandular cells of uncertain significance
AI	Aortic insufficiency
AI	Adrenal insufficiency
AI	Autoimmune
AIDS	Acquired immunodeficiency syndrome
AIMS	Abnormal involuntary movement scale
AION	Anterior ischemic optic neuropathy
ALK-P	Alkaline phosphatase
ALL	Acute lymphocytic leukemia
ALP	Alkaline phosphatase
ALS	Amyotrophic lateral sclerosis
ALT	Alanine transaminase
ALT	Alanine aminotransferase
AMA	Antimitochondrial antibodies
AMD	Age-related macular degeneration
AML	Acute myeloid leukemia
AN	Anorexia nervosa
ANA	Antinuclear antibody
ANC	Absolute neutrophil count
ANCA	Antineutrophil cytoplasmic antibody
ANP	Atrial natriuretic peptide
Anti-dsDNA	Anti-double-stranded deoxyribonucleic acid
Anti-GBM	Antiglomerular basement membrane
Anti-LKM	Antibodies to liver/kidney microsomes
anti-PL	Antiphospholipid antibodies
anti-Sm	anti-Smith
Anti-SMA	Antibodies to smooth muscle actin
Ao	Aortic
AOM	Acute otitis media
AP	Alkaline phosphatase
AP	Anterior posterior
APB	Abductor pollicis brevis
APC-resistance	Activated-protein C resistance
API	Arterial pressure index
APL	Abductor pollicis longus
aPTT	Activated partial thromboplastin time
AR	Aortic regurgitation
ARB	Angiotensin receptor blocker
ARDS	Acute respiratory distress syndrome
ARF	Acute renal failure

AS	Aortic stenosis
AS	Ankylosing spondylitis
ASA	Acetylsalicylic acid (aspirin)
ASAP	As soon as possible
ASC	Applied scientific concepts
ASCA	Anti-Saccharomyces cerevisiae antibody
ASC-H	Atypical squamous cell, cannot exclude HSIL
ASCUS	Atypical squamous cells of undetermined significance
ASD	Atrial septal defect
ASO	Antistreptolysin O
ASOT	Antistreptolysin O titer
ASPS	Advanced sleep phase syndrome
AST	Aspartate aminotransferase
AST	Aspartate transaminase
ASx	Asymptomatic
ATLS	Advanced trauma life support
ATN	Acute tubular necrosis
ATP	Adenosine triphosphate
ATPase	Adenosine triphosphatase
AUB	Abnormal uterine bleeding
AutoAb	Autoantibody
AV	Atrioventricular
AV	Arteriovenous
Avg.	Average
AVM	Arteriovenous malformation
AVN	Avascular necrosis
AVNRT	Atrioventricular nodal reentrant tachycardia
AVRT	Atrioventricular reentrant tachycardia
AxND	Axillary node dissection
AXR	Abdominal x-ray
B. burgdorferi	*Borrelia burgdorferi*
B. cereus	*Bacillus cereus*
b.i.d.	two times a day
BAL	Bronchial alveolar lavage
BAL	Bronchoalveolar lavage
BBB	Blood brain barrier
BBP	Biophysical profile
BBT	Basal body temperature
BC	British Columbia
BC	Bone conduction
BCC	Basal cell carcinoma
BCG	Bacille Calmette-Guerin
BG	Blood glucose
b-HCG	b-Human chorionic gonadotropin
BIPAP	Bilevel positive airway pressure
BMD	Bone mineral density
BMI	Body mass index
BMR	Basal metabolic rate
BN	Bulimia nervosa
BNP	Brain natriuretic peptide
BP	Blood pressure
BP	Bipolar disorder
BPE	Boiling point elevation
BPH	Benign prostatic hyperplasia
BPP	Biophysical profile
BPPV	Benign paroxysmal positional vertigo
BRAO	Branch renal artery occlusion
BRCA	Breast cancer
bs	Bowel sounds
B-S	Bernard-Soulier disease
BSO	Bilateral salpingo-oophorectomy
BUN	Blood urea nitrogen

BV	Blood volume
BV	Bacterial vaginosis
C&S	Culture and sensitivity
C.	Corynebacterium
C. albicans	*Candida albicans*
C. difficile	*Clostridium difficile*
C. glabrata	*Candida glabrata*
C. perfringens	*Clostridium perfringens*
C. pneumoniae	*Chlamydia pneumoniae*
c.a.	Carbonic anhydrase
C/S	Caesarean section
C_2LEO	Cultural-Communication Legal, Ethical, and Organizational
CA	cancer
CA	Carbohydrate antigen
Ca^{2+}	Calcium
CABG	Coronary artery bypass graft surgery
CAD	Coronary artery disease
CAEP	Canadian Association of Emergency Physicians
CAH	Congenital adrenal hyperplasia
CAH	Congenital adrenal hypertrophy
CAM	Cystic adenomatoid malformation
CAM	complementary and alternative medicines
cAMP	Cyclic adenosine monophosphate
c-anca	Cytoplasmic-staining antineutrophil cytoplasmic antibodies
C-ANCA	Cytoplasmic antineutrophil cytoplasmic antibodies
CAP	Community acquired pneumonia
CaP	Carcinoma of the prostate
CAS	Children's Aid Society
Cath	Catheterization
CB1	Cannabinoid receptor
CBC	Complete blood count
CBCD	Complete blood count with differential
CBC-D	Complete blood count with differential
CBF	Cerebral blood flow
CBS	Capillary blood sugar
CBT	Cognitive behavioral therapy
CCAM	Congenital cystic adenomatoid malformation
CCB	Calcium channel blocker
CCCT	Clomiphene citrate challenge test
CCD	Cortical collecting duct
CCR	Canadian C-spine Rule
CCU	Coronary care unit
CDH	Congenital diaphragmatic hernia
CDM	Clinical decision making
CEA	Carcinoembryonic antigen
CF	Cystic fibrosis
CFCP	Certified Functional Continuity Professional
CFCP	Certified Functional Continuity Professional
CFPC	College of Family Physicians of Canada
cGMP	Cyclic guanosine monophosphate
CHA	Canada Health Act
CHD	Coronary heart disease
Chemo	Chemotherapy
CHF	Congestive heart failure
CHL	Conductive hearing loss
Chr	Chromosome
Chron.	Chronic
CI	Contraindication
CIHR	Canadian Institutes for Health Research
CIN	Cervical intraepithelial neoplasia
CIS	Carcinoma in situ
CJD	Creutzfeldt-Jakob disease

CK	Creatinine kinase
CKD	Chronic kidney disease
Cl	Chloride
CL	Corpora lutea
CLL	Chronic lymphocytic leukemia
cm	Centimeter
CMA	Canadian Medical Association
CMC	Carpometacarpal
CME	Continuing medical education
CMI	Cell mediated immunity
CML	Chronic myeloid leukemia
CMPA	Canadian Medical Protective Association
CMV	Cytomegalovirus
CN	Cranial nerve
CNS	Central nervous system
CO	Cardiac output
CO	Carbon monoxide
CO_2	Carbon dioxide
CoA	Coarctation of the aorta
CO-Hgb	Carboxyhemoglobin
COPD	Chronic obstructive pulmonary disease
COX	Cyclooxygenase
coxibs	Cyclooxygenase-2-inhibitors
CP	Cerebral palsy
CPA	Cerebello-pontine angle
CPAP	Continuous positive airway pressure
CPB	Cardiopulmonary bypass
CPD	Cephalopelvic disproportion
CPDD	Calcium pyrophosphate deposition disease
CPP	Cerebral perfusion pressure
CPP	Chronic pelvic pain
CPR	Cardiopulmonary resuscitation
Cr	Creatinine
CRAO	Central renal artery occlusion
CRAO	Central retinal artery occlusion
CRAO	Central renal artery occlusion
CrCl	Creatinine clearance
CRF	Chronic renal failure
CRH	Corticotropic releasing hormone
CRP	Complex regional pain
CRP	C-reactive protein
CRPS	Complex regional pain syndrome
CRVO	Central renal vein occlusion
CRVO	Central retinal vein occlusion
CSF	Cerebral spinal fluid
CSF	Cerebrospinal fluid
CT	Computed tomography
CT	Connective tissue
CT/PE	Computed tomography for pulmonary embolism
CTA	CT angiogram
CTD	Connective tissue disease
CTG	Continuous cardiotocography
CV	Cardiovascular
CVA	Cerebral vascular accident
CVA	Cerebrovascular accident
CVA	Costovertebral angle
CVD	Coronary vascular disease
CVD	Cardiovascular disease
CVD	Cerebral vascular disease
CVD	Cerebrovascular disease
CVP	Central venous pressure
CVR	Cerebrovascular resistance

CVS	Cardiovascular system
CVS	Chorionic villus screening
CXR	Chest X-ray
d	day
Δ	Change
Δ	Difference
D&E	Dilation and evacuation
D/C	Discharge
d/c	Discontinue
D/O	Disorder
D2	Dopamine receptor subtype 2
D50W	50% dextrose in water
D5W	5% dextrose in water
DA	Dopamine
DB	Diabetes
dBP	Diastolic blood pressure
DC	Direct current
DCM	Dilated cardiomyopathy
DCT	Distal convoluted tubule
DDAVP	Desmopressin acetate
DDAVP	1-deamino-8-D-arginine-vasopressin (desmopressin)
DDH	Developmental dysplasia of the hip
DDx	Differential diagnosis
Derm	Dermatology
DES	Diethylstilbestrol
DHE	Dihydroergotamine
DHEAS	Dehydroepiandrosterone sulphate
DI	Diabetes insipidus
diastol.	Diastolic
DIC	Disseminated intravascular coagulation
DIP	Distal interphalangeal joint
DJ	Disco jockey
DKA	Diabetic ketoacidosis
DLCO	Diffusion capacity of carbon monoxide
DM	Diabetes mellitus
DM2	Type 2 diabetes mellitus
DMARD	Disease modifying antirheumatic drug
DMPA	Depot medroxyprogesterone acetate
DMSA	Dimercaptosuccinic acid
DOC	Deoxycorticosterone
DPL	Diagnostic peritoneal lavage
DPN	Diagnosis and Prevention Network
DRE	Digital rectal exam
DSM	Diagnostic and Statistical Manual of Mental Disorders
DSMIV	Diagnostic and Statistical Manual of Mental Disorders-IV
DSPS	Delayed sleep phase syndrome
DTaP-IPV	Diphtheria, tetanus, acellular pertussis, inactivated polio virus
DTR	Deep tendon reflex
DVT	Deep vein thrombosis
DWI	Diffusion weighted imaging
Dx	Diagnosis
DXA	Dual energy x-ray absorptiometry
dz	Disease
E	Estrogen
E.	Eustachian
E. coli	*Escherichia coli*
E. histolytica	*Entamoeba histolytica*
E.vermicularis	*Enterobius vermiculis*
EA	Efferent arteriole
EABV	Effective arterial blood volume
EBM	Evidence-based medicine
EBV	Epstein-Barr virus

EC	Emergency contraception
ECA	External carotid artery
ECF	Extracellular fluid
ECG	Electrocardiogram
ECHO	Echocardiogram
ECP	Emergency contraceptive pills
ECRB	Extensor carpi radialis brevis
ECRL	Extensor carpi radialis longus
ECT	Electroconvulsive therapy
ECU	Extensor carpi ulnaris
ECV	Effective circulating volume
ED	Emergency department
ED	Erectile dysfunction
EDC	Expected date of conception
EDM	Extensor digiti minimi
EDTA	Ethylene diamine tetraacetate
EDV	End-diastolic volume
EE	Ethynyl estradiol
EEG	Electroencephalogram
EENT	Eye, ear, nose, throat
EF	Ejection fraction
Eff	effusion
EFM	Electronic fetal monitoring
EFW	Estimated fetal weight
EGD	Esophagogastroduodenoscopy
EI	Extensor indicis
EKG	Electrocardiogram
ELISA	Enzyme-linked immunosorbent assay
emerg	emergency/ies
EMG	Electromyography
EMLA	Lidocaine + Prilocaine
EMS	Emergency Medical Services
ENG	Electronystagmography
ENT	Ears, nose, throat
EOM	Extraocular muscle/movement
EP	Electrophysiology
EP	Ectopic pregnancy
EPB	Extensor pollicis brevis
EPI	Epinephrine
EPL	Extensor pollicis longus
EPO	Erythropoietin
EPS	Extrapyramidal side effects
EPT	Estrogen progesterone therapy
ER	Emergency room
ER/PR	Estrogen/progesterone receptor
ERCP	Endoscopic retrograde cholangiopancreatography
ESR	Erythrocyte sedimentation rate
ESRD	End-stage renal disease
ESRF	End-stage renal failure
ET	Estrogen therapy
ETCO	End-tidal carbon monoxide
EtOH	Alcohol
ETT	Endotracheal tube
EWN	Edinger-Westphal nuclei
exam	Examination
exp	Expiratory
Ext.	Extension
F/P/T	Federal/Provincial/Territorial
F/U	Follow up
F:M	Female:male ratio
FA	fatty acid
FAI	Femoroacetabular impingement

FAP	Familial adenomatous polyposis
FAS	Fetal alcohol syndrome
FAST	Focused assessment with sonography for trauma
FB	Foreign body
FCR	Flexor carpi radialis
FCU	Flexor carpi ulnaris
FDMB	Flexor digiti minimi brevis
FDP	Flexor digitorum profundus
FDS	Flexor digitorum superficialis
FE	fractional excretion
Fe	Iron
FE_K	Fractional excretion of potassium
FENa	Fractional excretion of sodium
FEV	Forced expiratory volume
FEV_1	forced expiratory volume in 1 second
FFA	Free fatty acid
fFN	Fetal fibronectin
FFP	Fresh frozen plasma
FFS	Fee-for-service
FHA	Functional hypothalamic amenorrhea
FHR	Fetal heart rate
FHx	Family history
FHx	Family history
FiO_2	Fractional content of inspired oxygen
Fl	Femtoliter
Flex.	Flexion
Flu	Influenza
FMMSE	Folstein minimental status exam
FMP	Final menstrual period
FMR1	Fragile X mental retardation I
FNAB	Fine needle aspiration biopsy
FNAC	Fine needle aspiration cytology
FNIHB	First Nations and Inuit Health Branch
FNIHB	First Nations and Inuit Health Branch
FOB	Fecal occult blood
FOBT	Fecal occult blood test
FPB	Flexor pollicis brevis
FPD	Freeze point depression
FPG	Fasting plasma glucose
FPL	Flexor pollicis longus
FRC	Functional residual capacity
FRS	Framingham risk score
FSGS	Focal segmental glomerulosclerosis
FSH	Follicle stimulating hormone
FT4	Free T4
FTA-ABS	Fluorescent treponemal antibody-absorbed
FTP	Failure to progress
FTS	First trimester screening
FTT	Failure to thrive
FUO	Fever of unknown origin
FVC	Forced vital capacity
fx	Features
fxn	Function
g	Gram
G&S	Blood group and screen
G. vaginalis	Gardnerella vaginalis
g/L	Grams per litre
G6PD	Glucose-6-phosphate dehydrogenase deficiency
GA	Gestational age
GABA	Gamma aminobutyric acid
GABHS	Group A beta hemolytic streptococci
GAS	Group A streptococcus

GBM	Glomerular basement membrane
GBS	Group B streptococcus
GBS	Guillain-Barre syndrome
GC	Glucocorticoid
GCA	Giant cell artheritis
GCS	Glasgow Coma Score
GDM	Gestational diabetes mellitus
gen	Generation
GER	Gastroesophageal reflux
GERD	Gastroesophageal reflux disease
GFR	Glomerular filtration rate
GGT	Gamma-glutamyl transferase
GH	Growth hormone
GH	Glenohumeral
GI	Gastrointestinal
GIFT	Gamete intrafallopian transfer (immediate transfer with sperm after oocyte retrieval)
gluc.	Glucose
GLUT5	Glucose trasnporter 5
GMC	General medical conditions
GN	Gram negative
GN	Glomerulonephritis
GnRH	Gonadotropin releasing hormone
GPe	Globus pallidus externa
GPIIb	Glycoprotein IIb inhibitors
GRE	Gradient recalled echo
GSI	Gonadosomatic index
GTC	Generalized tonic-clonic
GTD	Gestational trophoblastic disease
GU	Genitourinary
h	Hour/s
H&N	Head and neck
H. ducreyi	*Haemophilus ducreyi*
H. flu	*Haemophilus influenza*
H. flu	*Haemophilus influenzae*
h/a	Headache/s
H/H	Hemoglobin and hematocrit
H1	Histamine receptor subtype 1
H2	Histamine receptor type 2
H_2	Hydrogen gas
H2 blockers	Histamine 2 receptor blockers
H_2O	Water
H2RA	H2-receptor antagonist
H_2S	Hydrogen sulphide
HAV	Hepatitis A virus
Hb	Hemoglobin
HbA_{1c}	Glycosylated hemoglobin
HBcAg	Hepatitis B core antigen
HBIG	Hepatitis B immunoglobulin
HBsAg	Hepatitis B surface antigen
HBV	Hepatitis B virus
HCC	Hepatocellular carcinoma
HCCA	Health Care Consent Act
hCG	Human chorionic gonadotropin
HCl	Hydrochloric acid
HCO_3	Bicarbonate
Hct	Hematocrit
HCV	Hepatitis C virus
HD	Hemodialysis
HDL	High density lipoprotein
HEENT	Head and neck
HELLP	Hemolysis, elevated liver enzymes, low platelets

HEME	Hematology
Hep B	Hepatitis B
HepBsAg	Hepatitis B surface antigen
Her2/neu	Human epidermal growth factor receptor 2
HERS	Heart and estrogen/progestin replacement study
HF	Hydrofluoric acid
Hgb	Hemoglobin
HHS	Hyperglycemic hyperosmolar state
HiB	Haemophilus influenza type B
HIDA	Cholescintigraphy hepatobiliary iminodiacetic acid
HIDS	Hospital Insurance and Diagnostic Services
HIT	Heparin-induced thrombocytopenia
HIV	Human immunodeficiency virus
HL	Hearing loss
HLA	Human leukocyte antigen
HLA	Human leukocyte antigen
HLA-B27	Human leukocyte antigen B27
HMD	Hyaline membrane disease
hMG	Human menopausal gonadotropin
HMG-CoA	3-hydroxy-3-methylglutaryl coenzyme A
HN	Hydronephrosis
HNPCC	Hereditary nonpolyposis colon cancer
HOCM	Hypertrophic obstructive cardiomyopathy
HONK	Hyperosmolar nonketotic syndrome
HPA	Hypothalamic-pituitary-adrenal
HPF	High powered field
hPL	Human prolactin lactogen
HPO	Hypothalamic-pituitary-ovarian
HPV	Human papillomavirus
HR	Heart rate
HRCT	High-resolution computed tomography
HRCT	High-resolution computed tomography
HRT	Hormone replacement therapy
HS	Hypernychthemeral syndrome
HSD	Hydroxysteroid dehydrogenase
HSG	Hysterosalpingogram
HSIL	High-grade squamous intraepithelial lesion
HSP	Henoch-Schönlein purpura
HSV	Herpes simplex virus
HTg	Hypertriglyceridemia
HTN	Hypertension
HU	Hounsfield unit
HUS	Hemolytic uremic syndrome
Hx	History
i.e.,	that is
I:G	Insulin to glucose ratio
I−123	Iodine-123
IA	Intermittent auscultation
IABP	Intraaortic balloon pump
IADL	Instrumental activities of daily living
IBD	Inflammatory bowel disease
IBS	Irritable bowel syndrome
ICA	Intracerebral artery
ICB	Intracranial bleed
ICD	Implantable cardioverter defibrillator
ICD-10-CM	International Classification of Diseases, Tenth Revision, Clinical Modification
ICF	Intracellular fluid
ICH	Intracerebral hemorrhage
ICH	Intracranial hemorrhage
ICP	Intracranial pressure
ICSI	Intracytoplasmic sperm injection

ICU	Intensive care unit
ID	Identification
ID	Infectious disease
IDDM	Insulin-dependent diabetes mellitus
Ig	Immunoglobin
IgA	Immunoglobulin A
IgE	Immunoglobulin E
IGF-1	Insulin-like growth factor 1
IgG	Immunoglobulin G
IgM	Immunoglobulin M
IGT	Impaired glucose tolerance
IHD	Ischemic heart disease
IL	Interleukin
IL-4	Interleukin-4
IL-5	Interleukin-5
ILD	Interstitial lung disease
IM	Intramuscular
IM	Intermedullary
IMB	Intermenstrual bleeding
INO	Internuclear ophthalmoplegia
INR	international normalized ratio
INR/PTT	International normalized ratio/partial prothrombin time
insp	Inspiratory
Insp + exp	Inspiratory plus expiratory
IO	Inferior oblique
IOP	Intraocular pressure
IP	Interphalangeal
IPF	Interstitial pulmonary fibrosis
IPF	Idiopathic pulmonary fibrosis
IPS	Integrated prenatal screening
IQ	Intelligence quotient
IR	Inferior rectus
ISLD	Interstitial lung disease
ISS	Insufficient sleep syndrome
IT	Iliotibial
ITP	Idiopathic thrombocytopenic purpura
IU	International units
IUD	Intrauterine device
IUFD	Intrauterine fetal demise
IUGR	Intrauterine growth restriction
IUI	Intrauterine insemination
IV	Intravenous
IVC	Inferior vena cava
IVC filter	Inferior vena cava filter
IVDU	Intravenous drug user
IVF	In vitro fertilization
IVF	Intravenous fluid
IVFA	Intravascular fluorescein angiography
IVH	Intraventricular hemorrhage
IVIG	Intravenous immunoglobulin
IVIg	Intravenous immunoglobulin
IVP	Intravenous pyelography
Ix	Investigation(s)
JGA	Juxtaglomerular apparatus
JIA	Juvenile idiopathic arthritis
JNC	Joint National Committee
JVD	Jugular venous distension
JVD	Jugular venous distention
JVP	Jugular venous pulse
K	Potassium
Kallmann's Syndrome	Congenital deficiency of GnRH associated with craniofacial midline defects and/or anosmia.

KDOQI	Kidney Disease Outcomes Quality Initiative
kg	kilogram
KGV	Lymphogranuloma venereum
KOH	Potassium hydroxide
KUB	Kidney, ureters and bladder
KUB	Kidney-ureters-bladder (x-ray)
L	Left
L.pneumophila	*Legionella pneumophila*
L/E	Lower extremities
LA	Left atrium
lab	laboratory
LABA	Long acting beta agonist
LAD	Lymphadenopathy
Lat	Lateral
LBBB	Left bundle branch block
LCAT	Lecithin-cholesterol acyltransferase
LCL	Lateral collateral ligament
LDH	Lactose dehydrogenase
LDH	Lactate dehydrogenase
LDL	Low density lipoprotein
L-Dopa	Levadopa
LEEP	Loop electrosurgical excision procedure
LES	Lower esophageal sphincter
LES	Lambert-Eaton syndrome
LET	Lidocaine + Epinephrine + Tetracaine
LFT	Liver function test
LGA	Large for gestational age
LGV	Lymphogranuloma venereum
LH	Luteinizing hormone
LLDP	Left lateral decubitus position
LLQ	Left lower quadrant
LLSB	Left lower sternal border
LMCC	Licentiate of the Medical Council of Canada
LMN	Lower motor neuron
LMP	Last menstrual period
LMWH	Low molecular weight heparin
LNG-IUS	Levonorgestrel intrauterine system
LNMP	Last normal menstrual period
LOC	Loss of consciousness
LOC	Level of consciousness
LP	Lumbar puncture
LPA	Left pulmonary arterial
LPD	Luteal phase defect
LPS	lipopolysaccharide
LR	lateral rectus
L-R	Left-right
LRT	Laryngeal reaction time
LSD	Lysergic acid diethylamide
LSIL	Low grade squamous intraepithelial lesion
LT	Leukotrienes
LUQ	Left upper quadrant
LUTS	Lower urinary tract symptom
LV	Left ventricle
LVEDP	Left ventricular end diastolic pressure
LVH	Left ventricular hypertrophy
Lytes	Electrolytes
m	Meter
M	Multiparous
M&M	Morbidity and mortality
M. catarrhalis	*Moraxella catarrhalis*
M. furfur	*Malassezia furfur*
M. genitalium	*Mycoplasma genitalium*

M. hominis	*Mycoplasma hominis*
M. pneumoniae	*Mycoplasma pneumoniae*
M1	Muscarinic receptor subtype 1
MAHA	Microangiopathic hemolytic anemia
MAOI	Monoamine oxidase inhibitor
MAP	Mean arterial pressure
MAT	Multifocal atrial tachycardia
max	Maximum
Mayer-Rokitansky-Kuster-Hauser Syndrome	Vaginal atresia with variable müllerian duct abnormalities
MB	Myoglobulin
MBP	Major basic protein
MCA	Middle cerebral artery
MCC	Medical Council of Canada
MCCQE	Medical Council of Canada Qualifying Examination
MCH	Mean corpuscular hemoglobin
M-CHAT	Modified Checklist for Autism in Toddlers
MCL	Medial collateral ligament
MCP	Metacarpal phalangeal joint
MCQ	Multiple choice questions
MCV	Mean corpuscular volume
MCV	Mean cell volume
MD	Medical doctor
MDAC	Multidose activated charcoal
MDD	Major depressive disorder
MDE	Major depressive episode
MDI	Metered dose inhaler
MDMA	3,4-methylenedioxymethamphetamine
MDRD	Modification of diet in renal disease
ME	Metaphysis + epiphysis
med	Medical
meds	medication
MEN-1	Multiple endocrine neoplasia type 1
Men-C	Meningococcal C conjugate
MetSyn	Metabolic syndrome
Mg	Magnesium
MG	Monoglyceride
MG	Myasthenia gravis
MGUS	Monoclonal gammopathy of uncertain significance
MH	Malignant hyperthermia
MHA-TP	Microhemagglutination for Treponema pallidum
MI	Myocardial infarction
mL	Milliliter
MM	Multiple myeloma
mm Hg	Millimeters mercury
MMR	Measles, mumps, rubella
MMSE	Minimental status exam
mo	Month
MOD	Myocardial oxygen demand
MOM	Milk of magnesia
MONA	Morphine, O_2, nitroglycerine, aspirin
MP	Metacarpophalangeal
MPA	Medroxyprogesterone acetate
MPGN	Membranoproliferative glomerulonephritis
MPSS	Methylprednisolone sodium succinate
MR	Mitral regurgitation
MR	Medial rectus
MR	Magnetic resonance
MRA	Magnetic resonance angiography
MRCP	Magnetic resonance cholangiopancreatography
MRI	Magnetic resonance imaging
mRNA	Messenger ribonucleic acid

MRV	Magnetic resonance venography
MS	Mitral stenosis
MS	Multiple sclerosis
MSAFP	Maternal serum AFP
MSDS	Material safety data sheet
MSE	Medical supplies and equipment
MSG	Monosodium glutamate
MSH	Melanophore-stimulating hormone
MSK	Musculoskeletal
MSS	Maternal serum screen
MTP	Metatarsal phalangeal
MTX	Methotrexate
Musc	Muscle
MVA	Motor vehicle accident
MVA/MVC	Motor vehicle accident/motor vehicle collision
MVC	Motor vehicle collision
Mx	Management
N	Nulliparous
N	No
N. gonorrhea	*Neisseria gonorrhea*
N. gonorrhoeae	Neisseria gonorrhoeae
N. meningitides	*Neisseria meningitides*
n/a	Not applicable
N/S	Normal saline
N/V	Nausea and vomiting
NA	Nasogastric aspiration
Na	Sodium
NAAT	Nucleic acid amplification test
NAC	*N*-acetylcysteine
NACI	National Advisory Committee on Immunization
NaOH	Sodium hydroxide
NASCIS	National Acute Spinal Cord Injury Study
NASH	Nonalcoholic steatotic hepatitis
NCS	Nerve conduction study
NE	Norepinephrine
NEC	Necrotizing enterocolitis
NG	Nasogastric
NG/NJ	Nasogastric/nasojejunum
NGT	Nasogastric tube
NICU	Neonatal intensive care unit
NKF	National Kidney Foundation
NKH	Nonketotic hyperglycemia
NMJ	Neuromuscular junction
NMS	Neuroleptic malignant syndrome
NO	Nitric oxide
No.	Number of
NPJT	Nonparoxysmal junctional tachycardia
NPO	Nothing by mouth
NSAID	Nonsteroidal anti-inflammatory drug
NSCLC	Non-small cell lung cancer
NSERC	Natural Sciences and Engineering Research Council
NST	Nonstress test
NSTEMI	Non-ST elevation myocardial infarction
NSx	Neurosurgery
NT	Neurotransmitter
NTD	Neural tube defects
NTHI	Nontypable haemophilus influenza
NTUS	Nuchal translucency ultrasound
O&P	Ova and parasites
O/E	On exam
O_2	Oxygen
OA	Osteoarthritis

OA	Occiput anterior
OA	Occiput anterior
OB/GYN	Obstetrician/gynecologist
OC	Oral contraceptive
OC	Obsessive compulsive
occ. lobe	Occipital lobe
OCD	Obsessive compulsive disorder
OCP	Oral contraceptive pills
OD	Overdose
ODP	Opponens digiti minimi
OG	Osmolar gap
OG	Orogastric
OGCT	Oral glucose challenge test
OGL	Orogastric lavage
OGTT	Oral glucose tolerance test
OHP	Hydroxyprogesterone
OHS	Occupational health and safety
OP	Occiput posterior
OP	Opponens pollicis
Op	Operative
OR	Operating room
ORIF	Open reduction internal fixation
ORS	Oral rehydration solution
os	Ostium of uterus
OS	Ostium of uterus
OSA	Obstructive sleep apnea
Osm	Osmolality
OT	Occupational therapy
OT	Occiput transverse
OTC	Over the counter
P	Progesterone
P	Progestin
p.v.	Per vagina
P/E	Physical exam
PA	Posterior-anterior
$PaCO_2$	Arterial pressure of carbon dioxide
pANCA	Perinuclear antineutrophil cytoplasmic antibody
P-ANCA	Perinuclear antineutrophil cytoplasmic antibodies
PaO_2	Partial pressure of oxygen in arterial blood
PAO_2	Alveolar oxygen tension
PaO_2/FiO_2	Partial pressure of O_2 in arterial blood to fractional content of inspired O2 ratio
Pap	Papanicolaou
PAPP-A	Pregnancy associated plasma protein-A
PBC	Primary biliary cirrhosis
PCA	Posterior cerebral artery
PCI	Percutaneous coronary intervention
PCL	Posterior cruciate ligament
PCO_2	Partial pressure of carbon dioxide
PCOS	Polycystic ovary syndrome
PCOS	Polycystic ovarian syndrome
PCP	Phencyclidine
PCR	Polymerase chain reaction
PCT	Proximal convoluted tubule
PCWP	Pulmonary capillary wedge pressure
PD	Peritoneal dialysis
PD	Personality disorder
PDA	Patent ductus arteriosus
PDE(-5)	Phosphodiesterase(-5)
PE	Pulmonary embolism
PEEP	Positive end expiratory pressure
PEG	Polyethylene glycol

PEx	Physical examination
PF	Peak flow
PFO	Patent foramen ovale
PFT	Pulmonary function test
PG	Prostaglandin
PGE1	Prostaglandin E1
PGE2	Prostaglandin E2
PGF	Placental growth factor
PGME	Postgraduate Medical Education
pH	Hydrogen potential (measure of acidity of solution)
PHAC	Public Health Agency of Canada
Phos.	Phosphorus
PID	Pelvic inflammatory disease
PID	Pelvic inflammatory disease
PIH	Pregnancy-induced hypertension
PIP	Proximal interphalangeal joint
PKD	Polycystic kidney disease
PKU	Phenylketonuria
PL	Palmaris longus
Pl	Pleural
PLM	Periodic limb movement
PLMD	Periodic limb movement disorder
Plt	Platelet
PMDD	Premenstrual dysmorphic disorder
PMHx	Past medical history
PMI	Point of maximal impulse
PMN	Polymorphonuclear leukocytes
PMNLs	Polymorphonuclear leukocytes
PMPRB	Patented Medicines Price Review Board
PMR	Polymyalgia rheumatica
PMS	Premenstrual syndrome
PNa	Plasma sodium concentration
PND	Paroxysmal nocturnal dyspnea
Pneu-C	Pneumococcal conjugate
PNS	Peripheral nervous system
PO	Per os
PO	By mouth
PO_2	Partial pressure of oxygen
PO4	Phosphate
POF	Premature ovarian failure
POGG	Peace, order, and good governance
POMC	Proopiomelanocortin
POPQ	Pelvic organ prolapse quantification
Posm	Plasma osmolality
P_{osm}	Plasma osmolality
PP	Prone positioning
PPD	Purified protein derivative test/Mantoux test
PPG	Postprandial glucose
PPH	Postpartum hemorrhage
PPHN	Persistent pulmonary hypertension
PPI	Proton pump inhibitor
PPROM	Prolonged premature rupture of membranes
PPV	Positive predictive value
PR	Pulmonic regurgitation
PR	Per rectum
PRBC	Packed red blood cell
Prbc	Packed red blood cell
Prep	Preparation
Prev.	Previous
PRL	Prolactin
prn	As needed
PROM	Premature rupture of membranes

PS	Pulmonary stenosis
PSA	Prostate-specific antigen
PSC	Primary sclerosing cholangitis
Psych Hx	Psychiatric history
PT	Physical therapy
PT	Prothrombin time
pt	Patient
PTH	Parathyroid hormone
PTHrP	Parathyroid hormone related peptide
PTL	Preterm labor
PTSD	Post traumatic stress disorder
PTT	Partial thromboplastin time
PTX	Pneumothorax
PUD	Peptic ulcer disease
PulmHTN	Pulmonary hypertension
P_{urea}	Plasma urea
PUV	Posterior urethral valve
PUVA	Psoralen ultraviolet A
PV	Pulmonary ventricle
PVC	Premature ventricular complex
PVD	Peripheral vascular disease
PVR	Peripheral vascular resistance
PVR	Postvoid residual
PWI	Perfusion weighted imaging
Px	Physical exam
PYLL	Potential years life lost
P-Σ	Parasympathetic nervous system
q	Every (dose related)
q.d.	Every day (dose related)
q.i.d.	Four times a day
QBHCG	Quantitative beta-HCG
QT	QT interval
R	Right
R&M	Routine and microscopy
R/O	Rule out
RA	Rheumatoid arthritis
RA	Right atrium
RADT	Rapid antigen detection test
RAI	Radioactive iodine
RAPD	Relative afferent pupillary defect
RAS	Renin angiotensin system
RAS	Renal artery stenosis
RBBB	Right bundle branch block
RBC	Red blood cell
RCC	Renal cell carcinoma
RCM	Radiocontrast media
RCMP	Royal Canadian Mounted Police
RCPSC	Royal College of Physicians and Surgeons of Canada
RCT	Randomized control trial
RDS	Respiratory distress syndrome
RDW	Red blood cell distribution width
REB	Research Ethics Board
rehab	Rehabilitation
Resp	Respiratory
RF	Rheumatoid factor
RF	Risk factor
RF	Renal failure
RFT	Renal function test
RHA	Regional Health Authority
RhIg	Rh immunoglobulin
RI	Respiratory infection
RICE	Rest, Ice, Compression, and Elevation

RL	Ringer's lactate
RLQ	Right lower quadrant
RLS	Restless leg syndrome
ROH	Alcohol
ROM	Range of motion
ROM	Rupture of membranes
ROP	Retinopathy of prematurity
RORX	Radiation therapy
ROS	Review of symptoms
RPE	Retinal pigment epithelium
RPLND	Retroperitoneal lymph node dissection
RPR	Rapid plasma reagin
RR	Respiratory rate
RSV	Respiratory syncytial virus
RT	Radiotherapy
RTA	Renal tubular acidosis
RTI	Respiratory tract infection
RUQ	Right upper quadrant
RV	Residual volume
RV	Right ventricle
Rx	Treatment
Rx	Therapy
RXN	Reaction
s	Seconds
S	Superficial
S&Sx	Signs and symptoms
S. Aureus	*Staphylococcal aureus*
S. pneumoniae	*Streptococcus pneumoniae*
S. viridans	*Staphylococcus viridans*
S/E	Side effects
SA	Sinoatrial
SABA	Short acting beta agonist
SABD	Short acting bronchodilator
SAH	Subarachnoid hemorrhage
SANRT	Sinoatrial node reentrant tachycardia
SBE	Subacute bacterial endocarditis
sBP	Systolic blood pressure
sc	Subcutaneous
SC	Sternoclavicular
SCC	Squamous cell carcinoma
SCH	Subconjunctival hemorrhage
SCI	Spinal cord injury
Scl-70	Scleroderma-70
SCLC	Small cell lung cancer
SD	Standard deviation
SDH	Subdural hematoma
SDM	Substitute decision maker
SE	South east
SE	Status epilepticus
SERM	Selective estrogen receptor modulator
SFH	Symphysis fundus height
SGA	Small for gestational age
SGLT1	Sodium-dependent glucose transporter 1
SI	Stress incontinence
SI	Sacroiliac
SIADH	Syndrome of inappropriate antidiuretic hormone
SIDS	Sudden infant death syndrome
SIRS	Systemic inflammatory response syndrome
SJS	Stevens-Johnson Syndrome
SLAP	Superior labral anterior-posterior
SLE	Systemic lupus erythematosus
SLP	Speech language pathology

SMX	Sulfmethoxide
SNB	Sentinel node biopsy
SNc	Substantia nigra pars compacta
SNHL	Sensorineural hearing loss
SNr	Substantia nigra pars reticulata
SNRI	Serotonin-norepinephrine reuptake inhibitor
SNS	Sympathetic nervous system
SO	Salpingo-oophorectomy
SO	Superior oblique
SOB	Short/shortness of breath
SOGC	Society of Obstetricians and Gynecologists of Canada
SOI	Syrup of ipecac
SPEP	Serum protein electrophoresis
spp.	Species
SR	Superior rectus
ß	Beta
SSA	Sulfosalicylic acid
SSHRC	Social Sciences and Humanities Research Council
SSRI	Selective serotonin reuptake inhibitor
Staph epidermidis	*Staphylococcus epidermidis*
STD	Sexually transmitted disease
STEMI	ST elevation myocardial infarction
STI	Sexually transmitted illness
STN	Subthalamic nucleus
Strep pneumo	Streptococcus pneumonia
Strep. pyogenes	*Streptococcus pyogenes*
Subcut	Subcutaneous
SV	Stroke volume
SV	Supraventricular
SVC	Superior vena cava
SVC	Superior vena cava syndrome
SVD	Spontaneous vaginal delivery
sVEGFR-1	Soluble vascular endothelial growth factor receptor 1
SVR	Systemic vascular resistance
SVT	Supraventricular tachycardia
SW	Social work
SWU	Septic work up
Swyer's Syndrome	46XY gonadal dysgenesis
Sx	Symptom
Syst.	Systolic
T	Testosterone
T	Temperature
T&X	Type and cross match
T. mentagrophytes	*Trichophyton mentagrophytes*
T. pallidum	Treponema pallidum
T. pallidum	*Treponema pallidum*
T. rubrum	*Trichophyton rubrum*
T. vaginalis	*Trichomonas vaginalis*
t.i.d.	Three times a day
T3	Triiodothyronine
T4	Tetraiodothyronine
T4	Thyroxine
TA	Temporal artery
TAb	Thyroid autoantibodies
Tab	Tablet
TAL	Thick ascending limb of the loop of Henle
TAPVD	Total anomalous pulmonary venous drainage
TB	Tuberculosis
TBI	Traumatic brain injury
TBSA	Total body surface area
TBV	Total blood volume
TBW	Total body water

TC	Total cholesterol
TCA	Tricyclic antidepressant
TcB	Transcutaneous bilirubinometry
TCC	Transitional cell carcinoma
Td	Tetanus
TD	Transdermal
TD	Tardive dyskinesia
TEE	Transesophageal echocardiogram
TEF	Tracheoesophageal fistula
TENS	Transcutaneous electrical nerve stimulation
TET	Tubal embryo transfer
TG	Triglyceride
TGA	Transposition of great arteries
TH	Thyroid hormone
TIA	Transient ischemic attack
TIBC	Total iron binding capacity
TIG	Tetanus immunoglobulin
TIMI	Thrombolysis in myocardial infarction
TIPS	Transjugular intrahepatic portosystemic shunt
TLC	Total lung capacity
TMJ	Temporal mandibular joint
TMP	Trimethoprim
TMP-SMX	Trimethoprim and sulfamethoxasole
TMP–SMX	Trimethoprim-sulfmethoxide
Tn	Troponin
TNF	Tumor necrosis factor
TNF-a	Tumor necrosis factor alpha
TNM	Tumor size, node involvement, metastatic spread
TNMS	Tumor size, node involvement, metastatic, serum markers
TNMS	Tumor nodes metastasis staging
TOF	Tetralogy of Fallot
tox	Toxin
tPA	Tissue plasminogen activator
TPN	Total parenteral nutrition
TP-PA	Treponema Pallidum particle agglutination
TPR	Total peripheral resistance
TR	Tricuspid regurgitation
TRH	Thyrotropin-releasing hormone
TRS	TIMI risk score
TRUS	Transrectal ultrasound
TS	Tricuspid stenosis
TSB	Total serum bilirubin
TSH	Thyroid stimulating hormone
TSS	Toxic shock syndrome
TT	Thrombin time
TTD	Teletype/telecommunications devices
TTE	Transthoracic echocardiogram
TTKG	Transtubular potassium gradient
TTN	Transient tachypnea of newborn
TTNB	Transthoracic needle biopsy
TTP	Thrombotic thrombocytopenic purpura
TURP	Transurethral resection of the prostate
TVR	Target vessel revascularization
TVS	Transvaginal sonography
TVUS	Transvaginal ultrasound
Tx	Management
TXA2	Thromboxane A2
U/A	Urinalysis
U/E	Upper extremities
U/O	Urine output
U/S	Ultrasound
UA	Unstable angina

UA	Uric acid
UC	Ulcerative colitis
UDP	Uridine diphosphate
UDP-GT	Uridine diphosphate glucuronyl transferase
UFH	Unfractionated heparin
UGI	Upper gastrointestinal
UI	Urinary incontinence
UIP	Usual interstitial pneumonitis
UMN	Upper motor neuron
Uosm	Urine osmolality
U_{osm}	Urine osmolality
UPEP	Urine protein electrophoresis
UPJ	Ureteropyelic junction
URI	Upper respiratory infection
URTI	Upper respiratory tract infection
USPSTF	U.S. Preventive Services Task Force
UTI	Urinary tract infection
UV	Ultraviolet
UVB	Ultraviolet B
v.cholera	Vibrio cholera
V/Q scan	Ventilation perfusion scan
Var	Varicella
vb insuff	Vertebro-basilar insufficiency
VC	Vital capacity
VCD	Vocal cord dysfunction
VCUG	Voiding cystourethrogram
VDRL	Venereal Disease Research Laboratory test (for syphilis)
VEGF	Vascular endothelial growth factor
VF	Ventricular fibrillation
Vfib	Ventricular fibrillation
VIP	Vasoactive intestinal peptide
Vit	Vitamin
Vit	Vitamin
Vit B_{12}	Vitamin B_{12}
VLDL	Very low density lipoprotein
VMA	Vanillylmandelic acid
VSD	Ventricular septal defect
VT	Ventricular tachycardia
VTE	Venous thromboembolism
VUJ	Vesicoureteral junction
VUR	Vesicoureteral reflux
vWD	von Willebrand disease
VZIG	Varicella zoster immunoglobulin
VZV	Varicella-zoster virus
w/u	Work-up
WBC	White Blood Cell/Count
WBI	Whole bowel irrigation
WCB	Workers Compensation Board
WHI	Women's Health Initiative
WHIMS	Women's Health Initiative Memory Study
WHO	World Health Organization
wk	Week
Wt	Weight
XR	X-ray
Y	yes
y.o.	Year old
yr	Year
ZIFT	Zygote intrafallopian transfer
Σ	Sympathetic nervous system

Clinical Presentation Index